Report on the Staten Island Project

The Ibogaine Story

Dedication:
TO WILLIAM MOSES KUNSTLER

Acknowledgements:
Bob Sisko, Howard Lotsof, Norma Alexander, Spencer Rumsey, Bruce Sakow, Dhoruba Bin Wahad, Geerte F., Boaz Wachtel, Rommell Washington, David Goldstein, Carlo Contoreggi, Nico Adriaans, Jon Parker, Andrew Hoffman, Brother Shine, Eddie Ellis, Flo Kennedy, Kiyoshi Kuromiya, Marty Robinson, Robert Rygor, John Spacely, John Holmstrom, Stanley Glick, John Morgan, Patricia Broderick, Deborah Mash, Juan Sanchez-Ramos, Dennis Peron, Ben Masel, Mark Molliver, Stuart Hameroff, David Flattery, Robert Goutarel, James Fernandez, John Marks and Marty Lee, Hans–Georg Behr, Charles Kaplan, Steve Sifanek, Fred Gotbetter, Curtis Wright, Frank Vocci, Charles Gudzinskas, Rick Doblin, Norman Spinrad, Philip K. Dick, Ekang Ngongo, Hugh Schonfield, Noah Potter, Evan Camp, Kenny Toglia, Rob MacDonald, Dennis King, Allen Berkman, John Valadez, Sandra Blakeslee, Judith Hooper and Dick Teresi

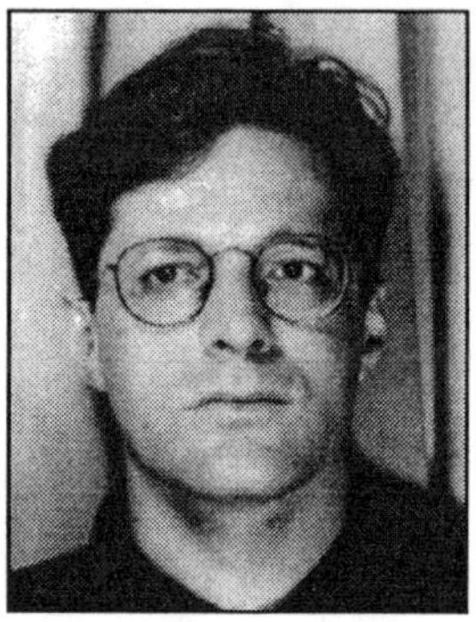

WBAI reporter Paul De Rienzo, who broke "Mena" (*Contra*–coke-for-guns in Mena, Ark) is a social historian of New York's radical Lower East Side as well as the Drug War.

Dana Beal, formerly of ACT–UP and the Yippies!, is a science writer, an AIDS activist, and one of the founders of the American Harm Reduction Movement.

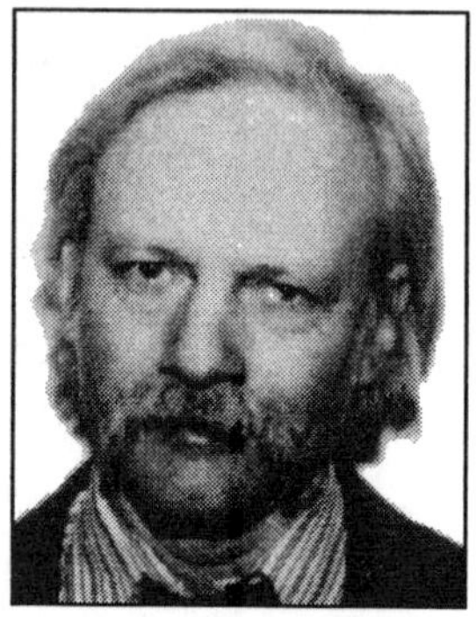

Autonomedia
POB 568 Williamsburgh Station
Brooklyn, New York 11211-0568 USA

Fax & Phone 718-963-2603

Printed in the United States of America

Report on the Staten Island Project

The Ibogaine Story

Paul De Rienzo, Dana Beal
& the Staten Island Project

Autonomedia

A WORD FROM OUR SPONSOR....

"I saw the best minds of my generation starving, hysterical, naked,
Dragging themselves through negro steets at dawn looking for an angry fix...
Allen Ginsberg, opening lines, "Howl," 1954

"What we're looking for is something we can spray over the Soviet trenches, and they'll march out whistling 'Yankee Doodle Dandy'."
—Ascribed to a CIA advisor, Defense Department, Pharmaco-Warfare Division

"Thus Spake Zarathrustra: 'Praise Be to Haoma!' "
—Yasna #3

"Deposition: Testimony Concerning a Sickness"

I awoke from the Sickness at the age of forty-five, calm and sane, and in reasonably good health except for a weakened liver and the look of borrowed flesh common to all who survive the Sickness... Most survivors do not remember the delirium in detail. I apparently took detailed notes on sickness and delirium...

The sickness is drug addiction and I was an addict for fifteen years. When I say addict I mean addict to junk (generic term for opium and/or derivatives including all synthetics from demerol to palfium). I have used junk in many forms: morphine, heroin, dilaudid, eukodal, pantopon, diocodid, diosane, opium, demerol, dolophine, palfium. I have smoked junk, eaten it, sniffed it, injected it in vein–skin–muscle, inserted it in rectal suppositories. The needle is not important. Whether you sniff it smoke it eat it or shove it up your ass the result is the same: addiction. When I speak of drug addiction I do not refer to keif, marijuana or any preparation of hashish, mescaline, *Bannisteria caapi,* LSD6, Sacred Mushrooms or any other drug of the hallucinogen group... There is no evidence that the use of any hallucinogen results in physical dependence. The action of these drugs is physiologically opposite to the action of junk. A lamentable confusion between the classes of drugs has arisen owing to the zeal of the U.S. and other narcotic departments.

I have seen the exact manner in which the junk virus operates through fifteen years of addiction. The pyramid of junk, one level eating the level below (it is no accident that the junk higher-ups are always fat and the addict in the street is always thin) right up to the top or tops since there are many junk pyramids feeding on people of the world and all built on basic principles of monopoly:

1—Never give anything away for nothing.

2—Never give more than you have to give (always catch the buyer hungry and always make him wait).

3—Always take everything back if you possibly can.

The pusher always gets it all back. The addict needs more and more junk to maintain a human form...buy off the Monkey.

Junk is the mold of monopoly and possession. The addict stands by while his junk legs carry him straight in on the junk beam to relapse. Junk is quantitative and accurately measurable. The more junk you use the less you have and more you have the more you use. All the hallucinogen drugs are considered sacred by those who use them—there are Peyote Cults and Bannisteria Cults, Hashish Cults and Mushroom Cults—"the Sacred Mushrooms of Mexico enable a man to see God"—but no one ever suggested that junk is sacred. There are no opium cults. Opium is profane and quantitative like money. I have have heard that there was once a beneficent non-habit-forming junk in India. It was called *soma* and is pictured as a beautiful blue tide. If *soma* ever existed the Pusher was there to bottle it and monopolize it and sell it and it turned into plain old time JUNK.

Junk is the ideal product... the ultimate merchandise. No sales talk necessary. The client will crawl through a sewer and beg to buy... The junk merchant does not sell his product to the consumer, he sells the consumer to his product. He does not improve and simplify his merchandise. He degrades and simplifies the client. He pays his staff in junk.

Junk yields a basic formula of "evil" virus: *The Algebra of Need.* The face of "evil" is always the face of total need. A dope fiend is a man in total need of dope. Beyond a certain frequency need knows absolutely no limit or control. In the words of total need: *"Wouldn't you?"* Yes, you would. You would lie, cheat, inform on your friends, steal, *do anything* to satisfy total need. Because you would be in a state of total sickness, total possession, and not in a position to act in any other way. Dope fiends are sick people who cannot act other than they do. A rabid dog cannot choose but bite. Assuming a self-righteous position is nothing to the purpose unless your purpose be to keep the junk virus in operation. And junk is a big industry. I recall talking to an American who worked for the Aftosa Commission in Mexico. Six hundred a month plus expense account:

"How long will the epidemic last?" I enquired.

"As long as we can keep it going... And yes...maybe the aftosa will break out in South America," he said dreamily.

If you wish to alter or annihilate a pyramid of numbers in a serial relation, you alter or remove the bottom number. If we wish to annihilate the junk pyramid, we must start with the bottom of the pyramid: *the Addict in the Street.* And stop tilting quixotically for the "higher ups," so called, all of whom are immediately replaceable. *The addict in the street who must have junk to live is the one irreplaceable factor in the junk equation.* When there are no more addicts to buy junk there will be no more junk traffic. As long as junk need exists, someone will service it.

Addicts can be cured or quarantined—that is allowed a morphine ration under minimal supervision like typhoid carriers. When this is done, junk pyramids of the world will collapse. So far as I know, England is the only country to apply this method to the junk problem. They have about five hundred quarantined addicts in the U.K. In another generation when the quarantined addicts die off and pain killers operating on a non-junk principle are discovered, the junk virus will be like smallpox, a closed chapter—a medical curiosity.

The vaccine that can relegate the junk virus to a landlocked past is in existence. This vaccine is the Apomorphine Treatment discovered by an English doctor whose name I must withhold pending his permission to use it and to quote from his book covering thirty years of apomorphine treatment of addicts and alcoholics. The compound apomorphine is formed by boiling morphine with hydrochloric acid. It was discovered years before it was used to treat addicts. For many years the only use for apomorphine which has no narcotic or pain-killing properties was as an emetic to induce vomiting in cases of poisoning. It acts directly on the vomiting center in the back brain.

I found this vaccine at the end of the junk line. I lived in one room in the Native Quarter of Tangier. I had not taken a bath in a year or changed my clothes or removed them except to stick a needle every hour in the fibrous grey wooden flesh of terminal addiction. I never cleaned or dusted my room. Empty ampule boxes and garbage piled to the ceiling. Light and water long since turned off for non-payment. I did absolutely nothing. I could look at the end of my shoe for eight hours. I was only roused to action when the hourglass of junk ran out. If a friend came to visit—and they rarely did since who or what was left to visit—I sat there not caring that he had entered my field of vision—a grey screen always blanker and fainter—and not caring when he walked out of it. If he had died on the spot I would have sat there looking at my shoe waiting to go through his pockets. Wouldn't you? Because I never had enough junk—no one ever does. Thirty grains of morphine a day and it still was not enough. And long waits in front of the drugstore. Delay is a rule in the junk business. The Man is never on time. This is no accident. There are no accidents in the junk world. The addict is taught again and again exactly what will happen if he does not score his junk ration. Get up that money or else. And suddenly my habit began to jump and jump. Forty, sixty grains a day. And it still was not enough. And I could not pay.

I stood there with my last check in my hand and realized that it was my last check. I took the next plane for London.

The doctor explained to me that apomorphine acts on the back brain to regulate the metabolism and normalize the blood stream in such a way that the enzyme system of addiction is destroyed over a period of four to five days. Once the back brain is regulated, apomorphine can be discontinued and only used in case of relapse. (No one would take apomorphine for kicks. *Not one case of addiction to apomorphine have ever been recorded.*) I agreed to undergo treatment and entered a nursing home. For the first twenty-four hours I was literally insane and paranoid as many addicts are in severe withdrawal. This delirium was dispersed by twenty-four hours of intensive apomorphine treatment. The doctor showed me the chart. I had received minute amounts of morphine that could not possibly account for my lack of the more severe withdrawal symptom such as leg and stomach cramps, fever and my own special symptom The Cold Burn, like a vast hives covering the body and rubbed with menthol. Every addict has his own special symptom that cracks all control. There was a missing factor in the withdrawal equation—that factor could only be apomorphine.

I saw the apomorphine treatment really work. Eight days later I left the nursing home eating and sleeping normally. I remained completely off junk for two full years—a twelve year record. I did relapse for some months as a result of pain and illness. Another apomorphine cure has kept me off junk through this writing.

The apomorphine cure is qualitatively different from other methods of cure. I have tried them all. Short reduction, slow reduction, cortisone, antihistamines, tranquilizers, sleeping cures, tolserol, reserpine. None of these cures lasted beyond the first opportunity to relapse. I can say definitely that I was never *metabolically* cured until I took the apomorphine cure. The overwhelming relapse statistics from the Lexington Narcotic Hospital have led many doctors to say that addiction is not curable. They used a dolophine reduction cure at Lexingon and have never tried apomorphine so far as I know. In fact, this method of treatment has been largely neglected. No research has been done with variations of the apomorphine formula or with synthetics. No doubt substances fifty times stronger than apomorphine[1] could be developed and the side effect of vomiting eliminated.

— William S. Burroughs, 1955
From the "Introduction" to *Naked Lunch*

[1] Alas, apomorphine is not accepted by most addicts because of unpleasant nausea, etc., compared with modern medications like buprenorphin, which can be given orally in a five-day detox. — Ed.

Contents

Appendices

Exhibits

CHAPTER I: The War With the Junkies

It never would have happened if Tom Forçade hadn't shot himself in the head. Forçade, who'd built *High Times* up to four million readers by being six months ahead on new trends, was the only one who could keep the functions of his sprawling Empire reconciled. But by October 1978, hounded by the DEA and acutely depressed by scheming, ambitious underlings as well as the death of his best friend Jack Coombs in a plane crash in Florida, the King was at the end of his tether.

He was also wired on coke, and dependent on valium. Which is a funny thing, since he had attended the opening of Howard Lotsof's film *Smoke-In,* and Howard always told important people about Ibogaine.[1] But Lotsof's odd factoid about Ibogaine interrupting his heroin/coke addiction in the early '60s had no tangible application for Tom. Lost in the din, Forçade could no longer pick out the one distant trend that could have saved him from his own bad habits. Tom Forçade had run out of time.

In one weekend, Tom committed suicide; Jim Jones snuffed himself out with a thousand followers; Dan White assassinated Harvey Milk and Mayor George Moscone in San Francisco. And the pendulum started to swing back. It was as if the CIA engineered a coup in a Third World country called the Counterculture.

High Times' motivating spark was extinguished. It began to drift. And there was this problem with the junkies in the art department.

A few years later John Lombardi would write in *Esquire* of his wife, Wendy, a talented photographer, strung out on smack. Down on Grand Street around the corner from the *Soho Weekly News,* Marcia Resnick and Johnny Thunders were living on the couch at Sunset Studios, doing up incredible quantities of smack, which they could afford because she was dealing it out of the back door of the *Soho* to a celebrity scene that included John Belushi. Both Marcia and Wendy were often employed by *High Times* art director Toni Brown, who was to end up in 1981 on Pat Robertson's Christian Broadcasting Network, denouncing her former employer and thanking Jesus for getting her off drugs.

With *High Times,* Forçade pioneered the true marijuana mass market. Before he died he tried to create the same acceptability for his other favorite drug, cocaine. But he always drew the line at heroin. He and Dana Beal had done the first YIPPIE march against CIA heroin on July 4, 1971. He knew, even though the William Burroughs groupies were dogging him the year before his suicide to do it, that this was one frontier the magazine should not cross.

It wasn't intolerance of drugs. After all, *High Times* stood for exuberant promotion of marijuana versus alcohol and cigarettes. And the '60s survivors clustered around Tom would have been horrified by the idea of

1 The "Lotsof Effect"— interruption of drug addiction — requires a heroic dose (15–18 milligrams per kilo of total body weight) or more than a gram, one hundred times the lowest dose effective as a stimulant (10–20 mgs per total body weight). According to Carol Realini, who worked for Forçade, Tom *was* familiar with the intermediate, "psycholytic" dose (and himself had taken doses of 250 mgs total body weight), as a "memory drug."

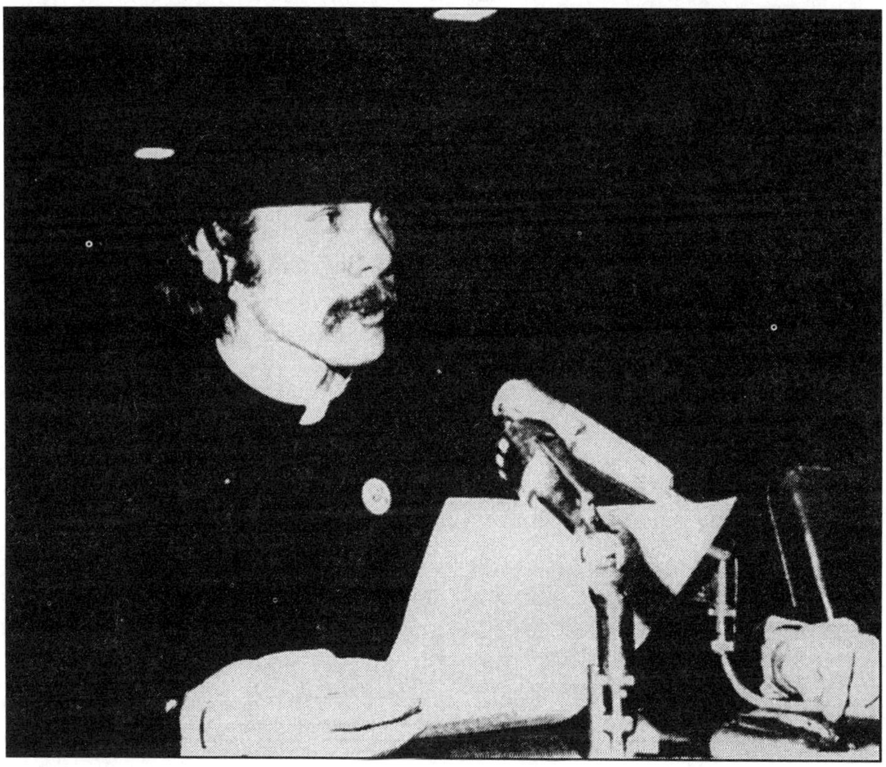
Blacklisted News

"FATHER" TOM FORÇADE TESTIFIES

turning in a friend just because they did problem drugs. But the deal was that junkies didn't proselytize. What '60s survivors all knew was that heroin equalled ODs and hepatitis. Except for coke, *High Times* editorial policy foreshadowed the Dutch "harm reduction" model of market separation of pot and hard drugs.

The trouble, as heroin began to come back at the end of the '70s and the Art Set got strung out, was that they only had two ways to pay for it on salaries that were minute compared to their prestige. Sell it, which meant turning on new people. Or — because the DEA would not seriously impede the flow of reefer for another five years — they could always set up a pot dealer for a rip off.

It worked like this: pot dealers had more marijuana and cash than they knew what to do with. But like all newly rich, they were starved for recognition. So some behind-the-scenes entrepreneur would be drawn to the minor glitterati at the *Village Voice, Soho* or *High Times*, and find they could gain entry to the scene, if they came bearing gifts. They would waive their usual built-in scruples when they discovered their new celebrity friends were dabbling in heroin. Soon their new friends would reveal that they also knew someone in need of a pot connection. After a couple of times, the artist would take a big front and "lose" it. Or report they had been "tied up and ripped off."

Scenario 2 came when credit was eventually cut off, and the celeb's bill with their junk connection got too high. Then that nice harmless photog or writer (now slightly tarnished) would do a Jekyll and Hyde, and "finger" their pot connection to some junkie stickup artists. For enough of the take to erase their bill and maybe keep themselves in smack for a month, they would send the gunman around to tie you up for real, pistol-whip you, and take everything you owned.

Wendy Lombardi had long since blown her credit when, on the night of Forçade's wake at the Windows on the World, her third old man (the disreputable one with the missing teeth) approached Dana Beal as he was going into his neighbor's place across Bleecker Street. This low-life followed Dana upstairs, where he tried in vain to persuade the neighbor to throw some business his way. After Wendy"s "friend" was brushed off and shown out, Dana turned to his neighbor and said: "That guy is setting you up for a rip."

Sure enough, the deadbolt downstairs had been reversed, leaving it unlocked. After locking it, the neighbor decided to miss the wake. Later that evening he heard people fooling around with the door downstairs, went to the window and yelled, and saw some people fleeing west up Bleecker Street.

Now in a heightened state of vigilance, the neighbor was ready the next day when two gunmen broke in next door and tried to get in via the roof. He chased two pistoleros away with his shotgun. The YIPS made sure the story was disseminated throughout the entire *High Times* scene. Wendy Lombardi's cover was blown.

About a month later, as Dana was knocking on the front door of the *YIPster Times* building at 9 Bleecker, he noticed Wendy and boyfriend bearing down on him from his left: Just as Ben Masel opened the door, a fist blind-sided Dana on his left jaw. But there happened to be almost fifteen people hanging around the ground floor. A tussle ensued, and in a twinkling, the authors of this unprovoked assault were hustled inside, where everything short of major bodily harm was done to get them to give up the identities of the two gunmen and the other gang members.

But such was the underlying non-violence of the YIPS that nothing was done to the two miscreants sufficient to get them to give up anything except one name Wendy blurted out in the beginning — "John." They were released into the night, minus a shoe.

And then a funny thing happened as the story circulated, especially in the art departments of the *Voice, High Times*, and the *Soho Weekly News*. It mutated into its opposite, and the intended victims of the armed robbery became a violent cult of YIPPIE breakaways (i.e., not Abbie Hoffman). This was right after Jonestown. The seed had been planted.

What it boiled down to was this: Unlike pot, the people's drug, heroin made people totally absorbed with their own jones. In a scene of junkies who considered themselves to be celebrities to begin with, the pot-smoking masses were despised, looked down upon as sheep fit only to be shorn of their cash. Junkie sympathies were with their friends, and their right *as an elite*[1] to rip off the YIPPIES.

1 Reminiscent of the medieval *"droit de seigneur,"* literally, the right of the lord to first use of a peasant woman on her wedding night. For more on this, see *Diary of a Dope Fiend*, by Aleister Crowley, the famous Black Magician of early twentieth-century England, who is still a cult figure among junkies today. Crowley was one of the "occult" influences on Hitler.

Related to this was another problem. *YIPster Times,* although the best underground paper in the country, had never gotten its ad-base on a regular footing. It was a party publication, known to be supported by a network of small and middle-sized contributors around the country. In late '78, because the YIP'S had just put every cent they could beg or borrow into a "Bring Abbie Home Benefit" at the Felt Forum (timed for the tenth anniversary of Chicago), the paper was in hiatus. Forçade had not been able to fund it for months before his death. Although socially contiguous with *High Times,* it was viewed as a tract instead of a "real" newspaper. When Tom died, the YIPS automatically became outsiders. Wendy depicted her misfortunes as a sinister attack on the journalistic establishment by political fanatics.

Still, 1979, when it came, was the year of the fall of the Shah and Somoza. *YIPster Times* resumed publication, better than ever, as *Overthrow.* In early '79, the YIPS also gathered in all the followers of all the smoke-ins and opened Studio 10 at 10 Bleecker. It was an instant success, with five bands a night for $3, dollar Heinekens, and free pot on the bar.

In March/April, with great fanfare, the Marijuana Coalition created Rock Against Racism (RAR) to have a legal concert in Central Park for the end of the annual pot parade in May.

Even the indictment of Beal on specious pot conspiracy charges out of Omaha, Nebraska, was dismissed in the fall without going to trial.

Professor Ansley Hamid of John Jay College studied the effect of the switchover from pot to crack in Jamaican communities in New York City in the early '80s, and described how with pot (which engenders no tolerance, and no significant dose-escalation in users) enough capital was retained in the community to start secondary businesses, restaurants, etc., while the coming of crack sucked those communities dry, enriching only the few at the top of the pyramid.

By early 1980 the New York pot scene's inner core was wired on coke and strung out on smack. It wasn't unusual to see a major dealer (himself coked to the gills) cursing out one of his boys who'd gotten so messed up on schmagoo that they couldn't finish paying off their last pot front. But if you didn't dip into the drugs, you found yourself shut out socially. And hard drugs were expensive, unless you dealt. Contributions to the legalization movement dried up.

WALKING HEADS

Cosmo's been cruising in from the Delaware Gap area of New Jersey for years now to celebrate National Marijuana Day. He was supposed to meet 39,999 other druggies in Washington Square Park on Saturday, but all but 1200 of them went to the beach instead. All right. 100 cops showed. A few Yippies brought a sound system. The Rock Against Racism gang had a truck and a band. But mainly it was just very young dopers with incredibly bad teeth, active acne and message T-shirts — about 1000 of them. That's who *really* cares about grass nine years after the first New York march to legalize marijuana.

Cosmo wasn't distressed, though. "Great day to get high," he said. He had designed the cardboard marijuana leaves that separated Aron Kay, the pie-throwing Yippie, from the junior druggies gathered around him. "The Pope smokes dope!" Aron boomed. A fat guy with Coke-bottle glasses, retarded-looking, got carried away and began a frenzied dance against nuclear power, against the draft, against racism, against disco and for cannabis. Aron, who is very hairy, leaned over. "Easy now," he said.

A sizable group of journalists,— including a reporter for *Noticias del Mundo,* a marijuana virgin who spoke no English — tried to get photos, but Cosmo refused to pose. "I don't know what I'll be doing in my future," he explained. But he had his present all worked out: "I just smoke dope and, you know, climb mountains. I can't remember anything, but in a way, that's great. My friends tell me the same joke 50 times, and each time it's like a new joke to me."

Cosmo and his buddies struggled through the roller skaters in the park and fell in behind the mounted police, the motorcycle police, a battalion of policemen on foot and the noisy Rock Against Racism truck, to begin the long hike up Fifth Avenue.

"Aren't you going to bust anybody?" wondered two clean young women in midtown.

"On National Marijuana Day?" one cop answered. "Nobody's getting busted." In fact, the cops were models of restraint. They carried nightsticks, just in case, and wore bulletproof vests under their shirts. Mostly they seemed as embarrassed as the black street musician who was doubled over on the corner of 42d Street. "Reefers!" he laughed. "Marching for reefers!"

Aron did his best to keep spirits high. "Nazis are no fun!" he screamed. "Remember Kent State!" But the protesters were too young to remember, or they just generally had memory problems, or like the guy in red shorts and a Santa Claus cap, they were too busy trying to keep from wandering into the side of a police van.

"This is a lousy assignment," said the cop. "I've been doing this every year, and we still don't get a meal break. The first year there were only five of us. Last year we had 150 cops. We had to bust a couple of people." For possession? "Nah, for being assholes."

Marilyn Johnson

Soho Weekly News

Up at *High Times,* which had gone through management changes, a far more ambitious solution to heroin's voracious appetite for money was in the works. Dean A. Latimer had come out on top in the latest management shuffle. His favorite drug after alcohol was always opium. And most of all, that powerhouse in the art department wanted to cross the line Forçade wouldn't: to solve the adverse equation of heroin tolerance versus money by vastly expanding their customer base — by using *High Times* directly to mass market smack, like marijuana before it.

A furious struggle ensued. Tom had packed the editorial side with New Left / YIP veterans of the underground press, who expended much of their waning influence stopping that story. This

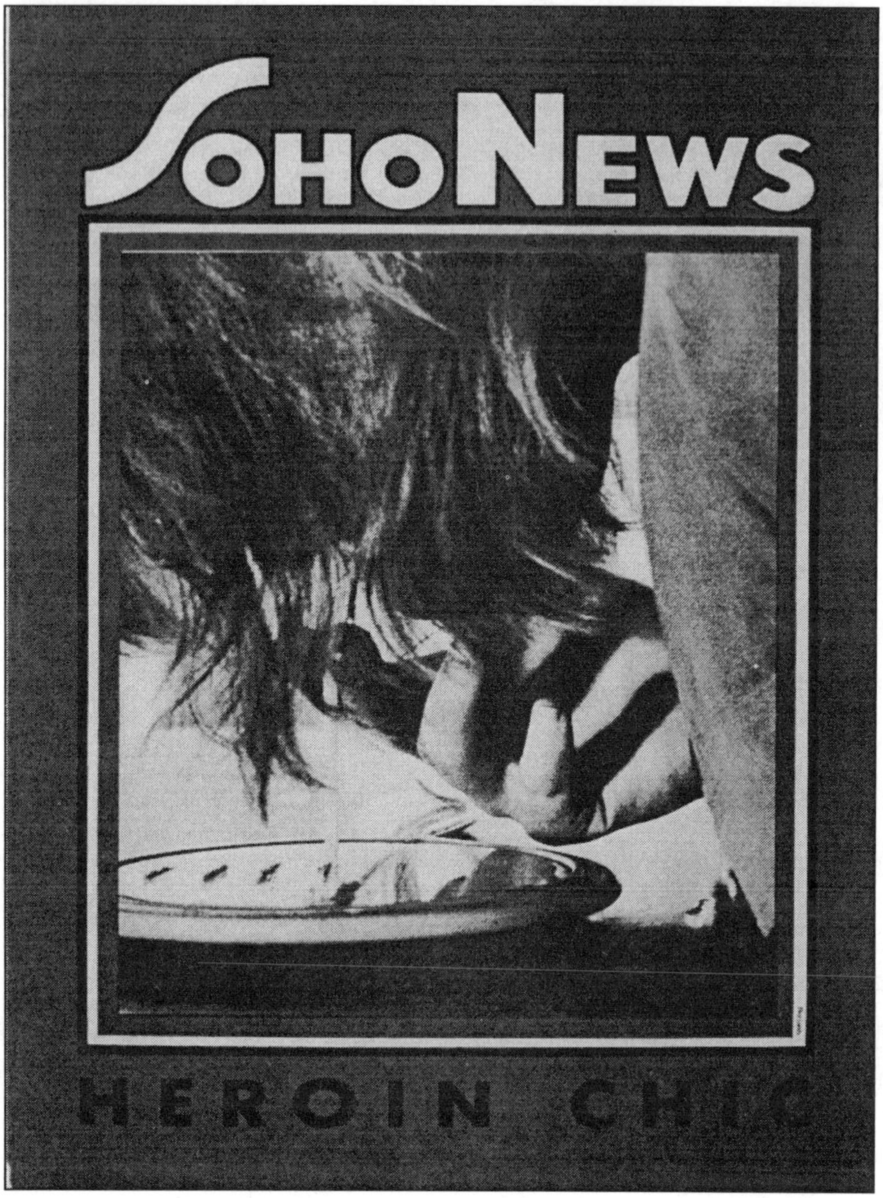

Soho Weekly News

left the junkies feeling embittered and discriminated against by a "politically correct" coterie that included *Overthrow*, the successor to *YIPster Times*.

The potheads, although they didn't yet know how to express it, knew the dispute went directly to the market separation of soft and hard drugs. The junkies got even: Pot-bashing became fashionable at the *Voice* for the whole first half of the next decade. Activism fell out of fashion at *High Times*. But the most interesting reaction came a few months later at the *Soho Weekly News*.

In early May, an article ran trashing the annual pot parade and heralding the death of the marijuana movement. The next week this poster went up advertising a new issue, showing a fashionable female snorting smack. Message: the new wave distinguish themselves from hippies by doing dope. And on the newsstand, emblazoned with the headline "NOW HEROIN," was an angelic blond peering from the cover of the *Soho* over a mirror with lines of what appeared to be cocaine, but was intended to represent heroin. The lead feature, with a big picture on the inside of a beautiful male torso injecting heroin, began with the story of Scott, driven, workaholic, trendy gallery owner, cooling out on weekends with smack.

The message was cleverly bracketed with *pro forma* warnings that heroin, like alcohol and cigarettes, could kill you. But that only added to the romance. The writers clearly felt they had to balance their personal misgivings with the pervasive acceptance of heroin on their immediate scene. The overwhelming thrust was that everyone was doing it. You could do it and not get addicted. They even told you where to cop the best stuff, and how to do it up (mix it with lemon juice).

Not a word about clean needles or serum hepatitis. (No one knew yet about AIDS, although it's now clear that this very scene, including Studio 10, was at the epicenter of the early epidemic.) It was the same damnable article that'd been axed from *High Times*. The radicals had kept it from going out across the country. But equivalent New York publication, by putting the physical survival of the local scene at risk, especially by influencing the bands of ROCK AGAINST RACISM and Studio 10, was a direct slap at New York YIP'S traditional role as trend-setter for the country.[1]

Once again, there was a furious brouhaha. The *Soho* received numerous complaints, calls, etc. RAR picketed. But the *Soho* staff, who considered the article "balanced," never acknowledged the central criticism to its subliminal thrust — especially the graphics. Most people don't read, they look at pictures. Consequently, the editors refused to print RAR'S letters objecting to putting heroin on the same footing as pot.

Now all the ugly rumors about RAR / YIP came back: that *YIPster Times* was not a "real" newspaper deserving of journalistic courtesy; that it was a top-down, violence-prone group; most of all, that mere pot

1 The contradiction became acute, for instance, when Columbus Yips had to run and find opiates for the drummer of the headline RAR band from New York. They were ex White Panthers who didn't even know where to get methadone.

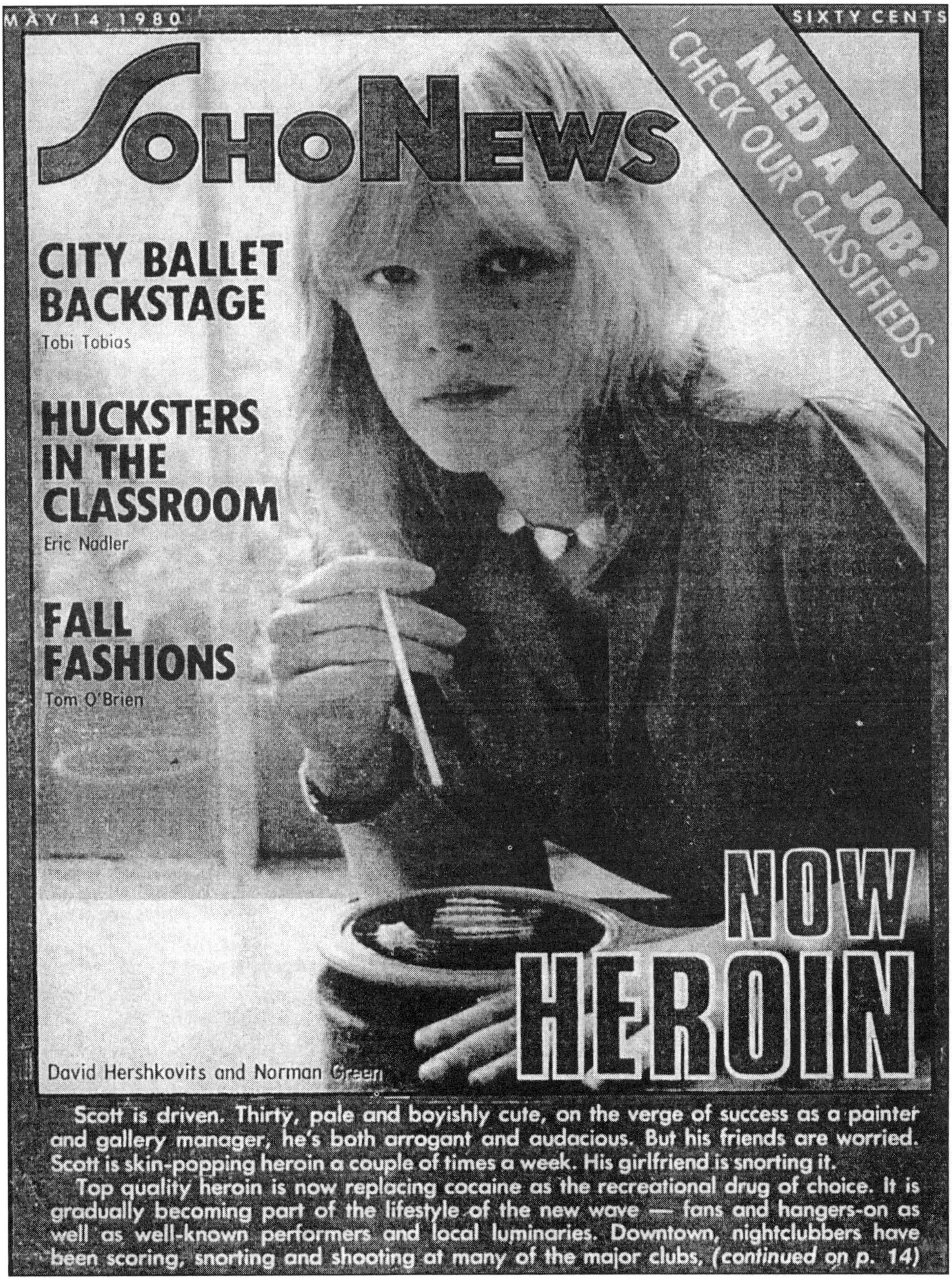
MAY 14, 1980

SIXTY CENTS

SohoNews

NEED A JOB? CHECK OUR CLASSIFIEDS

CITY BALLET BACKSTAGE

Tobi Tobias

HUCKSTERS IN THE CLASSROOM

Eric Nadler

FALL FASHIONS

Tom O'Brien

NOW HEROIN

David Hershkovits and Norman Green

Scott is driven. Thirty, pale and boyishly cute, on the verge of success as a painter and gallery manager, he's both arrogant and audacious. But his friends are worried. Scott is skin-popping heroin a couple of times a week. His girlfriend is snorting it.

Top quality heroin is now replacing cocaine as the recreational drug of choice. It is gradually becoming part of the lifestyle of the new wave — fans and hangers-on as well as well-known performers and local luminaries. Downtown, nightclubbers have been scoring, snorting and shooting at many of the major clubs, *(continued on p. 14)*

Soho Weekly News

advocates had no right — based on the bitterly learned lessons of collective experience — to criticize other drugs.

The nature of YIPPIE! is to thrive on symbiosis with the media. Such was the depth of upset amongst the junkie celebs of the interlocking art departments, that even though YIP did one of its best-ever rounds of protest

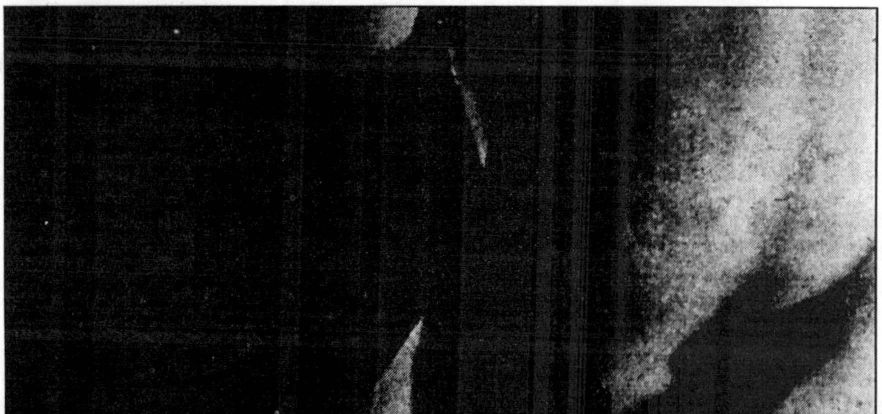
"Heroin is the
ultimate rebellion
when pot and coke
become middle-class
enjoyments."

Soho Weekly News

during the 1980 Democratic Convention, not a word of it appeared in the *Voice* and the *Soho Weekly News.* (To be fair, this also had something to do with the fact that Abbie — with friends on both papers — was in the process of re-surfacing from underground, and they were saving their column-inches for him. His close partisans always disdained the generation who came after him, and succeeded where he could not: in keeping the revolution alive after the collapse of the Antiwar movement, through the Smoke-Ins. For them, no one from the smoke-ins could ever be PC.)

On the neighborhood level most of the best bands playing Studio 10, through their management, were tied into Sunset Studios and the *Soho* scene. They were dabbling also, so the example they set for their fans undermined the YIP leadership. And into the scene came those willing to supply heroin together with the cheapest pot prices imaginable — freebooters like Bruce Brown, black sheep son of Liberty and David (producer of "Jaws") Brown. Bruce had the authority of a degree in Marxist economics, the prestige of a show on WBAI ("Psychoto-mimetic Radio"), and instant access to the dealing world due to the theory (untrue) that his dad would pay off his dealing debts as a last resort. With his bag of tricks, he made the rounds at the *Voice, High Times* and the *Soho* with the greatest of ease.

At first, he seemed a loyal friend. But gradually it became clear that to compensate for a feeling that he was a mere academic without a genuine background as a '60s organizer, he tended to disparage the self-discipline necessary for long-term accomplishment. Like all those who undermine freedom in the name of freedom, he instilled not genuine autonomy but self-destructive license, telling the kids the whole point of the revolution was to get as fucked up as possible. (Later he died of AIDS, after sharing needles and infecting almost everyone he turned on to smack.)

The YIP organization at the time was a direct successor of the "new" YOUTH INTERNATIONAL PARTY formed December, 1969, to replace SDS,[1] by merging the remnants of YIPPIE! and the WHITE PANTHERS. The Zippies had taken over from Abbie and Jerry in '72–'73 on the strength of WHITE PANTHER PARTY formations in New York, Ohio and Wisconsin. As former Field Marshall of the WPP, Dana was one of four or five recognized YIP leaders in the '70s. Therefore YIP ultimately derived part of its legitimacy from the charter granted by the Oakland Black Panthers to John Sinclair and the WPP.

Complicating matters, YIP (Zippie!) sympathized with the New York Panthers in their split with Oakland. So to the original White Panther dichotomy of *life drugs* (pot, psychedelics) versus *death drugs* (addictive white powders), the *YIPster Times* had added occasional articles all during the '70s on the movement against methadone, the use of accupuncture to treat addiction, and so on.

Pot was the only substance considered acceptable for heroin de-tox.

This core group did not start a smoke-in movement seeking to legalize pot explicitly to separate it from hard drugs — they did not

1 SDS, the Students for a Democratic Society, a mass-based organization with 100,000 members and chapters on every campus in the country, collapsed in June, 1969 into three factions, all of whom claimed to be SDS. Before Chicago, Yippies never numbered more than a few hundred; immediately afterwards a group styling itself the "Youth International Party for Self Defense" announced it was dissolving into its constituent collectives, cells, and affinity groups. In fact, the attempt to replace SDS with a new mass-based YIP only happened because the Chicago 7 Conspiracy Trial, which took up the second half of 1969 and the opening months of 1970, brought the Ann Arbor-based White Panthers into frequent contact with Abbie, Jerry and the nationwide effort going on around the Trial. The new YIP peaked in May, 1970, when the Yippie! flag flew on every campus during protests against Nixon's invasion of Cambodia.

build Studio 10 to give this movement a place to get together weekly instead of semi-annually — to turn kids on to smack.

So when they discovered kids were coming in from all over the country for the Demcon protests, only to be turned on to heroin, they freaked. And in retrospect, introducing heroin (whose dose/tolerance curve, unless you have $500-a-day, quickly leads from snorting to smoking to shooting) into a scene where passing the joint was a ritual (and info on clean needles nonexistent) was kind of like handing out firewater and smallpox-infected blankets to put down Pontiac's Rebellion.[1]

Yet YIP itself had been fatally weakened when Forçade and Peter Bourne[2] convinced them to make an exception for cocaine. So, a week after Carter's renomination, in the fall of 1980, when a novice writer at the *Soho Weekly News* wrote a review (actually, positive) of an anti-Reagan comedy skit at Studio 10, instead of seeming like the first step in breaking the media boycott, what grated was that they got Dana Beal mixed up with Dean Tuckerman. It seemed typical of a process where YIP would always be deliberately consigned to the blurry periphery of the picture instead of the focused foreground, "because they're only a bunch of publicity seekers."

Maybe it was the crash from coke done during the preceding week. Maybe it was just too much coffee and sugar. But all the frustration of watching the internal authority of the group ebb away so that he was powerless to stop the infiltration of heroin came to a head. Dana got on the phone to the *Soho,* reached Paul Slansky, and demanded a correction.

Slansky said: "Write a letter," and slammed the phone in Dana's right ear, the one with the painful earache.

Flashing on the fate of the never-published letter of protest against the "NOW HEROIN" issue, knowing for a fact that half the staff was "dabbling" and that Marcia Resnick was selling smack out of the back-alley door, some of which was reaching Studio 10.... Dana picked up a firecracker (not a bomb as later reported by the *Soho Weekly News,* but a short M-80 called an "M-60"), hopped on his bike, and went peddling over to the *Soho Weekly News,* three blocks away.

On the way he met David B., who offered to accompany him; and Alice Torbush, who told him it was the dumbest idea she'd ever heard. Disregarding this piece of wisdom, to his lasting detriment, he alighted on Broadway in front of the *Soho* and had David B. hold his bike. He went inside and told the receptionist he wanted to talk to Paul Slansky. Slansky wouldn't come out; and sent word for him to get lost.

Dana took out a match, lit it, and held it to the firecracker. "You're not going to light that in here?!" said the horrified receptionist. "Oh yes, I am," said he. The fuse caught fire. Dana turned toward the door, and carelessly tossed it back over his shoulder.

As he was passing out through the door cubicle, he glanced back through the intervening glass panel to see the innocent niece of some honcho at *Time* magazine (breaking her media teeth at the second most prestigious weekly in Manhattan) walk out from the back, just as the firecracker exploded next to a wastepaper basket.

The concussion stopped the clock on the back wall. It shut down production for the day. The staff felt like they'd been bombed. The niece (or maybe it was the daughter) of the *Time* exec was cut by a teeny, tiny bit of paper wrap from the firecracker, giving rise to the canard, later disproved before a jury, that it was a shrapnel-bearing device.

And Dana was plunged into the deepest shit of his life. On the *Soho* staff were good friends of Ed Koch. Charges were filed, which seemed especially unfair, coming just a month and a half after another set of junkies connected to the Sunset/*Soho* heroin scene had blown up the front door of 9 Bleecker with their own M-80, which detonated as Alice T. was answering their knock. But as a rule Yippies don't file charges.

Dana bided his time and planned how to turn himself in with maximum public support. The next time that could be was Halloween. The rank-and-file from the smoke-ins was still supportive, but much of the core organization had rotted out, and fell away. In the end, the only crew that would organize a protest on Dana's behalf was Howard and Norma Lotsof.

In nine days before the 1980 Halloween smoke-in, which was not a regular annual

[1] See Carl Waldman, *Atlas of the North American Indian,* p. 108; also, Alvin M. Josephy, Jr., *The Patriot Chiefs,* pp. 122–23.

[2] See Chapter Five, p. 45.

event at the time, they blanketed lower Manhattan with posters. Howard and his film crew had never been part of the YIPPIES proper; they were contract workers, making movies like *Smoke-In.* But they were close and loyal friends, and Howard credits that Halloween smoke-in with causing him to cross a key threshold in his own life.

Ever since Howard had been busted in '66, he'd never been a subject of the news. He'd always been behind the camera, not on-camera. But Dana was late to Washington Square Park. Dana wanted to make certain there were plenty of people, so that he could lead 600 people to protest outside the *Soho* and not get grabbed before he turned himself in at the Fifth Precinct five blocks south, on Elizabeth Street. So events forced Howard to get up and give a speech, to become a spokesperson, as he has been ever since.

Dana got out of jail after the weekend. The YIPS were almost broke. More protests at the *Soho Weekly News* seemed likely not to produce the same turnout. Escalating violence would only hurt innocent bystanders; anyway, it was out of the question once *Soho* contacts with the District Attorney produced a phony felony assault indictment on December 12. Then in early December, Howard and Norma came to Manhattan and proposed utilizing the one unique secret in the YIPPIES' possession.

Howard had always said that in 1962–63, out of twenty people who participated in an informal trial of Ibogaine, five of the seven using heroin, or heroin and cocaine together, had quit for six months or longer, without intending to. Why not *really* solve the problem — by dosing the junkies with Ibogaine?

Why not pay Howard's rent and food for two months so that he could do a literature search at New York University library, and figure out how it worked, whether it had mass application, and most important, if it could help the kids in the scene who'd fallen into bad habits?

RAR had $1,500 left over. What is more, Dana had originally been more interested in LSD than marijuana; and in the six years since Lotsof first told him of Ibogaine's effect, he had gradually worked the ramifications through in his own mind. So he said: "Why not?"

Like a stone kicked loose from a mountainside, picking up speed and knocking loose snowdrifts, that literature search began an avalanche.

Forçade always believed in discerning the "ultimate chaotic act," the one act that would overthrow the system perfectly, with no side effects. His favorite book was *Agent of Chaos,* by Norman Spinrad, who Dana met coincidentally just around the time of this sequence of events. Spinrad thought the only other significant chaoticist writing was Philip K. Dick. Spinrad told Dana and Alice they should pick up the hardbound edition of Dick's latest book, *VALIS,* which they did, since they were already big Philip Dick fans. Dana read it three times.

Perhaps because the Chaos Theory involved was much deeper than anything in *Agent of Chaos,* Dana found that months, even years afterwards, events would snap something from *VALIS* into exquisite, unforgettable focus. Besides, he considered parts of it evocative of the immediate situation, especially the part that read:

> *"The oppression lifted four years ago, and it will for a little while return. Be patient during this time..."* [1]

Since Dick had no way of knowing, when he wrote this in 1978, that Reagan would even be nominated (indeed, right up to the October debates, most people assumed Carter would be re-elected), Dana considered this to be a remarkable piece of prognostication — enough to pay attention, to see if the second half of the prediction would come true. It was indisputable that with Reagan, all the excesses and official lawlessness of Nixon were back. Yet would it last only a little while — say, two or three terms? Or half a lifetime?

Meanwhile, the concept that was animating Dana, as he sat writing a comprehensive review of *The Politics of Heroin in South East Asia,* and *The Great Heroin Coup,* on the role of fascist networks and covert agencies in maintaining heroin,[2] was that this time the outcome would be different, because this time the forces of resistance had something in reserve. They had begun development of a secret weapon. Definitely a long shot, but not just another protest. Ibogaine was more like the Manhattan Project.

Ibogaine would be the ultimate chaotic act.

1 See *VALIS,* p. 199.

2 "A New Heroin Conspiracy?" pp. 179–93, *Blacklisted News*

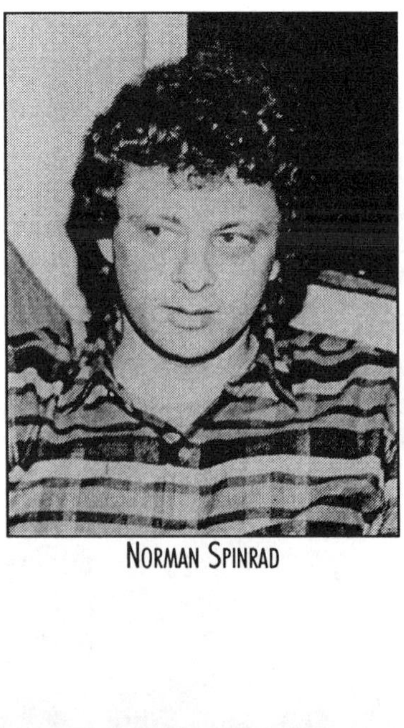

NORMAN SPINRAD

CHAPTER 2: Howard Lotsof

A conceptual split had occurred between a small group in New York, who knew about Ibogaine and had worked through its implications, and the conventional wisdom, which held that the next logical step after legalizing pot was to legalize cocaine. To outsiders, starting work on Ibogaine a month before Reagan was inaugurated might have seemed like embracing a lost cause. It was only a little more than ten years since prestigious academics tried, and failed, to stop LSD prohibition. The tightly-controlled research still allowed in humans was suspended altogether after 1975, even though it continued to show promise.[1] In fact, when asked about LSD by an interviewer in 1978, Keith Stroup of NORML said: "You want LSD, go talk to the YIPPIES."

But even as he was handing Lotsof the money, Dana remembered Leary had considerable success treating alcoholics and prisoners in the '60s. And in a way, the decision to develop Ibogaine to fight addiction harkened back even further, to the Manhattan Project,[2] and to the CIA experiments in psycho-pharmacologic warfare during the '50s. Because they did experiment with Ibogaine, and they refuse to this day to release the results.

In March of 1955 Eisenhower's special assistant for Cold War Planning, Nelson Rockefeller, was briefed by Allen Dulles on all covert CIA operations. The old Psychological Strategy Board of the National Security Council had been re-christened the Opera-tions Coordinating Board, designed to shield the President from direct knowledge of CIA "crown jewels" including Operation Bluebird and MK–ULTRA, later notorious for dosing unsuspecting Army personnel with psychedelics.[3] The CIA was looking for, among other things, a substance that could be put in the water supply or sprayed in an aerosol over Moscow, which would cause loyal Soviet citizens to wake up in the morning as patriotic Americans. You'd win without firing a shot. Unfortunately, they could never figure out a reliable delivery system, and they never found the right substance.

According to Marty Lee:

> "To conceal its role the Agency enlisted the aid of the Navy and the National Institutes of Mental Health (NIMH), which served as conduits for channeling money to Dr. Harris Isbell, a gung-ho research scientist who remained on the CIA payroll for over a decade. According to CIA documents, the directors of NIMH and the National Institutes of Health were fully cognizant of the Agency's 'interest' in Isbell's work and offered 'full support and protection'.
>
> "When the CIA came across a new drug (usually supplied by American pharmaceutical firms) that needed testing, they frequently sent it over to their chief doctor at Lexington, where an ample supply of captive guinea pigs was readily available. Over eight hundred compounds were farmed out to Isbell, including LSD and a variety of hallucinogens. It became an open secret among street junkies that if the supply got tight, you could always commit yourself to Lexington, where heroin and morphine were doled out as payment if you volunteered for Isbell's wacky drug experiments. (Small wonder Lexington had a return rate of 90%.) Dr. Isbell, a long-time member of the Food and Drug Administration's Committee on the Abuse of Depressant and Stimulant Drugs, defended the volunteer system on the grounds that there was no precedent at the time for offering inmates cash for their services."[4]

As early as 1955, at the virtual beginning of MK–ULTRA, Dr. Harris Isbell did try doses of up to 250 milligrams of Ibogaine hydrochloride on eight black ex-morphine addicts, at the Federal Narcotic Hospital at Lexington, Kentucky. The catch was that they'd been clean for six months, and 250 milligrams is a sub-therapeutic dose, so the interruption of an active addiction wouldn't have occurred. Isbell was investigating the potential of indole-alkylamines to "mimic" psychosis — according to the then-fashionable "psycho-mimetic" model championed by Dr. Paul Hoch of Columbia University.[5]

We know all this because in the '80s CIBA–GIEGY released to Howard a letter from

1 Experiments at Cold Harbor, Maryland continued to show clinical benefit in the treatment of alcoholism until the program was ended in 1976, ironically spurred by revelations of misuse of LSD by the intelligence community. In 1992, the FDA gave Donna Dryer and Richard Jenson the first IND in modern times sanctioning clinical use of LSD.

2 Harry Anslinger considered U.S. mind-control experiments with cannabinoids and other substances so sensitive that in 1943 he entrusted the research to the Manhattan Project, which made no sense, except that he had the clout as Bureau of Narcotics chief to put it there, and to know about the existence of the "Manhattan Engineering District" in the first place [!] Germany was busy experimenting with mescaline; their work became the basis of Canadian psychiatrist Cameron's "psychic driving" experiments during the '50s. Aldous Huxley, meanwhile, led a team of 200 British scientists looking looking for a way to use psycho-active chemicals to win WWII. In the early '60s a 24-year-old Austrian psychiatrist named Hans-Georg Behr cornered Huxley and asked: "You didn't really think you were going to be able to defeat the Nazi High Command by getting them high, did you?"
"No," said Huxley, "But we were able to keep 200 scientists from being sent to the front."

3 See the 1975 Church Committee Hearings. In 1993, a jury awarded Frank Olsen's family $4 million for his wrongful death due to being dosed with LSD with no warning as part of Operation Bluebird.

4 Martin Lee and Bruce Shlain, *Acid Dreams: The Complete Social History of LSD, the CIA, the Sixties, and Beyond*, pp. 24–25.

5 Dr. Hoch introduced chlorpromazine into the New York State mental hospital system.

Dr. Earl

Department of HEALTH, EDUCATION, AND WELFARE • Public Health Service
NATIONAL INSTITUTES OF HEALTH

IN REPLYING ADDRESS THE
National Institute of Mental Health
Addiction Research Center
U S Public Health Service Hospital
P O Box 2000
Lexington Kentucky

RECEIVED
DEC 5 [illegible]
A. E. E.

29 November 195[illegible] (1955)

file Ibogaine (Su 3772)

Dr. Jock Graeme
Research Dept., Div. of Clinical Investigation
Ciba Pharmaceutical Products, Inc.
Summit, New Jersey

Dear Dr. Graeme:

I thought you might be interested in hearing about the preliminary trials with Ibogaine. I am enclosing an extra copy of the letter which I would appreciate your passing on to Dr. Snyder since I feel he will be interested. I feel that this drug definitely is an hallucinogenic material and that further exploration will show that the Ibogaine psychosis will have both resemblances and differences to the LSD psychosis.

I have used 8 subjects, all adult, Negro male former morphine addicts. All of these patients were in good physical condition and none had any evidence of psychosis. Four had received LSD in past experiments, and 4 had not. None of the patients knew what the drug was, and were given no hints other than those inherent in a testing method of what subjective effects might be. Drugs were all given orally, procedure was double-blind, and every patient had a placebo control. Measurements included determination of blood pressure, pulse rate, respiratory rate, pupillary size, threshold for knee jerk, and subjective response as determined by LSD-questionnaire every half-hour for two hours prior to the drug and for eight hours after the drug. Short psychiatric interviews were conducted with each patient about 1-1/2 to 2 hours after taking the drug.

Three patients received 50 mg; 3, 100 mg; 4, 150 mg; 6, 200 mg; 4 had 250 mg; and 2 had 300 mg. Subjective effects with 50 and 100 mg. were negligible. At the 150-mg. level some reports of difficulty in sleeping and perception of colored lights were encountered. There were, however, no objective changes at this dose level. Doses of 200 mg. or higher found definite dilatation of the pupils, definite but mild increase in systolic blood pressure, but no significant effects on temperature, pulse rate or respiratory rate.

CIBA–Geigy

CIA–HARRIS ISBELL LETTER, PAGE ONE.

Isbell requesting Ibogaine for thirteen more subjects. And because one of CIBA's own researchers, named Schneider, discovered in 1956 that Ibogaine potentiates morphine analgesia (Ibogaine multiplies the painkilling effect of opiates), it is fairly certain Isbell checked it out further.

Since Isbell was also looking for an addiction cure, and experimented with many different psychoactive agents in all different dose regimens, both during and after withdrawal from morphine, the next logical step would have been to try to wean active addicts off opiates by substituting progressively more Ibogaine for their usual dose of heroin. And if he used a threshold dose, six milligram-per-kg., he would have started observing the Lotsof effect.[1]

"In addition to this role as a research scientist, Dr. Isbell served as a go-between for the CIA in its attempt to obtain drug samples from European pharmaceutical concerns which assumed they were providing 'medicine' to a US Public Health official. The CIA in turn acted as a research coordinator, passing information, tips, and leads to Isbell and its other contract employees so that they could keep abreast of each other's progress; when a new discovery was made, the CIA would often ask another researcher to conduct a followup study for confirmation. One scientist whose work was coordinated with Isbell's in such a manner was Dr. Carl Pfeiffer, a noted pharmacologist from Princeton who tested LSD on inmates at the Federal Prison in Atlanta and Bordentown Reformatory in New Jersey.

"Isbell, Pfeiffer, Cameron, West and Hoch — all were part of a network of doctors and scientists who gathered intelligence for the CIA. Through these scholar-informants the Agency stayed on top of the latest developments within the 'above-ground' LSD scene, which expanded rapidly during the Cold War. By the mid–1950s numerous independent investigators had undertaken hallucinogenic drug studies, and the CIA was determined not to let the slightest detail escape its grasp..."[2]

Did the CIA or Defense Department discover Ibogaine's ability to interrupt addiction? They "refuse to confirm or deny" that any file exists (even CIBA–GIEBY's reply to Isbell), not only in the face of Lotsof's Freedom of Information Act requests, but even to NIDA researchers. Evidence has surfaced, however, that the Addiction Research Center at Lexington, Kentucky continued to be on the CIA payroll from 1957 to 1962 — the years it would have taken them to check out Ibogaine and its probable impact. The record of payments (*see exhibits, pp. 20–22*) with entries spanning 1953 to 1961 (years during which Isbell was ARC director of research) — minus any additional descriptions of the disbursements or results of experiments carried out — came into Lotsof's hands when the CIA sent him documents related to someone else's Freedom of Information request. He forwarded it to the proper recipient, a private group in Washington, DC called the National Security Archive. And they sent back four pages showing that Isbell continued to be on the CIA payroll during the crucial five years it would have taken to check out Ibogaine and its probable impact.

1 For description, see p. 22.

2 Martin Lee and Bruce Shlain, *Acid Dreams: The Complete Social History of LSD, the CIA, the Sixties, and Beyond*, pp. 25–26. Isbell also believed that cocaine was not addictive, according to Stanley Yolis, then head of the National Institute of Mental Health. That would make Isbell a likely key disseminator of this idea through the psychedelic movement of the 1960s.

If they did discover something, they didn't follow it up. In Africa, the ritual use of the plant of which Ibogaine is the principal alkaloid, *tabernanthe iboga,* forms the basis of a religion called Bwiti. To become fully initiated, all Bwiti must eat enough iboga rootbark to induce intense visions and enable them to "meet their ancestors" — including a kind of universal African ancestor (the Bwiti).

In *Bwiti, An Ethnography of the Religious Imagination in Africa,* Princeton University anthropologist James W. Fernandez recounts an unforgettable first encounter, soon after arriving in Gabon in 1958:

> "Late one evening about three months after I had taken up residence in Assok Ening... there was a loud knocking at the door....The open door revealed in the light of the pressure lamp a man of about 35 with a beard, a long flowing robe, and a red cord about his waist. "Monsieur," he said addressing me in French, "I am Metogo Zogo, Nganga Bwiti, and I must speak with you." He fixed me with an unrelenting gaze. "You seek the truth here but you will not find it." As I stepped back, he made a dramatic entrance, sweeping himself and robes into the center of the room. "You do not know me but I am no stranger. I am a child of this village just returned from a long spiritual journey. I have been following the truth! You will not find it in this village talking to these old men. You must come to the Bwiti Chapel in my father's house...
>
> The nganga could not contain himself..."You want to know the 'old things.' But none here know them. They have not seen them. We Banzie see them when we eat eboga. We see the 'old people' there. We know the 'old things' through them.
>
> "Now you want to know why the condition of this village and of the Fang is desperate. None of this village execept we Banzie can tell you that. The people here are lost in sin. They have not paid the price of those sins. They have not died for their sins. But we Banzie have died and paid the price. We die and return, die and return, each time more purified...
>
> "...You should dance with Bwiti. You have heard the harp at night. While all these villagers are asleep we dance and journey far. They go nowhere here. They wander around in confusion. They don't know where to go. But we go far." He took hold of the red-woven cord around his waist. "You see this cord? This is the Path of Birth and Death. We follow this path. We know life. We know death."[1]

Dr. Graeme
Summit, N. J.
Page Two

Subjective effects were varying greatly in intensity from individual-to-individual, and were spectacular with doses of 200 to 300 mg. They included anxiety, fear of dying, confusion, perception of colored lights and patterns with eyes both open and closed, development in some cases of true hallucination, depersonalization, depersonalization phenomena, and difficulty in thinking and in concentration. These phenomena occurred with a clear sensorium and with insight. Visual perceptual distortion, if it occurred at all, was not prominent, and in this sense the Ibogaine psychosis may differ sharply from the LSD psychosis.

As mentioned above, there was a marked variation in the response of different individuals to the drug. Severe reaction was observed in one 60-kg. man with as little as 200 mg. of the drug, whereas one 80-kg. man had only a mild reaction to 300 mg. of the substance. Another 80-kg. man had marked reaction to only 200 mg. Not only does the reaction vary from person-to-person, but varies in the same individual. In one man, severe reaction was seen 30 minutes after ingestion of 200 mg. On another trial, the reaction was not apparent for 1-1/2 hours. These irregularities suggest that possibly absorption of the drug may be somewhat slow and irregular.

Pressure of other work means that I must lay Ibogaine aside for the moment, but I hope in the future to explore it further with the following objectives in mind;

1. Elimination of the irregularity in the action by using the material parenterally,
2. Detailed evaluation of the reaction in 15 men on all of the measures that have heretofore been used,
3. Detailed neurological study, with special attention to vision,
4. Electroencephalographic study,
5. Direct comparison of the Ibogaine reaction with the LSD reaction in the same group of patients,
6. Psychological tests, particularly the Minnesota Multiphasic Personality Inventory.

Could you supply enough parenteral material for about 15 men, estimating about 250 mg. for each man?

Yours very sincerely,

AB0492 410

Harris Isbell, M.D.
Director

HI:tkh

CIBA-Geigy

CIA—HARRIS ISBELL LETTER, PAGE TWO

The red cord represents the umbilicus which connects each of us back, generation through generation, to the original Mother. Initiates are advised that in the visions red is the color of the true road that leads to the Ancestors. In some versions of Bwiti, the Creator God is properly accessed only through the Mother.[2] Bwiti is the only native religion that has successfully resisted the inroads of Islam and Christianity. Lotsof's explanation, simply, is that it's very hard to get into a belief system with a sacrament as powerful as Iboga and ever forsake it afterwards for another. Despite being split up into 200 dialects by the rainforest, Bwiti unified the Gabonese Independence movement of the 1950s.

In the '50s, the United States was still in

1 James W. Fernandez, *Bwiti: An Ethnography of the Religious Imagination in Africa* (Princeton: Princeton University Press, 1982), pp. 291–292.

2 See also footnote, p. 125 of this report, ibid.

the thrall of segregation, of the racist police state of J. Edgar Hoover, nemesis of Marcus Garvey and Malcolm X. The highest-level person briefed on MK–ULTRA results was Presidential assistant for Cold War Planning — Nelson Rockefeller or his sucessor. The Cold Warriors equated African de-colonialization with international communism. The last thing they wanted was a drug treatment which would, through the population of Black junkies, release another force that could unify and electrify the Black movement in this country.

But in *In Search of the Manchurian Candidate,* John Marks poses a simpler explanation. Basically, the CIA concluded that the LSD conversion experience "wore off" with the drug. CIA researchers had great familiarity with LSD, which had acquired as yet no stigma, having dosed each other with it many times. This casual familiarity may have inclined them to underrate the strength and potential impact of other, more exotic substances which agents never bothered to try for themselves — even as they were vastly accelerating the introduction of psychedelics into US academia, according to Marks.[1]

When, at the beginning of the '60s, Tim Leary gave Allen Ginsberg acid, Ginsberg immediately flashed that an indole alkylamine of some kind could free the junkies, (although he was thinking more along the lines of substitute drugs.) Then, when the Harvard Administration cracked down, Leary issued a call for his Great Leap Forward: for undergraduates everywhere to continue and broaden paraclinical research into all the indole-ring psychoactives, with one goal being to find a cure for addiction *(See Leary–Ginsberg article, pp. 23–25, continued pp. 36–38).*

One of those who responded was a smart 19-year-old named Howard Lotsof, who was living with his parents in New Jersey after a childhood spent in the Bronx and Queens. His introduction to psychedelics was Aldous Huxley's *Doors of Perception,* which he read when he was 15. His interest was part illumination-seeker, part lay scientist. His hero was Einstein.

In the movement from the very repressive decade of the '50s, to the release and coming-together in the '60s, Howard sided with those who were dissatisfied, and who believed that if chemistry could be the means to resolve some of their questions and find some answers, they should use it. In those days it was possible to start your own chemical company with nothing more than a letterhead, and order all kinds of neat substances that were later controlled.

One day Howard was having breakfast with a chemist he knew who had been active in the small underground LSD scene of the '50s. The chemist offered him a dose of Ibogaine that he had in the freezer. Lotsof asked him what he could tell him about it. "Well, it's a thirty-six-hour trip," said the chemist.

A thirty-six-hour trip was the last thing Howard could imagine himself wanting to do, so he gave it to a friend and asked him to check it out. A month later, at 12:20 at night,

Drug experimentation, Narcotics, Hallucinogens, Drug addiction, --Citations for 1953-1957
Page: 1
REQNUM: F82-0212
PUBDATE: 1957-08-16
DECAL: CIA*DDA*OF MEMO 580956
TITLE: TRANSFER OF FUNDS FOR CONTINUATION OF A RESEARCH PROJECT AT THE ADDICTION RESEARCH CENTER PUBLIC HEALTH SERVI CE HOSPITAL LEXINGTON KY PROJECT 1 JULY 1957

SUBJECTS: ADDICTION RESEARCH CENTER; HOSPITAL; LEXINGTON KY; RESEARCH PROJECT; TRANSFER OF FUNDS

REQNUM: F82-0212
PUBDATE: 1957-08-16
DECAL: CIA*DDA*OF MEMO 580956
TITLE: TRANSFER OF FUNDS FOR CONTINUATION OF A RESEARCH PROJECT AT THE ADDICTION RESEARCH CENTER PUBLIC HEALTH SERVI CE HOSPITAL LEXINGTON KY PROJECT 1 JULY 1957

SUBJECTS: ADDICTION RESEARCH CENTER; HOSPITAL; LEXINGTON KY; RESEARCH PROJECT; TRANSFER OF FUNDS

REQNUM: F82-0212
PUBDATE: 1958-07-18
DECAL: CIA*DDA*O: MEMO 59 899
TITLE: TRANSFER OF FUNDS FOR CONTINUATION OF A RESEARCH PROJECT AT THE ADDICTION RESEARCH CENTER PUBLIC HEALTH SERVI CE HOSPITAL LEXINGTON KY REQUEST 59 899

SUBJECTS: ADDICTION RESEARCH CENTER; HOSPITAL; LEXINGTON KY; REQUEST 59 899; RESEARCH PROJECT; TRANSFER OF FUNDS

REQNUM: F82-0212
PUBDATE: 1959-09-15
DECAL: CIA*DDA*OF MEMO 5867 60
TITLE: TRANSFER OF FUNDS FOR CONTINUATION OF A RESEARCH PROJECT AT THE ADDICTION CENTER SERVICE HOSPITAL LEXINGTON KY PUBLIC HEALTH

SUBJECTS: ADDICTION CENTER; ALLOTMENT; HOSPITAL; LEXINGTON KY; RESEARCH PROJECT

REQNUM: F82-0212
PUBDATE: 1960-11-07
DECAL: CIA*DDA*OF MEMO 61 13373 1
TITLE: TRANSFER OF FUNDS FOR CONTINUATION OF A RESEARCH PROJECT AT THE ADDICTION RESEARCH CENTER LEXINGTON KY PUBLI C HEALTH SERVICE HOSPITAL PROJECT USE LETTER 61 13 373 1 4 OCTOBER 1960

SUBJECTS: ADDICTION RESEARCH CENTER; HOSPITAL; LEXINGTON KY; RESEARCH PROJECT; TRANSFER OF FUNDS

REQNUM: F82-0212
PUBDATE: 1977-09-20
DECAL: CIA*DDA*OF MEMO 56 124

Drug experimentation, Narcotics, Hallucinogens, Drug addiction, —Citations for 1953-1957
Page: 2
TITLE: TRANSFER OF FUNDS FOR CONTINUATION OF A RESEARCH PROJECT AT THE ADDICTION RESEARCH CENTER PUBLIC HEALTH SERVI CE HOSPITAL LEXINGTON KY

SUBJECTS: HOSPITAL; LEXINGTON KY; REQUEST 56 124; RESEARCH PROJECT; TRANSFER OF FUNDS

REQNUM: F82-0212
PUBDATE: 1977-09-20
DECAL: CIA*DDA*OF MEMO 56 124
TITLE: TRANSFER OF FUNDS FOR CONTINUATION OF A RESEARCH PROJECT AT THE ADDICTION RESEARCH CENTER PUBLIC HEALTH SERVI CE HOSPITAL LEXINGTON KY

SUBJECTS: HOSPITAL; LEXINGTON KY; REQUEST 56 124; RESEARCH PROJECT; TRANSFER OF FUNDS

National Security Archive

CIA RECORD OF PAYMENTS TO LSD RESEARCHER HARRIS ISBELL

1 See *Manchurian Candidate*, pp. 70–7.

Howard got a phone call from the friend, who said: “You know that drug you gave me? It’s not a drug, it’s a food. We have to tell Congress!”

Howard was 19 at the time, living at home with his parents, so he said: “You woke my mother up. I’ll get back to you.” After succeeding in getting the house back to sleep, he decided the matter bore further investigation. It took his circle six months to get further supplies, and they still didn’t know what they had.

To discover the interruption effect, you need active addicts, and you need enough experience with LSD to know sub-optimal doses of indole-alkalamines can produce a bum trip where a larger dose will get you above the “tree-top” effect of getting tangled up in your own emotions. Only people seeking a high-dose, thirty-six-hour experience would do the amount — about a gram for a 150-pound person — that produces a therapeutic result.

Contrary to some published reports, Howard did not hand the stuff out to some friends at a party. (“Some party,” he says. “After the first hour it would consist of everyone lying around in a darkened room, not talking.”) It was administered one dose at a time, over eight months, to twenty people. Seven of them, including Howard, happened to be using heroin or cocaine.[1]

Howard’s own experience began in the cab of a truck, because he happened to take it as he was in the process of moving back New York from New Jersey. Perhaps because he was 19 and very busy, Howard was not overwhelmed by Ibogaine ataxia (usual slight loss of balance coupled with an overwhelming urge to lie down). He was dropped off in the West Village and managed to make it upstairs to his regular session with his psychologist, and told him to turn on the tape-recorder so that he could tell him what he was seeing. Despite doing only about half of the dose addicts get today (and perhaps because he was sensitized by amphetamine) he was having a “full-blown Ibogaine experience,” with the Freudian overtones of dreams, or of a birth visualization:

> “The first thing I saw was a pulsating yellow screwdriver, which disappeared abruptly. And the next thing I knew I was walking up a ladder leading to a 10-foot diving board over a pool. As I was walking up the diving board, my bathing suit disappeared and I was naked. As I dived into the pool, my mother appeared beneath me with her legs open, and I was diving into her vagina. As I got closer, she changed into my sister, who changed into an infant. Then I went into the water, and that was it. The vision turned into a new one.
>
> For three or four hours, the way the visualizations changed was always the same and different from any other hallucinogen. It appeared that you’d get one vision, and then a gold or silver web would carry it off and an entirely new set of visions would arrive.”

On another trip, he was watching a stage, and all of a sudden music started. The music was like, *BOMdidaBOMPdidaBOMdidaBOMP,* and pairs of cavemen and cavewomen came dancing onto the stage. The men were behind the women, and they were dancing with them. And then two more of them came onto the stage, rolling this giant *stone heart...* Later he

Page No. 1
08/24/92

CIA OFFICE CODES AND ABBREVIATIONS

Code	Comp.	Abbrev.	Office
U			
00041	DDO	AF	AFRICA DIVISION
00086	DDI	ALA	OFFICE OF AFRICA AND LATIN AMERERICA ANALYSIS
00043	DDO	CCS	CENTRAL COVER STAFF
00045	DDO	CIS	COUNTERINTELLIGENCE STAFF
00070	DDO	CMS	CAREER MANAGEMENT STAFF
00009	DCI	COMPT	OFFICE OF COMPTROLLER
00016	DDI	CPAS	CURRENT PRODUCTION AND ANALYTICAL SUPPORT (WAS OCO)
00020	DDI	CPAS	CURRENT PRODUCTION AND ANALYTICAL SUPPORT (WAS OCO)
00055	DDO	CPN	COUNTER TERRORISM PARAMILITARY NARCOTICS STAFF
00015	DDI	CPS	CENTER FOR POLICY SUPPORT
00093	DDO	CTC	COUNTER TERRORIST CENTER
00010	DCI	DCI	OFFICE OF THE DIRECTOR
00030	DDA	DDA	DEPUTY DIRECTOR ADMINISTRATION
00029	DDI	DDI	DEPUTY DIRECTOR INTELLIGENCE
00040	DDO	DDO	DEPUTY DIRECTOR OPERATIONS
00060	DDST	DDST	DEPUTY DIRECTOR SCIENCE & TECHNOLOGY
00048	DDO	EA	EAST ASIA DIVISION
00090	DDA	EEO	EQUAL EMPLOYMENT OPPORTUNITY OFFICE-UNDER OP
00051	DDO	EPDS	EVALUATION PROGRAM DESIGN STAFF
00047	DDO	EUR	EUROPEAN DIVISION
00089	DDI	EURA	OFFICE OF EUROPEAN ANALYSIS
00025	DDST	FBIS	FOREIGN BROADCAST INFORMATION SERVICE
00046	DDO	FRD	FOREIGN RESOURCES DIVISION
00003	DCI	HS	HISTORY STAFF
00004	DCI	ICS	INTELLIGENCE COMMUNITY STAFF
00075	DCI	ICS	INTELLIGENCE COMMUNITY STAFF --ALL RECORDS REASSIGNED TO OPI 04 -- 25 JULY 83
00053	DDO	IMS	INFORMATION MANAGEMENT STAFF (WAS INFORMATION SERVICES STAFF)
00057	DDO	LA	LATIN AMERICA DIVISION
00095	DDI	LDA	OFFICE OF LEADERSHIP ANALYSISCMSN
00024	DDO	NCD	NATIONAL COLLECTION DIVISION
00052	DDO	NE	NEAR EAST & SOUTH ASIA DIVISION
00087	DDI	NESA	OFFICE OF NEAR EASTERN AND SOUTH ASIAN ANALYSIS
00071	DDO	NFIB	NFIB COMMITTEE ON EXCHANGES
00092	DCI	NIC/NIO	NATIONAL INTELLIGENCE COUNCIL/NIO
00091	DCI	NIESO	NATIONAL INTELLIGENCE EMERGENCY SUPPORT OFFICER
00014	DDI	NIO	NATIONAL INTELLIGENCE OFFICERS
00019	DDST	NPIC	NATIONAL PHOTOGRAPHIC INTERPRETATION CENT
00077	DCI	NSC	NATIONAL SECURITY COUNCIL
00033	DDA	OC HQ	OFFICE OF COMMUNICATIONS (HQS)

National Security Archive

CIA CODES AND ABBREVIATIONS, PAGE ONE

[1] His future wife, Norma Alexander, participated in the study, but as a control.

Page No. 2
08/24/92

CIA OFFICE CODES AND ABBREVIATIONS

Code	Comp.	Abbrev.	Office
00008	DCI	OCA	OFFICE OF CONGRESSIONAL AFFAIRS - FORMERLY OLL WHICH REPLACED OEXA
00081	DDA	OCDF	OFFICE OF COMMUNICATIONS DOMESTIC FIELD
00012	DDI	OCR	OFFICE OF CENTRAL REFERENCE
00065	DDST	ODE	OFFICE OF DEVELOPMENT & ENGINEERING
00088	DDI	OEA	OFFICE OF EAST EASTERN ANALYSIS
00044	DDO	OED	OFFICE OF EXTERNAL DEVELOPMENT
00038	DDA	OF	OFFICE OF FINANCE
00036	DCI	OGC	OFFICE OF GENERAL COUNSEL
00018	DDI	OGI	OFFICE OF GLOBAL ISSUES
00013	DDI	OGI	OFFICE OF GLOBAL ISSUES
00027	DDI	OIA	OFFICE OF IMAGERY ANALYSIS
00007	DCI	OIG	OFFICE OF INSPECTOR GENERAL
00037	DCI	OIGAS	OFFICE OF INSPECTOR GENERAL (AUDIT STAFF)
00094	DDI	OIR	OFFICE OF INFORMATION RESOURCES
00034	DDA	OIS	OFFICE OF INFORMATION SERVICES
00063	DDA	OIT	OFFICE OF INFORMATION TECHNOLOGY
00035	DDA	OL HQ	OFFICE OF LOGISTICS (HQS)
00082	DDA	OLDF	OFFICE OF LOGISTICS DOMESTIC FIELD
00084	DCI	OMB	OFFICE OF MANAGEMENT & BUDGET
00039	DDA	OMS	OFFICE OF MEDICAL SERVICES
00032	DDA	OP	OFFICE OF PERSONNEL
00083	DDA	OP	OFFICE OF PERSONNEL CREDIT UNION
00066	DDST	ORD	OFFICE OF RESEARCH & DEVELOPMENT
00031	DDA	OS	OFFICE OF SECURITY
00017	DDI	OSI	OFFICE OF SCIENTIFIC INTELLIGENCE MERGED WITH OWI TO FORM OFFICE OF SCIENTIFIC WEAPONS RESEARCH-64
00061	DDST	OSO	OFFICE OF SIGINT OPERATIONS
00050	DDST	OSO	OFFICE OF SIGINT OPERATIONS (WAS DDO DIVISION D)
00085	DCI	OSTP	OFFICE OF SCIENCE & TECHNOLOGY POLICY
00064	DDI	OSWR	OFFICE OF SCIENTIFIC WEAPONS RESEARCH
00011	DDA	OT&E	OFFICE OF TRAINING & EDUCATION
00099	999	OTH	OTHER
00056	DDST	OTS	OFFICE OF TECHNICAL SERVICE
00076	DCI	PA	OFFICE OF PUBLIC AFFAIRS
00049	DDO	PCS	POLICY & COORDINATION STAFF
00022	DDI	PPG	PUBLICATIONS AND PRESENTATIONS GROUP NOW PART OF OFFICE OF CURRENT OPERATIONS-16
00042	DDO	PPS	POLITICAL AND PSYCHOLOGICAL STAFF
00006	DDA	RCD	REGULATIONS CONTROL DIVISION (WAS REGULATIONS CONTROL BRANCH)
00054	DDO	SE	SOVIET EAST EUROPEAN DIVISION
00026	DDI	SOVA	OFFICE OF SOVIET ANALYSIS
00067	DDST	SPS	SPECIAL PROJECTS STAFF (MAY BE ADDED TO O-DDST)

National Security Archive

CIA Codes and Abbreviations, page two

"had the sensation of slides opening up, and sliding downward at a tremendous speed, with all my experiences arranged, accessible like filing cabinets flashing past." He also experienced behavioral immobility, which wore off only when the visualizations ceased, leaving him in a strange, high energy state. Howard explains:

> "The hallucinatory period ends abruptly, and the first reaction generally is, 'What happened? I thought this was supposed to last for 36 hours.' Then all of a sudden you realize that it hasn't stopped, it's just changed. You're no longer watching this motion picture, but there are like giant lightning flashes and movements of light all over the place...but there's no waviness, things do not lose their normal form, as they do under heavy dosages of common hallucinogens like LSD or mescaline, where a wall will seem to wave.
>
> "Another difference was, with hallucinogens generally, if you were to move your hand you'd see a wave-like pattern. With Ibogaine, you don't get a continuous wave, you get distinct images, and I noticed it the first time, when I was walking on the street... I was on my way to the west side, and I turned around, there were seven distinct after-images of myself. And as I took a step, a new one would appear, and the last one would disappear.
>
> "During that second high-energy period, which lasts from six to twelve hours, you're seeing all these flashes of light, and what's happening is you're getting thoughts coming into your mind which support the deep symbolic material which came out in the initial three or four hour visualization phase. For instance you might be thinking that all people are playing roles, that the basic interaction of humans is on a sexual, nonverbal type of level. And these realizations slowly diminish, till after about twelve hours that phase is completely closed out. Apparently a secondary stimulation effect occurs, and that slowly curtails, somewhere between twenty-four and thirty hours, and the subject goes to sleep."

Says Norma: "I remember thinking, when is this going to end? I'm so tired. I couldn't imagine anyone doing it for fun."

Strangest of all, Howard awoke after three hours of sleep completely refreshed.

> "Ten steps out of my door it hit me: For the first time in months, I did not want or need to go cop heroin. In fact, I viewed heroin as a drug that emulated death; I wanted life. I looked down the street, at the trees, the sky, my house and realized that for the first time in my life, I didn't feel afraid."

Five out of seven of the twenty in the initial trial were addicts who quit heroin or cocaine, involuntarily, for six months or longer, says Lotsof. And after two days, five of the seven had not gone through withdrawal, and had no desire to use heroin, for periods ranging up to eighteen months — up to six months from a single treatment, and up to eighteen months from a series of five treatments.

The other two got up the next morning and began their routine of going out to cop junk. "Why?" Howard asked them.

"Because we're junkies," they said. "We like being junkies."

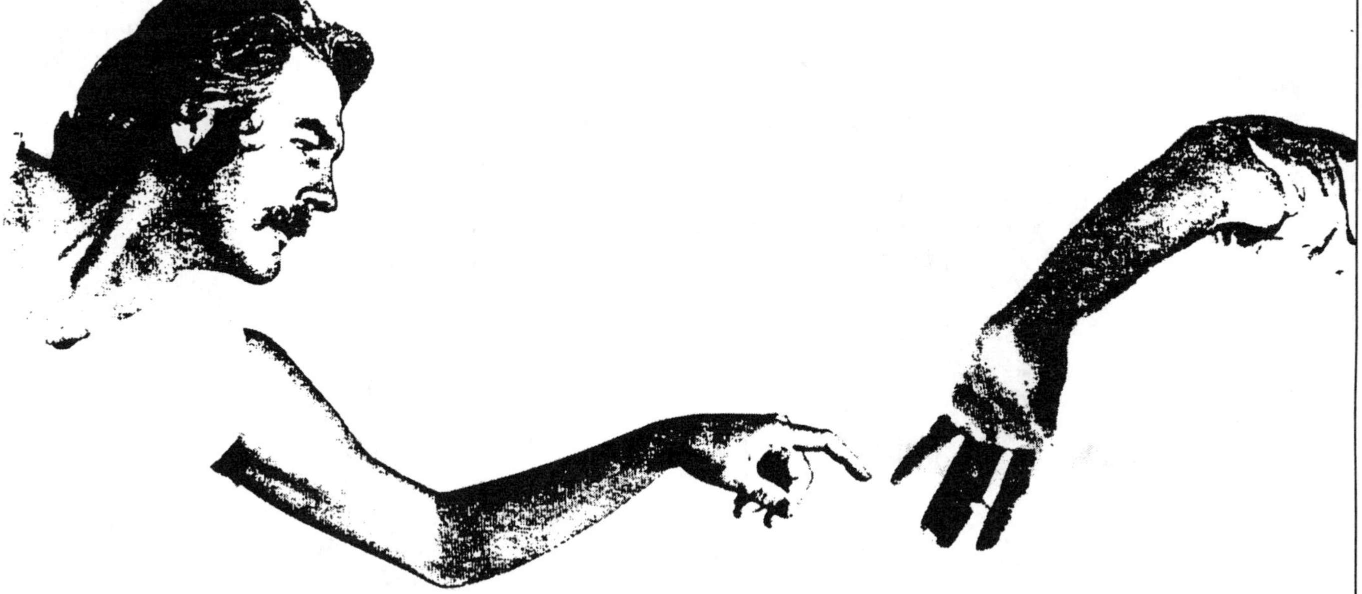

In the beginning, Leary turned on Ginsberg and saw that it was good....

by Timothy Leary

Genesis: Sunday, November 26, 1960 at Newton, Massachusetts

By the Fall of 1960 there was in existence an informal international network of scientists and scholars who had taken the psychedelic trip and who foresaw the powerful effect that the new alkaloids would have on human culture. The members of this group differed in age and temperament, and had varying ideas about tactics, but the basic vision was common to all—we believed these wondrous plants and drugs could free man's consciousness and bring about a new conception of man, his psychology and philosophy.

There was Albert Hofmann, who had invented LSD, who dreamed the utopian dream, but who was limited by the cautious politics of Sandoz Pharmaceuticals. What a frustrating web his genius had woven for Sandoz. How could a medical-drug house make a profit on a revelation pill?

Sandoz knew they had patented the most powerful mind-changing substance known to man. They expected to make millions when the psychiatric profession learned how to use LSD, and they were continually disappointed to discover that human society didn't want to have its mind changed, didn't want to touch a love-ecstasy potion.

In 1960 a top executive of Sandoz leaned across the conference table and said jokingly to me, LSD isn't a drug at all. It's a food. Let's bottle it in Coca-Cola and let the world have it. And his legal counsel frowned and said that foods still come under the jurisdiction of the Food and Drug Administration.

By 1966, when LSD was crowding Vietnam for the headlines, officials of Sandoz Pharmaceuticals were groaning, We wish we had never heard of LSD.

I do really wish to destroy it! cried Frodo. Or well, to have it destroyed. I am not made for perilous quests. I wish I had never seen the Ring! Why did it come to me? Why was I chosen?

—The Lord of the Rings

There were the detached philosophers—Aldous Huxley, Father Murray, Gerald Heard, Alan Watts, Harry Murray, Robert Gordon Wasson—who knew that the new drugs were reintroducing the platonic-gnostic vision. These men had read their theological history and understood both the glorious possibility and the angered reaction of the priestly establishment. They were not activists but sage observers.

Then there were the turned-on doctors—psychiatrists who had taken the trip, and came back hoping to fit the new potions into the medical game. Humphrey Osmond, witty, wise, cultured, had invented the name psychedelic and tolerantly wondered how to introduce a harmony-ecstasy drug into an aggressive-puritanical social order. Sidney Cohen, Keith Ditman, Jim Watt, Abram Hoffer and Nick Chewelos hoped to bring about a psychiatric renaissance and a new era of mental health with the new alchemicals.

And there was that strange, intriguing, delightful cosmic magician called Al Meyner, the rum-drinking, swashbuckling, Roman Catholic frontier salesman who promoted uranium ore during the Forties and who took the trip and recognized that LSD was the fissionable material of the mind and who turned on Osmond and Hoffer to the religious mystical meaning of their psychotomimetic drug. Al Meyner set out to turn on the world and flew from country to country with his leather bag full of drugs, claiming to have turned on bishops and obtained *nihil obstat* from Pope John. When the medical society complained that only doctors could give drugs, Meyner bought himself a doctor's degree from a Kentucky diploma mill and swept through northern California turning on scientists and professors and God seekers.

Right from the beginning this dedicated group of ring bearers was rent with a basic disagreement. There were those who said work within the system. Society has assigned the administration of drugs to the medical profession. Any non-doctor who gives or takes drugs is a dope fiend. Play ball with the system. Medicine must be the vanguard of the psychedelic movement. Any nonmedical use of psychedelic drugs would create a new marijuana mess and set back research into the new utopia.

The medical point of view made little sense to religious philosophers. Aldous Huxley called the psychedelic experience a gratuitous grace. His vibrant flame-colored wife, Laura, agreed. So, in gentle tones, did Huston Smith and Alan Watts and Gerald Heard.

And so did Allen Ginsberg, who had discovered the Buddha nature of drugs along with other writers.

I had been visited by most of the psychedelic eminences by this time and was under steady pressure to make the Harvard psychedelic research a kosher-medically-approved project. Everyone

Esquire

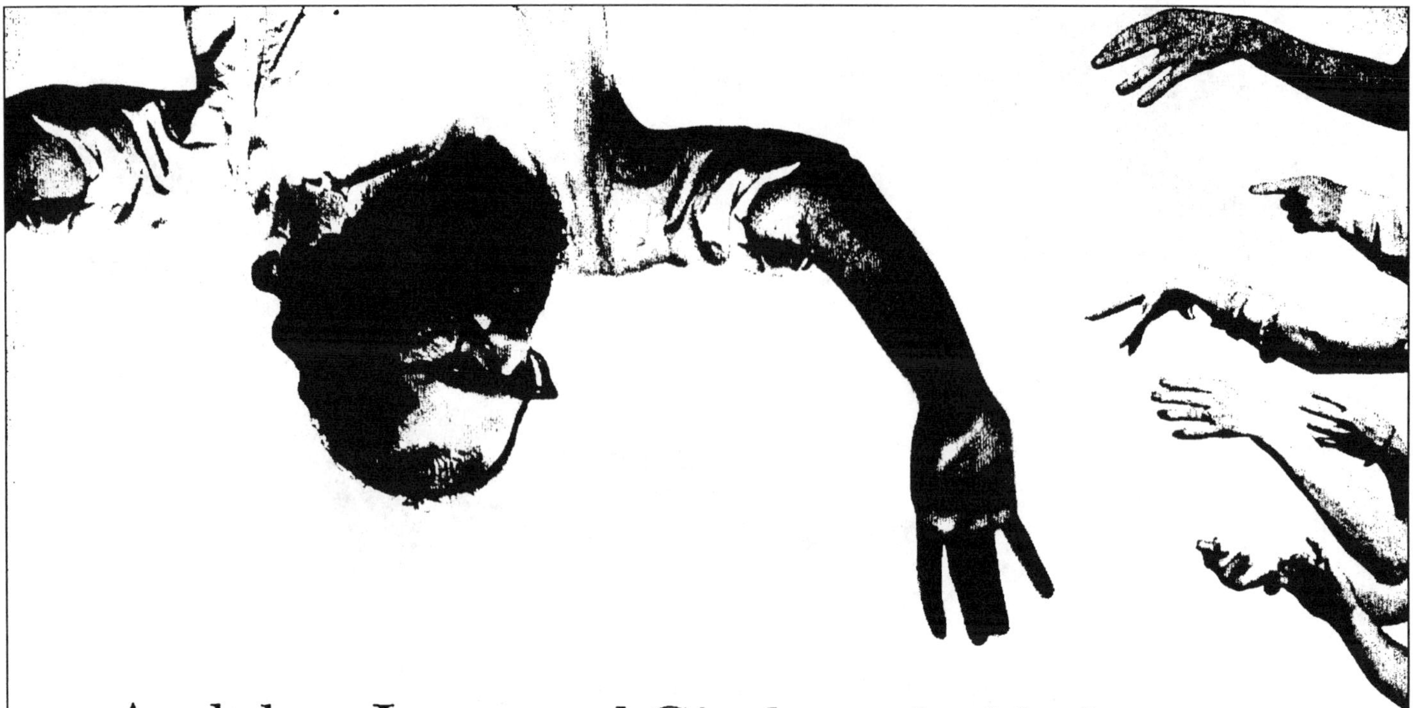

And then Leary and Ginsberg decided to turn on

Apostles: Sundry poets, painters and writers
Epistles: The letters of Allen to Timothy
Apocalypse: (Leary got busted)

was aware of the potency of Harvard's name. Timothy, you are the key figure, said Dr. Al Meyner; I'm just old deputy-dog Al at your service. But the message was clear: Keep it respectable and medical.

And now here was Allen Ginsberg, the secretary-general of the world's poets, beatniks, anarchists, socialists, free-sex/love cultists.

November 26, 1960, the sunny Sunday afternoon that we gave Allen Ginsberg the mushrooms, started slowly. First in the cycle of breakfasts at noon were my son Jack Leary and his friend Bobbie, who had spent the night. Bobbie went off to Mass. When I came down I found Donald, an uninvited raccoon hipster-painter from New York, solemnly squatting at the table gnawing at toast and bacon. Frank Barron, who was visiting, and the poets, Allen Ginsberg and Peter and Lafcadio Orlovsky, remained upstairs and we moved around the kitchen with that Sunday-morning hush, not wanting to wake the sleepers. Lafcadio, Peter's brother, was on leave from a hospital.

About twelve-thirty the quiet exploded into family noise. Bobbie was back from church where he had excitedly told his father about the party we had given the night before for the Harvard football team and how I had given the boys, Bobbie and Jack, a dollar each for being bartenders.

I toted up the political profit and loss from this development. The Harvard football team rang up a sale. But the boys bartending? Bobbie's father is Irish so that's all right. All okay.

Then wham, the door opened and in flooded Susan Leary, my daughter, with three teen-age girls, through the kitchen, upstairs to get clothes, down to make a picnic lunch, up again for records, out, and then back for the ginger ale.

By now the noise had filtered upstairs and we could hear the late sleepers moving around and the bathroom waters running, and down came Frank Barron, half-awake, to fry codfish cakes for his breakfast. And then, Allen Ginsberg and Peter. Allen hopped around the room with nearsighted crow motions cooking eggs, and Peter sat silent, watching.

Afterward the poets fell to reading The *Times* and Frank moved upstairs to Susan's room to watch a pro football game on TV. I told Allen to make himself at home and got beers and went up to join Frank. Donald the painter had been padding softly around the house watching with his big, soft creature eyes and sniffing in corners and at the bookcase and the record cabinets. He had asked to take mushrooms in the evening and was looking for records of Indian peyote drum music.

At dusk, Allen Ginsberg, hunched over a teacup, peering out through his black-rimmed glasses, the left lens bisected by a break, started telling of his experiences with ayahuasco, the fabled visionary vine of the Peruvian jungles. He had followed the quest of Bill Burroughs, sailing south for new realms of consciousness, looking for the elixir of wisdom. Sitting, sweating with heat, lonely in a cheap hotel in Lima, holding a wad of ether-soaked cotton to his nose with his left hand and getting high and making poetry with his right hand, and then traveling by second-class bus with Indians up through the Cordillera de los Andes and then more buses and hitchhiking into the Montaña jungles and shining rivers, wandering through steaming equatorial forests. Then the village Pucallpa, and the negotiations to find the *curandero* [guide], paying him with *aguardiente*, and the ritual itself, swallowing the bitter stuff, and the nausea and the colors and the drums beating and sinking down into thingless void, into the great eye that brings it all together, and the terror of the great snake coming. The old *curandero*, wrinkled face bending over him and Allen telling him, *culebra*, and the *curandero* nodding clinically and blowing a puff of smoke to make the great snake disappear and it did.

The fate of fire depends on wood; as long as there is wood below, the fire burns above. It is the same in human life; there is in man likewise a fate that lends power to his life. —I Ching

I kept asking Allen questions about the *curandero*. I wanted to learn the rituals, to find out how other cultures (older and wiser than ours) had handled the visionary business. I was fascinated by the ritual thing. Ritual is to the science of consciousness what experiment is to external science. I was convinced that none of our American rituals fit the mushroom experience. Not the cocktail party. Not the psychiatrist. Not the teacher-minister role. I was impressed by what Allen said about his own fear and sickness when-

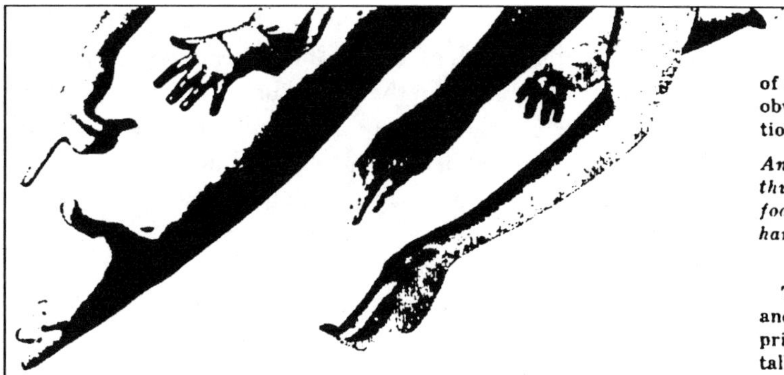

the world

ever he took drugs and about the solace and comforting strength of the *curandero*, about how good it was to have someone there who knew, who had been to those far regions of the mind and could tell you by a look, by a touch, by a puff of smoke that it was all right, go ahead, explore the strange world, it's all right, you'll come back, it's all right, I'm here back on familiar old human earth when you need me, to bring you back.

Allen was going to take the mushrooms later that night and he was shaping me up to help him. Allen was weaving a word spell, dark eyes gleaming through the glasses, chain-smoking, moving his hands, intense, chanting trance poetry. Frank Barron was in the study now, and with him Lafcadio Orlovsky.

A car came up the driveway and in a minute the door opened, and Donald, furry and moist, ambled in. He had brought his friend, an anthropology student from Harvard, to be with him when he tripped. Donald asked if his friend could be there during the mushroom session. I liked the idea of having a friend present for the mushrooms, someone to whom you could turn at those moments when you needed support, so I said, Sure, but he couldn't take the pills because he was a university student. Everyone was warning us to keep our research away from Harvard to avoid complications with the university health bureau and to avoid the rumors. He wasn't hungry so I mixed him a drink and then I got the little round bottle and pulled out the cotton topping and gave Donald 30 mg. and Allen Ginsberg 36.

Allen started bustling around getting his cave ready. I brought Susan's record player up to his room and he took some Beethoven and Wagner from the study and he turned out the lights so that there was just a glow in the room. I told him we'd be checking back every fifteen minutes and he should tell me if he wanted anything.

By the time I got downstairs Donald was already high, strolling around the house on dainty raccoon feet with his hands clasped behind his back, thinking and digging deep things. I stayed in the study writing letters, reading The *Times*. I had forgotten about the anthropology student. He was waiting in the kitchen.

After about thirty minutes I found Donald in the hallway. He called me over earnestly and began talking about the artificiality of civilization. He was thinking hard about basic issues and it was obvious what was going on with him—clearing his mind of abstractions, trying to get back behind the words and concepts.

And if he succeeds in assigning the right place to life and to fate, thus bringing the two into harmony, he puts his fate on a firm footing. These words contain hints about the fostering of life as handed on by oral tradition in the secret teachings of Chinese yoga.
—I Ching

The anthropology student was standing by, watching curiously, and Donald asked if he minded leaving so that he could talk to me privately. Anthro went back to the kitchen and Donald continued talking about the falseness of houses and machines and deploring the way man cut himself off from the vital stuff with his engines and structures. I was trying to be polite and be a good *curandero* and support him and tell him, great boy, stay with it and work it out.

Susan came back from her friends' about this time and went upstairs to her homework, and I followed her up to check on Allen. He was lying on top of the blanket. His glasses were off and his black eyes, pupils completely dilated, looked up at me. Looking down into them they seemed like two deep, black, wet wells and you could look down them way through the man Ginsberg to something human beyond. The eye is such a defenseless, naive, trusting thing. PROFESSOR LEARY CAME INTO MY ROOM, LOOKED IN MY EYES, AND SAID I WAS A GREAT MAN. THAT DETERMINED ME TO MAKE AN EFFORT TO LIVE HERE AND NOW. —Allen Ginsberg.

Allen was scared and unhappy and sick. And still he was lying there voluntarily, patiently searching, pushing himself into panics and fears, into nausea, trying to learn something, trying to find meaning. Shamelessly weak and shamelessly human and greatly classic. Peter was lying next to him, eyes closed, sleeping or listening to the record. I GOT NAUSEOUS SOON AFTER—SAT UP IN BED NAKED AND SWALLOWED DOWN THE VOMIT THAT BESIEGED FROM MY STOMACH AS IF AN INDEPENDENT BEING DOWN THERE WAS REBELLING AT BEING DRAGGED INTO EXISTENCE.

On the way downstairs I checked Susan's room. She was curled up on the carpet, with her books scattered around her and reading in the shadows. I scolded her about ruining her eyes and flicked on the two wall bulbs. Downstairs Frank was still at the study desk. Anthro was wandering in the living room and told me that Donald had gone outside. The rule we had set up was that no one would leave the house and the idea of Donald padding down Beacon Street in a mystic state chilled me. Out on the front porch I turned on the two rows of spotlights that flooded the long winding stone stairs and started down, shielding my eyes and shouting Donald. Halfway down I heard him answering back and saw him standing under an oak tree on the lower lawn. I asked him how he was, but he didn't talk, just stood there looking wise and deep. He was barefoot and higher than Piccard's balloon. I want to talk to you, but first you must take off your shoes. Okay, why not? I sat down to unlace my shoes and he squatted alongside and told about how the machines complicate our lives and how cold and hot were abstractions and how we didn't really need houses and shoes and clothes because it was just our concepts that made us think we needed these things. I agreed with him and followed what his mind was doing, suspending for a moment the clutch of the abstract but at the same time shivering from the November wind and wanting to get back behind the warm glow of the windows.

The young anthropology student was standing in the hallway. I told him that Donald was doing fine, great mystical stuff, philosophizing without concepts. He looked puzzled. He didn't want a drink or food. I walked upstairs and found the door to Allen's room closed. I waited for a while, not knowing what to do and then knocked softly and said softly, Allen I'm here now and will be back in a few minutes. *Paradise Lost*, A BOOK I'D NEVER UNDERSTOOD BEFORE—WHY MILTON SIDED WITH LUCIFER THE REBEL IN HEAVEN.

I GOT UP OUT OF BED AND WALKED DOWNSTAIRS NAKED, ORLOVSKY FOLLOWING ME, CURIOUS WHAT I WOULD DO AND WILLING TO GO ALONG IN CASE I DID ANYTHING INTERESTINGLY EXTRAVAGANT. URGING ME ON IN FACT, THANK GOD.

Susan was sitting cross-legged on her bed brushing her hair when there came a patter of bare feet on the hallway carpet. I got to the door just in time to see naked buttocks disappearing down the stairway. It was Peter. I was grinning when I went back to see Susan. Peter is running around without any clothes on. Susan

(Continued Page 36)

(Continued from p. 22)

Howard was energized:

> "I don't know if you know anything about heroin addiction, but one of the people that it worked on was a roomate of the other two that it didn't work on. He was living with those guys for six months, while they were shooting up every day, and he wasn't using it. Now, if you know anything about heroin addiction, you know how hard that is. So we knew we had something very unique here."

Early on, they sent a sample to Tim Leary, who didn't like it because it's not euphoric (no LSD mood swings, either). But Leary wasn't looking for *treatments,* but for something with a more universal, sacramental application; and he was tethered by his preference for a user-friendly party drug, whose therapeutic potential was supposed to sneak up on millions without them noticing *(See pp. 23–25, cont. 36–38).*

Howard procured a big supply of Iboga root and sent it to a dope chemist he knew. The chemist refused to do anything with it after producing a small initial sample. He was not a junkie and did not find the Ibogaine euphoric — and in 1963 underground chemists were were not interested finding cures for humanity's ills. They were looking for psychedelics they could market as great new highs. Howard was also puzzled by another now-familiar reaction: Instead of seeing Ibogaine as a Godsend for junkies who want to withdraw painlessly, some saw it as an affront to the myth, the potency of KING HEROIN — the "hard stuff." Howard says: "Dealers were not interested in selling anything that would cause people to quit doing drugs."

Through the years, though, the memory of one vision from his first Ibogaine experience resonated, and sustained him. At the end of the visions, he'd found himself in a darkened room, where a deep voice came to him, and said: "You will bring Ibogaine to the world, and set it free."

Still, it did not occur immediately to Howard and his circle to promote Ibogaine as an addiction interrupter, and events soon intervened to throw his plans into confusion. In 1963, the FDA was beginning to investigate hallucinogens, and they realized his laboratory was ordering large amounts of hallucinogens for experimentation. Before Lotsof could do much more than log his Ibogaine findings, he got a "visit" from the FDA enforcement unit responsible for tracking a shipment of 100 grams of mescaline, which had come in one or two days earlier and had already been disbursed.

"Where's the mescaline?" asked the two agents. At that time unauthorized use of mescaline on humans could only get you six months, but that was still enough to cause Howard to think fast: "It was used in rat experiments," he said.

"Where are the rats?" they asked. "They were destroyed in the course of the experiments," shot back Howard.

The agents eyed him for a moment; one said, "Good answer." It was, in fact, the only answer that could have gotten him out of trouble. In the search of his place, the agents unearthed two grams of the Ibogaine. "That's not mescaline," he said. "It's Ibogaine. You can't take that."

The agents' mouths formed an "O." They demanded to purchase the two grams as a sample and gave Lotsof a receipt. The feds now knew that he was involved in Ibogaine research. They cut off his supplies of all controlled substances.

If that didn't make Howard a marked man, events in Berkeley, where Howard and Norma felt it wise to relocate in late '63 and '64, certainly didn't endear him to the authorities. There they played a role in the Free Speech Movement of Mario Savio, which erupted in September of that year when the university administration sought to keep student civil rights activists returning from the South from setting up the traditional literature tables on Sproul Plaza.

Howard modestly describes himself and Norma as bit players in the drama, "mostly ferrying strikers around in our car."[1] But he does recollect a piece of "movement intelligence" about an FBI investigation of anti-war sentiment at Lawrence Livermore Nuclear Laboratories. Their report, which concluded that 90% of the staff at this top secret facility were using LSD, implicitly zeroed in on the flaw in the earlier CIA evaluation of LSD.

The Agency has dismissed its potential as a communist tool, one ex-analyst told John Marks, because under its influence "you tend

1 Howard now claims that he doesn't remember a story he used to tell in the '70s, of how someone smuggled a Bible into the local hoosegow, to the hundreds of kids being held after the takeover of Sproul Hall. A Bible soaked in LSD, whose pages were sacramentally consumed, thereby turning the Civil Rights Movement on to acid. But these oral histories can only be saved by diligent effort.

to have a more global view of things" — to be "more open to the brotherhood-of-man idea..." Or, as another put it,"I think everybody understood that if you had a good trip, you had a kind of above-it-all look into reality. What we subsequently found was that when you came down, you remembered the experience, but you didn't switch identities. You really didn't have that kind of feeling. You weren't as suspicious of people. You listened to them, but you also saw through them more easily and clearly. We decided that this wasn't the kind of thing that was going to make a guy a turncoat to his own country."[1]

But what happened if practically everybody in a group took LSD? What if the conversion effect was re-inforced by group feedback, and important government scientists started questioning the Vietnam war effort? The FBI's report, according to Lotsof, was forwarded to the Senate, initiating the campaign for total crackdown. "When the authorities realized their multi-million-dollar institution could be brought to a crashing halt with a few cents worth of chemicals, the decision was made to ban LSD."

It was the CIA's worst nightmare come true. One of their pharmaco-warfare genies had gotten out from government labs to the underground. In effect, "the communists had the Bomb," along with a mode of delivery the US wasn't willing to use.

Howard, who couldn't survive financially in Berkeley, accepted a free ride back to New York at the end of 1964, where he and Norma lived quietly in Brooklyn.

In 1965, the Senate held hearings, and Congress passed a law that became effective at the beginning of 1966. It established felony sentences for trafficking in a whole range of psychedelics including LSD and mescaline. At the same time a wave of media hysteria was loosed upon the country, intended to reprogram the populace to forget about therapeutic benefits and think broken chromosomes and acid-heads staring into the sun until they go blind.

Curiously, Ibogaine was not on the list, but the feds cut extraordinary corners to nail Lotsof — much more so than if he were the inconsequential acid dealer they claimed.

Howard was the very first person raided when the law took effect. Feds were waiting for Howard and Norma at their place in Brooklyn when they came back from a trip to Philadelphia. It was a typical case where there are no drugs — only conspiracy charges based on the word of an informant, because the drugs are gone. More curious still, the conspiracy was supposed to have taken place nine months earlier... before the new law had become effective.

All Assistant US Attorney Robert Morgenthau had was the word of a flaky kid that Howard Lotsof'd cut loose more than a year earlier, and who, upon getting busted, offered to give them... Lotsof. Howard was on some kind of priority list. His friends tried to get him the famous civil rights attorney Marvin Garbus, but that didn't work out. So with inadequate counsel, there came a point when the judge turned to Howard and said: "Mr. Lotsof, you claim to be a serious researcher. Name one thing you ever discovered."

"Well, your Honor, I discovered that Ibogaine can interrupt cocaine and heroin addiction with a single dose." The judge slammed his gavel down and barked, "The jury will disregard that testimony!" and cleared the courtroom for the day.

With that one decision not to allow Lotsof to testify into the court record, Ibogaine development was set back two decades — sacrificed to insure that the first-ever prosecution under a popular new law would not be derailed. Trial proceedings ground on to their foregone conclusion: Howard was found guilty on four misdemeanors and sentenced to eighteen months in federal prison.

Howard got the message: The U.S. certainly didn't want him around as an Ibogaine spokesman. He was in jail during the "Summer of Love" in 1967, when Dana got to know all the other local psychedelic luminaries. When Howard got out of prison in 1968, he decided to steer clear of further dissent. He travelled to Nepal, where for the first time in five years, eating opium, he became re-addicted. When he tried to find some Ibogaine to de-tox, in 1969, it was completely unavailable.

In 1968, State Police under Gov. Nelson Rockefeller informed the feds that Ibogaine was being used to cut heroin in the Syracuse area. (Syracuse was a Rockefeller stronghold).[2] Ibogaine soon became Schedule I, like LSD and heroin. Meanwhile, Rockefeller was busy

1 John Marks, *In Search of the Manchurian Candidate*, pp. 70–71.

2 Personal communication, Gerald Colby.

engineering public acceptance of his anti-crime brain-child, named Adolphine by its Nazi inventors — re-named "methadone" by the patent-holder, Rockefeller University.

Returning to New York, Howard and Norma enrolled in a methadone program, and got into New York University film school. But methadone withdrawal lasts about eight to ten times longer than kicking junk. It lingers in the tissues. The very long-acting quality that makes it socially preferable to smack (the addict can hold down a job because he doesn't have to do up every four hours) makes it a prison without walls. Addicts call it "the orange handcuffs." Still, Lotsof had one unique advantage over the average addict, who literally doesn't remember what it's like to be off drugs. From Ibogaine, Howard *remembered* that somewhere, the trap had an exit. Gradually, laboriously, five milligrams at a time (since methadone cold turkey can kill), he and Norma de-toxed themselves. On his own, Howard invented what is today the only standard method for methadone de-tox: several months of Hell.

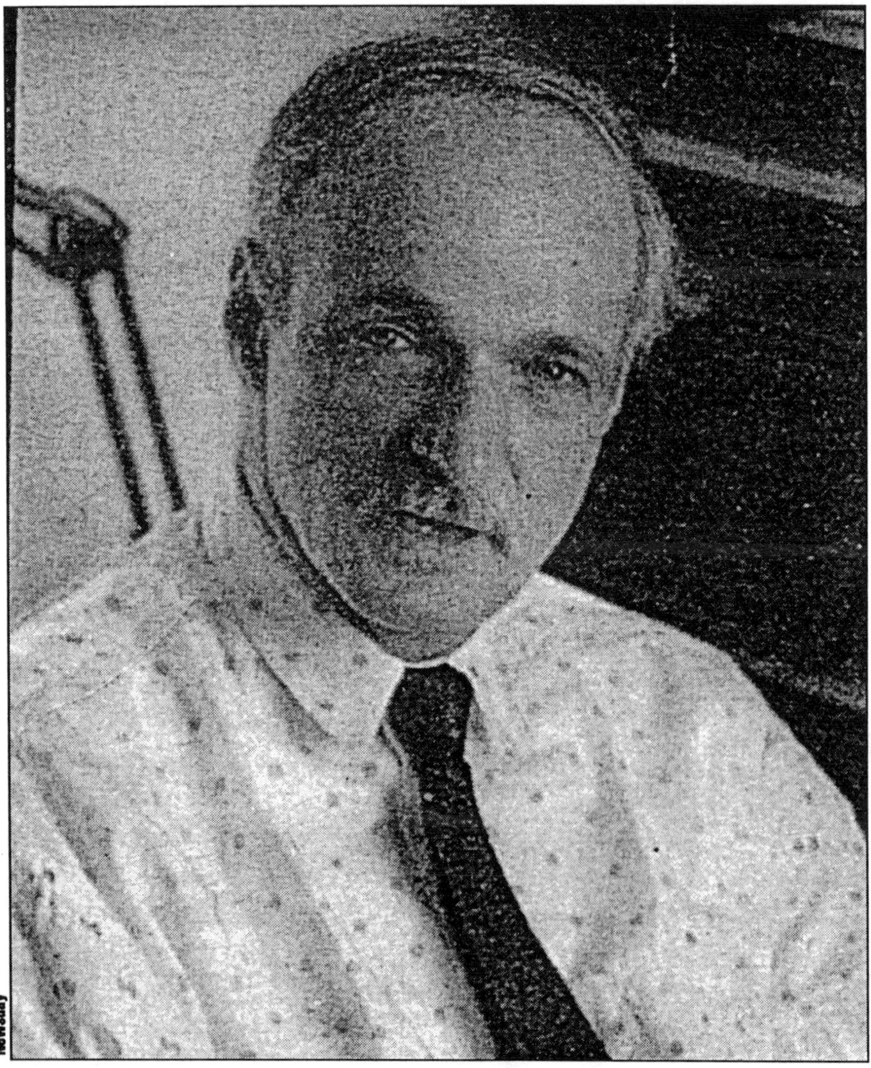

Newsday

HOWARD LOTSOF

A big factor in subsequent negative attitudes toward methadone later, among the initial supporters of the Ibogaine Project, came from Norma and Howard's recounting their own difficulties in getting off of it. They were just finishing getting off methadone in December 1973, when they were introduced to Dana Beal by a friend of pot guru Ed Rosenthal.

As final survivors of the psychedelic movement, they hit it off from the start. Soon Dana was making regular morning runs on the D train to hang out at their place in Brooklyn near Pratt Art Institute. One morning in early 1974, in the period of the gas lines after the first OPEC price hike, they were discussing which drug was "most psychedelic." Howard said it had to be Ibogaine.

"What's it like?" asked Dana.

"Kind of like harmaline," said Howard.

"Oh, you mean telepathine,"[1] said Dana, regurgitating the only thing (its synonym) he knew about harmaline.

"Yeah," said Howard. "But you know what? It stopped my heroin addiction."

The effect on Dana wasn't like a blinding flash of light — more like a bell going off. As the putative new leader of the YIPPIES, Dana was poking through the wreckage of the movement for anything that could be an asset. He filed this interesting fact away among the YIP crown jewels.

During the next six years, as they collaborated on a number of projects, including three films, Howard gradually regained the confidence he would need to become Ibogaine's spokesman. But to this day, Norma Alexander, a brilliant Afro-American woman who is chief financial officer of NDA International, refuses to go on camera as a spokesperson. She's still paranoid from the '66 bust — and from being Black in America.

Rockefeller capped off his successful installation of methadone maintenance with the toughest drug law in the country, named in his honor and still used to imprison substantial — and growing — numbers of young, Black men.

1 The whole extract of ayahuasca, *banisteria caapi,* telepathine, contains additional tryptamines that give it a different effect from pure harmaline.

CHAPTER 3: Dhoruba Moore

Sitting together in early 1974, Dana and the Lotsofs were not the first people to realize methadone has serious problems. Today Ron Fogel works with the Ibogaine Project, but he happens to be one of the researchers from the pilot study of methadone in 1965 with Drs. Robert DuPont and Janet Nyswinder. He says they knew it had serious liver and kidney toxicities almost from the beginning, but that Nixon and Rockefeller (and the patent-holder, Rockefeller U.) were hell-bent on solving the rising crime rate. To these serious concerns about methadone among early researchers, the word on the street soon added that it can rot your bones, make your teeth fall out, and cause ballooning of your joints.

(To be fair, many people tolerate it fairly well. Lotsof credits it with getting him off the street so he could put his life back together. But not all opposition is based, as proponents think, on moralistic objections against any addictive drug.)

In 1968–69, the Black Panthers participated in a movement in the Bronx that seized Lincoln Hospital Methadone Detox Unit, the pilot project for New York City and the country. They agitated, picketed and, after shutting it down, occupied it. Then they re-opened it as Lincoln Drug-Free Detox, using non-Western techniques such as accupuncture and "Social" re-education through the ideology of the Black Panther Party (BPP). Only much later would it become clear that one of the longest-lasting impacts of the Panthers was in this area — that many community health workers in the BPP in fact survived, minus guns, in the movement of Black acupuncturists.

The New York Panthers were never as well known outside the city as the Oakland bunch, who as the Central Committee controlled the party paper and apparatus. The one image from NYC that really made it out to white radicals across the country, though, was of Black Panthers waging a war against police-controlled heroin dealing in Harlem. It was all publicized during the three trials of Dhoruba Bin Wahad (then known as Dhoruba Moore) in the early seventies. His story left a lasting impression amongst the YIPs.

Born Richard Moore, Dhoruba grew up in the Southeast Bronx in the '50s, which he describes as a "time warp for Black people, who had not yet fully begun to struggle for their liberation." His father was a heroin addict. He was raised by his mother's side of the family. As a teenager, he joined a gang, the Sportsmen, and then the Disciple–Sportsmen. But because of his father he felt strongly enough about addiction that he resisted the pull of heroin, while the other gang members succumbed to addiction.

In 1962, he was sent to prison for five years for what he describes as "an act of self-defense." In prison he sharpened his mind with the works of various Black and revolutionary writers. His comrades gave him the name "Analye Zzliwani Dhoruba," which is Swahili for "He who is born in the storm." Dhoruba, or "Storm," for short. He was released in 1967, into the Vietnam protest era.

Wanting to become an artist, he began to frequent Manhattan's East Village. He had an apartment on East Third Street across from a jazz bar called Slug's. It was the Summer of Love, and he was a regular fixture at the happenings in nearby Tompkins Square Park.[1] But when the Provos marched off to tie up traffic, he would stay behind with his stock of knicknacks and pipes. He was in his hippie phase. It was not his protest.

He became politically active only after the assassination of Dr. Martin Luther King, on April 4, 1968. With the assassination of King, young Blacks everywhere felt that they had do something to make things happen faster — and that non-violence was not enough. Black Panther chapters popped up like mushrooms. Dhoruba decided to go by the Harlem office and check them out. Becoming a Panther meant a conscious decision to adopt a *persona* in some ways completely at odds with the East Village artist. A life-long commitment.

[1] See next chapter, p. 39.

Belying the guns and black leather, nine-tenths of the Panther program consisted of organizing rent strikes, community health clinics and free breakfasts for school children (liberally mixed with Black Consciousness education), as well as campaigning against hard drugs. This included both harassing local dealers and, as mentioned, the ground-breaking takeover of Lincoln Detox.

Introducing accupuncture or T'ai Chi was a logical extension of the community health focus and the Maoist ideology of the Panthers. (It's said that while the Oakland Panthers just sold Mao's *Little Red Book,* the New York Panthers actually read it.) And in fact the Lincoln Detox takeover was initiated by the Young Lords and Mutulu Shakur of the RNA[1] as well as Lumumba Shakur of the Bronx Panthers; and it came about after months of grumbling and protests about a perceived policy of over-medication combined with little therapy and no focus on jobs.

1 Republic of New Africa

Lincoln Methadone Detox was seized and re-opened as Lincoln Drug-Free De-tox in March, 1969 — a time when protests and insurgencies were multiplying in poor communities across America. Occupying buildings was a common tactic, pioneered in New York City by Jesse Grey, in rent strikes. But taking on the Feds' pet treatment initiative was guaranteed to get this coalition into a peck of trouble, even if the New York red squad and J. Edgar Hoover hadn't already had COINTELPRO (the Counter-Intelligence Program) to physically eliminate the Black Revolution. In a memo issued just forty days before the shooting of King, J. Edgar Hoover directed all agents to "prevent the rise of a Messiah" who could unify, and electrify, the militant black nationalist movement.[2]

2 See composite, inset p. 116.

The New York Police Department Red Squad (BOSS — Bureau of Special Services) had infiltrated spies into the Panthers from the beginning. On April 2, 1969 they made their move. Based on the actions of provocateurs among the ranks, twenty-one leading New York Panthers, including Dhoruba, were arrested on conspiracy charges of plotting to assassinate various public officials, blow up the subways, the Bronx Botanical Gardens, commit kidnappings, and so on.

Dhoruba, who'd advanced on his merits to Field Secretary of the New York Panthers, was visited in jail by BPP Chief of Staff David Hilliard, who — with Eldridge Cleaver exiled in Algiers and Huey Newton in jail — was running things in Oakland along with Bobby Seale and Field Secretary Don Cox. "The Oakland Panthers were what we called 'country'," recalls Dhoruba.

> "After their clashes with Ron Karenga's United Slaves, they rejected as 'cultural nationalists' many progressives who were into African consciousness. Hilliard, who was widely distrusted because of his shaky role in the shoot-out where Bobby Hutton was killed and Eldridge Cleaver captured, was afraid of the Chicago and New York Panthers, because of our African names.
>
> "Hilliard was ready to abandon the Panther 21, but then Bobby Seale was busted up in New Haven, and Don Cox said they couldn't do it. They needed a New York base. Harlem was too important to abandon, and besides, New York sold the most newspapers. But what Oakland really wasn't ready for was the massive outpouring of support for the 21, especially from white radicals. Leonard Bernstein threw a party."

"Ultimately, hundreds of thousands were raised — maybe more," says Dhoruba, although he adds that much of it was diverted to the West Coast by white radical minions of the Hilliard faction like Yippie Marty Kenner.

In early 1970 Abbie Hoffman donated his $20,000 advance from *Steal This Book,* enough for bond to bail out two of the 21. After joint consultations the 21 first obtained the release of Afeni Shakur, then of Dhoruba and Michael Tabor, the best public speakers, to represent them on the outside. In the next ten months Dhoruba displayed the kind of leadership that was only bound to get him in more trouble.

A charismatic speaker, he was released on March 28th, and immediately flew to Los Angeles, to do a forum with Angela Davis on police repression and to consult with the Central Committee.

A month later, on May Day, he joined Dave Dellinger and the rest of the Chicago 7 in New Haven, addressing tens of thousands gathered from all over the country to free Bobby Seale. Midway through, it was announced Nixon had resumed bombing North Viet Nam. On the fringes of the crowd Dana Beal was bumping into a guy in a stetson, dressed like a young Wyatt Earp, who had come with his own guerrilla sound system mounted on the roof of his car. It was Tom Forçade and his friend Jack Coombs from the New York White Panthers. Soon afterwards police opened up with tear gas on the stage and the crowd alike. They gassed people three times without dispersing the rally.

Dhoruba was fast becoming not only chief spokesman for the 21; in a situation where Huey and most of the original leadership were locked up or in exile, Dhoruba became the best, most forceful speaker the Panthers could field for rallies on the East Coast. By the next weekend, he was speaking to 100,000 massed on the Ellipse in Washington, D.C. to protest the killings at Kent and Jackson State. A wall of buses blocked the White House. Nixon feared they would seize it.[1]

The trial of the 21 commenced soon after that, so Dhoruba could only get out of New York on Friday, Saturday or Sunday.[2] As Field Secretary of New York, he was doing the job of Field Secretary for the entire East Coast, constantly travelling to set up new chapters from Baltimore to New England. Effectively he ranked just under Don Cox, the National Field Secretary, and his position required constant contact with David Hilliard, the BPP Chairman and virtually the last of the Central Committee who wasn't locked up. But while Dhoruba tried to mute criticism and coax support out of Hilliard and the National Office, at events like the BPP constitutional convention that June in Philly, Dhoruba became a lightning rod for complaints about Hilliard's regime —

"The party was totally different from the one that existed when we went into jail. Into the vacuum created by all the arrests had come all these police agents. One of them, Melvin 'Cotton' Smith, was put in charge of security by Hilliard, who controlled everything because he was the one who got to visit Huey in jail. Under the influence of these provocateurs, who fed his hatreds, Hilliard became a tyrant who slapped down anyone with initiative. I was demoted to 'member' after the convention in Philly, replaced by Thomas Jolly and Robert Bey. Except they weren't up to the job. And they weren't public speakers."

Dhoruba says he counseled folks to wait for Huey to get out and straighten up the mess. "There was this magical belief Huey would get out and make it right. Hilliard used to come to New York totally high on coke or acid — I knew because I arranged his security. But there was this magical belief in Huey. Then Huey got out sometime in August, and immediately fell into doing coke with Hilliard, so instead of being accessible to where he could mediate, Huey was only listening to Hilliard and things got worse," Dhoruba recalls—

"After that, I started securing all the mailing lists, changing all the safe houses — everything, without telling Oakland anything.

"This Melvin, who was an LAPD informer, got Hilliard to dispatch him to 'investigate' Geronimo Pratt's organizing in Texas. Geronimo Pratt was the hero of the military wing of the BPP because he fortified the LA Panther headquarters so that it withstood a full siege, including a bomb like the one that destroyed MOVE,[3] and they survived until dawn, when the community could come out and rally, and they could surrender alive.

"So when Geronimo and the entire Texas network got busted, this Melvin was the only one to 'escape,' and Hilliard accepted his story — that Geronimo was the informer, and denounced him on the front page of *The Black Panther* as an enemy of the people.

"This turn of events completely flipped out the military wing..."

Meanwhile, the Panther 21 trial dragged on for more than a year, the longest and most expensive in New York history. Taking a leaf from their successful elimination of Malcolm X, COINTELPRO next planted letters alleging that Dhoruba intended to assassinate Huey Newton. "It was crazy," says Dhoruba. "Huey didn't understand that because of what'd happened to Malcolm, in New York we didn't want people going around saying, 'The Black Panthers might have been something, but they killed their own leader.' Here I was trying to keep the 21 from issuing a letter supporting Eldridge in his dispute with Oakland; and I found out later the FBI was sending letters into prison, telling the 21 I was selling them out to Huey Newton.

"So the letter supporting Eldridge came out anyway, and then all hell broke loose." A

1 See the *Nixon tapes* – Watergate Hearings.

2 Many of the 21 were Muslim, and were able to get their Sabbath, Friday, off for the whole group.

3 In 1985 the Philadelphia police dropped a 4½-pound high-explosive device on the compound housing the Black anarchist back-to-nature group MOVE, shooting all but two of the women and children as they attempted to escape the resulting fire which quickly engulfed 41 blocks of Philadelphia.

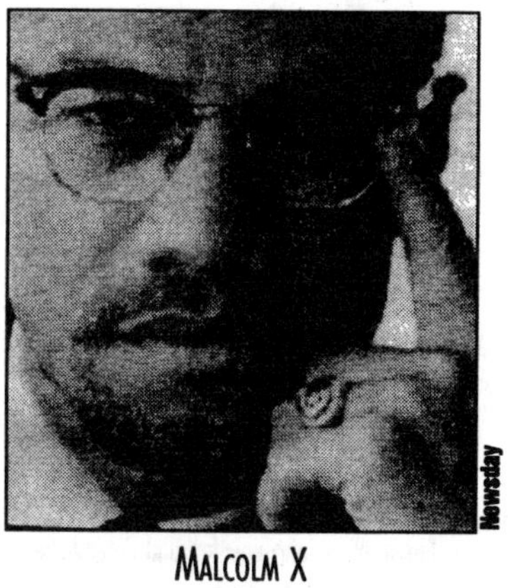

Malcolm X

CAPITALISM PLUS DOPE EQUALS GENOCIDE

By Michael "Cetewayo" Tabor (Political Prisoner, NY 21)
BLACK PANTHER PARTY, U.S.A.

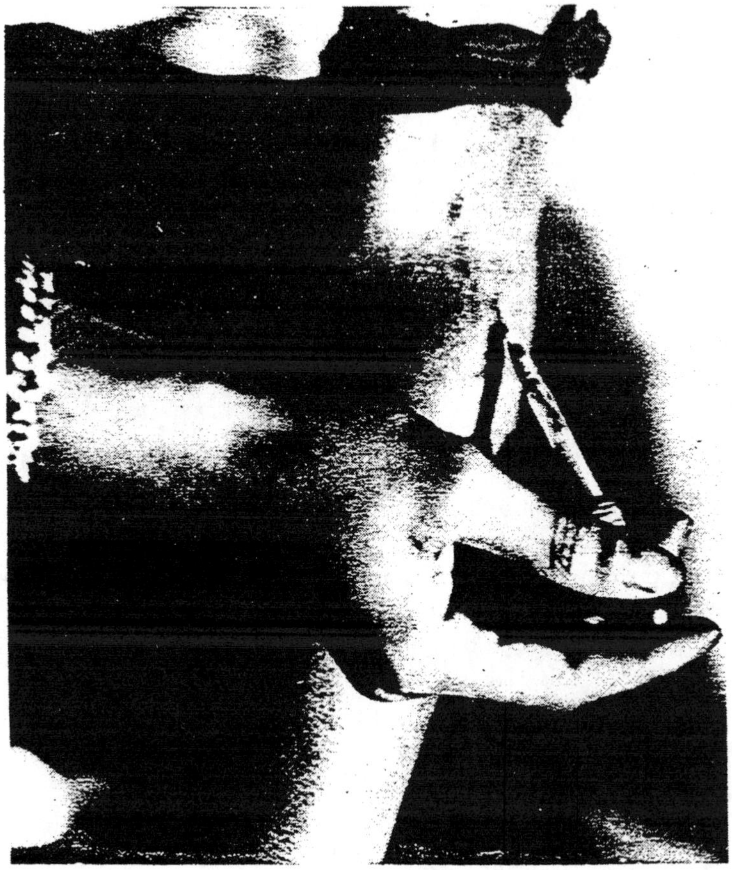

Black Panther Party

couple of people were shot. When Dhoruba got word that he was next, in February '71, he went underground; there was no choice. He and Michael Tabor were immediately denounced as "enemies of the people" on the front page of *The Black Panther.* The Central Committee said he did it to sabotage the defense of the 21. He was accused of ripping off defense monies.

The response of Dhoruba's faction was to escalate the struggle in the most creative way. NBC video footage still exists of heavily armed New York Panthers raiding a major Harlem dope distributor and dumping quarter-pounds of heroin into the gutter to be washed away by the rain.[1]

It was wildly popular with the Black Community. Even before he and Dhoruba were released on bail, Michael Tabor had published *"Capitalism Plus Dope Equals Genocide"* through the BPP, denouncing

> "the plague, poisonous, lethal... sold... to Black youths who are desparately seeking a kick, a high... anything that will help make them oblivious to the squalor, to the abject poverty, disease and degradation that engulfs them in their daily existence.... By weakening, dividing and destroying us, [the plague reinforces] the strength of the oppressor enabling him to perpetuate his dominion over us.
>
> "It is also the practice of... narcotics agents to seize a quantity of drugs from one dealer, arrest him, but only turn in a portion of the confiscated drugs for evidence. The rest is given to another dealer who sells it and gives a percentage of the profits to the narcotics agents.... In return for information, [informers who are dealers] receive immunity from arrest. The police cannot solve the problem, for they are part of the problem."

Tabor turned out to be right on — prescient even. Things had gotten so far out of control that New York police themselves were about to be busted, by the Feds. For all intents and purposes, the smack Panthers were dumping in the gutter *belonged* to the NYPD.

It's all a matter of public record, thanks to the Knapp Commission: how the heroin from the French Connection bust — the biggest haul in US history — had been systematically replaced with flour, spirited out of police evidence lockers downtown, and sold on the streets of Harlem. And that scam, which brought down the whole house of cards, was only the tip of the iceberg.

New York City was unique, because half the junkies in America lived in its five boroughs. All five Mafia families were represented in New York. According to Alfred McCoy's *The Politics of Heroin in Southeast Asia,* the Cosa Nostra had by then established new connections in Southeast Asia under the cover of the Viet Nam war, bypassing the now-too-well-known Turkish connection. And as documented by the Knapp Commission, the entire NYPD central narcotic squad (the Special Investigations Unit – SIU) was working hand-

1 *Passin' It On,* a one-hour PBS special by film-makers John Valedez and Peter Miller, now available on video.

in-glove with the five families, selling protection and dealing drugs. For the interlocking directorate of the CIA / SIU / Cosa Nostra, the French Connection heroin was only a tiny bit of a constant flow that kept a quarter million New York addicts in dope.

But that particular house of cards would not come crashing down until Nixon's second term — too late to do much good for Dhoruba and the Panthers. Dhoruba was already on the lam when word came out that the 21 had beaten their charges. In early May, 1971, the entire case was thrown out by the jury, a humiliating defeat for the criminal justice system.

Yet, for the Panthers staffing the Harlem office, waiting for the next move by the police, mere vindication by a jury was like the taste of ashes in their mouths. They might tweak the NYPD by expropriating police drug money and giving it away as breakfasts for school children, but that was a scant substitute for the ability to raise funds via mass organizing, which now seemed certain to expose them only to new conspiracy charges, or death.

Every Panther chapter in the country had members in jail, waiting trial, unable to make bail — and they were the lucky ones. Chicago police had assassinated Fred Hampton and Mark Clark in a fusillade of bullets as they lay sleeping. With the split with Oakland complete, there was no appeal, no process to reign in the snitches and provocateurs who were running wild in the organization. Dhoruba was rumored to be with Eldridge, in Algiers. For the New York Panthers, the waiting became unbearable. Many of them decided to stay one step ahead of the law, to go underground.

A new organization was formed, the Black Liberation Army (BLA). Jettisoning the community programs, its secret cells waged an armed struggle against the police, which of course they were bound to lose. The last Black guerrilla was wiped out by 1975. You can't win against atom bombs with a machine gun.

The very first action of the BLA freaked out the cops, though. Six days after the 21 were acquitted, someone machine-gunned two cops guarding DA Hogan's house — didn't kill them, but ruined them for life. A few days later, two more cops were shot, dead.

Now financially dependent on expropriating smack dealers, the underground continued the campaign of taking the money, destroying the dope, "punishing" the dealers. At a place called the Triple O Social Club in the Bronx, an after-hours club catering to dealers and their girlfriends, Dhoruba was caught. Somehow this dope den had pretty incredible police protection. He had just lined the patrons up against the wall, stripped them naked and was collecting their valuables, when the look-out came running upstairs and told Dhoruba the street was full of cops.

A day or so after the bust, a machine gun found at the scene was linked to the shooting of the two cops guarding DA Hogan. One of the patrons of the Triple O was trying to become a corrections officer; he was persuaded to tie Dhoruba to the machine gun. (Ballistics also matched that shooting to another gun later seized in California, but that was not disclosed for many years.) A fingerprint taken from a copy of the *New York Post* wrapped around the communique from the Hogan action was matched with Dhoruba's. (Unfortunately, it "had to be destroyed" to get it off the newsprint.)

The chief government witness was Pauline Josephs, a diagnosed paranoid schizophrenic who was on medication. Her first statement to the police was that they'd gotten the wrong man, because Dhoruba had been at her place with 3 friends until 9 PM. The shooting was at 9:08 PM — too soon for anyone to drive from the Bronx to Manhattan. But after holding her in protective custody for almost a year, the DA's men cooked her testimony until they got it just right. Nine PM became 7 PM.

Nonetheless, when she got on the stand there were so many inconsistencies that the first jury refused to convict. Was it 9 PM or 7 PM? After a second jury was selected with too many Blacks and Latinos, the Judge mysteriously caught a cold. Another mistrial. During trial number 3 the Judge refused to allow the Defense to question the Prosecution about an article by ex-Police Commissioner Robert Daley, which disclosed the existence of a tape of Pauline Joseph's original exculpatory phone call.[2] Finally, Dhoruba snapped, rose from the defense table and said, "I'm not going to listen any more to that lying bitch!" The display of temper alienated the jury. It took just forty-

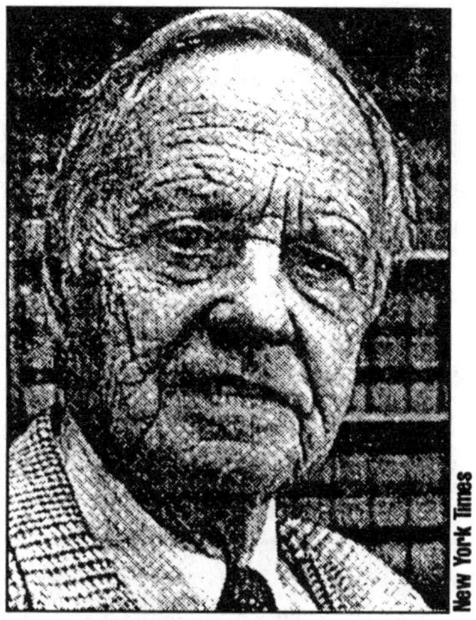

From 1972 to 1974 Whitman Knapp chaired the commission that investigated corruption in the New York Police Department. Narcotics Unit. Today, as a Federal judge who is "retired" but still handles cases, he refuses to preside over any narcotics cases — something that is within his perogative as a retired Federal judge. He believes that endemic corruption is inevitable under prohibition.

2 "The men you are holding are innocent. They did not do it!" was what the tape said, but the Judge characterized ex-Chief of Police Robert Daley — who leaked this juicy tidbit in exerpts of his book *Target Blue*, which appeared in *New York* magazine — as "just another reporter." The Prosecution admitted they had the tape — only it was too late to recall Pauline Josephs to the stand.

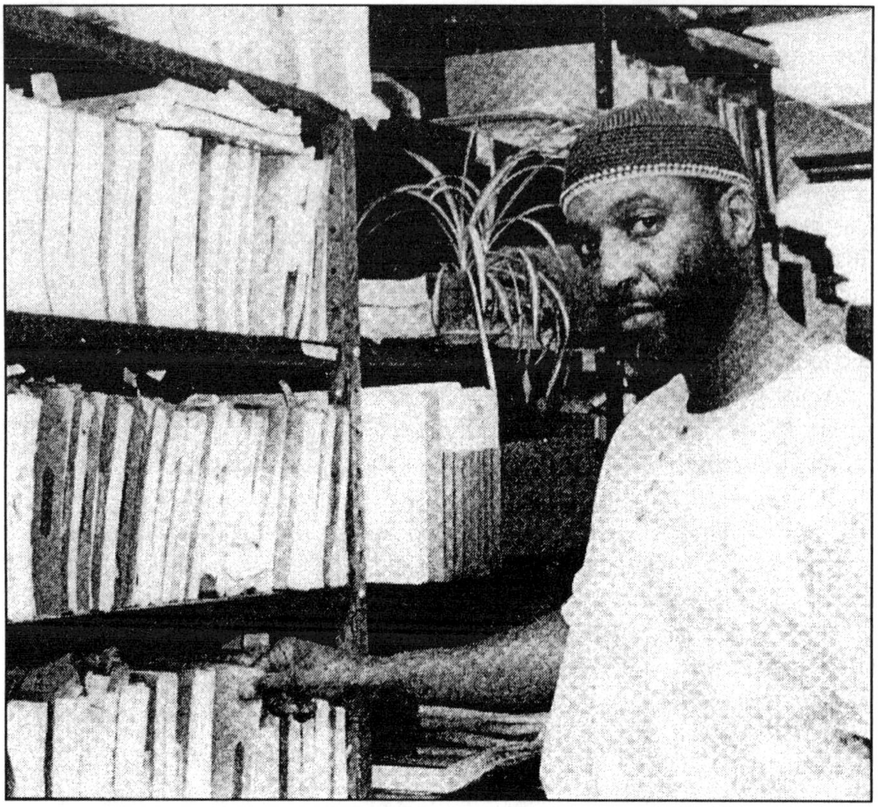

Counterspy

DHORUBA BIN-WAHAD WITH 300,000 PAGES OF FBI DOCUMENTS ON THE BLACK PANTHERS

five minutes for them to convict a man who had gone in four years from ex-con to contender for the mantle of Malcolm X.

He got nineteen years for a crime he didn't commit. For nineteen years he took whatever they threw at him and absorbed it, transformed it. By the end he saw that the problem wasn't just radicals being held political prisoner, but the 40 per cent of all black males in N.Y.C., enmeshed in jail, prison, the courts, or some other phase of the System. In a letter to his wife Tanaquil, dated September 7, 1989, he wrote:

> "I'm tired of being tired, and winters are the loneliest and worst times in prison. I remember the feeling of being "up north" in Clinton or Attica during the winter, so far away from the source of any care or love or warmth — not that anybody really loved me during those harsh, bitter times. In Clinton — it's on a mountain — it was so cold your hair would freeze, and the long, heated corridors of that dismal place made you feel like you were underground.
>
> "Clinton County is one of the poorest in the state, so it's always getting a new prison. Its major growth industry is the traffic in Black and Latino flesh..."

The new Involuntary Servitude.

The major, unintended side effect of putting Dhoruba on ice was that he survived to do something about it, while the BLA went down in flames, and even whites in the wing of the movement that were into armed struggle were finished off in 1981, in Rockland County, New York, in the Brinks job.

Dhoruba was freed in February 1990, through the diligence of his attorneys (and his own diligence) in combing through 350,000 pages of FBI documents released under the Freedom of Information Act, which proved conclusively he had been framed.

The narcs who sold the French Connection heroin in Harlem went down as well. Ninety-seven out of 100 members of the SIU resigned in disgrace, were convicted, or committed suicide.

When the U.S. later invaded Panama to snag Noriega, President Bush propounded an interesting doctrine, that whenever a government is so riddled with corruption, from top to bottom, the people have a right to rise up and rebel.

Much of the rest of the Panther serve-the-people program did survive, shorn of armed struggle, in community-based movements of the '70s and '80s such as the Black accupuncturists. In fact, *YIPster Times,* in 1977, ran a story about the mysterious death of the head of Lincoln Detox, Howard Taft, hours before he was to meet Carter Drug Czar Peter Bourne. He was found stuffed in a closet. The editor who solicited the story, Bob Sisko, attributed it to followers of Lyndon LaRouche,[1] who were vying to take the program over from ex-Panthers. In the fall-out, Dr. Michael Smith became the head of Lincoln Detox.

Later, Smith would confirm to writer Dennis King that a LaRouche supporter on staff at Lincoln had been feeding info on the Panthers to the New York Police Department. A public campaign emerged against the nest of radicals and Black Panthers at Lincoln Detox. As Ed Koch swept into office as Mayor of New York City, on a platform of cutting all city funding of drug treatment — a shortfall the State of New York was supposed to pick up, but never did — then-State Senator Charles Schumer and others questioned why any government funds at all were going to programs that promoted Black history and community

1 A.K.A. "Lyn Marcus" when still a member of the Students for a Democratic Society (SDS), in the late '60s originated the National Caucus of Labor Committe (NCLC), emulating the "worker–student alliance" politics of the overtly Stalinist Progressive Labor faction of SDS, in contradistinction to Weatherman/Yippie!/BPP, but with LaRouche as supreme leader. After NCLC's bludgeoning attacks on American Communist Party regulars in 1973 failed to estabish hegemony over the Left, LaRouche flipped 180 degrees to the right, bringing elements from the Ku Klux Klan to the National Renaissance Party of James Medole into an anti-Semitic alliance with his inner-city regulars, who had always constituted the more uptight, anti-pot element of the New Left. A would-be American Mussolini who ran for President several times, LaRouche began his decline in 1983 and was ultimately imprisoned by the Feds for massive credit-card fraud. But LaRouche is now out, and he recently issued an encyclical against "Chaos Theory."

activism as part of treatment.

Mutulu Shakur and the Panthers who had occupied Lincoln Detox without a break for almost 10 years were lured to downtown Manhattan, to a meeting that was supposed to decide their fate. When they returned to the Bronx, they found Lincoln Detox occupied by 500 police.

All of the radicals refused to accept the new regime, so they automatically didn't get their jobs back. Michael Smith decided to stay for the sake of some kind of continuity.

As for the LaRouchoids, after riding the National Anti-Drug Coalition (NADC) to mass-movement status in '76 and '77, LaRouche was denounced in '78 by then Black Muslim leader Wallace Muhammad, who called him "hateful." NCLC propaganda[1] (Queen of England dealing dope and all) turned out to be carelessly borrowed whole cloth from the rantings of Nazi propaganda chief Joseph Goebbels, with anti-Semitic references too bold even for the Black Muslims. But perhaps in return for ratting out Lincoln Detox, cooperation and support was unimpeded at the National Institute on Drug Abuse (NIDA), in the person of Dr. Thomas Gleaton and the "parents' groups" (including Sue Rusche of suburban Atlanta and Otto Moulton of Massachusetts) that NIDA had put together to publicize the anti-marijuana pseudo-science of one Gabriel Nahas.

In interviews much later with Dennis King, the name that LaRouche defectors linked to the eviction of the Panthers from Lincoln Detox was a Dr. Ned Rosinsky. With the Black movement against heroin neutralized, the Nahas group had no problem working closely with Dr. Rosinsky and LaRouche's "War on Drugs" Organization well into the '80s. They incorporated key LaRouche tenets into their "drug prevention" message, e.g., confounding addictive and non-addictive drugs, and the attitude that any drug-induced experience constituted a theft from society. They also co-sponsored conferences at NYU in '79 and Columbia University in '80, featuring supposed findings of Nahas (the student of the Nazi Stringaris[2]) first presented in 1978 at the University of Rheims, his alma mater.

Mutulu Shakur moved to Harlem and started BAANA — the Black Acupuncturists Association of North America— only to be caught up in the Brinks fiasco in Nyack, New York. BAANA fell apart when Mutulu and others drew long prison sentences. Acupuncture itself became politically suspect. Those were the years that LaRouche "Executive Intelligence" personnel had twice-weekly access to the White House — years when marijuana arrests returned from 25 per cent under Carter to the 50/50 parity with hard drug busts that had existed under Nixon. It took the crack epidemic of 1985–86 to get the public to wake up — and to rehabilitate acupuncture as well, since nothing else seemed to work for crack.

On August 22, 1989, Huey Newton was shot dead by a drug dealer who was tired of being shaken down for donations to Huey's crack habit. Ironically, Bobby Seale had been informed of Ibogaine earlier that year. But by May of 1989, Seale no longer had much to do with Newton, who apparently was difficult to deal with on coke.

Six months later, Dhoruba was released on a showing of gross prosecutorial misconduct during his trial. That day Dana Beal walked across town to the house of his lawyer, William Kunstler, who was also one of Dhoruba's lawyers. Dana found Dhoruba relaxing with his wife, Tanaquil Jones, on the second floor, and presented him with a summary of information on Ibogaine — so that he would never again need to confront the armed might of the State with a machine gun just to fight heroin.

Shunned by the BPP, with no bail money, Geronimo Pratt was convicted in 1972 of a 1968 murder, despite FBI wiretap logs showing he was 400 miles away at the time; he languishes to this day, with Leonard Peltier and 250 other American political prisoners, victims of a COINTELPRO that never ended.

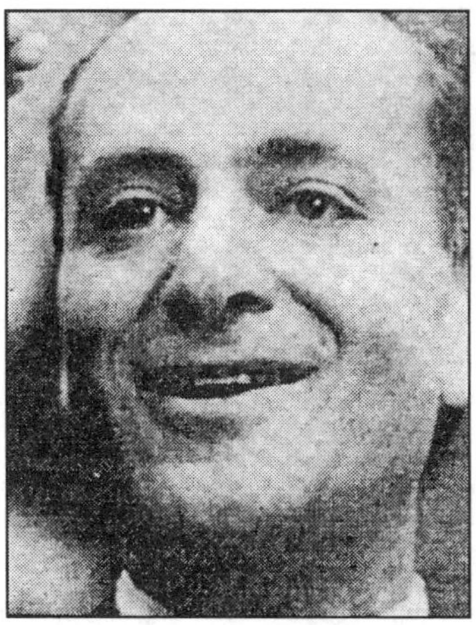

REP. CHARLES SCHUMER

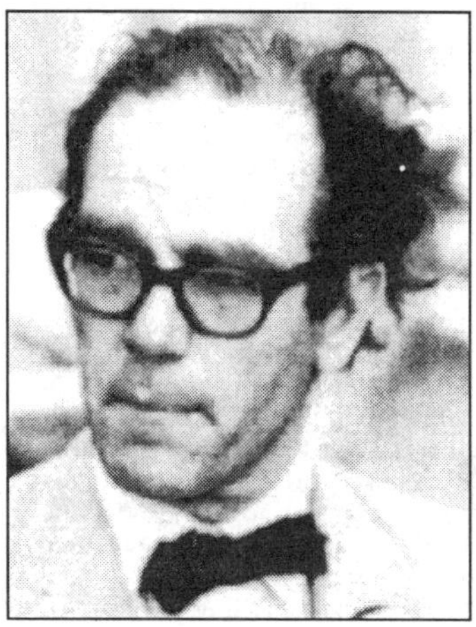

Newsday; Dennis King

LYNDON LAROUCHE

1 *Dope, Inc.*, a 500-page book written by three LaRouche aides, became a kind of underground bestseller. Cf. Dennis King's *Lyndon LaRouche and the New American Fascism*, p. 326.

2 Stringaris was a Greek national who found employ before and during World War II as Joseph Goebbels' drug expert, and as a professor in the '50s and '60s in Athens, only to die in disgrace for suppporting the Greek fascist colonels' coup. He compiled all the pseudo-scientific claims — e.g., that pot weakens the immune system, grows breasts on males, etc. — that Nahas later translated and presented as his own work in the 1950s. Nahas' UN-sponsored experiments in the '70s, trying to substantiate these claims, were pathetic in their inability to be replicated; but Nahas was much more circumspect than LaRouche in concealing the ultimate origins of his material. As NIDA's latest pronouncements show, Nahas and his ilk still have our government busily at work trying to prove that the Nazi doctors were right about pot. See footnote, pp. 216–17. Stringaris corresponded on behalf of Goebbels with Anslinger about the plan to intern Black U.S. jazz musicians. See Hans-Georg Behr's *Von Hanf Ist Die Rede*, and Larry Sloman's *Reefer Madness* (1979).

Continued from p. 25.

picked up her paraphernalia—curlers, brush, pins, and trotted up to the third floor. I headed downstairs.

When I got to the study Frank was leaning back in his chair behind the desk, grinning quizzically. In front of the desk looking like medieval hermits were Allen and Peter, both stark naked. I WENT IN AMONG THE PSYCHOLOGISTS IN STUDY AND SAW THEY TOO WERE WAITING FOR SOMETHING VAST TO HAPPEN, ONLY IT REQUIRED SOMEONE AND THE MOMENT TO MAKE IT HAPPEN—ACTION, REVOLUTION. No, Allen had on his glasses and as I came in he peered out at me and raised his finger in the air. Hey, Allen, what goes on? Allen had a holy gleam in his eye and he waved his finger. I'm the Messiah. I've come down to preach love to the world. We're going to walk through the streets and teach people to stop hating. I DECIDED I MIGHT AS WELL BE THE ONE TO DO SO—PRONOUNCED MY NAKEDNESS AS THE FIRST ACT OF REVOLUTION AGAINST THE DESTROYERS OF THE HUMAN IMAGE.

Well, Allen, that sounds like a pretty good idea. Listen, said Allen, do you believe that I'm the Messiah. THE NAKED BODY BEING THE HIDDEN SIGN. Look, I can prove it. I'm going to cure your hearing. Take off your hearing machine. Your ears are cured. Come on, take it off, you don't need it. AND GRABBED THE TELEPHONE TO COMMUNICATE MY DECISION—WANTED TO HOOK UP KHRUSHCHEV, KEROUAC, BURROUGHS, IKE, KENNEDY, MAO TSE-TUNG, MAILER, ETC.

Frank was still smiling. Peter was standing by, watching seriously. The hearing aid was dumped on the desk. That's right. And now your glasses, I'll heal your vision too. The glasses were laid on the desk too. ALL IN ONE TELEPHONE LINE AND GET THEM ALL TO COME IMMEDIATELY TO HARVARD TO HAVE SPECTRAL CONFERENCE OVER THE FUTURE OF THE UNIVERSE.

Allen was peering around with approval at his healing. But Allen, one thing. What? Your glasses. You're still wearing them. Why don't you cure your own vision. Allen looked surprised. Yes, you're right. I will. He took off his glasses and laid them on the desk.

Now Allen was a blind Messiah squinting around to find his followers. Come on. We're going down to the city streets to tell the people about peace and love. And then we'll get lots of great people onto a big telephone network to settle all this warfare bit.

Fine, said Frank, but why not do the telephone bit first, right here in the house. Frank was heading off the pilgrimage down the avenue naked.

Who we gonna call, said Peter. Well, we'll call Kerouac on Long Island, and Kennedy and Khrushchev and Bill Burroughs in Paris and Norman Mailer in the psycho ward in Bellevue. We'll get them all hooked up in a big cosmic electronic love talk. War is just a hang-up. We'll get the love-thing flowing on the electric Bell Telephone network. Who we gonna call first, said Peter. Let's start with Khrushchev, said Allen.

Look, why don't we start with Kerouac on Long Island. In the meantime, let's pull the curtains, said Frank. There's enough going on in here so I don't care about looking outside. Allen picked up the white telephone and dialed Operator. The two thin figures leaned forward wrapped up in a holy fervor trying to spread peace. The dear noble innocent helplessness of the naked body. They looked as though they had stepped out of a quattrocento canvas, apostles, martyrs, dear fanatic holy men. Allen said, Hello, operator, this is God, I want to talk to Kerouac. To whom do I want to talk? Kerouac. What's my name? This is God. G-O-D. Okay. We'll try Capitol 7-0563. Where? Northport, Long Island. There was a pause. We were all listening hard. Oh. Yes. That's right. That's the number of the house where I was born. Look, operator, I'll have to go upstairs to get the number. Then I'll call back.

Allen hung up the receiver. What was all that about, Allen? Well, the operator asked me my name and I said I was God and I wanted to speak to Kerouac and she said, I'll try to do my best, sir, but you'll have to give me his number and then I gave her the number of my mother's house. I've got Kerouac's number upstairs in my book. Just a minute and I'll get it.

Back at the phone, Allen was shouting to Jack. He wanted Jack to come up to Cambridge and then he wanted Jack's mother to come too. Jack had a lot to say because Allen held the phone, listening for long spaces. Frank was still sitting behind the desk smiling. Donald and the anthro student were standing in the hallway looking in curiously. I walked over to explain. Allen says he is the Messiah and he's calling Kerouac to start a peace and love movement. Donald wasn't interested. He went on telling me *(Continued on page 116)*

Messages from Ginsberg to

DECEMBER, 1960:

Here is a statement for Sandoz Pharmaceuticals. Is it okay?

"Have had experience with mescaline, LSD-25, and psilocybin. The mushroom synthetic seems to me the easiest on the body physically, and the most controllable in dosage. The effects are generally similar, subjectively. Psilocybin seems to me to be some sort of psychic godsend. It offers unparalleled opportunity to catalyze awareness of otherwise unconscious psychic processes. To widen the area of human consciousness. To deepen reification of ideas and identification of real objects. To perceive the inner organization of natural objects and human art works. To enter the significance and aesthetic organization of music, painting, poetry, architecture. It seems to make philosophy make sense. It aids consciousness to contemplate itself and serve some of the most delightful functions of the mind. As if, turning up the volume on a receiving set, background and FM stations can be heard. The effects are not unnatural.

"I have experienced similar things without use of chemical catalysts, and correspond to what I, as a poet, have called previously aesthetic, poetic, transcendental or mystical awareness. A kind of useful, practical cosmic consciousness. I think it will help mankind to grow."

JANUARY, 1961:

I spoke to Willem de Kooning yesterday, and he was ready to swing, too, so please drop him an invitation. I figure Kline, de Kooning and Gillespie are the most impressive trio imaginable for you to turn on at the moment, so will leave it at that for a while, till they can be taken care of. I won't send you new names and work trouble for a while. Hope you can get these three letters off.

I also wrote Osmond and Huxley asking them to connect Burroughs with Heim, or anyone in Paris. None of my business actually, but Koestler always struck me as a little <u>hard</u>hearted somehow. Hate myself to have him as a final <u>curandero</u>. That is, being an intellectual, he tends to organize a polemic-dogmatic-mental system around experience. As in his essay on Zen, which is very intelligent, but not so magnanimous. By all means send him batches to hand out.

So H.S. fears the perils of mind let loose. Well I agree with you generally. But I have had that experience of absolute fear. Suppose it decides not to keep the body going? --In Peru. It never recurred, but I can't guarantee it won't recur to me.

Send me a bill for the mescaline. No need for you to pay. No news yet from Cuba, so I think it safe to send psilocybin here. I'll call you before I leave, which may yet be another week--if at all at this rate.

Burroughs is in Paris. I wrote Huxley his address today with an explanatory note--but if you have any means of connecting him with Heim or anyone there--could you do so? Perhaps send him an academic letter of introduction which he could deliver to Heim? This got to be done soon, as Burroughs is on way East in a few weeks I think--not sure. He writes he had some LSD in London, as well as an injection of another drug. He writes--Don't flip pops is all. One must be careful of altitude sickness and depth madness and the bends. Hazards of the silent world. Space is silent remember, etc.

Anyway, I'll let you know before I leave to Cuba. Send me what you can, if you can, when you can. Been finished with proofs of my book this week and doing some writing.

FEBRUARY:

Been paralyzed making decisions, so forgive me not writing last week till I figured out what I wanted to do. Got letter and telegram from Corso in Athens summoning me to hurry up or he sez he'll take a boat to here. I replied I'd stand on Acropolis with him in a month if the gods please and he replied he'd wait then....

Meanwhile I've been conspiring with everyone I can reach

Leary on high

in New York the last weeks to do something about the general dope problem. Various other working on other different angles. Yesterday got on TV with N. Mailer and Ashley Montagu and gave big speech attacking Narco Dept. and recommending everybody get high--be on locally in New York Sunday after this, if they don't suppress the program. Montagu is an old woman, but he cooperated a bit. Maybe I'll go on Mike Wallace show. They asked me to. Also making an appointment with Eleanor Roosevelt to try to interest her in the social problem. Met her and Martin Luther King at Dorothy Norman's last night. Got lunch date with Reverend Norman Eddy of East Harlem Protestant Parish this Tuesday. He's the big dope do-gooder.

Didn't mention mushrooms in all of this, for tactful reasons. Best keep that on its own high level. I dunno, but I think it would help the mushroom atmosphere lots if there were a general U.S. rethinking (as The New York *Times* friend says) on the dope social problem.

Lindesmith and Indiana U. Press are putting out this joint report of interim committee of A.M.A. and American Bar Association. So I got in touch with all the liberal pro-dope people I know to have it publicized and circulated and have all of them inter-connect to exchange information.

I wrote a five-page summary of situation to this friend Kenny Love on The New York *Times* and he said he'd perhaps do a story (newswise) on the book, which could then be picked up on by U.P. friend on national wire.

Also gave copy to Al Aronowitz on New York *Post* and Rosalind Constable at *Time* and Bob Silvers on *Harper's* magazine and informed *Yugen*, *Evergreen*, *Big Table*, *Metronome*.

Meanwhile Indiana U. people are working on *Commentary*, *The Nation*, etc. Regular network. Also got a copy of La Guardia Report to Grove Press. They may republish it with additional stronger material. Maybe Dan Wakefield edit a book....

I don't know exactly when I'm leaving yet--but it's *got* to be around the first week in March. Peter and I will come up to Harvard for weekend before we leave though. Please don't be mad at me for taking off and leaving you holding the bag with so much on your mind. In the long run I do much better in anonymous goofing and writing than being Allen Ginsberg politicking.

I get the impression that the general psychic fog in the U.S. may be lifting....Do you want or need, or does the situation actually need, that I stay longer here and make the Harvard conference? I feel if I stay I'll just keep staying--Gregory is calling, etc. If he comes here it'll be a ball, but it'll be a year or half-year before we can go again.

Prison sounds great. Don't give mushrooms to junkies who are just in physiological process (first weeks) of kicking. Burroughs says in an article it would be pure hell....David Solomon is a good guy, but he is long-winded, an ex-political left-wing intellectual who's got humane.

All the young kids lately are shooting (needle) a drug called methedrine...an amphetamine semi-hallucinogen--haven't tried it yet. It's all the vogue.

See--I don't know if I should stay here and rave and scream politically and give big Carnegie Hall readings and Harvard readings--but I think a quiet silly trip to Greece would be better in the long run.

MARCH:

Still hoping to come up, but can't figure it till I settle other things--leaving arrangements, filing all papers, etc. Glad Burroughs will be back at Harvard.

It's hard trying to turn off faucet of correspondence. The F.C.C. complained to John Crosby about my TV speech and after network pressure Crosby let them play a seven-minute rebuttal last weekend, lots of crap. I also hear Paul Goodman and N. Podhoretz are forming some kind of committee for intelligent action which has as program various things such as sex freedom and drug freedom.

A young girl approached me and transmitted a suggestion from Goodman that I go to jail in passive resistance action on marijuana. Sounds like a good deal, actually. I told her I was going to Greece though, so couldn't. They're having a meeting tonight at Debs Hall--just like the Twenties.

The *Times* refused to run a series on Fed Narco Bureau but Harrison Salisbury is now lobbying to find why; and they did agree to run the Lindesmith-Ploscowe report in summary when it does come out and various Chicago and S.F. papers are now interested too.

I think people at Living Theatre and Goodman and others soon will prepare some sort of intellectual's petition to free pot from prohibition. I'll write Dr. Spiegel. Reverend John Snow of Gould Farm says he been reading up on subject and now wants to try LSD or mushrooms. Dave Solomon gave LeRoi Jones the mushrooms finally--very good results too.

APRIL:

I receive mail safely at American Express, 11 Rue Scribe, Paris, France. If you have a sufficient supply, I would like to have some mushrooms or LSD. I am looking for French connection, no success yet but have not looked intensively. Can use all you can send.

Burroughs is in Tangier, c/o U.S. Consulate. He or Brion Gysin et my mushrooms. I'll go down to visit Burroughs as soon as financially able....All three of us down to $80, but there will be loot coming in. We got offer from Girodias of Olympia to be editors of a big-time sexual magazine, free hand with vast salaries and print anything *mad* we want. Gregory wants to, I'm hesitating, Peter still wants India directly. If I accept it means being tied down here in Europe a year or two, but also weirdest century literary mag yet. I dunno. I'll probably be around here when you come in June. Send me forms to fill out as I gave mushrooms to Gregory. Gysin has filled out and will send you his.

Gysin has invented a *great* flicker machine. Dig this--cut out 10 apertures on a stovepipe hat or piece of cardboard and set it revolving on phonograph at 33 speed. It flickers and is homemade strobe. I looked in it--it sets up optical fields as religious and mandalic as the hallucinogenic drugs --literally....(look in with eyes closed)--it's like being able to have jeweled biblical designs and landscapes without taking chemicals. Amazing. It *works*. Gysin says the apertures have to be measured and adjusted right to get 16 flickers a second or something. He also paints the inside of the stove-pipe-cardboard. Of course, you have to drop an electric bulb I forgot it, in the center of it to flicker through apertures. I'll try to connect him with a toy manufacturer--homemade optic movies possible.

Can you send me a pack of psilocybin?--and also send the forms, they'll be filled out. Here is Peter, who a half-hour ago shot 250 of mescaline into his vein with a needle.

First, yes, also, I saw Michaux who has just finished a book on his experiments with mushroom pills too--nice old man--says it's all in *you* and no outside forces or gods too....

MARCH, 1962

Forgive my long silence. I received your chapter, read it: you are too nice about me, i.e., too grandiloquently respectful and in a way (as prose à la prose artistique) it's still over-written and maybe over-eager...naïveté. Nonetheless it's strictly you and I do "dig"/love you. I hear all sorts of laconic sounds (rarely) from Burroughs and he said he's written something (negative I take it) for *Evergreen*--didn't say specifically whether it dealt with your Harvard project ...about drugs--haven't seen the issue yet and hope he doesn't come on meanly. I will sit down and write you when I am settled--right now living out of knapsack and sleeping in *ashrams* (i.e. Hindu Y.M.C.A.'s) and railroad trains.

Peter here is fine--Gary Snyder real interesting on Zen technique. He'll try to arrange later in Japan for some bona fide guaranteed enlightened Zen masters to try pills out.

IN THE BEGINNING, LEARY TURNED ON GINSBERG AND SAW THAT IT WAS GOOD. . . . AND THEN LEARY AND GINSBERG DECIDED TO TURN ON THE WORLD

(*Continued from page 86*) about the foolishness of believing in hot and cold. It occurred to me that Allen and Peter were proving his point. The phone call continued and finally I walked back in and said, Hey, Allen, for the cost of this phone call we could pay his way up here by plane. Allen shot an apologetic look and then I heard him telling Jack, Okay, Jack, I have to go now, but you've got to take the mushrooms and let's settle this quarrel between Kennedy and Khrushchev. BUT NEEDED MY GLASSES—THOUGH HAD YELLED AT LEARY THAT HE DIDN'T NEED HIS EARPIECE TO HEAR THE REAL VIBRATIONS OF THE COSMOS. HE WENT ALONG WITH ME AGREEABLY.

Allen and Peter were sitting on the big couch in the living room and Allen was telling us about his visions, cosmic electronic networks, and how much it meant to him that I told him he was a great man and how this mushroom episode had opened the door to women and heterosexuality and how he could see new womanly body visions and family life ahead. BUT THEN I BEGAN BREATHING AND WANTING TO LIE DOWN AND REST. Peter's hand was moving back and forth on Allen's shoulder. It was the first time that Allen had stood up to Jack and he was sorry about the phone bill but wasn't it too bad that Khrushchev and Kennedy couldn't have been on the line and, hey, what about Norman Mailer in that psychiatric ward in Bellevue, shouldn't we call him.

I don't think they'd let a call go through to him, Allen. Well, it all depends on how we come on. I don't think coming on as Allen Ginsberg would help in that league. I don't think coming on as the Messiah would either. Well, you could come on as big psychologists and make big demanding noises about the patient. It was finally decided that it was too much trouble.

Still *curandero*, I asked if they wanted anything to eat or drink. Well, how about some hot milk. IF I ATE OR SHIT AGAIN I WOULD TURN BACK TO MERE NON-MESSIAH HUMAN. Allen and Peter went upstairs to put on robes and I put some cold milk in a pan and turned on the stove. Donald was still moving around softly with his hands behind his back. Thinking. Watching. He was too deep and Buddha for us to swing with and I later realized that I hadn't been a very attentive *curandero* for him and that there was a gulf between Allen and him never closed and that the geographic arrangement was too scattered to make a close loving session. Of course, both of them were old drug hands and ready to go off on their own private journeys and both wanted to make something deep and their own.

Anthro's role in all of this was never clear. He stood in the hallway watching curiously but for the most part we ignored him, treated him as an object just there but not involved and that, of course, was a mistake. Any time you treat someone as an object rest assured he'll do the same and that was the way that score was going to be tallied.

We ended up with a great scene in the kitchen. I bustled around pouring the hot milk into cups, and the poets sat around the table looking like Giotto martyrs in checkered robes. Lafcadio came down and we got him some food and he nodded yes when I asked him about ice cream and Allen started to talk about his visions and about the drug scene in New York and, becoming eloquent, wound up preaching with passion about the junkies, helpless, hooked, lost, thin, confused creatures, sick and the police and the informers. I SAW THE BEST MINDS OF MY GENERATION DESTROYED BY MADNESS, STARVING HYSTERICAL NAKED, DRAGGING THEMSELVES THROUGH THE NEGRO STREETS AT DAWN LOOKING FOR AN ANGRY FIX. And then we started planning the psychedelic revolution. Allen wanted everyone to have the mushrooms. Who has the right to keep them from someone else? And there should be freedom for all sorts of rituals, too. The doctors could have them and there should be *curanderos*, and all sorts of good new holy rituals that could be developed and ministers have to be involved. Although the church is naturally and automatically opposed to mushroom visions, still the experience is basically religious and some ministers would see it and start using them. But with all these groups and organizations and new rituals, there still had to be room for the single, lone, unattached, non-groupy individual to take the mushrooms and go off and follow his own rituals—brood big cosmic thoughts by the sea or roam through the streets of New York, high and restless, thinking poetry, and writers and poets and artists to work out whatever they were working out.

Allen Ginsberg hunched over the kitchen table, shabby robe hiding his thin white nakedness, cosmic politician. Give them the mystic vision. They'll see it's good and honest and they'll say so publicly and then no one from the police or the narcotics bureau can put them down. And you're the perfect persons to do it. Big serious scientist professors from Harvard. That's right. I can't do it. I'm too easy to put down. Crazy beatnik poet. Let me get my address book. I've got lots of connections in New York and we'll go right down the list and turn them all on.

Now Allen Ginsberg, stooping over the kitchen table peering at his address book. There's Robert Lowell and Muriel Rukeyser, and LeRoi Jones. And Dizzy Gillespie. And the painters. And the publishers. He was chanting out names of the famous and the talented. He was completely serious, dedicated, wound up in the crusade. I'M NEARSIGHTED AND PSYCHOPATHIC ANYWAY. AMERICA, I'M PUTTING MY QUEER SHOULDER TO THE WHEEL.

And so Allen spun out the cosmic campaign. He was to line up influentials and each weekend I would come down to New York and we'd run mushroom sessions. This fit our Harvard research plans perfectly. Our aim there was to learn how people reacted, to test the limits of the drug, to get creative and thoughtful people to take them and tell us what they saw and what we should do with the mushrooms. Allen's political plan was appealing, too. I had seen enough and read enough in Spanish of the anti-vision crowd, the power-holders with guns, and the bigger and better men we got on our team the stronger our position. And then, too, the big-name bit was intriguing. Meeting and sharing visions with the famous.

It was around midnight. Donald still seemed high and would walk in and out of the room, silently, hands behind his back, Talmudic raccoon, studying the kitchen crowd seriously, and then padding out. The anthropology student had joined us around the table. We had given him something to drink and he was listening to the conversation and saying nothing. He made some comment about schedules back to Cambridge and it was time for him to make the last train, so I drove him down to the station. He asked some questions about the scientific meaning of the mushroom research and it was clear that he didn't understand what had happened and what we were doing. There wasn't time to explain and I felt badly that he had been dragged into a strange situation. We had made the rule that people could bring their friends when they took the mushrooms and this seemed like a good idea for the person taking the mushrooms but it was just beginning to dawn on me that the problem never was with the person taking the drug but rather the people who didn't. Like Brother Toriblo, the Spanish monk, who talked about cruelty and drunkenness caused by the Sacred Mushrooms. It's okay to bring a friend, but he should take the mushrooms with you. And poor Anthro, it turned out, wasn't even a friend of Donald's and as it turned out didn't like him and was clearly bewildered by and critical of what he had seen and heard and the nakedness of the poets. His train was about due and I was too preoccupied by what Allen had been saying to feel like explaining to Anthro. The uneasy feeling persisted and I suggested that he not tell people about the mystic visions and the naked crusaders because this might be misunderstood and he said he wouldn't talk about it and we shook hands and he left.

That was Sunday night. By Monday afternoon the rumors were spreading around Harvard Yard.

Beatniks. Orgies. Naked poets. Junkies. Homosexuality. Drug parties. Tried to lure a decent naïve graduate student into sin. Wild parties masquerading as research. Queers. Beards. Criminal types.

The chairman of my department called me. What the hell is going on, Tim? Two graduate students have come to me indignant—demanding that your work be stopped.

I laughed. I'll send you the reports from the session as soon as they are typed. It was a good session. God would approve. We're learning a lot.

The disapproving gaze of the establishment was on us. You should fear the wary eyes of the servants of Sauron were the words of Elrond. I do not doubt that news . . . has already reached him, and he will be filled with wrath. —The Lord of the Rings

In the months that followed we began to see ourselves as unwitting agents of a social process that was far too powerful for us to control or more than dimly understand. A historical movement that would inevitably change man at the very center of his nature, his consciousness.

We did sense that we were not alone. The quest for internal freedom, for the elixir of life, for the drought of immortal revelation was not new. We were part of an ancient and honorable fellowship which had pursued this journey since the dawn of recorded history. We began to read the accounts of earlier trippers—Dante, Hesse, René Daumal, Tolkien, Homer, Blake, George Fox, Swedenborg, Bosch, and the explorers from the Orient—tantrics, Sufis, Bauls, Gnostics, hermetics, Sivaites, sadhus.

From this moment on my days as a respectable establishment scientist were numbered. I just couldn't see the new society given birth by medical hands, or psychedelic sacraments as psychiatric tools.

From this evening on my energies were offered to the ancient underground society of alchemists, artists, mystics, alienated visionaries, dropouts and the disenchanted young, the sons arising. ##

Esquire

CHAPTER 4: Dana Beal

As Dhoruba said a few months later, June 22, 1990, just before he embraced Nelson Mandela at a rally in Harlem on 125th Street, every movement needs a "symbol" to inspire it. The final unintended side effect of all those trials, all that political agitation by Dhoruba's supporters, was that a single television image escaped from New York in 1971. Black Panthers had tried to drive heroin out of Harlem with guns. Dana had heard about it / seen it on TV in New York, where he was living just before he returned in July to be arrested in Madison, Wisconsin, and the memory lingered with him in jail afterwards.[1]

Dana Beal was born in the same hospital in Ravenna, Ohio, where the dying students were later taken from Kent State. He counts among his formative experiences shaking hands with Jack Kennedy when he campaigned in East Lansing in 1960, and hitchhiking in August '63 at age sixteen to Washington, D.C., in order to be near the foot of the Lincoln Memorial for the "I Have a Dream" speech. Two months later he organized his first demonstration of 2,000 people, in Lansing, Michigan, after the Klan blew up four little Black girls in a Birmingham, Alabama church on Sunday.

The next year he did a brief stint in a state mental hospital because of his mercurial temper. But that kept him from being drafted in January '65, a month with the highest proportion of casualties in Viet Nam. He also became a lifelong critic of thorazine and prolyxin. He escaped, got a job in New York, saved his money, and legalized his status in late 1965.

On Christmas Day, 1966, to continue his study of epistemology and metaphysics, he tried LSD for the first time. His reaction: Kant was right, it's all phenomena. But after the first few times (including one session with a friendly psychologist who helped him plumb distressing episodes of his early childhood), he found that more and more of the acid was being compounded with a speed base such as ritalin to get twice as many hits out of a gram — thereby demonstrating the flaws of an underground market. People were no longer getting a genuine LSD effect. Reinforced by speed or ritalin, the ego-structures wouldn't let go.

Because of the furious controversy surrounding CIA sponsorship or involvement in psychedelics,[2] speculation was rife that all this was deliberate — part of a program to keep the psychedelic revolution under control. When Dana got real LSD again, he had a vision:

> "I flashed that all of us in the psychedelic movement were like voluntary guinea pigs in some kind of CIA experiment that had gotten out of control. The White Light was flashing across us like searchlights on a World War I no-man's land. All around me, we were taking casualties. But *some of us would make it to the other side;* and someone would bring back something wonderful."

He decided the first battle should be for the least threatening, most popular drug: marijuana. Inspired by a *Village Voice* article on the Dutch Provos, he started the New York Provos with Greg Hill and A. J. Weberman, and called a smoke-in for Tompkins Square Park. The smoke-ins got bigger and bigger, and after a judge ruled a roll-your-own cigarette seen from a distance wasn't grounds for arrest, the Feds moved in an informer who wheedled Dana's personal acid stash out of him. When he was busted in late August of 1967, 3,000 people marched from a Fugs concert at Union Square to the federal holding pen on West Street. It was Dana's first fifteen minutes of fame.

In October, New York Provos gave out four pounds of joints at the "Levitation of the Pentagon."[3] Then in December, the Provo Free Store on First Street was raided, and Dana was framed for a pot sale he didn't do. Panicked, he fled to Mexico, then Canada, where he had to watch the Chicago '68 Democratic Convention on television.

One day, sitting in a Vancouver community center, he read an *Esquire* article by Tim

1 For some idea of the impact, see three essays on community organizing in the "How to Revolt Handbook," *Blacklisted News*, especially pp. 670–74.

2 By early summer, '67, Dana learned about the CIA connection from, among others, Wendy Allen, who heard it from Margaret Mead, who found out as a consequence of being head of the American Anthropological Society—an occasional conduit for CIA funds. Because of her involvement with various CIA fronts, Mead's name comes up in *In Search of the Manchurian Candidate*, whose author comments: "In 1969 the Federal Bureau of Narcotics and Dangerous Drugs published a fascinating little study designed to curb illegal LSD use. The authors wrote that the drug's 'early use was among small groups of intellectuals at large Eastern and West Coast universities. It spread to undergraduate students, then to other campuses. Most often, users have been introduced to the drugs by persons of higher status. Teachers have influenced students; upperclassmen have influenced lowerclassmen.' Calling this a 'trickle-down phenomenon,' the authors seem to have correctly analyzed how LSD got around the country. They left out only one vital element, which they had no way of knowing: That somebody had to influence the teachers and that up there at the top of the LSD distribution system there could be found the men of [the CIA's] MK–ULTRA."—pp. 119–120, *In Search of the Manchurian Candidate*, by John Marks.

3 Mistakenly identified by Kirk Sale in *SDS* as Yippies; Yippie! would not be invented for another two months, around Christmas, 1967, by Paul Krassner, Abbie Hoffman, Bob Fass and Jerry Rubin, tripping during a storm in the Bahamas. Its first incarnation did not outlast the Chicago Convention. Immediately afterwards, a "Youth International Party for Self Defense" announced Yippie! was disbanding. See footnote, p. 14.

Leary and Allen Ginsberg on the early days of the psychedelic movement. What stuck in his mind, for years, was a passage about using psychedelics to cure heroin addiction. (Of course, LSD doesn't stop withdrawal symptoms. If every junkie could kick with five dollars worth of acid, they'd do just that every time they wanted to cut back on their habits and start over. Ginsberg was thinking of it more as a *substitute* for hard drugs; he writes Leary that Burroughs said that it would only make withdrawals worse.) (*See p. 37.*)

In April of '69, Dana filtered back into the United States on a Canadian ID, living in Milwaukee, Wisconsin. Unable to stay away from organizing, he became involved with the White Panther Party (WPP), and, in a psychedelic manifesto, *"Right on, Culture Freaks"*,[1] expanded on William Burroughs' insight that all forms of social control resemble addiction because the same "backbrain" reflex component involved in addiction underlies everyday work routine.

In September Dana travelled to Ann Arbor, where he was appointed Field Marshal of the WPP, based on his reputation from New York.[2] But that didn't last past the merger of the White Panther Party and YIPPIE in December. (The Ann Arbor folks were really organizing mostly to get John Sinclair out of ten years in prison for two joints.)

When, in the aftermath of Kent State, Abbie Hoffman, Jerry Rubin and the Ann Arbor crew cancelled the first D.C. July 4 smoke-in, Dana got Rennie Davis to call it back on. Nixon, emboldened by reports of hard hats beating up peaceniks in New York City, had called his supporters to Washington for a July 4th "Honor America Day." The smoke-in wound up with three times as many people as Nixon, and when Billy Graham on the steps of the Lincoln Memorial saw 4,000 protesters marching up the Reflecting Pool in a spontaneous act of self-baptism, he stopped his sermon.

It took a second July 4 smoke-in, in 1971, where Beal and Forçade added a march against CIA/Vietnam heroin (and which got airplay on CBS Evening News) to motivate the authorities sufficiently to snag Beal on his old warrant. Ten days later he was busted in Madison, Wisconsin. It was Bastille Day, July 14th. In September, 2,000 people held a smoke-in outside the jail, giving Dana his second fifteen minutes of fame.

Dana was not freed of his legal entanglements until five days before the '72 Demcon. But he reached Miami in time to walk into the vicious split between the Yippies (Abbie, Jerry) and the Zippies (Forcade and the ex-White Panthers, minus Ann Arbor, who'd faded out since Sinclair was released). Four days later, when McGovern sought to soften his stance against the war on the morning of his nomination, Beal was one of the leaders of the Zippie/SDS takeover of the lobby of the candidate's campaign headquarters at the Doral Hotel.

Dana was the one who caught McGovern, live on prime time, just hours before he was nominated, with a trick question. First he got McGovern to confirm that the CIA and the Saigon regime were deeply involved in pipelining heroin into the U.S. from Vietnam. Then he asked the follow-up: "How can we protect 26 million Americans who just smoke pot from all this heroin unless we 'control' pot like alcohol, by legalizing it and selling it over the counter?"

McGovern ducked the question!

For Democrats — including Abbie's people who were wooing the Democrats — this was more like fifteen minutes of infamy than fifteen minutes of fame. Never mind it was the first mass-media confirmation that hard drugs had fatally corrupted the U.S. Intelligence Community — a view that became conventional wisdom by the mid-'80s. Beal made McGovern look bad, on prime time. For a long time after that, everything he did had to draw its support from the street people. Twenty years later, he's still blackballed in some quarters, because of that five-minute exchange.

Then, a year later, Abbie was busted selling three kilos of cocaine. When he went underground, the Zippie wing took over. Their smoke-ins mobilized thousands, but they did lots of other things, most notably publicizing the pictures of Hunt and Sturgis on the grassy knoll — i.e., the theory that a CIA/Mafia conspiracy coordinated by Richard Nixon killed Kennedy.[3] (At the end of the decade, *YIPster Times* staffers even worked closely with the House Committee on

[1] "Right on, Culture Freaks." See *Blacklisted News*, pp. 501–13.

[2] The WPP Central Committee, consisting of Sinclair's relatives plus Skip Taub and Pun Plamundon, had convened a national party-building conference that attracted most of Ben Morea's Up Against the Wall Motherfuckers, for whom Dana was already a legend.

[3] See A. J. Weberman, *Coup D'Etat In America*, for pictures, with acetate overlays, of JFK's assassins.

Assassinations, which concluded there had been a second gun.)

In reaction to the leadership style of Abbie and Jerry, Yippies were at this time more concerned about their own faithful internal practice of formal democracy than what was happening in Washington, DC. In July, 1974, as the Impeachment of Nixon unfolded, Dana spent weeks preparing a second issue with better comparison photos of the tramps and Hunt and Sturgis, with a story attached revealing for the first time Nixon's presence in Dallas until just hours before the assassination. Then he got on a plane to Washington state, where YIPs were having a conference at Spokane. On the plane he sat next to the only woman who looked vaguely hip and showed her *"House to Probe Nixon Death Squad."*

She surprised Dana by not only knowing of the story, but adding information with a personal twist — the focus of the conspiracy that killed JFK was a cell of high-level drug dealers in the Coast Guard, Customs, and the Office of Naval Intelligence. They were centered on Long Island and in Philadelphia. They could never be busted because the Navy, conveniently, was in charge of investigating itself.[1] Their only Achilles heel was that people on the inside had access to huge quantities of dope, and sometimes became strung out. She herself was the daughter of an officer in the Navy or Coast Guard, and she was being shipped out to Spokane to dry out because she'd become totally addicted. Dana urged her to come to the conference, to tell her story to the other YIPs, but she was met at the airport and whisked away.

At the time, Dana discounted her story, but years later, after seeing the autopsy scene in the movie "JFK," the one with all of the admirals standing in the back of the room, it came flooding back. It was still very much on his mind the next day, just two weeks before Nixon resigned, when everyone at the Spokane conference did ALD-52 (5-acetyl-LSD, which was represented to them as "LSD put through an additional step of purification") in a Provo-style attempt to "get everyone on the same trip."

Robert Goutarel, the father of Ibogaine research, says indole-alkylamines of the LSD series are fundamentally different from the iboga-harmala group — "clear and angelic" as opposed to oneiric (REM-generating). Nonetheless, ALD-52 turned out to be ten or twenty times more psychedelic than LSD. That is, its effects lay far more in the direction of Ibogaine than a mere LSD "fishbowl effect," the "apprehension of the oneness of experience" often referred to as "seeing God."

Philip K. Dick, writing about his own celebrated religious or Near-Death Experience (NDE) in early 1974, described the phenomena of "laminate personality," of being several personalities millennia apart at the same time. Aron Kay, who also took the ALD, confirms that he had flashes of the same thing, the definite sensation of co-existing at several points of time simultaneously: 2,000 years ago, in the present, and some time far up ahead in the future. It was Beal's second vision.

> As we came down to the river, it was like this other personality was in my mind with me, a dominant personality, who looked at the water, saw the twentieth-century pollution, and thought: "The water in this river is totally unacceptable for performing Baptisms." And this other person was kind of daydreaming, not even conscious of the me there, until I looked at the litter along the streambank and thought — "But of course, they didn't have non-biodegradable plastics back then" — and the other personality kind of noticed I was there, and who I was, and thought: "Oh, a Baptist (I had attended Baptist Sunday School)... well, just make sure you don't get your head cut off this time!"

After puzzling it out ("Who *was* that masked man?"),[2] Dana decided this meant he was supposed to avoid taking any unnecessary risks until his mission, in the unknowable future, was accomplished. Aron says they sat looking at that river for hours.

Dana consulted with Lotsof when he got back to New York: "Ibogaine was more psychedelic than that!?"

"On Ibogaine, you would have visualized the other personality as sitting there talking to you," was Howard's cryptic reply.

The ALD-52 affected the others who took it — Bionic Bob, Ben Masel, etc. — similarly. It changed the political trajectory of YIP's inner core. For five more years, until the Brink's job fiasco in '81, various fringe elements continued to fall for the idea that membership in some

1 This state of affairs was not reformed until the presidency of George Bush.

2 See Hugh Schonfield, *Those Incredible Christians,* footnote # 4, p. 77. J. Klausner, *From Jesus to Paul,* pp. 324–30, quotes a letter from the mystic Rabbi Moses Luzzatto (dated 1730) describing revelations made to him by a "messenger from heaven." "I saw nothing of him," he wrote, "but I heard his voice speaking out of my own mouth."

kind of secret armed underground vanguard was hipper than building a mass movement using weapons of consciousness and information. That year, 1974, the romantic attachment to the Symbionese Liberation Army (SLA) — which had kidnapped Patty Hearst, and whose leader, Donald DeFreeze, was probably a police provocateur — had seriously competed among the YIPs with the less glamorous organizing around Nixon's impeachment. After Spokane that was never a problem.

Within three years the new generation of YIP leaders like Ben Masel had gotten into Tai Chi, the "passive" martial arts form based on throwing blocks, not striking blows — and on side-stepping your opponents' blows. Typical of the time was the YIP action the day after Carter's inauguration: YIPs were arrested for chaining themselves to the White House fence to draw attention to several hundred Nixon-era political prisoners still being held, long after COINTELPRO was exposed. Yet Carter never extended his amnesty from draft dodgers to political prisoners — hundreds, including Dhoruba, continued to sit in captivity.

Meanwhile, the YIPs really didn't care if they were blacklisted in some circles, or dismissed as "the marijuana movement," because *High Times* was opening up access to millions of people. By July 4, 1977, they could assemble the same number of people for a smoke-in in front of the White House — 10,000 — as laid siege to Chicago in '68. All from a series of ads in *High Times.* In early 1978, YIPPIE published the *Soft Strategy,* a major course-correction. You could say it was based on the Tai Chi concept "soft on the outside, hard on the inside" — but why did they get into Tai Chi in the first place?

Instead of the knock 'em, sock 'em, blow 'em up approach of the Weather Underground, they had turned to the tough, self-disciplined task of maintaining a more ingratiating exterior while digging in for the long run. They even tried to make peace with the other wing of the Yippies, earning Abbie's personal gratitude with a Bring Abbie Home benefit at the Felt Forum, although not all of Abbie's people *wanted* to be friends.[1]

When racial clashes dogged New York smoke-ins, it was only a hop, skip, and a jump to start ROCK AGAINST RACISM (RAR). And RAR

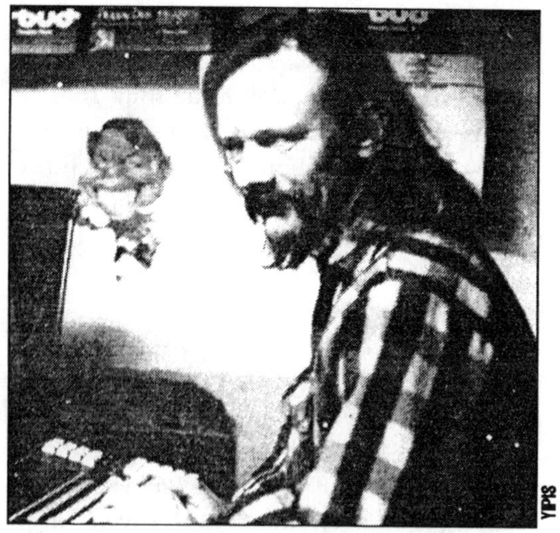

YIPS

DANA BEAL AFTER HIS RELEASE, IN EARLY '82

was something Howard and his Afro-American wife Norma Alexander could comfortably join. As veterans of the Free Speech Movement, they'd always been a little too grown-up for the Yippies.

The stage was set. In the early '60s, when Lotsof had tried to initiate an Ibogaine Project without a support structure in place, it came to nothing. It was like an egg fertilized at the wrong time, coming down the fallopian tube and finding the womb is not ready for it.

This time Howard had the support of his personal network as well as Dana, *Overthrow,* Rock Against Racism,[2] and the activist Yippie wing of the marijuana movement in practically every state of the Union. And somewhat in reaction to Abbie's coterie siding with the *Soho Weekly News* against Dana, the younger YIPs — the real '70s activists — now took a turn toward a more closed decision-making process, making it very hard to unseat the Ibogaine Project once it got going.

In December 1980, Dana Beal was mad as hell, and he wasn't going to take it anymore. He was willing to "pay any price, bear any burden" to win the war against addiction — including use of psychopharmaco-chemical weapons from the CIA's closet.

But there's a postscript:

In September '81, Dana was acquitted of felony assault at the *Soho Weekly News* after the judge ruled it was a firecracker, not a bomb. The jury convicted him of recklessness, a misdemeanor which netted him thirty-five days on Riker's Island.

While he was waiting to be sentenced,

1 After the benefit, Abbie's cousin Sam Leff dismissively told Ben Masel that his turnouts, no matter how large, could never equal the impact of what they did in the '60s. Ben continues to gather 20–30,000 people every year for the Great Midwest Harvest Fest in Madison, Wisconsin, on the first Saturday in October.

2 The need was mutual, considering the many musicians with heroin problems in the rock world.

Dana and Alice Torbush attended one of the first showings of *Prince of the City* (much of which was shot a few blocks away from 9 Bleecker, on Mulberry Street). It's the story of Danny Ciello, the narc who narked out the SIU (NYPD Central Narcotics Unit) in the early '70s. The story had two morals:

1.) Even if police were 100 percent incorruptible, heroin can't be wiped out, because to penetrate above the street level, agents must either deal it themselves or maintain a number of dealers as informers. But that gives a crucial edge to dealers with police connections; soon *they* dominate the trade. Organized crime consists of dealers who can buy a cop, an Assistant District Attorney, a judge, or secure protection through the federal intelligence community.

Cops themselves are damaged by this; in the movie Danny Ciello is moved to act because his own brother, strung out on smack (the methadone is not working), begs him for a connection. That night he returns to Manhattan to supply one of his own snitches after the smack he gave him earlier turns out to be bogus. So he has to go out in the rainy night, to rip off another junkie to take care of his informant.

2.) Drugs are impossible to prohibit, but police will not give up drug prohibition because junkie snitches are their eyes and ears in the community. Without snitches, they lose control. Moreover, by fostering constant rip-offs, addiction breaks down solidarity, breeds paranoia, and saps the community's potential for social revolution. The Panthers were on to something, all right.

But if Black Panthers couldn't stop heroin with machine guns, neighborhood support, and no need for search warrants, neither can the police with all the prisons, armed might, and sophisticated technology of the State. (Nor can there be redress through the courts, as shown later in the '80s when the Christic Institute tried to sue elements of the Intelligence Community for bringing 500 tons of cocaine into the country to fund the Nicaraguan Contras. The federal judge fined *them* $1.2 million for general chutzpah.)

As Dana and Alice left the theatre, another layer of reality fell into place:

Fighting addiction with a War on Drugs is worse than useless. It's misleading.

What we need is a cure, not a war.

Under Reagan, we got the war, not the cure. As the war dragged on, the proponents of the Dutch harm-reduction approach became officially despised, their advice relegated to the sidelines of public discourse. Only when widespread doubt set in after revelations of gross government complicity in the Contra arms-for-drugs affair was it possible for respectable opposition, beginning with Mayor Kurt Schmoke of Baltimore, to emerge.

The real *coup de grâce* was self-inflicted, however, as the Reagan boom collapsed, spectacularly, on Black Monday, October 19, 1987. Four days earlier, just before noon on Thursday the 15th, Dana pulled together four yippie sympathizers to hold a banner in front of the New York Stock Exchange that said "JUMP!" Dana and co. were assailed by irate stockbrockers, but in the next three days, the market fell 650 points. Later he talked to someone who'd worked inside, who told him the crash was really just a matter of the market's collective coke habit catching up with it. *In the picture below Dana is second-from-the-left, head bent behind the banner* (*Newsweek*).

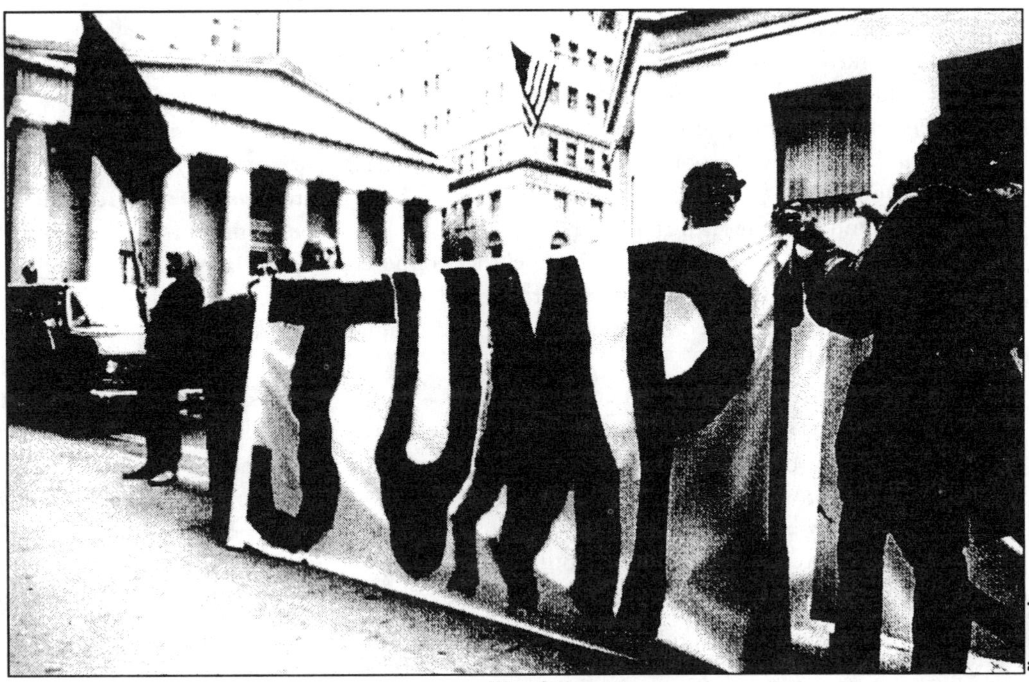

WALL STREET DEMONSTRATORS

Meanwhile, in the commodity marts of Chicago, Richard Denis was also betting the market would crash. The difference was that Denis, a gay libertarian with a strong belief in drug legalization, walked away with market futures profits variously estimated from $40 to $400 million. He teamed up with Arnold Trebach and Kevin Zeese of the Drug Policy Foundation to begin a serious drive to legalize drugs. In autumn of 1988, there were hearings in front of Congressman Charles Rangel's Select Sub-committee on Narcotics, and ABC News convened the most American of institutions, an electronic town meeting:

Getting the Last Word — The Ted Koppel Town Meeting on Drug Legalization, September 8, 1988

Cong. Rangel: I'm asking you — you say that the 13-year-old can't get it, as if you have some scheme as to who can get it. Would you have to be an addict to get it?
Hugh Downs: Anybody can get drugs now.
Cong. Rangel: I'm asking — under legalization — would the pharmacist be able to give it? Would you have to go to a doctor to get it?
Hugh Downs: Wouldn't he be able to do the same kind of thing as with liquor, and determine somebody's age?
Cong. Rangel: You're asking *me* questions. I'm asking — what kind of control would it *be?!*
Ethan Nadelman: I would think that the first thing to do would be to make marijuana legally available — and fairly readily available.
Ted Koppel: To everyone...
E. Nadelman: To adults. Like alcohol and tobacco, but with stricter controls. We know right now that sixty million Americans in this country have smoked marijuana. Between twenty and thirty million are smoking it right now. We have *zero* overdose deaths. We know that the vast majority of people who smoke marijuana have not gone on to harder drugs...
Cong. Rangel: Get to cocaine.
E. Nadelman: Last week the Administrative Judge of the DEA, in a suit which asked whether or not marijuana should be made legally available for medical purposes to deal with chemotherapy–
Cong. Rangel: What happened to crack cocaine and heroin?
E. Nadelman: You know the polite thing to do would be to let me at least finish what I'm saying.
Cong. Rangel: You'll be for legalizing cigarettes next.
E. Nadelman: Listen — everybody on this panel that's opposed to legalization is opposed to legalizing marijuana. Now the DEA Judge said that compared in toxicity to aspirin, marijuana is overwhelmingly safer.
Bob Stutman: It's foolish to legalize marijuana.
E. Nadelman: He said that marijuana is perhaps one of the safest psychoactive substances ever known to man.
Outburst in the audience!
Ed Koch: Everybody believes–
E. Nadelman: When Mayor Koch talks about throwing users in jail, when Mayor Koch says that sixty million Americans...
Ed Koch: Everybody believes that the drugs that have to be addressed now are cocaine and heroin and crack, and when we've addressed those, even though most of us believe that marijuana ought to not be legalized, that's the *last* one on the list...
Outburst in the back of the hall!
Cong. Rangel: He didn't answer the question!
Ed Koch: ...and what he has done is to dodge the issue.
E. Nadelman: Ted, it's the first one. You start with marijuana. Marijuana of all the illicit drugs is the safest...
Ted Koppel: Hold it! Just all of you hold it one second — *turning to the audience, calling on the source of the outburst* — the gentleman behind you who was yelling...
Dana: My name is Dana Beal, I've been...
Ted Koppel: I don't care what your name is, what were you yelling about?
Dana: Okay. The exact quote from the Federal Judge was "the safest, therapeutically active substance known to mankind." That means safer than caffeine, safer than aspirin...
Ted Koppel: Yeah —
Dana: That means you're putting people in jail for basically doing something that's completely harmless.
Ted Koppel: Let me turn to —
Dana: How can you talk about locking people up in work camps? How can you talk about taking people's...
Ed Koch: We're talking about cocaine and heroin.
Dana: ...taking people's *homes* away from them, evicting people *in New York City.* Why don't you want to go after the worst first? And this is the real point — how can you justify a situation where you've *eliminated* pot, but crack — and heroin — are *four times* more available, *four times* cheaper than at the beginning of the Reagan War on Drugs. All you've done, is design a system that *gets rid of marijuana,* leaving hard drugs! That's all you've done.
Ted Koppel: I think...
Dana: And *that's* to the guy from the DEA.
Ted Koppel: ...if we can cut that mike over there for a minute now, Dr. Jaffe, you are one of our most distinguished experts here....I would like to address the question to you, when that Judge — I must confess I didn't read the decision, I read reports of the Judge's decision — true? marijuana really the safest–what was the phrase — "therapeutic drug, the safest therapeutic drug?"
Ed Rosenthal: The safest therapeutically active substance known to humankind.
Ted Koppel: What do you think Doctor?
Jerome Jaffe: I think it's nonsense.

CHAPTER 5: The Staten Island Project

In 1981 the marijuana movement was divided between NORML ("the suits") and a larger group of activists who did smoke-ins. Today's Drug Reform Movement (the Drug Policy Foundation and its offshoots) was still a glimmer in the future. NORML was in eclipse, having lost its Capitol Hill clout when Carter Drug Czar Dr. Peter Bourne got caught writing a phony script for quaaludes. That activated a little tidbit about Bourne doing coke at a NORML party, planted with columnist Jack Anderson by NORML head Keith Stroup. Stroup thought of this as insurance in his running feud with the White House; not realizing Bourne was the best negotiating partner he was going to get. (Some of Stroup's own judgment was missing due to coke.)

The DEA became the lead agency for U.S. drug policy for ten years until, exasperated with the results, Congress re-established the Drug Czar office by statute in 1988.

After Reagan came in, federal agencies were forbidden even to deal with NORML. Prohibitionists wouldn't appear with them on the same television panel. But the marijuana movement of the smoke-ins was unfazed. For five years, until Howard Lotsof started NDA International and achieved self-sufficiency in '86–'87, tremendous resources were secretly diverted from legalizing pot to jump-starting Ibogaine. Like some Third World country developing nuclear weapons, up to half of the YIPPIE political expenditures went either to the Project or to corollary organizing like RAR and the GREENS, in order to gain access and build support in the Black and environmental movements.

After Howard and Norma moved to Staten Island from Brooklyn, it was only a matter of time before people in the loop started calling it "the Staten Island Project." And there was the same degree of secrecy as the Manhattan Project. At first it was based on assumptions that forces within the government would once again stop Ibogaine in some way. Once Howard decided to go for patents, it became vital to protect the secret from being pirated and suppressed by hostile corporate interests.

Initially, in '81, Ibogaine was a research project tucked away in a RAR task force innocently called Citizens Against Heroin. Other activities included publication in *Overthrow* of the aforementioned report on complicity of World Nazism and the Intelligence Community in the rising heroin influx (*"A New Heroin Conspiracy?"*), and a demo against blatant police corruption in the Ninth Precinct. By April, however, Howard was already moving to put the Ibogaine Project on independent footing to spare it from intra-YIPPIE feuding. Then everyone ran out of money, at once.

As 1981 wore on, though, Howard found that a back injury made it impossible to continue as a film-maker, or to pursue his backup gig as a plumber. His options were narrowing. In December, he landed the first large-scale contribution from an outside source: $4,000. At a Christmas party he ran into a woman he knew who said she had a boyfriend who was an addict, and she would be very interested in treating him. He told her he needed money for more basic research, and she put him back at work in the libraries until mid-'82.

From the original RAR-sponsored literature search of New York University Library, Howard had several books and about two hundred articles on Ibogaine and *Tabernanthe iboga.* These he studied while he continued to scour other sources for additional materials mentioned in the footnotes. Then for about six months he again ran out of money. When he could resume, at the end of 1982, his next move was to get everything translated from French, and to document every paper ever done on Ibogaine. That took another six months, with the help of a research librarian. What he was looking for was a clearly demonstrable relationship between the biochemical mechanisms of action of Ibogaine and the biochemical mechanisms of action of the opiates. So after he reviewed about a century of work on Ibogaine, he reviewed the last twenty-five years of biochemical research on the opiates.

What he found was that every system the

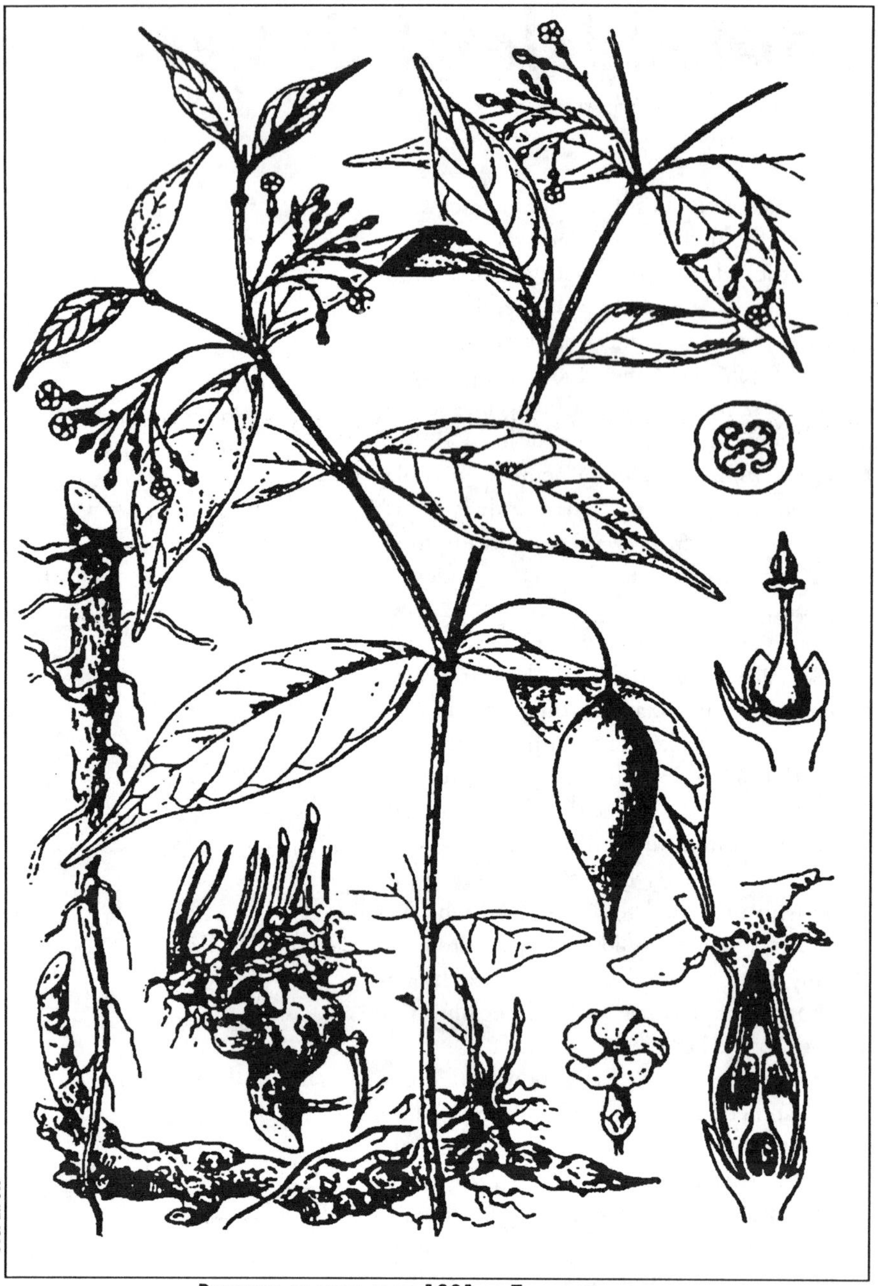

Overthrow

BOTANICAL DRAWING FROM 1901 OF *TABERNANTHE IBOGA*, THE MAJOR SOURCE OF IBOGAINE AND RELATED ALKALOIDS.

opiates work on Ibogaine works on — like the neurohormonal system in the brain, the central nervous system, the production of proteins relating to RNA templating. Virtually every system where the opiates were active, Ibogaine also was active. Additionally, he ran across the 1956 paper by Jurg Schneider, who was working at CIBA–GEIGY at the time, but went on to become president of Dupont's Biochemicals Division. It said Ibogaine potentiates morphine analgesia. It wasn't analgesic itself, but combined with morphine, it could reduce by fifty percent (!) the amount of morphine used to maintain a certain level of freedom from pain.

The state of Howard's understanding of Ibogaine at the end of 1983 can pretty much be seen in the original patent for treatment of morphine addiction (U.S. #4,499,096), filed November 18, 1983, in the section reproduced here, with asides:

Historical Background

Ibogaine is one of at least twelve alkaloids found in the *Tabernathe iboga* shrub of West Africa. The indigenous peoples have used the drug as a ritual, ordeal or initiation potion in large dosages and a stimulant in smaller doses. One of the first European references to the drug was made by Professor Baillon at the March 6th, 1889, session of the Linnean Society in Paris during which he described samples obtained by Griffon de Bellay from Gabon and the French Congo.

Early isolation and identification of Ibogaine was accomplished by Dybrowski and Landrin (Compt. rend. ac. sc. 133: 748, 1901); Haller and Heckel (ibid. 133: 850); Lambert and Heckel (ibid. 133: 1236) and Landrin (Bull. sc. pharm. 11: 1905).

Interest in the drug seemed to lie fallow until it was picked up by Raymond-Hamet and his associates. E. Rothbin and Raymond-Hamet published *The Effect of Ibogaine on the isolated Rabbit Uterus* in 1938 (Compt. rend. soc. biol. 127: 592–4). Raymond–Hamet continued to study the drug for twenty-two years. He himself published nine papers: *Pharmacological Action of Ibogaine* (Arch. intern. pharmacodynamie, G3: 27–39, 1939), *Two Physiological Properties Common to Ibogaine and Ephedrine* (Ibid. 134: 541–4, 1940), *Difference Between Physiological Action of Ibogaine and That of Cocaine* (Ibid. 211: 285–8, 1940), *Mediate and Intermediate Effects of Ibogaine on the Intestine* (Compt. rend. soc. biol. 135: 176–79, 1941), *Pharmacologic Antagonism of Ibogaine* (Compt. rend. 212: 768–771, 1941), *Some Color Reactions of Ibogaine* (Bull. soc. chem. biol., 25: 205–10, 1943), *Sympathicosthenic Actions of Ibogaine on the Vessels of the Dog's Paw* (Compt. rend. 223: 757–58, 1946), and *Interpretation of the Ultraviolet Absorption Curves of Ibogaine and Tabernathine* (Ibid. 229: 1359–61, 1949).

D. Vincent began his work on Ibogaine by a collaboration with I. Sero: *Inhibiting Action of Tabernathe Iboga on Serum Cholinesterase* (Compt. rend. Soc. Biol. 136: 612–14, 1942).[1] Vincent participated in the publication of five other papers: *The Ultraviolet Absorption Curves*

[1] This effect may be a key the to "behavioral immobility" often experienced during the first 3–4 hours of treatment.

of Ibogaine and Tabernathine (B. Brustier, D. Vincent and I. Sero, Compt. rend. 216, 909–11, 1943), *Detection of Cholinesterase Inhibiting Alkaloids* (D. Vincent and Paul Beaujard, *Ann. pharm. franc.* 3: 22–26, 1945), *The Cholinesterase of the Pancreas: Its Behavior in the Presence of Some Inhibitors in Comparison with the Cholinesterases of Serum and Brain* (D. Vincent and P. Lagreu, *Bull. soc. chem. biol.* 31: 1043–45, 1949); and two papers, which he and Raymond-Hamet worked on together: *Action of Some Sympathicosthenic Alkaloids on the Cholinesterases* (*Compt. rend. soc. biol.* 150: 1384–1386, 1956) and *On Some Pharmacological Effects of Three Alkaloids of Tabernathe Iboga: Ibogamine, Iboluteine and Tabernathine* (*Compt. rend. soc. biol.* 154: 2223–2227, 1960).

The structure of Ibogaine was investigated by Dickel et. al. (J.A.C.S. 80, 123, 1958). The first total synthesis was cited by Buchi et al. (J.A.C.S. 87, 2073, 1965 and J.A.C.S. 88, 3099, 1966).

In 1956 Salmoiraghi and Page elucidated Ibogaine's relations to serotonin (*J. Pharm. I. expt. ther.* 120(1) 20–25, 1957–9). About the same time J.A. Schneider published three important papers. The first, *Potentiation of Ibogaine on Morphine Analgesia,* was done in collaboration with Marie McArthur (*Experientia* 12: 323–324, 1956).[1] The second was *Neuropharmacological Studies of Ibogaine: An indole alkaloid with Central-Stimulant Properties* (Schneider, J.A. and Sigg. E.B., *Annals of the NY Academy of Sciences,* Vol. 66, 765–776, 1957) and third was *An Analysis of the Cardiovascular Action of Ibogaine HCI* (J.A. Schneider and R.K. Rinhard, *Arch. int. pharmcodyn,* 110 92–102, 1957).[2]

Ibogaine's stimulant properties were further investigated by Chen and Bonner in *A Study of Central Nervous System Stimulants* (*J. Pharm. and Expt. Ther.,* 123 (3): 212–215, 1958.[3] Gershon and Lang published *A Psychological Study of Some Indole Alkaloids* (*Arch. intern. pharmacodynamic,* 135: 31–36, 1962).

In 1969, Claudio Naranjo reported on the effects of both Ibogaine and harmine in human subjects in his paper: *Psychotherapeutic Possibilities of New Fantasy-Enhancing Drugs* (*Clinical Toxicology,* 2(2): 209–224, June 1969).

H.I. Dhahir, in his 1971 doctoral thesis, published *A Comparative Study of the Toxicity of Ibogaine and Serotonin* (University Microfilm International 71-25-341, Ann Arbor, Mich.).[4] His paper gives an overview of much of the work accomplished with Ibogaine.

Additional studies of interest include: *The Effects of Some Hallucinogens on Aggressiveness of Mice and Rats* (Kostowski et al., *Pharmacology* 7: 259–263, 1972), *Cerebral Pharmacokinetics of Tremor-Producing Harmala and Iboga Alkaloids* (Zetler et al., *Pharmacology* 7(4): 237–248, 1972), *High Affinity 3H Serotonin Binding to Caudate: Inhibition By Hallucinogens and Serotonergic Drugs* (Whitaker, P. and Seeman, *P., Psychopharmacology* 59: 1–5, 1978 Biochemistry), *Selective Labeling Of Serotonin Receptors by d-(3 H) LSD in Calf Caudate* (*Proc. natl. acad. sci, USA,* Vol. 75, No. 12, 5783–5787, Dec. 1978, *Biochemistry*) and *A Common Mechanism of Lysergic Acid, Indolealkylamine And Phenthylamine Hallucinogens: Serotonergic mediation of Behavioral Effects In Rats* (Sloviter, Robert et al. J Pharm. & Expt. Ther., 214 (2): 231–238, 1980).

While Howard harvested data, Dana was still looking for vindication. On St. Paddy's Day, 1981, a small but real bomb had gone off outside 9 Bleecker in the faces of two bomb squad officers. The *Soho Weekly News,* already gunning for a felony conviction for the firecracker, promptly ran a full page charging that if Beal himself hadn't done it for publicity, he should be locked up anyway as "the leader of a violent cult" — a danger to the community who "attracts violence." They called him *"Jim Jones on Bleecker Street."* The real perpetrators were never caught, although all indications are it was one of two people on the fringes of the *Soho Weekly News* itself.[5] But coming after four days of mass media hysteria about the martyrdom of the two cops (who were not maimed, although one lost part of his eyesight), such character assassination made an impression that long outlasted the trial.

So in the summer of 1981, dead broke, Dana found himself handing John Spacely, ex-publisher of *Punk* magazine, $20 bills for info about the Marcia Resnick/Johnny Thunders/John Belushi connection which Bill Kunstler might be able to use during the firecracker trial. Spacely was making a movie about punks on junk with Lech Kowalski, who'd already chronicled the fall of Sid Vicious in the film *DOA: A Rite of Passage.* Spacely was strung out, and when the junk need was in him, he'd talk freely. Kunstler never used most of Spacely's information, however, because he firmly believed no one should be denounced for their private habits, even to save a client.

But Dana's trial and partial acquittal had so shifted the debate on heroin that by

1 The earliest clue to Ibogaine's unique interaction with opiates.

2 Which showed Ibogaine's temporary cardiovascular stimulant effect is independent of the central nervous system, the first indication that caution should be observed in giving it to people with weak tickers.

3 The first indication Ibogaine is a healant; rats pretreated with Ibogaine recovered from electroshock twice as fast as those treated with saline (i.e., nothing).

4 In which he established that Ibogaine is less toxic than the common neurotransmitter serotonin. No damage upon microscopic examination of brain, liver or kidneys of rats after 30 days of daily adminiustration of 50 mgs/kg.

5 The cops' main suspect was in effect part-owner of Sunset Studios. The Yippies suspected either a Secret Service informant, later arrested in a shootout with the JDL, or a "crank caller from Brooklyn" (see pp. 113–14, and pp. 214–15) who was one of two primary sources for Doug Ireland's "Jonestown on Bleecker Street."

Christmas, when Dana was released from 35 days in prison on Riker's Island — where he wrote much of *The Secret History of the '70s* — Abbie Hoffman was busily publicizing his own benefit for Veritas, a residential program specializing in treatment of heroin addiction. Benefit organizer Jill Seiden had convinced her friend DA Robert Morgenthau that Abbie was such an important counter-culture figurehead that having him publicly affirm that heroin was much more serious than grass, or acid, or even coke, would make a difference to millions of people. Such a difference, in fact, that Abbie's sentence on the 1973 cocaine rap should be reduced. In January, 1982, Dana, Howard, Norma and virtually everyone they knew attended Abbie's first benefit for Veritas.[1] All of a sudden, anti-heroin was hip. And so Abbie Hoffman succeeded in maintaining his radical credibility while securing a substantial reduction in his imprisonment.

[1] Not an especially left-wing group.

Dana's trial also caused *Soho Weekly News* owner Robert Maxwell to check into rumors that his paper had a heroin problem. He discovered a $1.2 million deficit, and folded the *Soho* in 1982. Covering up to the bitter end, one staffer wrote in the *New York Times* Op-Ed that the *Soho Weekly News* had been shut down by a bomb.

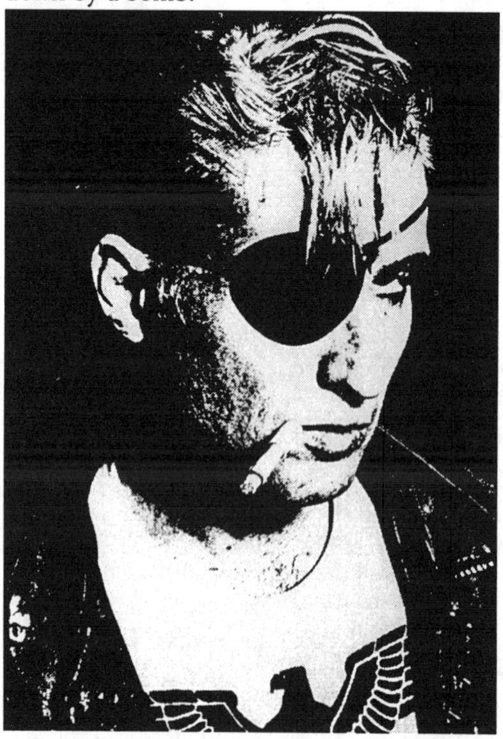

JOHN SPACELY

So Dana was motivated. He kept asking when there would be an Ibogaine story *Overthrow* could publish, and more to the point, when there would be some Ibogaine, since Spacely was only the most prominent of scores who it seemed had become strung-out in the early '80s. Spacely, a former member of the STP family, had no problems with a 36-hour trip, and volunteered repeatedly to do Ibogaine once the shooting on his movie, *Gringo,* was finished.

But Howard's experiences had led him to a somewhat different set of conclusions. Most important — he realized the goal was not to treat a few hundred addicts, underground, only to be shut down again by the DEA. His goal was to make Ibogaine a viable alternative, and treat millions. He had to get patents, which could be challenged if any premature leaks in the press undermined his claims of originality. Fortunately, when Dana tried to pull an end-run in May of '83 by getting a mention in *High Times,* now staffed with ex-*Soho*-ites, Dean Latimer was unsympathetic. His response: "Why would anyone want to quit drugs?"

High Times was interviewing representatives of the British, French and German marijuana movements, assembled for the '83 World Cannabis March on the UN on the first Saturday of May — the first US appearance of the original hemp proponent, Dr. Hans-Georg Behr, author of *Von Hanf Ist Die Rede.* But Latimer was unwilling to run anything new on the US movement, either Ibogaine or the pioneering work of Boston's "Doc" Humes, whose Unidentified Flying Idea was successfully using black hash for heroin detox, in conjunction with acupressure massage at 45-minute intervals. Harold Humes' views on the historic clash of Persian enlightenment and Babylonian obscurantism never got the exposure to the *High Times* audience they probably deserved.[2]

[2] See Dr. Harold Humes, *The City,* et al. Humes also started *The Paris Review,* with George Plimpton and others.

That year Howard informed Dana he was resigning as producer of the annual May Central Park Rock Against Racism Concert to work full-time on Ibogaine. "With RAR, it's fight the same battle every year. Your problem is that the Black and Jewish groups don't *want* to work together," he told Dana (who never again found anyone as competent to put on the concert). "I'd rather be a healer." Howard continued. "I want to do something permanent."

Howard and Norma did come in for the publication party of *Blacklisted News,* held on the fifth anniversary of Tom Forçade's wake. Jill Seiden had booked it at the Limelight, a new club which was supposed to be scandalous because it was in a de-consecrated church. Everyone was there, including John Spacely, who informed Dana he'd run out of patience waiting for the Ibogaine, and quit the old-fashioned way, cold turkey. Outside, a severe culture clash erupted between doormen and Yippies who didn't meet the dress code. Mitch "the Bitch" Blotter, sometimes of David Peel's band,[1] and several others were arrested before Ben Zippie came out and stopped everything by stripping naked.

Meanwhile, inside the church, Howard Lotsof was engrossed with Hans-Georg Behr, himself a psychiatrist/addictionologist, swapping the most advanced secrets of the US and German undergrounds — the secret of Ibogaine for hemp information. Georg, who was back in the US trying to find a publisher, never succeeded in getting his book out in English. Instead, a summary prepared the next year for another publisher and several thousand dollars worth of research were turned over to Jack Herer of the California Marijuana Initiative to use to bring out a White Paper.

But Hans-Georg stayed at 9 Bleecker for another month and a half, sharing reminiscences with Les Ledbetter, who was in the process of quitting the *New York Times* after being found with two joints in his locker. This was unfair, since Les was being fired for the very credentials which got him hired in the first place, including being a White House page at age 18, in which capacity Les procured pot for John Kennedy, who used it medicinally for back pain.[2] Later, at the height of the Vietnam war protests, Les was hired by the *Times* because they had no one inside the counter-culture. Les soon became part of Forçade's Capitol Hill "Underground Press Syndicate" network, around the time Tom pied the US Commissioner of Pornography. In twelve years, Les graduated from the youth beat to edit the night edition, until *Times* security illegally searched his locker.

Ironically, Les died less than two years later, carried off by a flu because years of alcohol and cocaine (which he would do in the wee hours, after getting off work as night editor) had left him with only seven per cent of his liver. A victim of *cocaethylene* poisoning,[3] busted for trying to use something less toxic, Les edited *Overthrow* for a couple of issues with Georg's friend Tom Todd, who hung around after Georg left.

Behr went back to Germany a few weeks after the 1983 NORML Formal,[4] where he met Eric Sterling, staffer to U.S. Congressman Robert Drinan, who was about to be reassigned to the House Judiciary Committee. Eric was able to arrange for Georg to "testify"

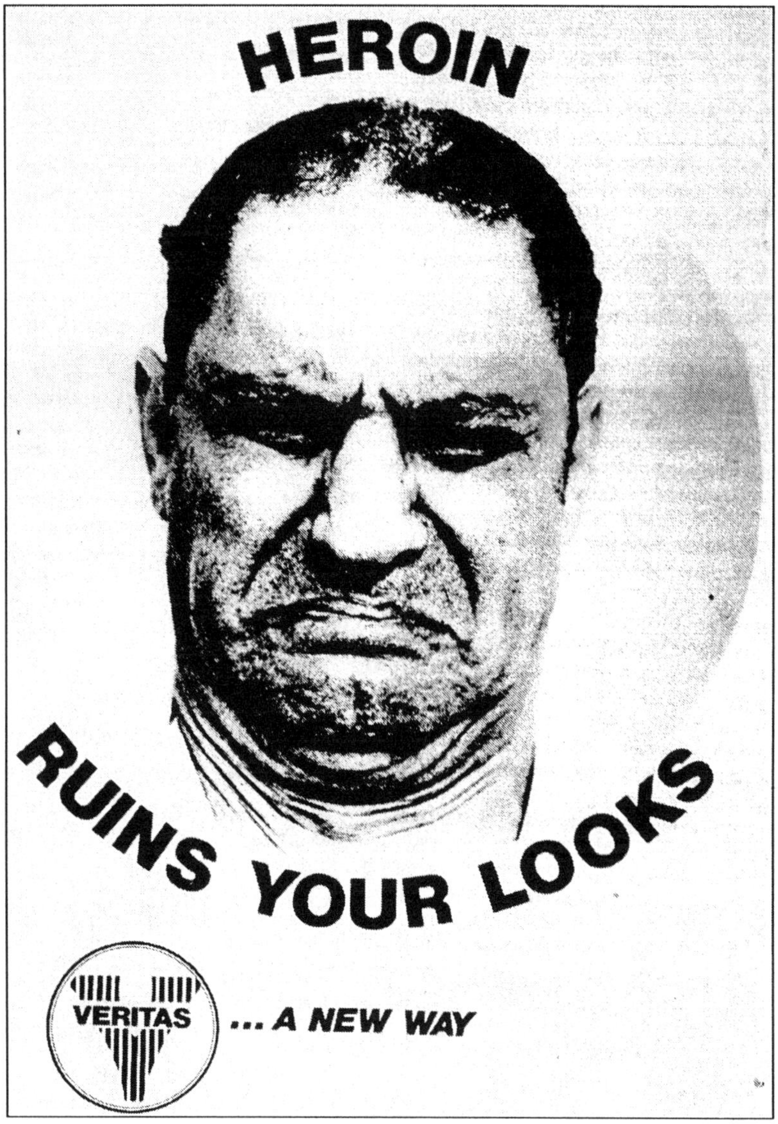

MODEL ABBIE HOFFMAN POSES FOR VERITAS POSTER

1 David Peel, one-time confidant of John Lennon, is universally known in the marijuana subculture due to the album *Hava Marijuana* and the song "The Pope Smokes Dope."

2 Les insisted that he wrote "I Was J.F.K.'s Dealer," which appears in *The Best of High Times.*

3 See the beginning of Chapter 12, on discovery by Deborah Mash, p. 113.

4 The annual NORML national conference.

about the Dutch system of separating cannabis and hard drugs — but only to two staffers, one of whom only came to denounce the Greens *à La*rouche.

By the end of 1983, Howard Lotsof realized he needed help from real professionals. He made the first of many approaches to the National Institute on Drug Abuse (NIDA), where he found that this part of the government, at least, was not about to shut him down. They just wouldn't take him seriously. The '60s hysteria about psychedelics might be a fading memory, but everyone at NIDA immediately pigeon-holed Lotsof's account of a twenty-year old Ibogaine experiment with the LSD claims of Tim Leary. And despite Leary's original record of success treating prison recidivism, or Richard Yensen's LSD work in the '70s confirming efficacy against alcoholism, the tide was running strongly against anything "liberal," and NIDA-crats could fall back on the fact that the risk/benefit ratio with LSD had already been reckoned unacceptable by a higher authority — the U.S. Congress.

No one was paying any attention to Lotsof's real point: that the interruption of addiction was due to a distinct pharmacologic effect of the Ibogaine itself, and not interaction with a good therapist — as with LSD. But when he was reviewing the opiate literature, he'd come across a paper by Dr. Doris Clouet, who had reviewed 256 other medical projects relating to opiates, and classified and catalogued them. Howard ended up giving her a grant to study his data and explain it to him. For a number of years other NIDA researchers laughed at her behind her back. They called Ibogaine "Clouet's folly."

In her report to Howard in 1984, Clouet stated:

> "I am not certain...that one should expect or wish that Ibogaine should act like an opiate."

And:

> "I will discuss some of my thinking about possible mechanisms of action... I am not adverse to positive clinical studies...with certain precautions concerning Ibogaine toxicity, especially in "at risk" groups, clinical settings, double-blind tests, etc. because your invention is a new approach to the treatment of addiction...
>
> "There is no data on toxicity in man... There is no information on the setting in which the trials took place and no information on the presence of a physician at the trials. The data probably does not exist in part because interest in the mechanisms of action underlying hallucinogenic action has been desultory. Therefore, it is not possible... to make any definitive statement about the relationship between the opiates and [Ibogaine]. It should be mentioned that many therapeutic successes arise empirically and not as the result of a well-defined research program."

Subsequently Clouet confirmed the fact that Ibogaine abolishes *tonic extensor seizure* (rigidity of the muscles, as during withdrawal [see Chen, Bonner[1]]); that it inhibits intestinal contractions; and that it's a nor-adrenalin antagonist — all were specific mechanisms that might interfere with withdrawal.

To get Ibogaine to addicts, in 1983 Howard and Norma had begun setting up a charity, the Dora Weiner Foundation. Lotsof named the foundation after his grandmother and put Norma in charge of fundraising. But when she went looking for funding for Ibogaine research, the response was even more dismal than the one at NIDA. They were up against "Just Say No!"

"Ninety percent of the anti-drug abuse foundations were only interested in education," says Lotsof.

"When it comes to solving addiction, I found no sympathy for any disease people think is self-induced," Norma recalls. "The reaction was: 'Oh, you're addicted — serves you right, suffer!' That's what they said."

Even if the eventual harvest of ignoring Ibogaine was more death and addiction, rehabilitation of an obscure illicit drug didn't square with the strategy of intolerance that was afoot in the land.

[It was also some time in mid-1983 that Dana remembers his upstairs roommate Mitch Halberstadt coming in fuming about new reports of a 'Gay-Linked Immune-Deficiency Disease': "It's blatant homophobia!" said Halberstadt. "They're saying that just being gay causes a fatal disease."

Mitch was a member of Gay–Lesbian Anti-Discrimination (GLAD); in the late '70s, 9 Bleecker functioned for a couple of years as a back office in putting on annual Gay Pride

[1] Chen, Bonner, in the text of Lotsof's first patent. See p. 47.

Day. Many of the kids whom Dana tried and failed to keep from turning on to heroin at Studio 10 were bisexual or gay. He ran into them again later in ACT UP.]

The Dora Weiner Foundation managed in just under two years of activity to accrue $4,000. Howard continued to be dependent on handouts from friends and supporters in the movement. But he did get one thing: On February 12, 1985, the U.S. Patent Office granted him patent protection for the use of Ibogaine to interrupt narcotic dependency.

Described as "an improved method for interrupting the physiological and psychological aspects of the heroin addiction syndrome," Howard's invention was said to consist in "its high degree of success, the absence of great pain or discomfort accompanying earlier treatments, the ease and convenience of application, the absence of undesirable or persistent side effects and the persistent effectiveness of the treatment." It was "based on the discovery... that Ibogaine hydrochloride and other non-toxic salts of Ibogaine, possess the unexpected unique ability to disrupt... all the symptomology demonstrated by addicts in their use of and search for heroin."

The patent covered the method of treating heroin addiction via oral administration of between 6 mg./kg. and 19 mg./kg. body weight, or between 400 and 1,000 milligrams, either once or more than once, but with successive doses being separated by a number of days. In other words, the claim was that it wasn't a maintenance drug.

Howard was ecstatic when he heard his patent had been reported in the *New York Times.* Imagine his distress when he learned that the *Times* patent reporter, a genial drunk, had gotten it wrong, and said the ENDABUSE procedure involved intravenous administration — a method that is ten times more toxic than the proper oral route Lotsof uses.

Howard quickly followed up on this by filing for U.S. Patent #4,587,243, for the rapid interruption of cocaine and amphetamine abuse syndromes. And he did one thing more: He furnished an excellent story to *Overthrow.* In the fall of '85 the paper published a world scoop, information known to YIP's inner core but only the inner core until that time. Ibogaine, a psychedelic drug from the African rainforest, had been secretly developed by the movement as a miracle cure for hard drugs.

Now Lotsof was in a position to approach major drug companies. But when he and Norma approached Dupont, Eli Lilly and CIBA–GEIGY, once again they were met with crashing indifference.

"While the indication for narcotic addiction withdrawal is almost certainly worthwhile, it has not been identified as a strategic commitment for our company," wrote Gerald F. Sieschio, licensing manager of CIBA, which held a patent for Ibogaine as a "tonic stimulant" ("Lambarene") up until 1970. They were so uninterested, in fact, that they turned over all their files (the equivalent of a million dollars in research) to Lotsof, gratis. That's how he got the Isbell letter.

That same year Du Pont's associate diretor of product licensing, Hermann S. Weissman, told Lotsof, "Our Research and Marketing groups have come to the conclusion that Ibogaine does not fall within the priorities of our developmental pharmaceutical program."

Lotsof learned the majors had no interest in developing a natural alkaloid they could not call their own. "The type of patent protection the pharmaceutical companies prefer is one in which they actually own the molecule," he says.

> "Our patent protection is use protection — we own the rights to use Ibogaine pursuant to drug dependency. They could earn a million dollars distributing it but their board of directors would say, 'What's a million dollars to us?' That's why our company has its own special niche.
>
> "The second reason they're not interested is the stigma of drug dependency, and I'll give you an example: clonidine. A group of researchers at Yale discovered that clonidine, an anti-hypertensive, was useful in ameliorating withdrawal. They got a patent for that use, and Boehringer-Ingleheim, which was the initiator of clonidine, bought up that patent and sat on it. The last thing they wanted was for the middle-class hypertensive to walk into the pharmacy with a clonidine script and be pegged as an addict. They don't consider that profitable.
>
> "The third reason is that Ibogaine is a Schedule I Drug. It takes three to six months for the paperwork to clear the DEA just to move it around the country."

The big drug companies were not interested, but Howard had one more move before he started his own company. He called the Director of Clinical Research at NIDA, Barry Brown, who gave him introductions to Herb Kleber, Richard Resnick and Arnold Washton — all prominent drug researchers. He managed to get several of them to serve on his foundation's advisory board: Doctors Kleber, Resnick (one of the developers of naltrexone), and Robert Milman (director of the Substance Abuse Unit at New York Hospital).

Next Howard contacted various persons within the government: Charles Rangel, Chairman of the House Select Committee on Narcotics; Nancy Reagan, Alphonse D'Amato, Guy Molinari, Mario Cuomo and Ed Koch. Rangel was the first to respond, asking NIDA Director William Pollin to evaluate the procedure. Howard followed this up with a letter asking Pollin *how* he intended to evaluate it, and if he had the money to do so.

Pollin's reply cited Doris Clouet's conclusion that there was no evidence in the existing literature that Ibogaine could act as a substitute narcotic — missing her point that this wouldn't be desirable in an addiction interrupter anyway.

"She further expresses concern about toxicity. She refers specifically to changes in blood pressure, but we would in addition worry about longer term neurological and psychological effects, including the potential for Ibogaine like other hallucinogens becoming a drug of abuse...."

"Perceptual problems, visual hallucinations, motor difficulties..." suggested to Dr. Pollin a "potential for brain damage."

In his next letter Pollin mentioned the need for FDA approval and sufficient funding to carry out the research, suggesting that Lotsof submit an application for a grant from NIDA. Lotsof replied that in designing an investigational new drug application (IND) for the FDA, he'd come across data "relating to the 'potential for brain damage'" in Dhahir's 1971 paper: "No brain damage was evident after thirty-day chronic studies at fifty milligrams per kilogram day. The average dose for our protocol is about *nine* per kilogram day in a single-administration treatment."

What Howard did next was to write to Rangel and say, "Look, I've got Herb Kleber, Richard Resnick and Robert Milman, the top people in the field, ready to evaluate this."

When he sent copies of all this correspondence to Kleber, Milman and Resnick, they resigned. They resigned because he was using

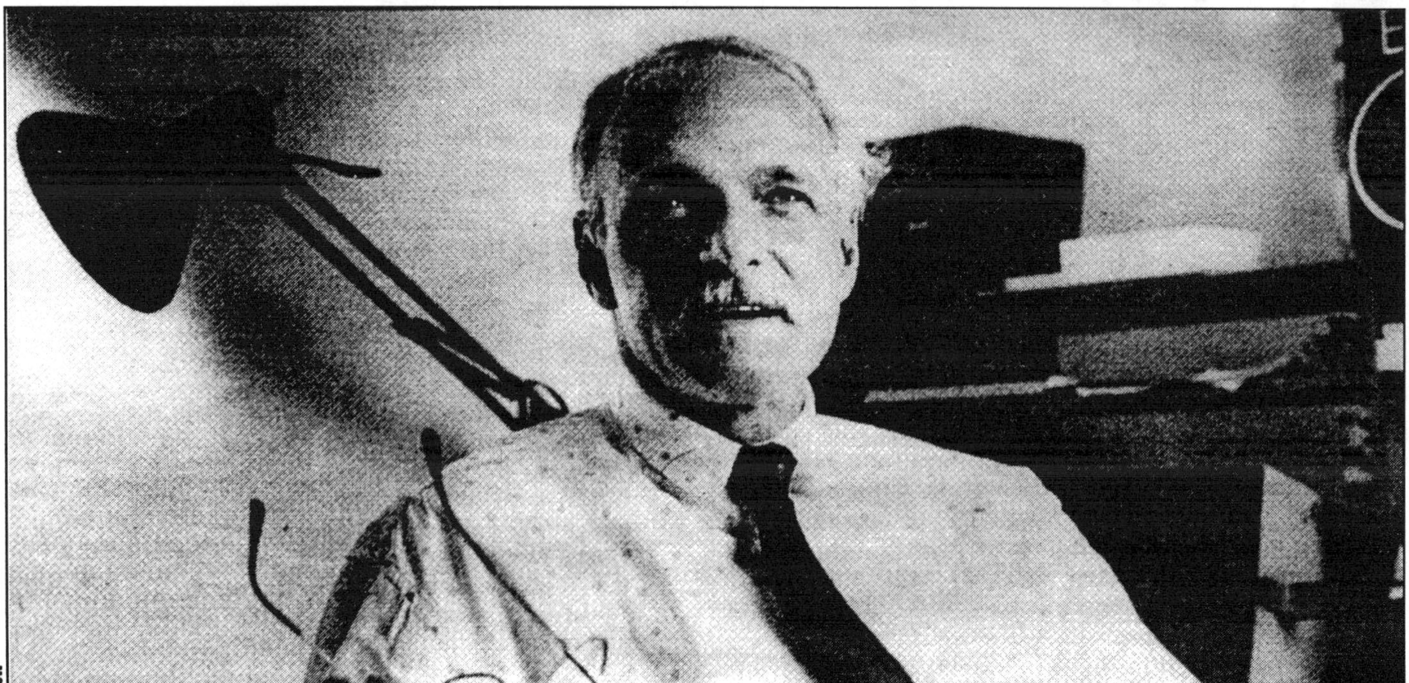

Overthrow

HOWARD LOTSOF

them not for research, but *to attract money* to do research.

"He said money was not an issue," Kleber recalled. (And Howard truly believed money would not be an issue, once he made his case.) "Then I got calls from across the country. Howard was using my name to raise money to do this research." Kleber was interested in keeping tabs on Ibogaine, but all three experts wanted $110 an hour apiece just to meet — $2,000-a-day, which Howard didn't have. And when the advisory board names were used in a letter to Rangel to get that funding from Congress, Kleber, Resnick and Milman all resigned from the board. Kleber told Howard he'd crossed the line by using the names "pro-actively," i.e., in a way that undermined his reputation for scientific objectivity.

Howard wondered what the hell an advisory board is good for if you can't put it on the letterhead of your foundation. But Herb Kleber had mixed motives. He was working closely with Yale University psychiatrist Dr. Thomas R. Kosten, who has called Ibogaine "snake oil! It works for everything — nothing works like that."

They were deep into preliminary studies on their own drug, buprenorphine, an opiate "agonist/antagonist" that seemed to show promise as a treatment for crack. That promise didn't hold up in subsequent studies, unlike Ibogaine, which does work for crack (a big problem in '86), and (unlike buprenorphine) is not a maintenance drug. Buprenorphine is somewhat useful as a maintenance, or as a detox, for opiates (withdrawal is mild compared to methadone). But since, psychoactively speaking, the only failing buprenorphine might have is that some junkies find it so euphoric they actually *prefer it* to heroin,[1] it seemed a much safer bet to pass the regulatory hurdles than Ibogaine — even if it didn't ultimately work out. And if Ibogaine worked, it would make buprenorphine obsolete before it got off the ground. Millions of dollars in research grants might be jeoparized!

"My issue is not with Ibogaine but with Howard Lotsof," says Kleber, who later became Bush's Deputy Drug Czar for Demand Reduction, his treatment expert. "I don't want to tar a chemical with the personality of the person pushing it."

Today, buprenorphine is near completion of Phase III trials — the last stage before approval. The Medications Development Division of NIDA didn't really start evaluating Ibogaine until Kleber was on his way out of the White House New Executive Office Building Annex to his current job — heading up the Substance Abuse Division at Columbia University.

1 See *Scottish Journal of Addiction Medicine.*

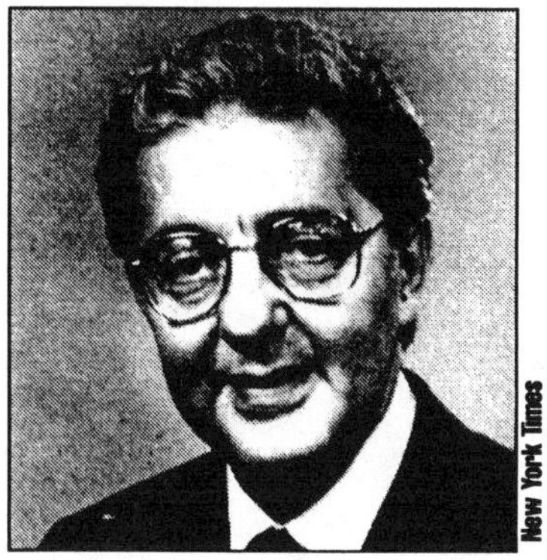

Dr. Herbert Kleber

CHAPTER 6: Bob Sisko

Before their falling out, Kleber did introduce Lotsof to Louis Harris, a very prominent biochemist in the opiate field. Harris maintained colonies of addicted animals at the Medical College of Virginia. He and Mario Aceto started designing studies to test Ibogaine on those animals. Harris told Lotsof about another person he should check with. Arthur Jacobson, at the National Institute of Mental Health's Committee on Problems of Drug Dependency (CCPD) was willing to run and pay for additional studies on any potential for abuse with Ibogaine.

One bit of information Howard did get from Pollin was that the Director of the Addiction Research Center, Jerome Jaffe, was interested. Jaffe was about to replace Pollin as head of NIDA. Howard called him, and he put Howard in touch with Dr. Robert Lange. Lange introduced him to a chemical company. He also put him in contact with a lab in Massachusetts competent to do FDA work that agreed to design and budget studies. But he was still $50,000 short of the money it would take to produce and refine the first Ibogaine.

In 1986, Lotsof formed NDA International and with a small band of friends, lawyers and investors, secured the worldwide use patents for Ibogaine. The second patent (#4,587,243) — for coke and amphetamine — came through May 6th. Three months later, as if to punctuate the urgency of the situation, Mitch Blotter of the Blotter brothers OD'd in one of the new squats on East 8th St. He was celebrating a settlement from the city for his illegal arrest at the Limelight three years earlier. Mitch was not a junkie, just another casualty of the idea that heroin is okay as a rare treat. To stop OD's and fires, the squatter movement banned hard drugs, but that was hard to enforce. Support for Ibogaine seemed logical.

Howard's first important investor was Leo Zeff. One of the Grand Old Men of Ibogaine, Dr. Zeff had given Iboga alkaloid compounds to more than 500 of his psychiatric patients when psychedelic research was still respectable. The famed Chilean psychiatrist Claudio Naranjo, who is much better known because he published *The Healing Journey* in the late '60s, was Zeff's protege. When Lotsof contacted Zeff in Los Angeles, Zeff was transfixed by Howard's explanation of Ibogaine's effect as an addiction interrupter. He immediately reviewed all his files, and came up with only three who'd had substance abuse problems.

"They all quit drugs!" he said, when he got back to Howard, "but there were only three who were drug abusers, so I never noticed. When it worked, you see, the Ibogaine always transformed the patient completely."

"What do you mean?" asked Howard. "What were the effects?"

"With Ibogaine, we got the most wonderful effects." Zeff immediately withdrew $25,000 from his life savings and invested it in the company. Howard took the money and sponsored the first international Ibogaine symposium in Paris on January 6, 1987. He brought together the twelve foremost experts in the world, including Zeff, Robert Goutarel, Otto Göllnhofer, H. Deportere, and William Gladstone.

"The common denominator is Iboga," explained Professor Otto Göllnhofer in his opening remarks, placing Lotsof's discovery in perspective: "If we have cancer and AIDS against which we are struggling, another of the evils of our era is 'drugs,' which may have more victims than any other. The stakes are enormously high."

Lotsof addressed the conferees, giving a detailed account of Ibogaine effects at the therapeutic dose before patients finally fall asleep. Upon awaking, Lotsof explained, "patients… no longer possess the desire to use cocaine or other drugs."

The experts, skeptical of this claim, began to grill Lotsof, probing and challenging. The onslaught began when Goutarel, honorary director of the French National Center for Scientific Research (CNRS), asked, "If the pateint is cured, why do you have to repeat the treatment six months later?"

"The effects of the treatment are not permanent," Lotsof responded.

Goutarel fired back, "What is the status of the patient when he leaves the hospital?"

"Completely drug free." Lotsof went on to explain that Ibogaine's effects are only temporary, and the same drives and forces that lead patients to use drugs in the first instance gradually return. Under fire, Lotsof was cool and professional, displaying knowledge and expertise on a par with, if not greater than, many of those present.

Professor Portier, Director of the Natural Substance Division of the CNRS, quizzed Lotsof like a headmaster would a sophomore: "Can you define what you mean by 'anxiety'?"

"I define anxiety in these terms: an increased adrenergic activity which begins to create a state of discomfort in the patient." As the probing continued, Lotsof passed each test put to him, winning the respect and acceptance of those present. As a peer, he had been put through a sort of scientific 'rite of passage.' Acknowledged as an expert by the experts, Lotsof sat down and shared his insights and experiences of 25 years with Ibogaine.

The upshot was a call for an international research initiative. "We must put forth all of the information we have on the subject from every field," said Professor Göllnhofer, calling for the creation of an interdisciplinary team to conduct Iboga research.

Among the attendees was Dr. Peter Baumann, a Swiss psychiatrist from Zurich. Baumann had been influenced by Naranjo, and Naranjo's whole approach to Ibogaine grew out of his experience with harmaline, which is like a stripped-down Iboga molecule.[1] To get his patients to verbalize — they tended to withdraw and even doze on harmaline — Naranjo customarily administered it with amphetamines, a practice he extended to Ibogaine. Hence his descriptions of Ibogaine as "engendering unique rage." [Quips Howard: "Patients on Ibogaine and speed, mad as Hell, because he was trying to distract them from their visualizations in order to grill them about what they were seeing!"]

All of the other experts present blamed the "unique rage" phenomenon on Naranjo's technique. And they were all being deferential to Zeff, who had given Ibogaine to many more people than Baumann,[2] who was somewhat in the minority in feeling psychiatric intervention during the actual Ibogaine experience was the key to successful therapy, as with LSD.

"That was not my experience," said Zeff. "Of everything we tried, Ibogaine achieved the most profound personal transformation of the patient — which after all is the goal and purpose of psychiatry. When it worked, the therapist was just a bystander."

Baumann berated him. "What do you know, old

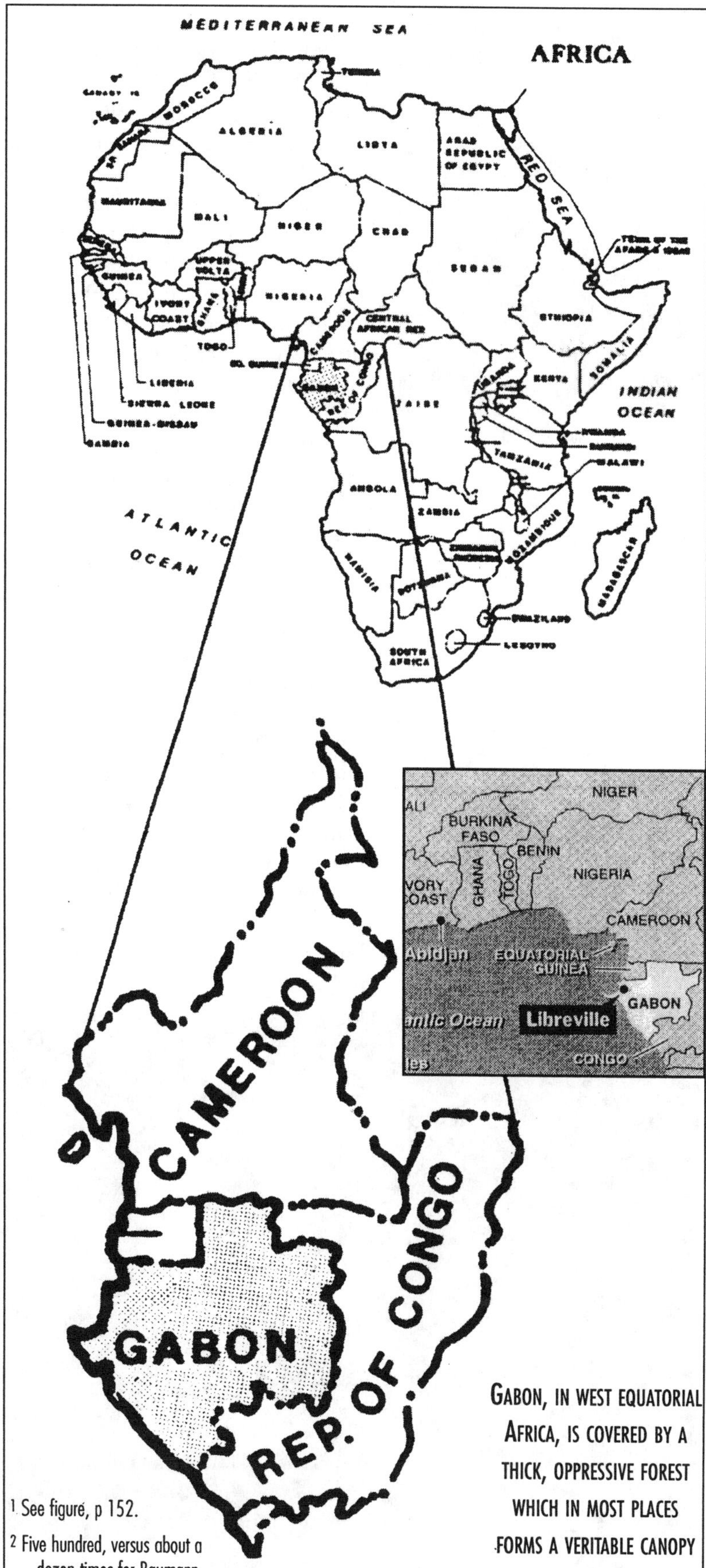

1 See figure, p 152.

2 Five hundred, versus about a dozen times for Baumann.

Gabon, in West Equatorial Africa, is covered by a thick, oppressive forest which in most places forms a veritable canopy of vegetation.

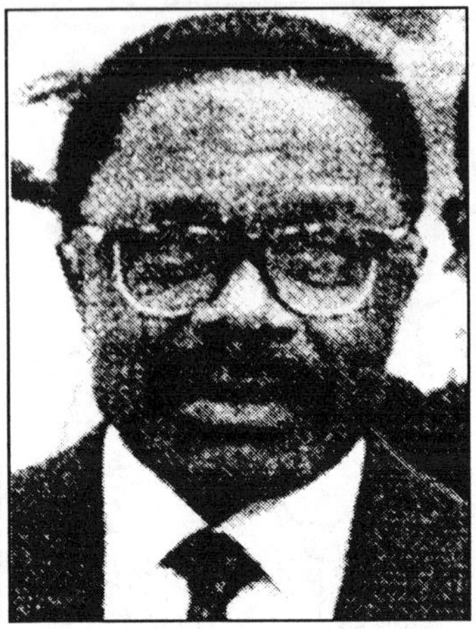

New York Times

OMAR BONGO

man. I was Claudio Naranjo's protegé."

"Ah yes, Naranjo. He was a student of mine." Everyone present was embarrassed by Baumann's attempt to humiliate the older man.

[Baumann, however, nursed a grudge, and in 1990 blamed Ibogaine for the death of one of his patients, during a group therapy session at his villa in France, where his Swiss license was not valid. It may well have been caused by Baumann's intrusive badgering technique. The patient had a weak heart; but death was inconsistent with Ibogaine overdose — it occurred not at onset but four hours after administration, when it should have begun to wear off, and only 400 mg. were given. Baumann, however, was mostly interested in "clearing" his drug of preference, MDMA, several doses of which turned up missing in the ensuing investigation. Swiss regulatory authorities and the French medical examiner refused to release full autopsy results for many years. But Howard had long since informed all of his collaborators, world wide, and established a procedure for administration of an antidote.]

From Paris, Howard and Norma flew to Libréville, Gabon, accompanied by Bob Sisko and their translator Bill Gladstone. The four of them met with President Omar Bongo and his science adviser, Dr. Jean-Noel Gassitta, who spent two weeks probing Howard's sincerity. In Gabon, *Tabernathe iboga,* the plant of which Ibogaine is the main alkaloid, is the sacrament of the national religion, Bwiti. Once in a lifetime, most often at puberty, initiates are given enough of the bark of the plant's roots to "split the head" and induce the four to five hours of visualizations necessary to "meet their ancestors." Possibly they may "meet the Bwiti," a kind of universal African ancestor "between man and angel" equivalent in their religion to the Holy Spirit in Christianity.

Both Omar Bongo and his predecessor Leon M'ba, the father of Gabonese independence, were Bwiti. Their sacrament was persecuted by French Catholic (Dominican) colonial authorities. Gabonese are extremely sensitive about being bamboozled by Western druggies and the adverse international regulatory consequences that might ensue from bad press. Export of the root to the outside world is embargoed.

And here was Howard, asking for supplies:

> "Your Excellency, America and all the 'advanced' countries are in the grip of a terrible epidemic of addiction. Many of the victims in my country are African-Americans — kidnapped perhaps from this very land. But we believe the antidote exists, here in the sheltering rain forest. We believe the anti-toxin for this terrible plague is iboga, the plant which heals the spirit. We implore you to release emergency medical research supplies of iboga, so that testing can begin to demonstrate to our Food and Drug Administration that iboga is safe —"

"I know iboga is safe," replied President Bongo. "I myself have eaten *iboga.*"

Howard looked him in the eye and said: "I too have eaten *iboga,* and I know it is safe."

President Bongo's jaw dropped. Howard was an initiate! The President agreed to release forty kilos of root bark to NDA. He said: "This will be Gabon's gift to America." He thought a minute. The irony of the so-called Advanced World coming asking for technical assistance was palpable. President Bongo said: "This will be Gabon's gift to the world."

He flew them in his private plane to Ombway, south of the Equator, where they were personal guests of the Binkt Maktar and other parliamentary notables. Dr. Jean-Noel Gassita took them into the densest forest, to see the giant 35-foot *iboga* trees, which no westerner had seen for sixty years. In the village, they also saw it under cultivation, and were presented with seeds, which did not, unfortunately, germinate later when supplied to a botanical garden.

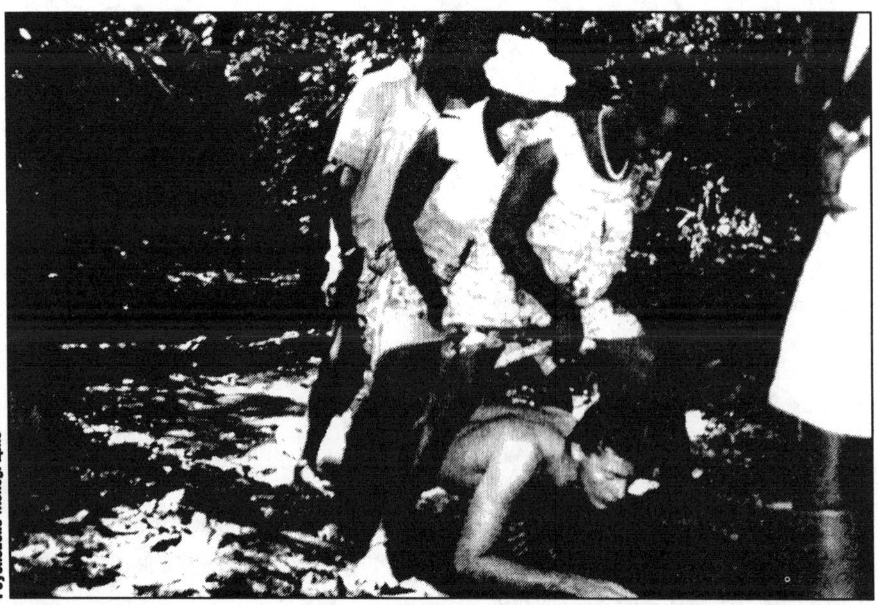

Psychedelic Monographs

WESTERNER IS INITIATED INTO CHAPEL

Viewing the old videotape of the trip you can see that Howard and Norma's travelling companion, Bob Sisko, is not his current self. He's almost skeletal. He was *de facto* the addict representative on the trip, since he had a bad coke habit. He would be the first person treated. He would also be the next great architect of Ibogaine development. In the next two to three years, in new human trials involving two dozen addicts, he would replicate and expand Howard Lotsof's original results, with far closer measurements and greater understanding.

Bob Sisko returned to New York City from Woodstock in 1976 when he divorced his wife Pauline. He moved in on the Yippie ground floor (literally, rebuilding the ground floor of 9 Bleecker). He did a stint in D.C. YIP, putting on the Jimmy Carter Counter-Inaugural at the Warner Theatre and recruiting political commissar Alice Torbush into the organization. He drove the bus on the smoke-in tour, and became tight with Howard during the making of *Smoke-In*. He appears in the film with his girlfriend and their horse, introducing the actual footage of the July 4, '77 march and protest — grinning while she talks. Even when he left for a while, he'd be back. [Down in Florida, the same girlfriend stole his horses, and left him.]

In '79–'80, he organized the eighteen months' resistance to the eviction of Studio 10 from the groundfloor of 10 Bleecker St., which became the prototype for a squatter's movement on the Lower East Side. He led CITIZENS AGAINST HEROIN in 1981, producing a White Paper correlating recurrent crackdowns on soft drugs with upsurges in heroin, and characterizing pot as the "thin green line between society and addictive drugs." He did the RAR concerts with Howard, and assisted him somewhat during the early Staten Island Project years.

But during the first half of the '80s, his major human rights focus was the American Clemency Committee. The Clemency Committee helped convince Governor Charles Robb to free Roger Davis, a Black man sentenced in Virginia to forty years for possession of eight ounces of pot. Sisko's celebrated "Clemenaid" concert and postcard campaign forced New York's Governor Mario Cuomo to free Gary McGivern, a convict accused of killing a guard when McGivern was actually handcuffed in the back seat of a police car. Then, after the Clemency Committee went into hiatus, Dana asked him: "Why don't you do more on Ibogaine?"

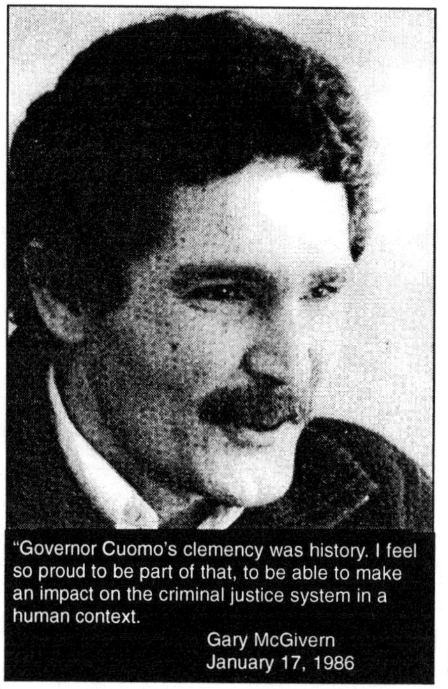
"Governor Cuomo's clemency was history. I feel so proud to be part of that, to be able to make an impact on the criminal justice system in a human context.
Gary McGivern
January 17, 1986
ICASH

GARY MCGIVERN "CLEMENAID" POSTCARD

Sisko, whose new thing was a public relations company in midtown Manhattan, responded by putting together the first corporate package for NDA International. He wrote the first product information. He coined the name for the product: "ENDABUSE."

His PR firm shared space with a Black architect's office housing the defense committee for the "New York 8," Black radicals who were successfully fighting off a police frame-up on weapons charges. Later they organized with Al Sharpton. They were never that keen on Ibogaine, despite its RAR pedigree and African origins. They associated it with YIPPIE marijuana decrim. And its representative, as far as they were concerned, was Sisko. While others on the scene were quitting coke after the '70s, Sisko continued to do it every day. He was also doing in excess of a liter of vodka a day.

Sisko was accompanying Howard to Gabon because his Israeli contacts would be important for running the first experiment in rats to determine efficacy in treating alcohol dependency.[1] By the time they made the trip, though, Sisko was free-basing an eighth of an ounce of coke a day.

The first batch of root bark was bogus — low alkaloid concentrations. The Gabonese had to be massaged into providing a second shipment — the real thing. In the summer of 1987, Omar Bongo visited President Reagan. Unbeknownst to the White House, Lotsof and Sisko also arranged to meet with Bongo during his official stay in Washington, D.C. So circumspect was Bongo's security detail in ushering the Ibogaine representatives upstairs, where Bongo received them in shirtsleeves, that the Secret Service didn't even know they were there. Sisko and Howard were almost detained on the way out by flustered feds, until their status as Omar Bongo's honored guests was confirmed by Gabonese security.

President Bongo arranged to have forty kilos of primo grade *iboga* delivered by diplomatic pouch to his embassy in Ottawa, where

[1] See the beginning of the next chapter, p. 66

it was not illegal, and Howard Lotsof could take possession. From Canada the forty kilos of root bark scrapings moved back to the Centre National du Recherche Scientifique (CNRS) in France, for extraction and reduction into 99.7% Ibogaine hydrochloride, in collaboration with Goutarel and others — the first fruit of the conference in January. Then it had to be shipped back to Canada. The first Ibogaine wasn't ready until December.

Meanwhile, Sisko's business was falling apart.

"Everyone who knew him was afraid that one day we'd call Sisko," says Howard, "and no one would be alive to answer the phone. Or that we'd get the call. And he'd be dead."

Finally, the Ibogaine was ready. Based on Howard's '60s experience, it was decided not to bring it into the United States. Holland, due to its reputation for having the most rational drug policy in Europe, became the site for the first human experiments with Ibogaine in twenty-five years. Bob Sisko arrived in Holland on December 10, 1987, a few days after a friendly U.S. physician.

"I was in the public relations business," he says,

> "and I was surrounded by cocaine — my clients, the people I worked with. They either wanted it, expected it, or they procured it and put it in front of me.
>
> "What I'd do when I'd travel abroad, is I'd buy a couple of Afrin bottles, you know, and I would empty the Afrin out, and pour the cocaine in. I would fill it up with water, and I would shake it up. Being in the public relations business, you have to be cool. But if you're in a meeting with a straight client, you can always reach in your pocket and take out a bottle of nasal spray. Tilt your head back. And nobody knows.
>
> "Before taking Ibogaine, I was sitting around waiting and drinking a great deal, and doing this coke I had in the Afrin bottle, smoking a lot of cigarettes. Finally, the doctor said, 'Yeah, we can do it in the morning,' and then I realized I had only three cigarettes left, and I said, 'This drug — I've been told — takes thirty-six to forty-eight hours. I'll be damned if I'm going to sit here for thirty-six hours without cigarettes.'
>
> "Somebody had to go out for me, in the middle of the night, to get me a pack of Camels. And I took the Ibogaine. And the whole time I didn't smoke. And then I looked up, and I saw the doctor take out a cigarette and light it, and I saw him cough. I saw his body violently react to it, with a tremendous heave-ho. And I said to myself, 'How is it possible that this brilliant man can continue to ingest small amounts of toxin — twenty, thirty times a day — when he knows it to have a cumulative effect?'
>
> "I haven't had a cigarette since that day."

Here was the first new discovery, one quite unexpected. Ibogaine can interrupt nicotine addiction. A few years later US Surgeon General C. Everett Koop got on TV and informed us cigarettes and heroin share a common narcotic receptor. Since most addicts smoke cigarettes, Sisko and Howard realized right away this was a big bonus.

But there was more. In the time before and after their trip to Gabon, they had immersed themselves in literature about the African religious version of the experience. Chapter 18 of James Fernandez's *Bwiti— An Ethnography of the Religious Imagination in Africa*[1] became part of their orientation package for addicts they were treating. Consider Bob's account of his first treatment:

> "Within an hour of taking it, you start to get wobbly, and say, whoa, I have to lay down. And then time passes, and all of a sudden you look up and a movie screen appears [like a "Windows" program]. You find a place, either a wall or a ceiling — and what happens is your subconscious and all of your repressed memories come forth, and you're able to view it in a totally impartial manner. In the same way as if you were viewing a motion picture. It's just like watching TV. And this is the stuff that might normally get released fifteen-to-twenty-minutes a night while you're in REM sleep.
>
> "Then what happens is you go through another stage where you ask questions about what you've experienced, and you come up with answers. And then you go through a third period. You gain access to the information stored in your individual hereditary archive. You meet your ancestors. It was a very spiritual experience for me.
>
> "It is a wonder drug. It's like a re-set button, and it clears and re-sets all the neurotransmitters to operate at maximum efficiency, so that everything becomes crystal clear to you. It's a miracle."

Although he was wary of expressing it for a long time, like many who have the experience, Sisko met the Bwiti — the very avatar of the African religion — a very definite, highly energetic though discorporate entity.

When he saw Howard, though, soon after he got back to New York, they had their first

[1] See Appendix 1, p. 219.

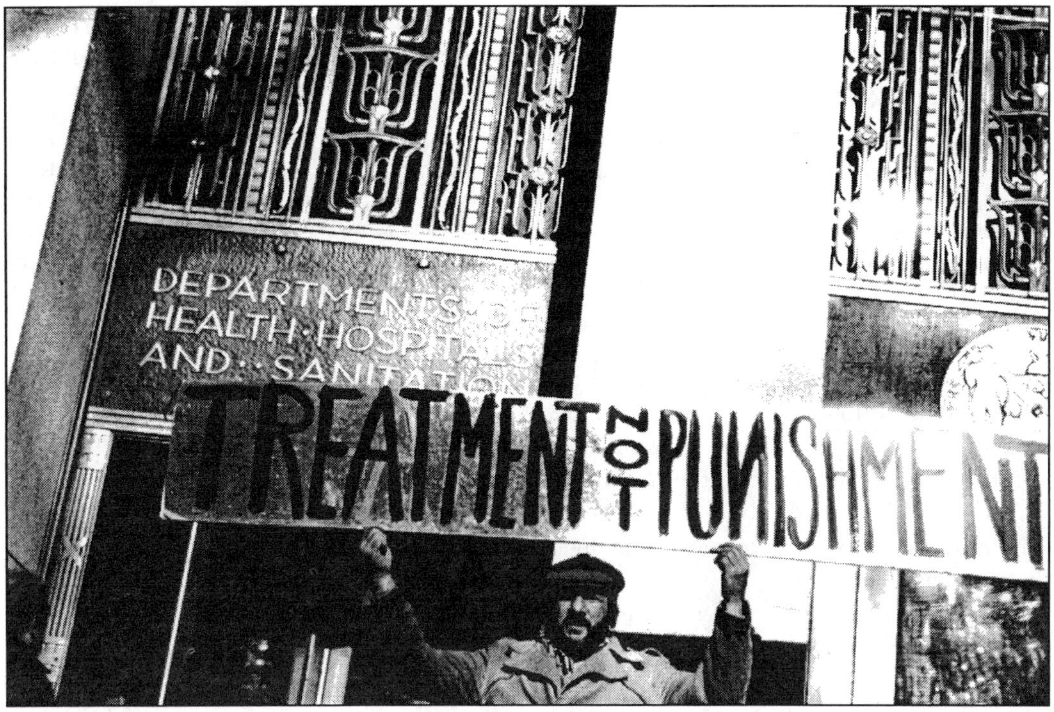

Bob Sisko at Centre Street

big dispute. Sisko told him, "The Ibogaine really works! I never experienced anything like it. We've got to start treating people — real, live addicts — now."

"As president of a corporation engaged in legitimate pharmaceutical development, I can't get NDA involved in anything that would run afoul of the laws or regulations of the U.S. or any other country where we intend to do business," said Howard. "I really sympathize — and I'm interested in sharing your findings. But I can't jeopardize our entire development schedule just to treat a few individuals."

"Howard, people are dying," Sisko objected. "I know dozens of people personally who need Ibogaine. It's not right to withhold it any longer."

The argument raged all winter. By spring relations were icy. It took almost a year, using connections he had established with the head of the Chemistry Department of a large university in Western Africa, for Sisko to get his own Ibogaine.

Among the first to be treated was Fred from New York, a hardcore fiend known to Dana from Studio 10 days. He'd been in and out of jails and Odyssey House since becoming addicted to heroin in 1981. Fred was never a perfect success. But like the patient who can keep his cancer under control with recurrent chemotherapy, Fred's improvement after his first treatment in April 1989 was so visible that Dana, completely startled, stopped paying attention to the parade he was marshalling for ten whole minutes.[1] This was long enough for a rival faction to divert the entire back half of the parade to Central Park from its original target, Congressman Charles Rangel's office at 125th Street in Harlem.

1 The annual Fifth Avenue Pot Parade, held the first Saturday in May.

Dana had started going to ACT UP meetings in early '88 because he thought the whole Dutch harm reduction ("safe drugs") model was essential to stop AIDS; now he got up and plugged Ibogaine at ACT UP meetings. The change in Fred was so dramatic, Dana also decided the time had come for the drug reform movement to give Ibogaine equal priority with legalizing pot or clean needles. He staked all his prestige as founder of the smoke-ins on it, and split the pot movement for three years. Ibogaine prevailed in the end.

Fred even moved into 9 Bleecker. With the re-treatments, he became the most Ibogainized person in the world. And like a scientist puzzling over moon rocks, with each treatment Dana gleaned more data.

"I met Bwiti the first time," said Fred.

"All of a sudden this 300-pound Black Buddha a lot like Fats Domino pops into the room and says "What are you waiting for? Let's go!" He took me on a journey to a pyramid or mountain of light, and on it were arranged a Star of David, a cross, a star and crescent, all the symbols of the religions. But from the top of the mountain, shining through all of them but superior to all of them, was this blinding light. And I recognized it as the light Moses saw through the burning bush."

Five months later, feeling strong pre-addictive anxiety, Fred contacted Howard for a re-treatment. During it, he re-experienced the Holocaust through the eyes of his mother, a survivor of the camps. Later he was able to describe to his uncle, perfectly, the faces of relatives who'd died in the Nazi death camps, whom he had no way of knowing. His uncle started crying.

[How do you know if you're having a true religious experience, and not just crazy? Philip Dick says that if you come into information you have no way of knowing, and it later turns out to be true, then perhaps you have had a genuine revelation (a "theophany," he calls it). The catch, of course, is acting in time on it. Yet if it turns out to be true, the initiate is transposed into realms of freedom — i.e, freedom to act on truth previously unsuspected — realms that would not exist without *iboga*.]

Now of everyone connected with the Project, Sisko's scene overlapped most with the original YIPPIES; he is good friends with YIPPIE founder Bob Fass, for instance. Bob lobbied heavily for the treatment of the wife of his friend Joe the Gentle Giant, a 34-year-old woman named Linda T. He had to lobby, because Linda didn't seem like a good candidate for treatment. "Not only was I a drug addict," she said, "I was an unrepentant one."

> "Everybody kept saying 'oh, you gotta quit drugs! You gotta quit drugs!' And I kept saying 'Yeah, yeah, yeah, yeah,' but I didn't really want to, because — let's face it — I could afford it. I spent $300 a day on my habit — $300! I'd been doing heroin since I was 14 years old. When I wasn't doing it I was taking pills of some sort.
>
> "I didn't think Ibogaine was going to work. The reason why I got it was because I was addicted to Dutch heroin."

Sisko wanted to respond to the Dutch doctors who argued that Ibogaine might work on weak American smack, but not real Dutch quality stuff. But Linda had a job that required her to commute to Holland, so she had learned to smoke it there, in the Dutch manner, on tinfoil.

"From what I know," she continued,

> "the Ibogaine I took was from the Gabon Republic. It looked like a big gelatine capsule. It had this white-silvery powder in it that had been adjusted to my body weight. I just put it in my mouth and took it. There were other people in the room, and in the other room outside, but I preferred to be alone throughout the whole thing. They kept asking me how I felt. My hands were still shaking four days later.
>
> "At seventy minutes, it started hitting me. Then I started getting dizzy. And then I said 'I think I'm going to lay down.' And then I went to my bed and lay down... My eyes... my eyelids... when I closed them, turned into a TV screen. And I'm watching a stage."

She met the Bwiti:

> "I came before the Throne, and his face was a mask with which he gestured 'Yes' and 'No' very emphatically — and he had incredibly deep eyes, so deep I kept thinking they must hurt. He spoke only simple words. He said, *'Go Back!'* At first I thought he meant go back to the beginning of the Ibogaine, which I wanted to do because I was resisting it, but then I understood what he meant when I was jet-propelled back to the beginning of time. And I witnessed the beginning of the earth and how it was formed. Century after century. How it was put together. I saw behind me and past me. I saw from the beginning of time. I had my life handed back to me, here... finish it.
>
> "Immediately after the treatment, my heroin use stopped. It worked immediately. With no heavy withdrawals. Just chills. It changed the way I think — even my personality."

She found her Catholic religious convictions were strengthened; she never again doubted the existence of an afterlife, for example.

> "It totally changed my life. I [didn't] have a habit anymore. I experienced chills, but not bad ones. And I was an experienced drug addict, one that had been through jonesing many times, not always of my own volition. I was still on heroin before I took the Ibogaine. At first, I took the drug, and I thought that I still wanted to get high, what's wrong? And then, you know, as time wore on, and the Ibogaine wore on, it took it out of me — the urge. I had been a junkie for many years, so this, to me was something totally new."

Linda provided dramatic confirmation of Lotsof's original '63 finding, that Ibogaine can interrupt addiction even in people who neither particularly want nor expect it to work: "I sort of took it to appease everyone," she said, "and the fucking drug worked. I couldn't believe it. It worked." For the next six months she remained drug free, and used the money she saved to invest and start a business manufacturing gaming equipment, which she was soon shipping all over to new places that were opening up legal gambling. After six months she notified Sisko she was beginning to feel the urge to use heroin again, and needed re-treatment. She had, on three occasions during the previous thirty days, taken quaaludes. But she'd remained junkfree. Within a month, she was re-treated.

Now Linda was something of a social lion of the Manhattan Bohemian set. She was good friends with the "Pope of Pot" Mickey Cesar, leader of the breakaway a few months earlier from the Parade to Congressman Charles Rangel's office. Linda actually appeared in two videos with Mickey around this time while he was out of jail for a spell. So for anyone in the Pope's retinue to pretend Ibogaine didn't work after that was really a matter of focusing on the relapse and ignoring Linda's business success. She also happened to be a card-playing buddy of Herbert Hunke, the man who turned William Burroughs on to heroin. He's one of the folks who's just as happy as can be on his daily 100 mg. of methadone. But according to Hunke, Ibogaine is the closest thing yet to the cure Burroughs and the beats were looking for in the '50s: "Howard Lotsof found the first thing that actually helps you to quit — if you want to."

In October, 1989, Bob Sisko treated the first Dutch addicts — Ron and Geerte F. of the squatters movement. Geerte — back in Holland after opening up the Umbrella House squat on Avenue C around the corner from Sisko's place on East 3rd Street — had found out about Ibogaine in New York. She was anxious to get a treatment for Ron, her multiply-addicted boyfriend.

Both treatments were a success, even though Geerte tried to resist the Ibogaine's effects.[1] Bob went back to New York, leaving Geerte and Ron enough Ibogaine to treat ten additional Dutch junkies. "At first," she says, "everyone was totally cynical. No one is more cynical than a junkie. But by the end, they were banging on my door, saying, 'Treat us, treat us!' And there wasn't enough Ibogaine. She adds, "Ibogaine is not the solution in itself, although it takes away withdrawal completely. Ibogaine helps you to realize that all power is available to cure yourself through will power."

What first convinced all her junkie friends Ibogaine was for real was that Ron, her boyfriend, was selling his 65 milligram daily dose of methadone, and spending the money, not on coke or smack, but on camping gear for their upcoming trip to Nepal. The powerful purgative action of Ibogaine (prized by the Africans) had flushed the methadone right out of Ron's system.

Ibogaine interrupts *methadone* addiction. In thirty-six hours. Same as heroin. No more two to six months of excruciating withdrawal. This was the second great unexpected finding of Sisko's paraclinical research. It would reverberate powerfully back through the anti-methadone movement, especially the ex-Black Panther acupuncturists.

When Sisko got back from Holland, he was heavily lobbied by Dana and Fred on behalf of Jeff — a friend of Charles Kritsky, who'd known Howard and Sisko since the days his wife Joan set type for *YIPster Times,* circa '77–'78. A big fan of Spinrad and a New York survivor of Forçade's Chaoticist circle, Charlie was a half-German, half-Puerto Rican from the Lower East Side. Most of his childhood friends had become junkies except he and his friend Ric, who just smoked pot and did coke. When they were teenagers, they took four of their buddies up to the country for a detox. After sitting up for 48 hours without sleep trying to help four junkies kick cold turkey, they developed a profound respect for addiction, but were no closer to getting even one of their friends off junk. Once in the city, one by one, they relapsed.

Charles, a zealous student of the Ultimate Chaotic act, had consciously followed the progress of Ibogaine since the late '70s. He was a font of reassurance and support for the project amidst indifference; he tried to use his connections on the club scene to line up publicity and endorsements. Charles needed a treatment for his friend Jeff, a talented interior designer who, in between being on the nod, did little carpentry jobs at the World, a club on East Houston. Charles had a dream that if

[1] See Chapter 11, pp. 101–102.

he could just get Jeff off dope for a litle while, they could turn the cinderblock front of his carriage house on East 5th St. into a store for his rock 'n' roll accessories.

Jeff was an industrious addict, working long hard hours to maintain $80–$100 daily heroin and almost daily cocaine use. Charlie went along for the treatment. But there was only about a gram of Ibogaine for Jeff, who was almost six feet tall and needed more. "He was laying there saying 'Charlie it isn't working'," Charles said later, "But I asked him — so how come you don't get up and go cop?' He couldn't!" Ten hours after taking the Ibogaine, he requested a hot fudge sundae.

Following treatment, Jeff begain to complain bitterly about his back. The symptoms were not related to detox, but rather to a back injury which the detox had unmasked. A work-related injury had gone undiagnosed for sometime, with Jeff in effect self-medicating for a slipped disc.

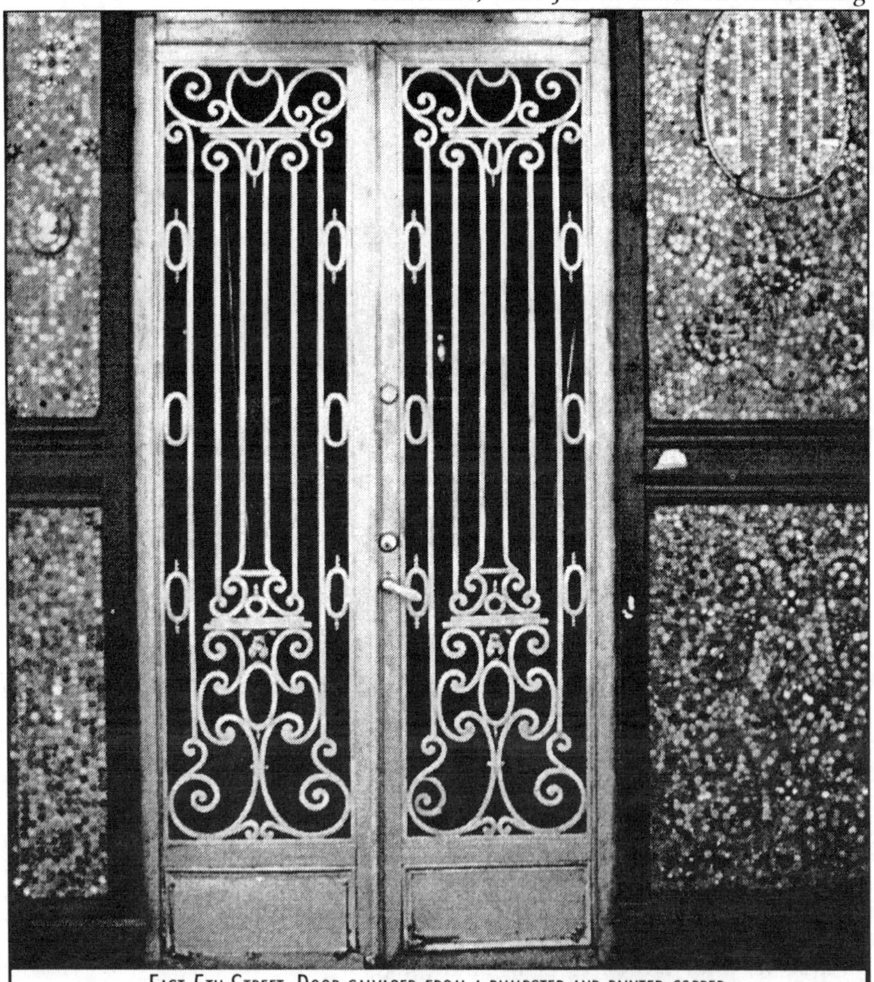

EAST 5TH STREET. DOOR SALVAGED FROM A DUMPSTER AND PAINTED COPPER. WALLS COVERED WITH PENNIES EMBEDDED IN CLEAR URETHYENE.

The difference Ibogaine made in Jeff was electric — the "Xanadu effect." Jeff was one of those junkies who is constantly knick-knacking, pulling antique grills and window-frames out of dumpsters and bringing them home only to have them pile up, unused. Now, in several weeks of feverish construction, all the opium dreams stopped up in Jeff's head were actualized. [*See photo of storefront.*] When the showroom was unveiled — a veritable pleasure dome — Sisko and Dana realized this was the first of a subtle new class of effects: the "Ibogaine artifact."

Perhaps as result of unmasking the back injury, or perhaps as a result of his age — 41 — the post-treatment recovery period was markedly longer than most. But it was useful to find that a heroin habit could mask an underlying injury; and Sisko also noted that the recovery period seemed notably shorter the younger the individual. Jeff's alcohol consumption did decrease markedly at first; personal appearance and hygiene improved. But Jeff's loyalties were sufficiently tangled by the contempt many of his junkie friends had for the whole YIP trip, that after two months he relapsed, ripping off Charles in the process. Still, a single Ibogaine treatment had put the store over the hump, and Kritsky attired stars, including Madonna, Billy Idol, Hall & Oates, and Lisa Lisa & Cult Jam.

What would the effect be in the inner city, if all creative people currently impaired on heroin and coke were unleashed, and started small businesses?

Among the last of nine initial treatments done by Sisko in Amsterdam were a Greek theatrical couple — a director and his mate, a costume designer — who'd read a reprint of the original *Overthrow* article in the journal of the Greek YIPPIES. "M," the director, was addicted to both heroin and methadone. He used 50-mg.-a-day of methadone, as well as ¼ of a gram of heroin, but rarely drank and had ceased once-frequent mushroom and LSD use.

The treatment began with routine initial Ibogaine symptoms. After an hour, though, "M" began vomiting. Despite the beginnings of the visionary stage, he complained of physical discomfort. Two-and-a-half hours later, he asked for methadone. He was not exhibiting any signs indicating physical withdrawal, however. Under the pretext of using the bathroom, he phoned his *fiancee* "A" and insisted she bring him methadone at once.

When she arrived, she surreptitiously slipped the methadone to "M," who renewed his request to Sisko for methadone. Sisko refused. "M" persuasively argued he was in great discomfort — that the therapy was not working. Sisko debated the pros and cons of aborting treatment. "M" was displaying high anxiety, but still no physical symptoms of withdrawal. He continued to campaign to end the treatment. Sometime thereafter, "A" returned and slipped him 25 mg. Halcion, which he took and promptly threw up, before finally drifting off to sleep hours later.

Upon awakening, he again summoned "A" to his side and took an additional 30 mg. of methadone. Sisko, upon learning of this, decided to terminate the treatment. In the next days, in conferences with both "M" and "A," "M" came to see that what he had experienced was an anxiety reaction, not physical withdrawal from narcotics. Sisko agreed to try again, but as soon as he was done treating "A."

"A" had been living in Athens, sniffing one gram of smack a day for months. She'd been using continually for three years. She had been able to observe what Ibogaine was like in "M," and was most cooperative. Her Ibogaine dose was given in two administrations, one-and-a-half hours apart. At no time did she vomit or feel nauseous. Nor did she experience any discomfort of withdrawal. She recovered quickly, and went home to join "M," who had continued to shoot heroin and do methadone. For a week she refrained from using heroin, despite being around "M's" continued use. At the end of the week, she accompanied him for his second treatment attempt, ten days after the first one.

Sisko had observed about half of his subjects become nauseous, and half of these vomit at some time during the treatment. Therefore, "M" began by taking two dramamine. An hour later "M" ingested his dose of Ibogaine, and within 35 minutes was beginning to feel the effects. Seventy minutes after ingestion, he reported the onset of nausea.

A booster dose of Ibogaine was administered, but "M" vomited immediately, losing the booster and some Ibogaine ingested earlier. Sisko determined that emergency measures were in order. By prior consent of "M," a rectal aqueous solution had been prepared. It was administered. Within an hour "M" was experiencing the full Ibogaine effect, being characteristically "overwhelmed." The balance of the treatment was uneventful. "M" recovered within three days, declared the procedure an overwhelming success, and moved with "A" to another city.

These treatments pin-pointed problems — such as coping with "enabling behavior" in a couple where the one who isn't being treated is slipping drugs to the one who is, as well as the urgent requirement for a better anti-nausea medication — that would have to be overcome to perfect the procedure. And there was another discovery here — Ibogaine might work, but only on the second or third try — a result that would be confirmed in animals, as we learn in the next chapter.[1] There was one follow-up phone interview of this couple. "M" told Sisko that he'd used heroin on just two occasions; "A" told him she had remained completely heroin-free.

All of these initial treatment episodes became the basis for Sisko's *Interrupting Drug Dependency: A Summary of Nine Case Histories.* With publication of *Nine Case Histories,* Sisko set the stage for his next big idea — making freedom from addiction a reality for those, specifically the Dutch Junkie-bond, who'd initiated the struggle for addict rights.

Without Ibogaine, "Freedom from addiction" is just a slogan. But Sisko knew that not using Ibogaine once he had it would mean acquiescence in slavery and the perpetuation of slavery.

It was a challenge Sisko couldn't resist.

Once he was sure the interruption of addiction was real, Bob Sisko knew that he had to form an organization to make freedom from addiction a reality for addicts everywhere. The name he chose was the International Coalition for Addict Self Help (ICASH). The first ICASH treatment was of the founder of the Junkie-bond, Nico Adriaans.

Yet it was through the cases of Nico and his girlfriend Josien that Sisko came to know as well the limits of Ibogaine — that Ibogaine is not the cure it was first hoped to be, but a treatment. In time, both Nico and Josien relapsed into addiction, and required re-treatment. On a tape made

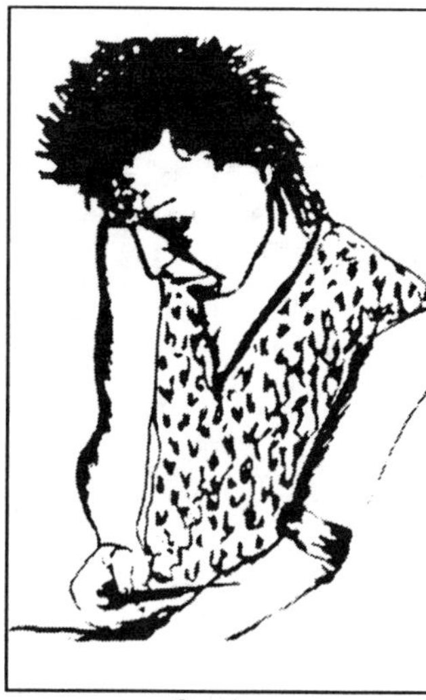

SID VICIOUS

I.C.A.S.H. INTERNATIONAL COALITION FOR ADDICT SELF HELP
POB 20882
TOMPKINS SQ. STA.
NEW YORK, NY 10009
TEL: (212) 228-5427
FAX: (212) 677-1963

ICASH LOGO

[1] See Chapter 7, p. 67.

ten months after his treatment, Nico gave a much clearer description than before to an American junkie of the religious quality of his first experience;[1] and Dana upon seeing this later, asked Sisko: "How could some one relapse after such an experience?

[1] See "Chapter 8: Nico Adriaans" — p. 78, where the Voice comes and says, "So if you know, act like it."

Sisko thought a minute and said: "He forgot. On Ibogaine he will *remember* again."

Josien Harms recounted how she became re-addicted to heroin in another tape made in February, '91, during that later round of treatments:

> "The Ibogaine gives you a feeling that you want to use your brain. You want to be occupied. You want to do things. After Ibogaine, it really gives you a sense like 'Wow — what possibilities you have,' and with heroin, it's just not possible. It puts some [vise] grip on your brain, and you're not able to use your brain fully. Maybe four months after I had taken the Ibogaine, I tried it one time and I thought, 'Oh yeah, now I remember why I don't want to use any more.' But somehow, I just tried it a few times, and six months after I took the Ibogaine I was back on, using daily again. I thought I had it under control, and that I could do that. Just take it once in a while. And now, if I do the Ibogaine again, I don't want to play around with it any more. I don't want to try, even try, if I can do that — to use once in a while. I just want to stay away from it this time. It costs too much money. And it's just not nice."

So even though it's not a perfect cure, through a kind of Ibogaine learning curve the possibility of freedom exists for each individual. Because through Ibogaine, unlike the ordinary addict, they have learned how to quit — later, without Ibogaine.

What is more, information made available during the experience may lay around, and then, under the stimulus of a disinhibiting situation, snap into focus months afterward.

During the spring of 1991, for instance, an ex-Israeli Army medic who was working with

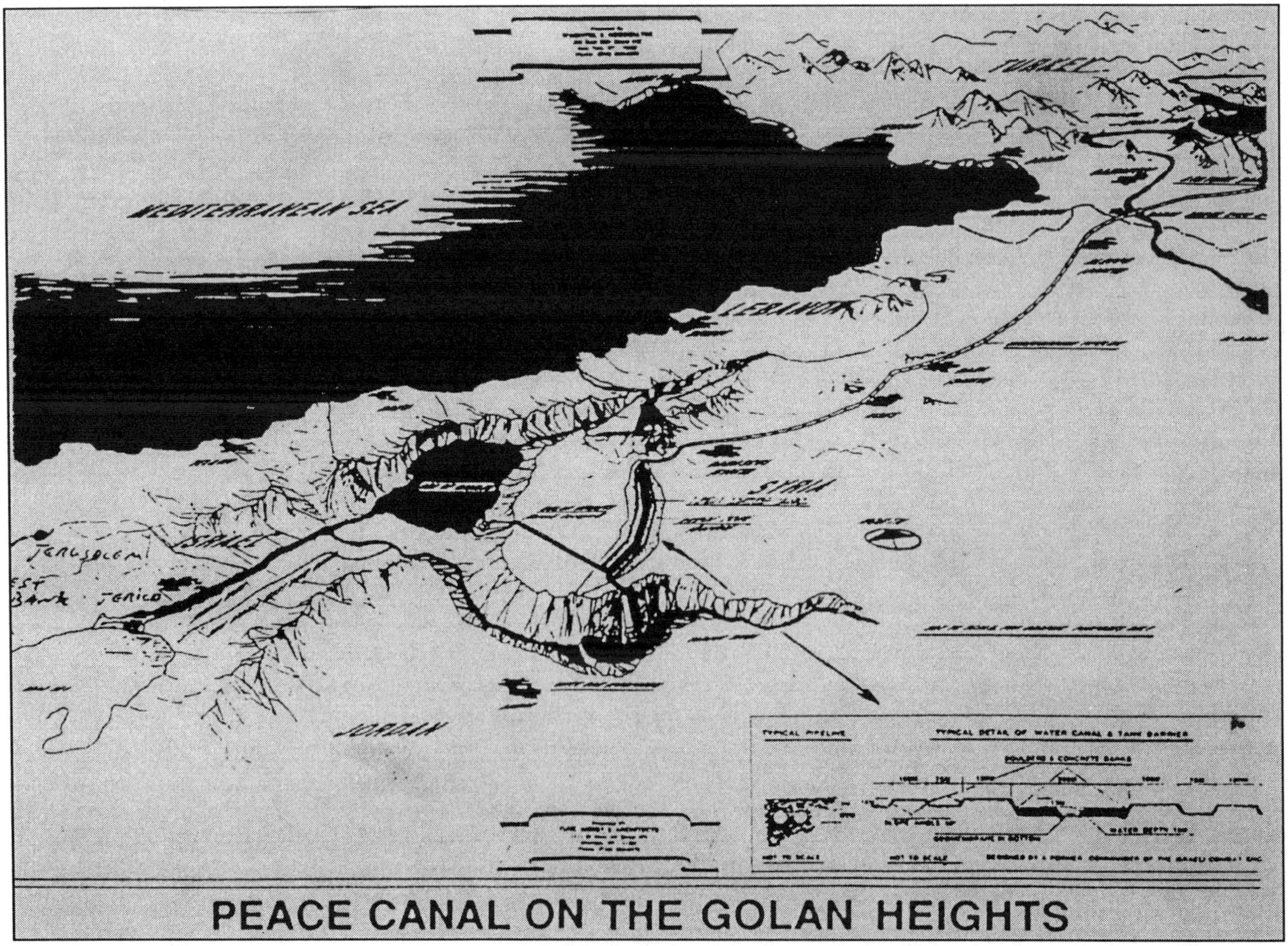

PEACE CANAL ON THE GOLAN HEIGHTS

Sisko and Howard, named Boaz Wachtel, succeeded in wheedling a treament for his cigarette addiction. The treatment worked; but on Ibogaine Boaz experienced being present, 4,000 years earlier, at the offering of the Tablets, and then wandering in the desert for forty years.

In August of '91, when Bob Sisko re-treated himself because his drinking had gotten too heavy again, Bwiti instructed him to go to a certain *schul* on East First Street. There he met someone with contacts in Czechoslovakia and access to an investment house with several million dollars to invest. The ICASH clinic in Prague didn't work out; the new Czech government was too beholden to Bush and James Baker to grant approval. But soon after the initial contact in the *schul*, in the Lower East Side apartment of the Czech contact, Boaz experienced one of those moments where everything seems to re-arrange — and information made available to him months before, on the Ibogaine — snapped into focus.

They were talking about a tank ditch on the Golan, between Israel and Syria, when Boaz remembered a fragment from his visions: the greening of Israel, Syria, Palestine, Jordan, even Saudi Arabia by bringing water down from lakes in Eastern Turkey via a series of aquaducts. A review of elevation maps showed it was eminently feasible. Boaz credits Ibogaine for strengthening his conviction to act on the vision, the sense that peace in that particular corner of the world remains somehow essential in the design of things. He went to work, and today his water-for-peace plan forms one of the few really solid bases for peace negotiations with Assad. The region has dangerously depleted its aquifers; everyone in the area needs an agreement that will let them share in the potential water from the north, if agreement with Syria can be reached.

One night not long after Boaz first got his Great New Idea, after he was done explaining how he felt it related to his Ibogaine experience, Sisko conceded that his own recent re-treatment "really refreshed my memories of the first time I did it. The reality of it. When you don't do it for awhile, you really forget what it's like. Did you know that I traveled anywhere in the world in a blink of an eye? It was like Astral Projection."

He went on to speculate that the effect may be somewhat dependent on place. Sisko wants to take Ibogaine at Mt. Sinai, to see if he might be able to talk to *Moishe Rebbineu.* After another six months or so, he told Dana about a story from *Numbers,* Chapter 12, Verses 1–16, about Moses and Moses' sister, a story Jews are supposed to study once a year.

"It really supports the idea that *dreaming* was the usual medium for religious experience and prophecies," said Sisko.

Moses was married to an Ethiopian — a Black woman. And Miriam, his sister, and Aaron started making a stink,[1] saying "Hath the Lord indeed spoken only with Moses? Hath He not spoke also with us?" — Sisko paused for dramatic effect — "And the Lord heard it."

So God called Moses, Aaron, and Miriam to the Meeting Tent, and descended on a pillar of cloud and said, "If there be a prophet among you, I the Lord do make Myself know unto him in a vision, I do speak with him in a dream.

"My servant Moses is not so; he is trusted in all My house; with him do I speak mouth to mouth, even manifestly, and not in dark speeches; and the similitude of the Lord doth he behold" — in other words I talk to this guy face to face, not in dreams at night like any run-of-the-mill Prophet.

Then God said, in effect: "You have grievously hassled my Man, Moses. You want White? I'll give you White."

And he turned Miriam into a leper. But because God is merciful, after a week He turned her back.

"Jews don't talk about this story a lot," Sisko said, "because it involves racism, even though Miriam's primary offense was to undermine the Project, by dissing Moses."

"But the story seems to say God is against racism. That he views it as spiritual leprosy."

Since his second treatment, Sisko religiously dons his skull-cap and strolls over to *schul* every Friday night. He is unavailable on Saturdays. His gadfly role, in hassling the feds for proceeding so ponderously with Ibogaine development, is in the highest tradition of confronting complacent, Pharonic authority, and speaking truth to power.

Also, for seven years, he hasn't smoked a cigarette.

1 Saying Moses was losing interest in sex because Zephirah, his wife, was Black; whereas Orthodox Jews teach that such loss of appetites is the natural result of adopting a receptive [i.e., female] attitude to *Torah.* The real offense here was interference with Divine Disclosure to Moses.

CHAPTER 7: Stanley Glick

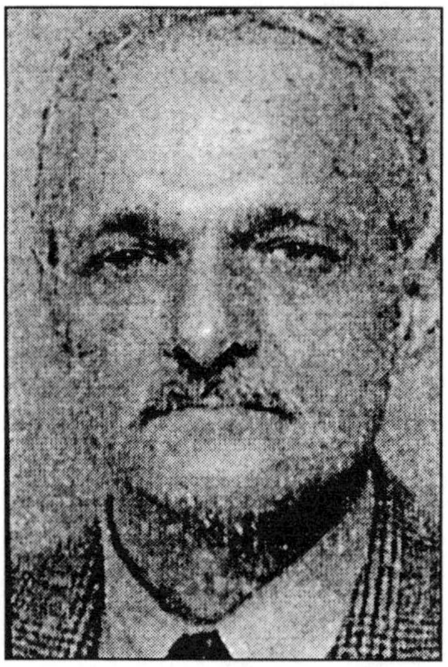

Albany Times Union

HOWARD LOTSOF

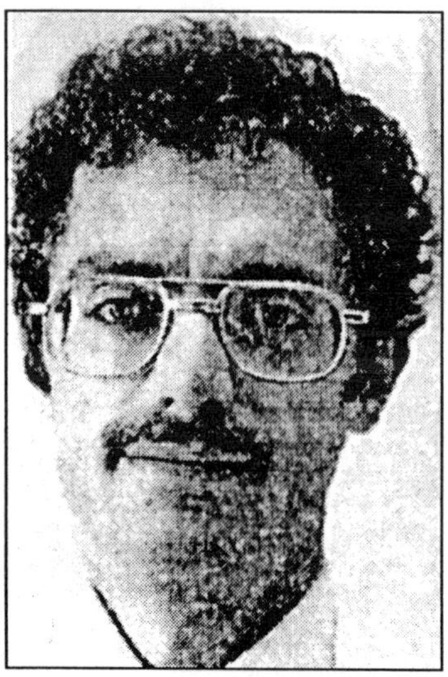

Albany Times Union

DR. STANLEY GLICK

In 1986, Howard Lotsof again approached the National Institute on Drug Abuse (NIDA) and asked them to put Ibogaine to the hardest test. "Have your doctors," he said, "give it to subjects you pick, double-blind."

"We don't really believe you," they replied, "and any way, you have to demonstrate it in the animal model."

"Animals are animals and people are people," he objected. But he realized the work would have to go forth, and he set out to do it. First Lotsof would have to get Ibogaine, and none of the European pharmaceutical giants would sell him any, unless he got European patents. So while he obtained patents in fourteen countries other than the United States, he made the trip to Libreville so he could manufacture his own Ibogaine.

When he finally got his first Ibogaine nine months later, Howard began working on data for attenuating the alcohol dependency syndrome. Here he was venturing beyond his original '62–'63 trials, so he contracted with a professor through a graduate student at McGill University in Montreal to check out Ibogaine's effect on alcoholic rats. The professor turned the real work over to the same graduate student — who turned out to be simply incapable of performing the analysis to recognize the trend that was clear in his experimental data. Says Howard:

> "This kid could have published the first scientific paper showing Ibogaine's efficacy. Instead, he went with me to the bank, where I withdrew every cent I had and gave it to him. Then he said, 'You know, you really fucked me over.' And quit. Fortunately, our contract specified that I owned the data from his experiment. When I looked it over, the attenuation of alcohol consumption was clear. This guy was simply unwilling to see it."

Howard filed the patent (U.S. #4,857,523) for attentuation of alcohol dependency syndrome, July 18, 1988. It was granted the next year, August 15, 1989.

Upon getting supplies, Howard had fired off a sample to the Drug Testing Program of the College on Problems of Drug Dependency at the National Institute on Mental Health in Maryland. In January of '88 he got back a letter from Dr. Arthur E. Jacobson, the Chairman of the Program, reporting that the Dr. James H. Woods of the University of Michigan Medical School in Ann Arbor had determined Ibogaine is not a substitute narcotic.

Using *in vitro* (i.e., in glass, not in living animals) preparations of the brains of rats and the brain stems of mice, Woods showed Ibogaine "did not exhibit significant opioid activity."

Howard next furnished Ibogaine to researchers in the Pharmacology Department at Erasmus University, Rotterdam. E.D. Dzoljic, Charlie Kaplan and M.R. Dzoljic had developed a method of direct injection into the ventricles (little spaces) of rat's brains, so that they would get the effects of regular IV or interperitoneal administration with a thousandth of the usual amount. For them, fifty grams was like fifty kilos.

In '88, the Dutch group was the first to publish a full paper, *Effect of Ibogaine on Naloxone-Precipitated Withdrawal Syndrome in Chronic Morphine Dependent Rats.* Live rats were addicted by implanting them with morphine pellets, then thrown into withdrawal with naloxone (the morphine "blocker" developed in the '60s, prototype of today's longer-acting naltrexone). By injecting Ibogaine into the brain (intercerebroventricularly) fifteen minutes before the naloxone, withdrawal was lessened, especially signs related to locomotion (rearing, digging, jumping) — as well as head-hiding, chewing, teeth-chattering, writhing and salivation — which showed withdrawal was being blocked. The rats also had less desire to hide and to escape; the only withdrawal sign that increased was penile-licking(!). Kaplan and the Dzoljics noted studies showing Ibogaine simultaneously stimulates sleeping (acetylcholine) and fight-or-flight (noradrenalin) brain pathways.

Now in the world of pharmaceutical giants, NDA International was an amoeba among whales ("Three officers and nine lawyers," says Norma). It was Norma, Howard and Bruce Sakow, a commercial screen writer who was their first investor ("I've known Howard since the eary '70s," says Sakow. "When I put my money in I thought I was throwing it away. I didn't think he would get as far as he has.")

Lotsof ran out of money in 1989, after he had contracted with Dr. Stanley Glick, the head of the Department of Pharmacology and Toxicology at Albany College of Medicine, to test whether Ibogaine would depress long-term intake of morphine in rats.

To find out, Glick trained his rats to self-inject about 75 milligrams (mg.) of morphine a day, enough to feel pleasure but not enough to be addicted. He took them off morphine on weekends: These were "casual user" rats. Each time a rat would press a lever, they'd get .04 mg. morphine per kilo (mg/kg) of body-weight.

Ibogaine in doses ranging from 2.5 to 80 mg/kg was given either before or after the morphine on day one of the experiment. Immediately, 5 mg./kg. of Ibogaine cut morphine intake 40 percent; 10 mg. cut it in half; 20 mg., 60 percent; and 40 mg. cut it to one-tenth of what it was at the beginning of the experiment. But since Ibogaine causes behavioral immobility, in the first twenty-four hours water intake was also severely depressed by the time the dose run-up reached 40 mg./kg.

What grabbed Glick's attention was the *after-effect.* Ibogaine goes out of the body in a few hours, but doses of 40 to 80 mg./kg. depressed morphine intake — up to several weeks! Moreover, after several weekly treatments, this after-effect kicked in with some rats who were initially resistant. Not only that, this after-effect was not aversive (a simple conditioned negative response) because it happened whether Ibogaine was given before or after the morphine on day one of the experiment.

Although Ibogaine was shown in 1956 to double the painkilling effect of morphine, that only happens for the few hours that both are in the body. Ibogaine couldn't be an antagonist, because the rats would just have bar-pressed more morphine. Anyway, most researchers thought indole-alkaloids aren't supposed to interact with the morphine pathways at all. Glick speculated that either a long-lasting Ibogaine metabolite or some lesioning of the brain might be involved.

Now under the terms of their contract, Dr. Glick had to send Lotsof a preliminary report. But researchers don't like to circulate anything before formal publication in a scientific journal; and to Glick's embarrassment, he says, Lotsof "sent the data to two dozen people around the world!" On a certain level Glick was actually relieved when Lotsof couldn't pay him in full. It allowed him to break the contract, but continue Ibogaine research with his regular block grants from NIDA.

His next experiment (summarized in *Interactions between Ibogaine, a potential anti-addictive agent, and morphine: an in vivo microdialysis study,* with I.M. Maisonneuve and R.W. Keller, Jr.) used probes set in the skulls of living rats to collect minute amounts of a neurotransmitter called dopamine (DA), to track the effect of Ibogaine on the morphine high.

Dopamine (DA) makes your "pleasure centers" do their thing; when one neuron fires off dopamine to the next neuron, it feels good. It also stimulates locomotion; in Parkinson's disease the dopamine system shuts down, causing paralysis.

Cocaine produces a surplus of DA in the intersynaptic space by occupying a slot on the protein "transporter" that carries DA back into the neuron for re-use.[1] Morphine, nicotine, and booze increase the neuronal firing rate. Amphetamine increases DA release directly. But take away your usual drug (except for marijuana, which keys into completely different [anandamide] receptors throughout the brain, including the grey matter, the cerebrum), and you'll feel listless, anhedonic (no pleasure), and even the pangs of acute withdrawal.[2]

The common denominator effect of all hard drugs is chronic dopamine surplus in the mesocortical and mesolimbic system — the three sites of the "common narcotic receptor" — i.e., where dopamine pathways project either into the prefrontal cortex (decision-making) from a little bulb called the nucleus accumbens (sexual pleasure, movement), or further back in the occiput, into the striated cortex, the striatum (visualization). In the standard model of addiction, visualization in the striatum (a) triggers craving in the nucleus accumbens, (b) which sets up a dopaminergic cascade of further visual-

1 See illustration, Chapter 8, p. 75.

2 Researchers have found that with hard drugs, DNA in nerve cells eventually express less receptor protein, which explains tolerance. On the other hand, anandamide receptors of mice exposed to THC congeners for two weeks in a 27-fold run-up experiment exhibited no down-regulation of receptor protein, and the mice exhibited the same psycho-motor stimulation measured in an activity box through the entire experiment. See Abood, Sauss, et al., "Development of Behavioral Tolerance to Delta-9 THC Without Alteration of the Binding or mRNA Levels in the Whole Brain," *Pharm. Biochem. and Behavior*, Vol. 46, pp. 574–579, 1993.

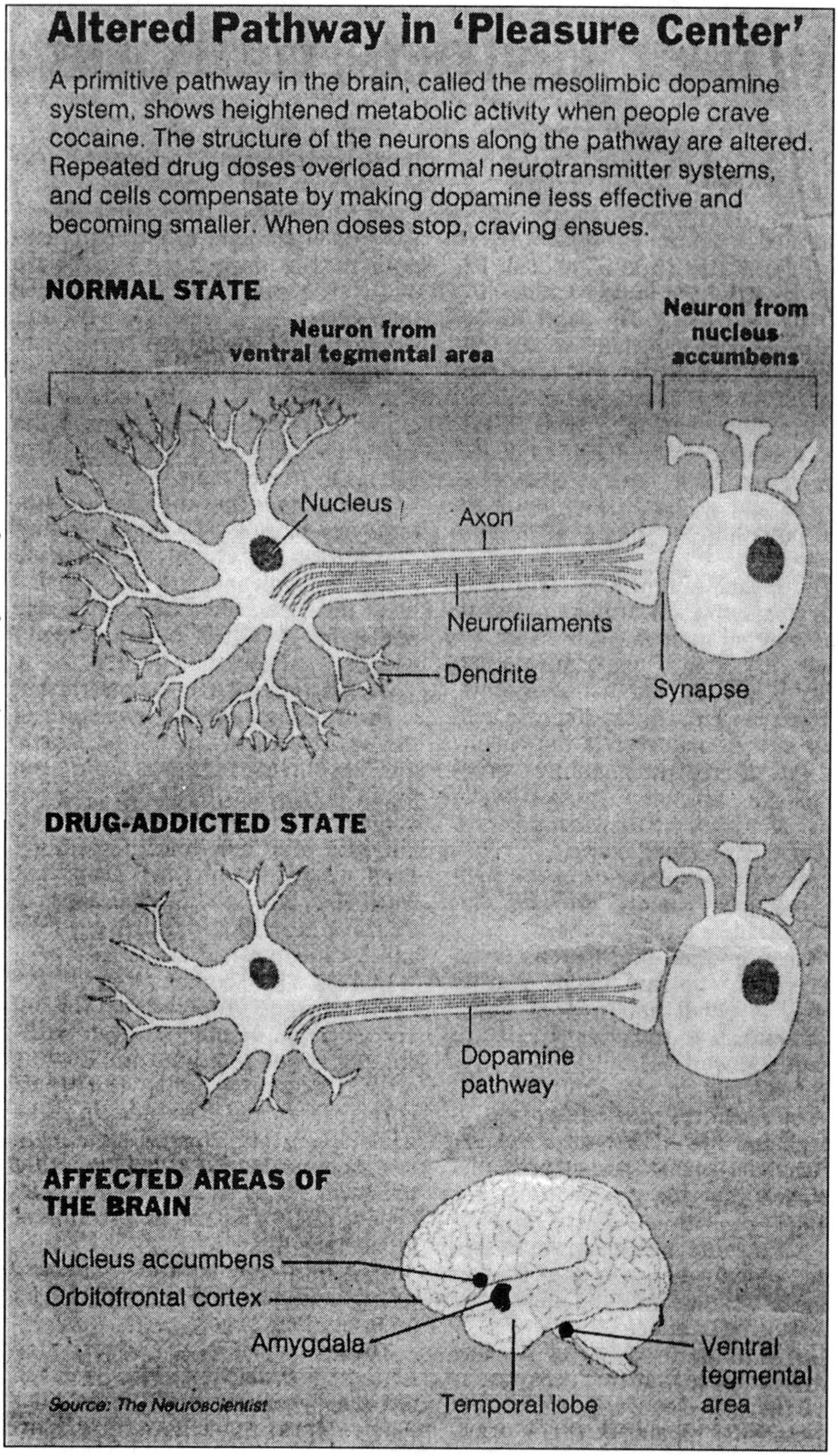

New York Times, Illustration by Al Granberg

izations and cravings that finally trip the dopamine switch in the pre-frontal cortex, (c) initiating drug-taking.

Glick, Maisonneuve, et al. sought to determine: first, what does Ibogaine alone do to extra-cellular DA and its metabolites, DOPAC (3,4 dihydroxyphenacetic acid) and HVA (homo-vanillic acid)? Next, how does morphine by itself, five mg. and thirty mg., effect all three regions? Finally, what does Ibogaine pre-treatment 19 hours prior to five mg. of morphine (by which time the Ibogaine — with a "half life" in the body of one hour, according to Dhahir — is certainly gone) do to the dopamine release and behavioral change that normally come with a five-milligram-per-kilo dose of morphine?

Acutely (i.e., right away) Ibogaine decreased DA in the striatum, increased it in the pre-frontal cortex, had no effect in the nucleus accumbens.[1] But the metabolite DOPAC increased in all three areas; HVA increased in the striatum and nucleus accumbens.

On the other hand, the lower five mg. dose of morphine kicked up DA and its metabolites in all three regions; while thirty milligrams increased not dopamine but the metabolites. [On the graph it looks like the entire increase shifts into metabolites.[2]]

After Ibogaine pre-treatment, five milligrams of morphine failed to raise DA levels in the three areas. Instead there was a rise in metabolites similar to thirty millligrams of morphine with no Ibogaine pre-treatment (except in the neo-cortex, where DOPAC stayed flat and HVA increase was delayed and smaller).

Likewise, five milligrams of morphine by itself inhibited motor activity for forty minutes, followed by a burst of excitement. But in pre-treated rats there was no excited period, just an inhibitory phase (of two hours) much like the effect of thirty milligrams of morphine (three hours). Was a long-lasting metabolite of Ibogaine potentiating the morphine, so that a five-milligram dose had the same effect as a thirty-milligram dose? Or was a neurotoxic effect damaging some DA neurons while boosting the firing of the remaining ones? The second possibility seemed ruled out by Dhahir's '71 study, in which rats treated for thirty days with ten to thirty mg./kg. of Ibogaine showed no neuronal damage.

With five milligrams of morphine, increased motor activity matched a rise in striatal dopamine (80% of DA receptors are in the striatum). Glick concluded that at the thirty mg./kg. dose somehow additional opioid

1 See Fig. 1, next page. The graph actually shows a slight effect from Ibogaine.

2 See Fig. 4, next page.

receptor sites were being activated, *blocking* striatal DA release.

With Ibogaine treatment, DA release was also down. Since Glick maintained the same morphine level (5 mg./kg.) in the control group, this meant neither Ibogaine nor a long-lasting metabolite was prolonging morphine half life. Morphine was still firing off DA, but it was turning into metabolites DOPAC and HVA instead of hanging out. Glick did know that by preventing a DA surplus in the nucleus accumbens, Ibogaine ought to decrease morphine's "reinforcing effect."

Glick's group followed this up with the most complex set of tests yet, trucking in radioactive samples (radio-ligands) of Ibogaine and its closest relatives to find out whether the reduction of morphine intake was specific to Ibogaine, or if previous psychedelic researchers had missed a general effect of a number of indole-ring compounds. Glick chose Ibogaine hydro-chloride, ibogamine, tabernanthine, corinaridine, harmaline hydrochloride, harmane hydrochloride, and harmine hydrochloride.

Published later as *Mechanisms of action of Ibogaine and Harmaline cogeners based on radioligand binding studies,* the experiments aimed to answer three questions: Was Ibogaine locking into one of the opiate receptors? Does the hallucinogenic effect involve the serotonin (5HT) receptors? And third, iboga and harmala alkaloids produce tremor (slight shaking) — how? For comparison purposes, drugs were used with known affinities for thirty different kinds of brain receptors including dopamine, serotonin, adrenaline and opiates, but also GABA, cannabinoid, Cl (since Ibogaine HCl is a chloride salt), benzodiazapine (BZD), etc. *(See Table 1, next page.)*

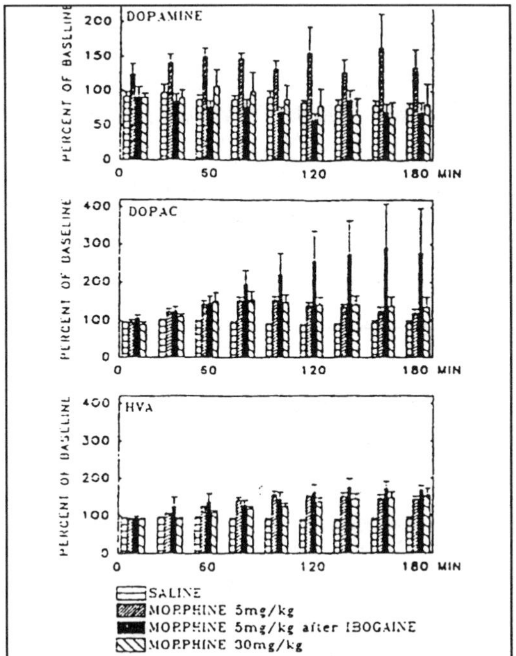

Fig. 4. Time course of extracellular DA, DOPAC and HVA levels in the nucleus accumbens after administration of morphine (5 mg/kg n = 6, and 30 mg/kg, n = 6) in naive rats and morphine (5 mg/kg n = 6) in rats pretreated with ibogaine (40 mg/kg) the day before. Samples were collected at 20 min intervals. Data are expressed as percent (± S.E.) of baseline values.

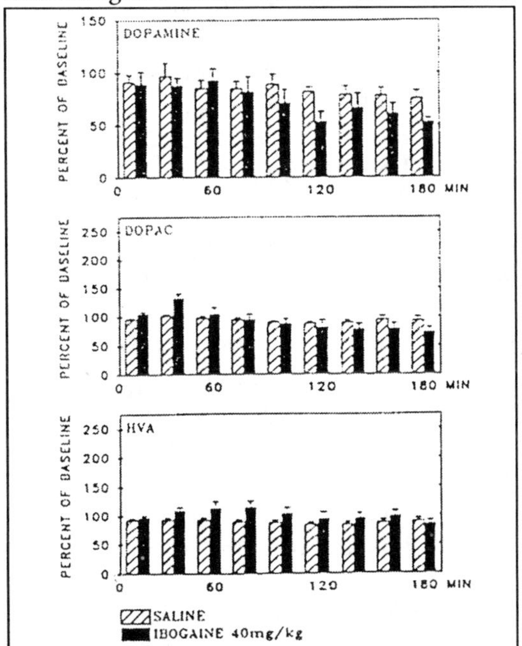

Fig. 1. Time course of extracellular DA, DOPAC and HVA levels in the nucleus accumbens after administration of saline (n = 6) and ibogaine (40 mg/kg, n = 6). Samples were collected at 20 min intervals. Data are expressed as a percent (± S.E.) of baseline values.

There were some big surprises. Lack of affinity for serotonin receptors showed that iboga and harmala indolealkalamines — even though they share an indole ring — are fundamentally different from the LSD series. As for tremor, it wasn't happening in the GABA receptor; nor was chloride uptake being blocked at the BZD (valium) receptor. Instead all the harmala and iboga compounds were conductively — i.e, neuro-electrically — firing via the sodium channels.

But the real find was that all iboga compounds — and none of the harmala — had a transient affinity for the *kappa* opiate receptor. But only transient — one rinse of the homogenized brain tissue used in the experiment freed it up for any competing chemical. By comparison, buprenorphine, which cannot be blocked by naloxone once it is administered, gives up its hold on opiate receptors most

TABLE I

Survey of receptor affinity for ibogaine and harmaline using radiolabeled binding assays.

Assay conditions followed references cited; all data are representative of triplicate determinations from 3 experiments using different membrane preparations.

Receptor	*[^{3}H]Ligand*	*Tissue*	*Refs.*
Adrenergic			
α_1	prazosin	rat cortex bovine cortex	13
α_2	*p*-amino- clonidine	rat cortex calf cortex	30
β_1	dihydro- alprenalol HCl	rat cortex calf cortex	18
Cannabinoid	CP55,940 Win5212-2	calf cerebellum calf cerebellum	11
Dopamine			
D_1	SCH23390	rat striatum calf caudate	14 31
D_2	*N*-methyl- spiperone	rat striatum calf striatum	19
GABA			
A	muscimol	bovine cortex bovine cerebellum	3
BZD	flunitrazepam	rat cortex bovine cortex	6
Cl^- channel	$^{36}Cl^-$	mouse synaptoneurosome	5
Muscarinic	QNB	bovine cortex bovine hippocampus	37
Nicotinic	methylcarbamyl- choline	bovine cortex	1
Opiate			
μ	carfentanil	bovine cortex	35
δ	DPDPE	bovine cortex	7
κ	U69,593	bovine cortex	17
Serotonin			
1_a	DPAT	Rat hippocampus	33
1_b	5-HT	rat striatum	33
1_c	mesulergine	rat cortex	33
1_d	5-HT	bovine caudate	8
2	ketanserin	rat cortex	34
3	GR65630	area postrema	22

reluctantly. Ibogaine's long-lasting effect doesn't come by *locking out* opiates. It does just enough to block withdrawal 95 percent, but leaves the addict something to overcome. Once again it was shown to be neither a substitute narcotic nor an antagonist (blocker).

Glick was now completely hooked on Ibogaine research. He converted one-third of his lab to his own mini-Staten Island project, spending a few hundred thousand in NIDA block grants.

Next Glick studied Ibogaine and D-amphetamine (remember "dexies"?[1]), since amphetamine produces dopamine surplus via the most straightforward route (increased release, versus increased neuronal firing rate on morphine, etc.). Rats will inject amphetamine directly into the nucleus accumbens. Also, lesioning there decreases amphetamine-induced DA release and hyperactivity.

Nineteen hours after the pre-treatment, dopamine levels were back to normal; but both metabolites (DOPAC, HVA) were still down. When D-amphetamine was given, DA levels were *doubled* in both the nucleus accumbens and striatum of pre-treated rats, while metabolites decreased. Pre-treatment also increased locomotion across a broad range of doses, and after the first hour, made it peak *sooner.*

How, if pre-treatment doubled DA release, and DA is the transmitter of brain reward we sense as pleasure, how could Ibogaine interrupt amphetamine abuse? The answer lies in the well-known unpleasant "wasted" feeling produced by *too much* amphetamine. As Glick said later in *Interactions of ibogaine and D-amphetamine: in vivo microdialysis and motor activity in rats* (with I.M. Maisonneuve and R.W. Keller, Jr.), released DA activates other autoreceptors, so that one too-high dose can produce an *averse reaction* to subsequent low doses.

How? Glick proposed Ibogaine might do this by sensitizing the neurons, or via his elusive "long-lasting Ibogaine metabolite."

Next Glick's group went back to measure, more exactly, what happens with dopamine and behavior when morphine is given one hour, nineteen hours, one week and one month after Ibogaine pre-treatment. As explained in *Acute and Prolonged effects of Ibogaine on brain dopamine metabolism and morphine-induced locomotor activity in rats,* they first recorded the effects of morphine on locomotion. Then, instead of teasing traces of DA and its metabolites from between the neurons with dialysis, this time they killed the rats and determined total DA tissue content.

The first mystery solved was how DOPAC and HVA are depressed nineteen hours after pre-treatment: within an hour of Ibogainization, dopamine fell a whopping 54% in the prefrontal cortex, 51% in the nucleus accumbens, and 42% in the striatum (where 80% of DA receptors

1 Dexamphetamines, a stand-by for generations of college students cramming for exams. Two days later you would remember nothing.

reside). Nineteen hours later, DOPAC was still at 85% of normal in the nucleus accumbens and 83% in the striatum; the prefrontal cortex was normal. A *week* after Ibogaine, striatial DOPAC was still 90% of normal. (Glick was so surprised he checked this finding twice.) After a month, everything was normal.

Now Ibogaine itself inhibits motor activity, but only during the first hour. A week after Ibogaine Glick's rats were *more* active, which indicates the initial DA drop wasn't a result of simple lesioning — say of the nucelus accumbens. But even after a week, Ibogaine (40 mg./kg.) depressed morphine's behavioral stimulation, except at the high dose of 30 mg./kg. Since his second study *(Interactions between Ibogaine and Morphine)* found standard morphine-induced DA release was depressed in the striatum (where vision/visualization occurs), but not the nucleus accumbens (which is thought to govern movement), Glick could only speculate the absence of stimulation might result from striatally-induced morphine rigidity. [The alternative explanation — inhibition of visualization in triggering craving — is hard to check out in rats. But he was also inclined to see visualizations as an undesirable side-effect of Ibogaine therapy.] At one month, the inhibition of morphine effect finally wore off.

Yet if the second study recorded no 50% DA release, and only moderate metabolite increase (HVA), where was the dopamine going? Ibogaine action on voltage-dependent sodium channels could release a little, and block re-uptake a bit, but that doesn't account for 50%! Perhaps DOPAC decrease at nineteen hours might be the result of new DA being diverted into storage pools. To fully explain it, Glick was left either with his elusive, and now *very* long-lasting, metabolite or "persistent neuronal change."

Finally, Maisonneuve and Glick tried out Ibogaine on cocaine. Repeating the combo of micro-dialysis and measurement of behavioral stimulation, they found that cocaine challenge (i.e., fresh administration) nineteen hours after Ibogaine pre-treatment boosted and lengthened the usual DA release in the nucleus accumbens, and to a lesser extent, in the striatum. Behavioral stimulation was increased only in the second hour, but that might be because the rats were not yet *habituated* to cocaine. They could only begin to be habituated in the second hour, when the motor enhancement would correspond to the first point of the cocaine "crash," where the user typically becomes uncomfortable and hyperstimulated.

In *Interactions between ibogaine and cocaine in rats: in vivo microdialysis and motor behavior,* Maisonneuve and Glick noted the effect would be the same as a higher-than-intended dose of cocaine — anxiety-producing, ergo, aversive. Just like amphetamine. Of course, how Ibogaine pre-treatment could increase DA release with amphetamine while blocking DA re-uptake with cocaine, was as big a mystery as how pre-treatment could work at all when Ibogaine is completely out of the body after nineteen hours.

Glick now leaned toward the "long-lasting metabolite" hypothesis. If he could find it, and patent it, it might do everything Ibogaine does *sans* psychedelic effect. And as Dr. Marvin Snyder of NIDA told a *Newsday* reporter in the summer of 1990: "We're not looking at any drugs with psychedelic effects [for treatment of drug dependency]."

To be fair, as a veteran NIDA grantsman, Glick knew Ibogaine had powerful adversaries in high places. He was aware Ibogaine had been plugged in the first draft of a 1989 Senate Judiciary Report on new medications for drug dependency, only to be dropped from the final draft because Dr. Thomas Kosten and another doctor from Yale wrote a letter objecting that "it's an herbal." (Actually, Howard now gets synthetic 99.7 percent pure Ibogaine from Omnichem in Belgium.)

The centerpiece of the report? Buprenorphine, which it was admitted doesn't work that well, and is addictive... *but* which was developed by Kosten and Herb Kleber. So where Glick told *Newsday* in 1990 that "lying on your back for two days would be a small price to pay" if Ibogaine worked, by October 16, 1991, he told the *Albany Times Union*, "It is doubtful Ibogaine could ever be marketed because of its psychoactive properties and the muscle tremor." He opined that they'd probably wait ten years to develop a synthetic. But Glick needed NIDA grants to do *anything;* and, until the end of 1990, Herb Kleber was Deputy Drug Czar.

To Lotsof and his supporters, the "waking REM" (Rapid Eye Movement, as in dreaming)

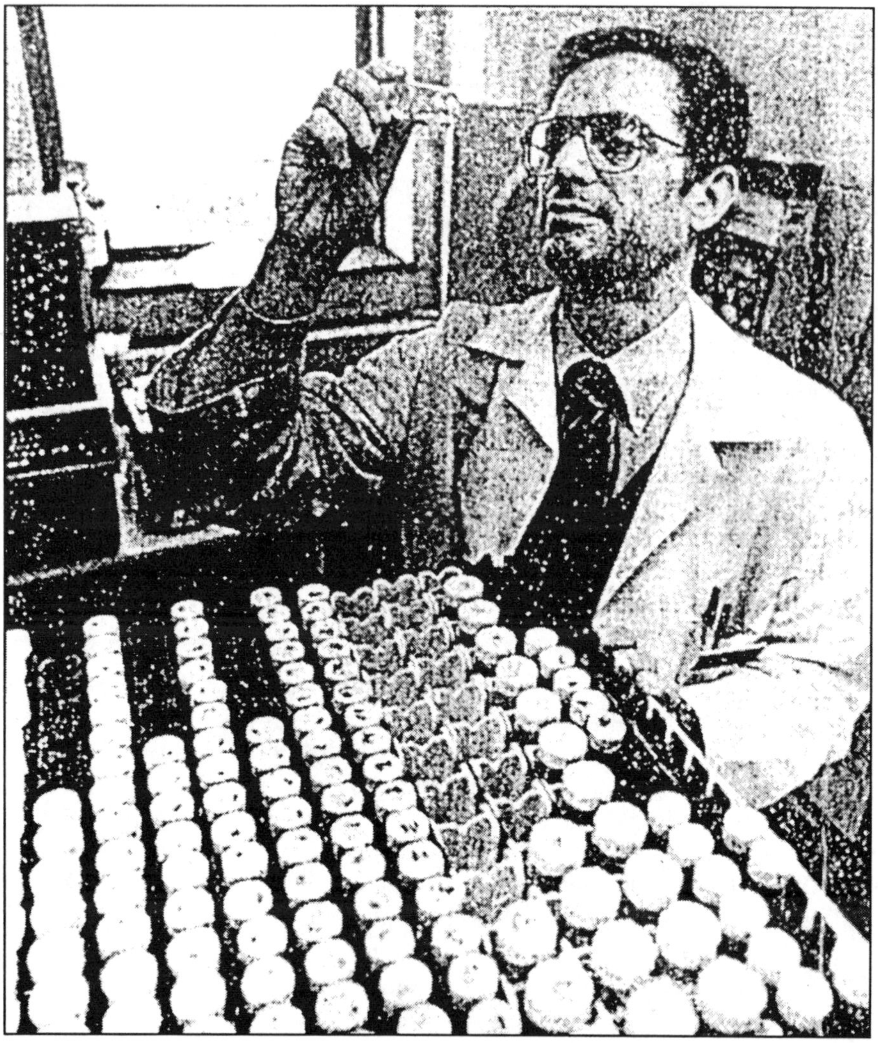

DR. STANLEY GLICK IN HIS LAB

effect is integral to Ibogaine's efficacy. The incessant array of pictures "like a movie," "an onslaught of pictorial gestalts" which lasts four-to-five hours, enables the addict to dredge up all kinds of traumatic material while in a "neutral cognitive state," and is essential to their "maturing out of addiction."[1] Certainly, there's no way to learn how important lucid REM is by studying rats, mice, or monkeys.

"Originally our critics told us no medication can get at the deep psychological roots of addiction," says Howard. "Well, you certainly can't affect those roots without getting at them.

"They want crops without plowing up the ground... rain without thunder and lightning. They want the Ocean without the awful roar of its many waters."

Gradually, though, Lotsof has become reconciled with Glick. In February 1990, when he got more good news from Jacobsen of the Committee on Problems of Drug Dependence, he made certain Glick was first to know. Drs. Aceto, Bowman and Harris of the Medical College of Virginia had performed research showing that Ibogaine does not cause significant physical dependence. Here was independent confirmation Ibogaine had at least one characteristic of a true addiction interrupter.

On April 30, 1991, Dr. Stanley Glick gave a one-hour lecture, with slides, at Mt. Sinai Hospital — as a courtesy, since personnel there had been instrumental in introducing him to Lotsof in 1986. As a courtesy, Howard, Bob Sisko, Boaz Wachtel and Dana Beal were all invited. They sat there as Glick presented a slide show on his phase of the Staten Island Project — an overwhelming profusion of charts, graphs, and statistics. But his principal findings were simple:

§ Ibogaine is neither a substitute narcotic nor a crude mechanical blocker like naltrexone.

§ The iboga group, but not other indoleakylamines, temporarily binds to the *kappa* opiate receptor, enough to ameliorate withdrawal, but not so much that the addict feels no or almost no withdrawal whatsoever.

§ Ibogaine depressed morphine intake in all but one of twelve rats who were not addicted, but were self-injecting for pleasure. Ibogaine decreases, but does not extinguish, pleasure response.

§ Through the same mysterious mechanisms Ibogaine boosted amphetamine and cocaine effect in a way that could be anxiogenic, "aversive" in addicts upon first trying coke or amphetamines after treatment.

When the hour was up, and Glick was done, Howard Lotsof walked up to him and said: "Listening to your presentation, viewing your data, I felt like I was present when Enrico Fermi initiated the first nuclear reaction under the Stadium at the University of Chicago."

[1] The theory that addicts naturally "mature out" of their addictions was coined by Charles Winnick, in "Maturing Out of Narcotic Addiction," (*Bulletin on Narcotics,* 6:1), to account for the high proportion— 85% — of veterans returning from Vietnam who were able to quit using back home — data that defied conventional wisdom about heroin invariably addictive, and virtually impossible to quit on your own.

CHAPTER 8: Nico Adriaans

At the beginning of Glick's presentation, he threw on a slide he considered to be a gag: a headline from an article in the *Village Voice,* entitled: *Miracle Cure? Advocates say Ibogaine Ends Craving for Dope.* The article was Dana's first big score in a new role: public point-man for Ibogaine. It had taken him thirteen months of prodding the *Voice* to get it printed, since the day in late May 1989, when a hotshot freelance writer named Max Cantor walked in to 9 Bleecker, aiming to do a big exposé on the furious controversy in the annual pot parade between Dana's people and a faction of Lower East Side squatters who'd been in the news a lot since the police riot in Tompkins Square Park the August before. They claimed to speak in the higher interest of the Parade/Movement, but due to entanglement with a 12-step faction in the squat scene vehemently opposed to Ibogaine, and the fact some of them now owed their apartments to the eviction of addicts,[1] their opposition to making Ibogaine an issue had hardened. They would rather evict junkies than turn 'em into non-addicts. But they didn't feel confident to pull off such a bald-faced coup without a figurehead — Michael Cesar, the self-styled "Pope of Pot."

For ten years, the "Pope" had a simple but effective way of glomming all the column inches available for pot coverage in the New York papers: open up a marijuana delivery service. Offer all the younger anarchists jobs (without the political discipline they'd be subjected to at 9 Bleecker, where they were *forbidden* to deal pot). Let 'em do hard drugs (Fred was the Pope's chief lieutenant; all his earnings went into his arm.) Then go public in unfriendly media like the *New York Post,* get busted, and take all the delivery boys to jail with you.

So Dana said to Max: "Why write the same stupid article the *New York Post* has run four times already, when you can do a real scoop? Let me tell you about the real issue behind the split — Ibogaine."

The roots of the split actually went back to 1987, when Dana was sitting in the DC NORML office talking to the new National Director, Jon Gettman. "Can't you do something about Charlie Rangel?" asked Gettman, referring to the head of the House Select Sub-Committee on Narcotics. "We can't budge him."

"Well," said Dana, "the only time we have enough people to do anything is the annual pot parade. It's a schlep up fromWashington Square Park, but we could take a rest in Central Park, and have it end up at Rangel's office on 125th Street."

When the first Saturday in May, 1988 rolled around, though, the bulk of the parade wouldn't go past Strawberry Fields at 72nd and Central Park West. Legalizing pot wasn't really a political goal for them. The parade was an annual occasion to party.

When the political vanguard of the parade did get to Rangel's office at 125th, they were confronted by a fat white lady police community relations officer and about eight mostly elderly black activists she'd assembled, who were fuming over this invasion of their turf. In a twinkling Dana saw they wouldn't be into a hemp rap. But except for the white lady cop, they were all *very* interested in an African rain forest cure for addiction.

The problem was that Dana was implementing a "paradigm shift" here before most of the movement even *knew* about Ibogaine. By the time he finished revising a book on environmental hemp in February '88 (which started out in 1983 as Hans-Georg Behr's *Von Hanf Ist Die Rede — "When the Subject is Hemp"* — and metamorphosed along the way into *The Emperor Wears No Clothes,* by Jack Herer), he'd realized a purely environmental approach left out all the really good public health arguments. After all, there was now the experience of twelve years of de-crim in Holland to go on. So he phoned Georg in Germany, who told him all drug reform during the next period was going to be driven by the AIDS crisis.

So Dana started going to ACT UP.

As far back as 1986 Beal and the grassroots caucus recommended to the Greens that

[1] See Chapter 9, pg. 88, Chapter 11, pg. 112. The ones who owe their current apartment to such ethnic cleansing are understandably unenthusiastic about Ibogaine access as an alternative.

they approach AIDS activists *re* medical marijuana, since Chinese medicine, which calls cannabis "The Empress of Herbs," specifies it for treating immune disorders. For his trouble, Dana was denounced within the New York Greens in three letters sent in early '87 to 200 people, including three City Councilpersons. [A few months later Dana was busted for pot. All the files of the Impeach Reagan/Bush Campaign were confiscated by a joint federal-state task force. This aborted the protests outside Oliver North's appearance before the Iran–Contra committee, leaving the field clear to *pro*-Ollie demonstrators.

To add insult to injury, Abbie Hoffman was then forced to tell Dana the same environmentalists who'd snitched him out were pressuring Abbie not to work with Dana publicly, scotching any kind of coordination with Abbie's network of anti-CIA activists[1] on the last impeachment protest, October 3rd. Beal was placed on five-years probation on marijuana charges in August 1987. He never talked to Abbie again longer than to say "Hello."]

Dana attended his first ACT UP (AIDS Coalition to Unleash Power) meeting in early April '88 as an unabashed "Safe Drugs" advocate of what the Dutch call "harm reduction," i.e., "reducing the harms involved with drugs." Ever since the '60s, he'd backed legalizing pot as a means of *market separation* of pot and hard drugs. By 1988, though, he'd also come to see

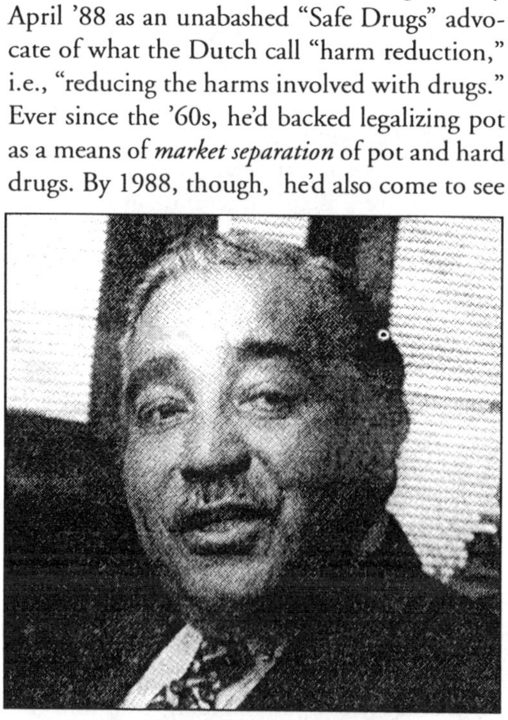

New York Times

REP. CHARLES RANGEL — D., N.Y.

the Dutch model of separate hash cafes as more do-able than outright legalization. He came to ACT UP hoping to get some ACT UP participation in the annual May parade. But he was shocked to see how many people in ACT UP he knew from Studio 10 days. The whole Bruce Brown generation was starting to drop dead of AIDS. Yet to ACT UP cynics, all the well-reasoned "Safe Drugs" manifestos for market-separation (which decreased the growth of new hard drug addiction in Holland 40%[2]) and clean needles (which kept AIDS among intravenous drug users there at 2%, versus 67% in New York City and Newark) only confirmed Dana's status as an outsider who just wanted to push pot.

In 1988, the ACT UP IV-drug user interest group wouldn't even intervene to save NYC's pilot needle exchange program. It was firmly under the control of twelve-step drug-free types led by Richard Elovitch. When Chuck Eaton of the pilot Koch program came to them begging for support against Dinkin's order shutting him down, they told him they considered clean needles to be "enabling addiction." After his experience in the Greens, Dana made a mental note: For the next two years he would furnish no pot to anyone he met through ACT UP; he advised them to grow their own.

Anyone can join New York ACT UP by coming to three general meetings on Monday nights at 208 W. 13th Street. If you don't cultivate the support of a substantial portion of the floor, though, your proposals don't go anywhere. Because a former roommate of Mitch Halberstadt named Steve Ault had vouched for YIP's service in the gay movement, Dana was befriended by ACT UP founder Marty Robinson. But the first time Dana brought up Ibogaine to the floor as a means of interrupting addiction and the spread of AIDS, Marty came to him and warned him he could get ejected if he did it again. Ibogaine was much more offensive to the twelve-step faction than methadone. Methadone had no credibility: it's addictive, whereas with just one treatment Ibogaine offers a 40 percent chance of complete recovery without dependency on a twelve-step group for the rest of your life. Just one treatment.

But Dana was stubborn. In 1989, in the aftermath of Abbie's suicide (due to a combination of cocaine and Prozac), he decided to bypass Central Park and go straight up Fifth Avenue to Rangel's office. Pope Mickey, backed by anarchists who charged Dana had forsaken pot legalization in favor of mere de-crim,

1 Which included Amy Carter. A few weeks earlier Abbie and student anti-CIA protestors had been acquitted by a Massachusetts jury on a necessity defense, a result that was nationally reported, and drew nationwide support. An abortive Impeachment demo was organized by NOW and the Christic Insitute August 12th, but the Christics — who wouldn't deal with "pot activists" — were only willing to work through Abbie, who'd missed out on the Nixon Impeachment, and didn't care. The movement blew its main chance when Ollie testified in July, supported by 50 rightwing pickets, and opposed only by D.C. activist Rupert Chapelle.

2 See Gail Collins, *New York Daily News,* March 8, 1989, on the mayor of Amsterdam at Ed Koch's Mayors' Conference on Drugs: "Amsterdam, which has 700,000 citizens, now has 7,000 addicts — down from 12,000 in 1982... Nearly two-thirds of the remaining 7,000 are in regular touch with health clinics. The drug-related crime rate is dropping five per cent a year. [Mayor] van Thijn attributed this good news to get-tough law enforcement, an aggressive effort to extradite foreign drug addicts, and a legal distinction between hard drugs like heroin and cocaine and soft drugs like marijuana and hashish."

Ethnographic research by Charles Kaplan, et. al. confirmed that new, young junkies were not being recruited from the coffeebar scene because of this market separation—a finding borne out by statistics showing that the mean age of the 7,000 addicts was 10 years older than the original cohort of 12,000.

[allegedly because he owned stock in Ibogaine!?] diverted the first one-fourth and the last half of the parade to the Sheep's Meadow,[1] a "quiet zone" where there couldn't be any sound equipment anyway — no rally. But the Pope had promised to give away a pound of good weed if they could divert the parade to Sheep's Meadow, because he was only interested in passing out business cards with his phone number.

Dana responded by getting more into ACT UP, publishing a pamphlet entitled *What Is the Safe Drugs Movement?*[2] which introduced Ibogaine into the context of Dutch harm reduction. But Ibogaine detractors made him so controversial that people from the Parade and ACT UP both were afraid of being blackballed for working with him. So when, in December 1989, Dana and Marty Robinson co-sponsored a "Safe Drugs" Conference up at 137th St. at City College with Dr. John Morgan, nobody from ACT UP came, and only a few people attended from the marijuana movement. (There was also a cold snap that weekend, and power on the IRT Subway went out.)

The conference did endorse a new plan: the May 1990 Parade would start at Rangel's Spanish Harlem offices (at East 109th) and come *down* town, stopping at the Partnership for a Drug Free America at 666 Third Avenue,[3] and ending up at Washington Square Park. But

[1] This is the same incident referred to in Chapter 6, pp. 59 and 61.

[2] With Mitch Halberstadt & Father Frank Morales, the Squatter Priest.

[3] To evade sonorous mentions of 666 Third Avenue in every hemp rally, the PDFA relocated around the block at the Chrysler Building on Lexington Avenue. However, their parent group — the Advertising Association of America — continues to occupy the original offices at 666 Third, with ominous implications for the truth of any ads we see on TV.

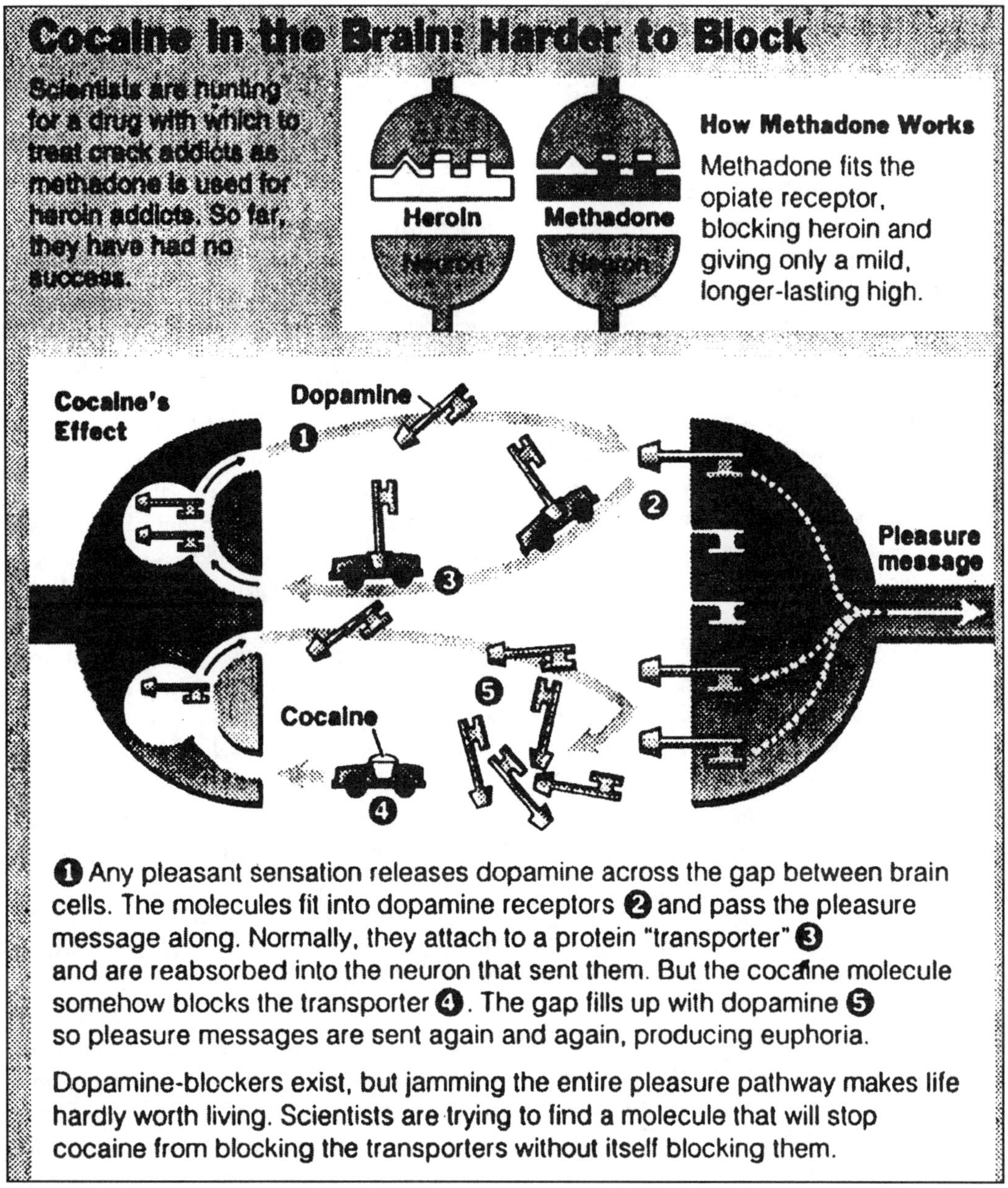

THIS ILLUSTRATION, WHICH APPEARED IN *THE NEW YORK TIMES* "WEEK IN REVIEW," IS ACCURATE AS FAR AS THE "DOPAMINERGIC" DRUGS — AMPHETAMINE, COCAINE, HEROIN, NICOTINE AND ALCOHOL — ARE CONCERNED. HOWEVER, CANNABIS HAS ITS OWN (ANANDIMIDE) RECEPTOR, AS DOES VALIUM (THE "BZD" RECEPTOR). CANNABIS IS *NOT* ACTIVE AT THE DOPAMINE RECEPTOR.

the confab produced another, unanticipated benefit: Dr. Morgan was Chairman of the Pharmacology Department of the City College of New York. He gave the assignment of seeing if Ibogaine would in fact interrupt drug dependency to his workaholic colleague Patricia Broderick, a crack rat scientist.

Now cocaine makes you high more by blocking out negative feedback (perhaps this is related to blocking dopamine re-uptake, *see illustration, preceding page*) than by sensitizing you to positive feedback, as LSD does. This is a tremendous problem when you get into a syndrome like sex-for-crack, because crackheads become numb to useful negative feedback — like soreness in the mucous membranes of the genitals. As old hippies say, "Numb is dumb."

With re-uptake blocked, your neurons have trouble producing another squirt of dopamine; and soon a couple of other neurotransmitters, nor-epinephrin (which makes you irritable and paranoid) and serotonin (which in the presence of nor-epinephrin makes you more awake — aware of how paranoid and irritable you are) come crashing back, just when you feel like your plug has been pulled because your synapses can't get up another squirt of DA.

Presto: the cocaine crash. You can solve this, temporarily, with another hit of crack. But each time makes it worse. Women who trade sex for crack may do it with twenty different partners a night, and because their negative feedback loops are out, they're indifferent to the need for condoms. Anyway, a condom *costs* more than a hit of crack.

This is very bad for the AIDS crisis.

In a little more than a year, Dr. Broderick would come back with tantalizing news: in her lab rats, Ibogaine was bringing dopamine in cocaine-habituated rats back down to normal levels, without depressing them completely, which would cause anhedonia (no pleasure at all) and paralysis.[1]

[1] See illustration, p. 130.

Dana's next move, just after Christmas '89, was to fly to Hamburg. Hans-Georg Behr had been keeping abreast of Ibogaine since he stayed at 9 Bleecker in late 1983, trying to find a publisher for his hemp book. Now Beal told Georg it was time to move Ibogaine to the top of the agenda in Germany.

Georg's political party, the Green Alternative List, controlled the Hamburg state government in coalition with the socialists. In Germany, like Holland and Switzerland, doctors have the right to use experimental therapies without government approval. Georg agreed to try to get the Hamburg Health Ministry to sponsor clinical trials. But somehow with the fall of East Germany (where Georg discovered indications the communists did their own Ibogaine trials in humans from '85–'88) approval was held up on the *federal* level, perhaps under US prodding in the context of the overall trade-off for the absorption of the Eastern states.

Back in the US, Dana kept trying to get the *Village Voice* to publish Max Cantor's article. As the months went by, Max had to write three major updates. One that was never used was devoted to an attempt to get the badboy of Rock 'n' Roll, Johnny Thunders, to take Ibogaine. Thunders had approached Dana about doing his new single on the homeless at the annual RAR concert. But Dana, who was in touch with that whole scene of junkie musicians through John Spacely, refused to barge in and change the schedule unless Johnny backed Ibogaine — say, by being treated.

Thunders said yes, at first. But at the initial meeting with Sisko and Howard, he balked — he thought Ibogaine would be too much like LSD, which he didn't like. He and Stiv Bators and Cheetah Chrome were all on mucho methadone. By exaggerating his heroin habit, Cheetah claimed to have talked a program into giving him enough to get a full opiate high.

Spacely, on the other hand, was totally off smack, doing great on pot. His giant cartoon likeness, with eyepatch, smoking a cigarette, was on a wall on St. Mark's place — an ad for Lech's movie, *Gringo,* which had premiered in the mid-'80s. Spacely constantly encouraged John Holmstrom and the other *Punk* magazine alumnae who now put out *High Times* to run more about Ibogaine.

But the *Voice* still wouldn't print Max's story. To ratchet up the pressure, Beal had his friend Charlie Kritsky (whose sumptuous showroom had just opened up in record time, thanks to Jeff's successful treatment) get an Ibogaine story published by the competition — *The Village Beat.* And knowing a different *Voice* writer was pushing yet another story (the same tired story) on Pope Michael, and that the *Voice* prefers to throw coverage to advertisers, Dana thoughtfully purchased a large ad for the Safe Drugs Parade for May 5, 1990. He knew Pope Mickey was only interested in *free* advertising for his dial-a-joint. The ad specified the parade began with an Ibogaine rally at Rangel's office.

Yet the real breakthrough came from one of the synchronicities that crop up regularly when Ibogaine is involved. On the morning of May 5, 1990, a few hours before the Safe Drugs Parade (going downtown) passed the Marijuana Parade (going uptown) at 42nd Street, Bob Sisko began his most important treatment yet: Nico Adriaans, the founder of the Dutch junkie liberation movement.

And videotaped it.

One day some months earlier, Nico, a community field worker for the Addiction Research Center, had been talking to Charlie Kaplan, the head of the center, which is part of Erasmus University in Rotterdam. And Kaplan mentioned Ibogaine. A little later, Nico was putzing around Kaplan's desk, and he came across *A Summary of Nine Case Histories,* by Bob Sisko. Nico was fascinated because, besides being a salaried government worker, he was also an addict, doing three-fourths of a gram of high-grade Dutch heroin a day. In fact, Nico was the founder of the Dutch Junkie-bond (junkie union), with a role parallel to Dana's as founder of the marijuana movement in the United States.

So he asked Kaplan, What about this Ibogaine? Can you get any? Do you have to go to the States? And one day at the end of April 1990, he had an appointment with Sisko, which he didn't know about, but was made by Charlie. And he told Sisko the story of how, after the Dutch had achieved civil rights for potheads in 1976, the mayors of the four big cities in Holland — Amsterdam, Rotterdam, the Hague and Utrecht — in 1979 came up with a proposal for forced therapy for heroin addicts. When they had to back down because of the outcry from civil liberties advocates, the mayors amended their proposal to lock up only the kids who were using.

Nico's background was organizing other kids when he was in the orphanage, so he was against this plan. He and some other friends on the junkie street scene put out a leaflet

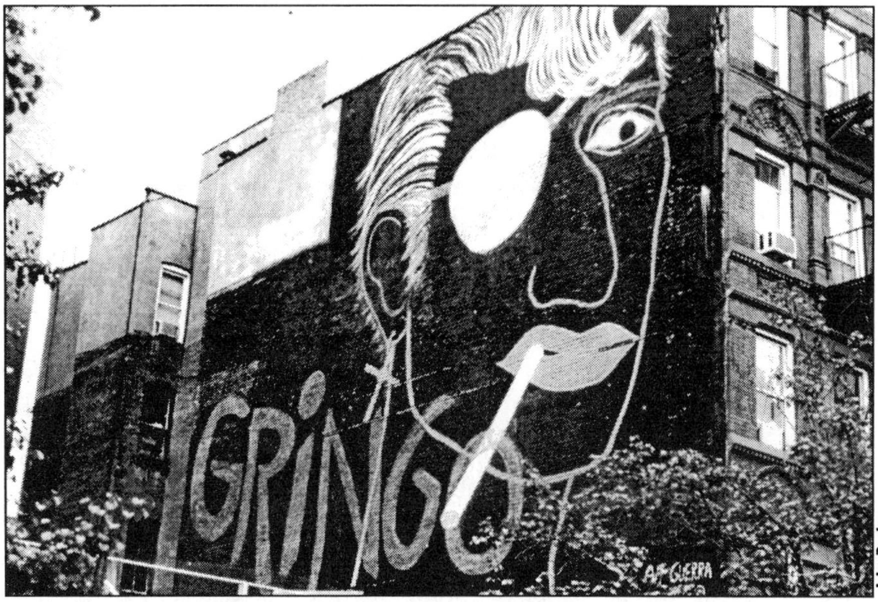

John Pandey

JOHN SPACELY LIVES! — ON THE WALL ON ST. MARK'S PLACE.

and got almost one hundred addicts together for the founding meeting of the Junkie Bond. At the meeting they wrote down ideas for a manifesto for junkie liberation, and a separate bill of rights. And they composed a telegram, which they sent to the mayors, telling them the plan for civil commitment of users was unacceptable.

They began to crash meetings and hearings, to pressure city councils and the Health Ministry. But the cops still harassed the junkies, because in those days the dominant idea was still, as in the United States today, that you have to hound the addict, so he can't feel safe and secure. First you have to break them down so they're on the street as prostitutes or thieves — so they will "bottom out" sooner — and *then* they will accept your therapy (which is so lame to begin with that it's the last thing they would choose to do voluntarily).

Yet unlike junkies in the United States, who have historically aligned themselves with wealth or power or at least a cop in order to make individual deals for themselves, the Junkie-bond made an alliance with the squatters movement. The squatters were very knowledgeable about real estate. They had found out certain members of the Dutch criminal underworld had made a lot of money on heroin, and decided to get out of "the business" and into real estate. To wash the money, white as snow, they employed the services of a certain Schlauffenberg's Bank.

So the junkies and the squatters got together and xeroxed the brightly colored Dutch currency in black and white (black money), and made up little bags of salt and talcum powder, which looked just like bags of dope. After tipping off the media, about one hundred people went to the headquarters of the Schlauffenberg's Bank and went running through the lobby and the halls throwing the little bags and the black money up in the air.

A funny thing happened. A few days later there was a big police raid on the headquarters building of the Schlauffenberg's Bank. The cops found all sorts of illegal things, double books, proof of money-laundering. The Bank officers were all busted, but of course, not one of them did a single day in jail. After that, however, someone told the police to lay off the street junkies, and life became somewhat more tolerable.

At a certain point there were about twenty-five Junkie-bond locals in Holland, and a few in Germany, in Frankfurt and so-on. The first needle-exchange was set up by these groups, in 1981, to fight the spread of hepatitis. The first AIDS education in the world was done by these groups. They formed an organization of parents of users. They formed the Broad Front for the Reform of Drug Policy, for all the clergy, lawyers and social do-gooders who became involved.

The government even gave the Junkie-bond a subsidy of 25,000 guilders a year. But as Dutch government employees, they were of course expected to get off dope. Because of international pressure, Dutch authorities still sought to de-tox methadone clients instead of giving them as much as they wanted. One of the first things the Junkie-bond did was to write a Black Book of the experiences of thirty-six methadonians, how they were forced to cut down, etc. The struggle of the '80s was pretty much to get the freedom to use.

Why, in this most liberal of all societies, would Nico Adriaans be looking for a better way to quit?

Because cold turkey is the junkie's regular companion. Just as junk sickness is a part of their mornings. When the monkey on your back turns into a 600-pound gorilla, you have to cold turkey just to be able to afford your habit. Nico had tried to quit many times, but he couldn't get through withdrawal: "First you go on a holiday; then you think, 'Just five more minutes,' then you say, 'Shit, it's for the fishes.'"

By the time he saw Sisko's *Nine Case Studies* he was simply tired — really tired — of dope. "It's not the running, because I hardly run. It's not the stealing; I didn't steal. It's not the dope, 'cause I liked the dope — I had good times with it, bad times — but *I just don't like it anymore.*"

So that he would know what to expect, Sisko had him read *Bwiti: An Ethnography of the Religious Imagination in Africa,* by James F. Fernandez, especially Chapter 18, on the normal experience of initiates who eat the raw root bark of the *Tabernanthe iboga* bush in Gabon.

The night before Nico's treatment, he did up his last shot, about 150 milligrams of 50%-pure Dutch heroin. Then he didn't eat anything in the morning, just had a little tea. Soon after the allergy dose (10 mg.), Nico did the first half of his Ibogaine, and within ten minutes recognized (as an LSD veteran) the first faint vibrations. After the second half of his dose, thirty minutes later, he became aware that he no longer had any junk sickness. He noticed the edges of objects beginning to oscillate. He was just asking for a cup of coffee when he became slightly confused; then suddenly his mind cleared: he *knew.*

"Certain sounds would suddenly become like synthesized voices," he said later, "and I felt sea legs. So I went to bed, behind the curtain, trying to meet my ancestors... And then at a certain moment I lost all control of time, and it really *banged* into my head."

He experienced the sensation of cosmic impact (but not pain) that the Bwiti call "the splitting of the skull." And the visualizations began: "On the surface of my eyes, the moistures, like on the surface of a bubble, started running all over each other, becoming blue, yellow, depending on how thick the tears were. And I laid down on the bed — very easy — and the people around me were very encouraging, understanding."

But the rush was the most overwhelming of his life: "There you are — O God, O God, O God, God, God. Oh, man! What an experience, Ibogaine!" Behind the curtain, the treatment team had darkened the room. "On the walls I saw things that could remind me of the original tradition, as how I have read it: in the images I saw, [archetypes[1]] like the woman in the tent, the Priest... and it's hard to explain, because you don't *know* [in the Gnostic sense] anything any more [now that you've come down] but I am certain... I be introduced by, by — shit! — by the Bwiti..."

Just to Whom he had difficulty even articulating, until interviewed again, nine months later, in Feb. '91:

> "At the end of the visions, I really had, the only way how I can describe it is I had a meeting with God, or the Supreme Being.
>
> "There was clouds. And it was blue. And then, up there somewhere, some sort of a rectangle opened up. And there came a lot of light... And all the time increasing, increasing, increasing... And it felt like, you know, there's something impressive there.
>
> "And then a Voice came to me, and said to me, asked: *'Do you KNOW, now?'*
>
> "And I only could say [lowering voice]: 'Yes, I *KNOW* now.'
>
> "And then the Voice said: 'So you *KNOW*!' in a way it would say, like, 'So you *KNOW*; *ACT* like it!' "

Then there came a long phase where the visualizations were less and less, but he still thought a lot about those things; and then a period of nausea, but not like cold turkey, "which feels like your stomach is being scratched out," but more like the purgative effects of the Ibogaine.

Finally, when the trip was mostly over, he experienced a bit of withdrawal — hot and cold flashes, sweat — but no running nose, no diarrhea, intestinal contractions or muscle cramps. Said Nico: "You're still not totally in control of your body, your legs don't want to move; you have to turn around in your bed all the time; you want to be left alone, you still don't want to talk."

Most of all Nico is amazed, when Sisko interviewed him on video just afterwards, when he realizes two and a half *days* have gone by and he feels no need to go out and score dope.

He relishes the taste of a cup of coffee. He's been up for forty-eight hours, and yawning, so he tries to steady himself with a cigarette. But after one drag, he tries to spit the taste out of his mouth and throws it out the window!

The tobacco tastes terrible. It's sickening. Nicotine and heroin, remember, have exactly the same effect on dopamine receptors (*increased rate of neuronal firing* — Glick). With Nico's tobacco "tolerance" stripped away, the nicotine effect is sickening enough to overwhelm any pleasurable tobacco taste.

His pattern of rolling a cigarette whenever he starts to fiddle with his hands is undisturbed. The nicotine lives up to his expectation that it will "focus" him enough to finish the interview (indeed, with a single drag, much less than usual). But Nico has inadvertently kicked cigarettes, despite only intending to quit heroin.

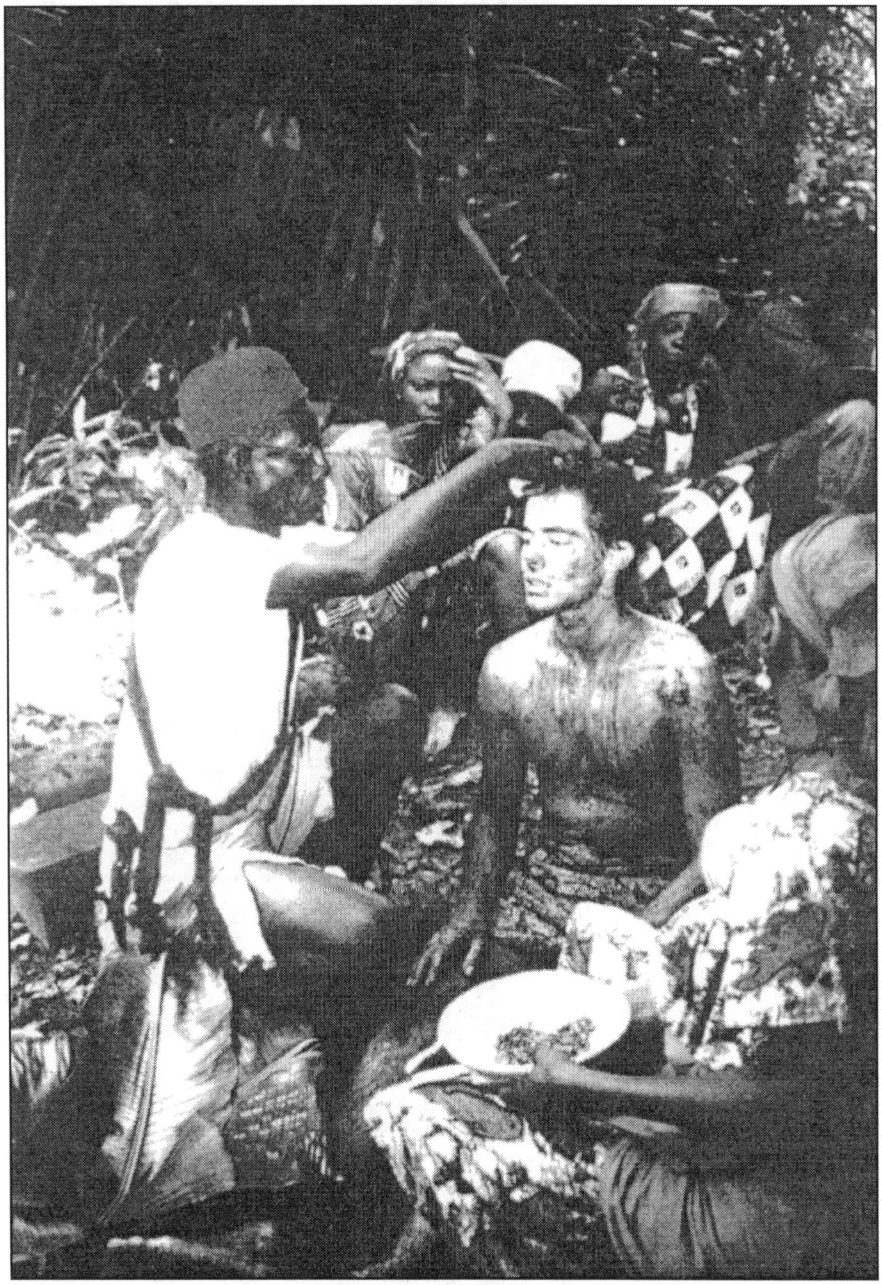

INITIATION OF YOUNG FRENCH MAN

1 See Carl Jung, *Archetypes and the Collective Unconsciousness,* (c. 1935). Fernandez catalogues them to some extent. There is some affinity to the Platonic Idea, i. e, "a clear glass woman who came out of the wall" was typical.

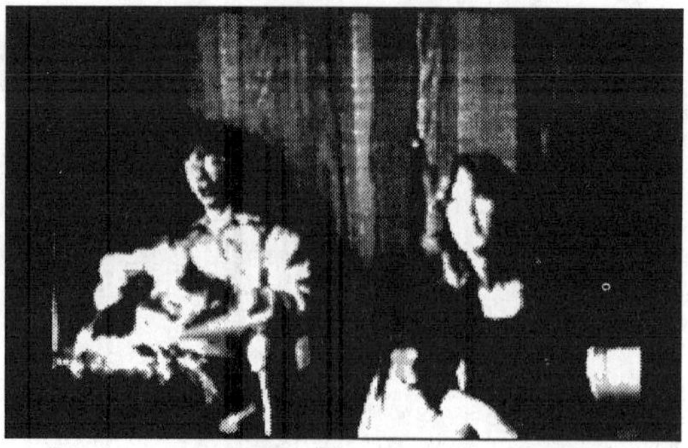

1 NICO ROLLS A CIGARETTE...

Not only that, during his truncated withdrawal, his girlfriend came, and they made a date for him to slip out and do some dope. But at the appointed time he couldn't summon up that familiar craving he'd been using to organize his daily existence for all his adult life: "The Ibogaine let me stay in the bed... I *couldn't* want to go out."

Four times he repeats parts of a poem, by Ginpo Zenzi, which exactly expresses the futility of fighting withdrawals with dope:

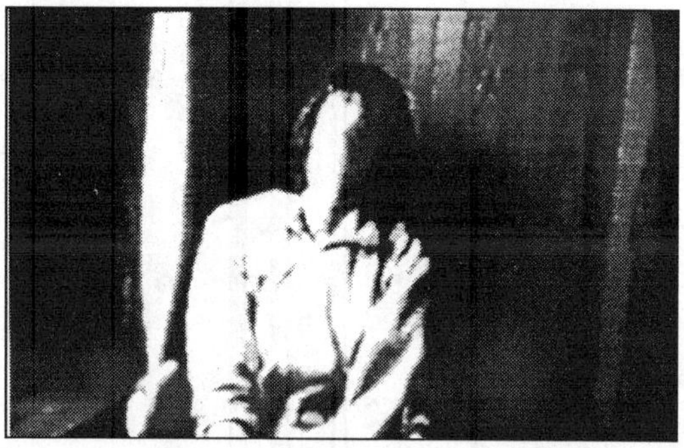

3 ...BUT AFTER JUST ONE DRAG...

It is a simple fact:
Whatever you resist, will persist.
If you are resisting suffering, you suffer more.
If you are trying to deny your confusion, you remain confused.
If you are striving for Peace, you find yourself constantly disturbed.

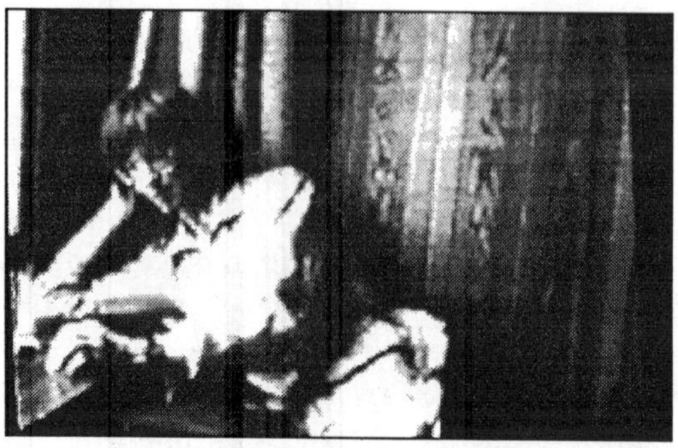

5 ...AND FLICKS IT OUT THE WINDOW.

If you are seeking after clarity, you are in a muddle.
If you do not want to be angry, you are going to walk around angry.
If you do not mind being angry, you will never be bothered by anger.
Because you will constantly be pushing it away.
Having no options, For or Against,
Just being open to whatever comes,
You are free.

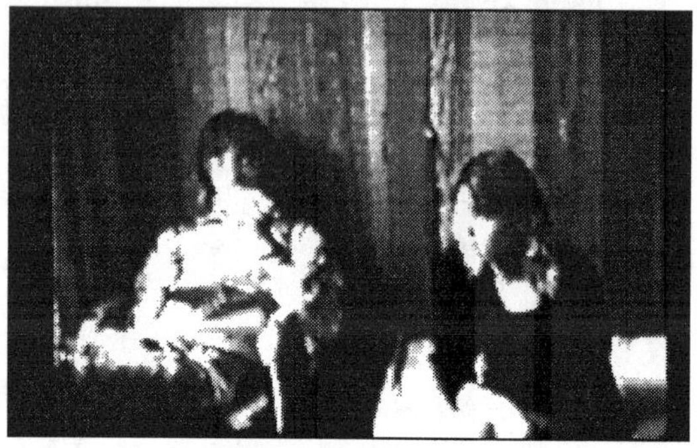

2 ...LIGHTS UP...

He cautioned that Ibogaine is an *ordeal;* but as to whether it should be developed as a cure for addiction, Nico said: "Yes."

"I think that drug use... is a part of humanity. Throughout the history of mankind, over the whole globe, all continents, every people, every nation — has, have had — and is developing new drugs, or mind-altering states. And so I think it is very important, what you have done now here in my case, to write a good report, about how you recruited, who you met, what the problems were."

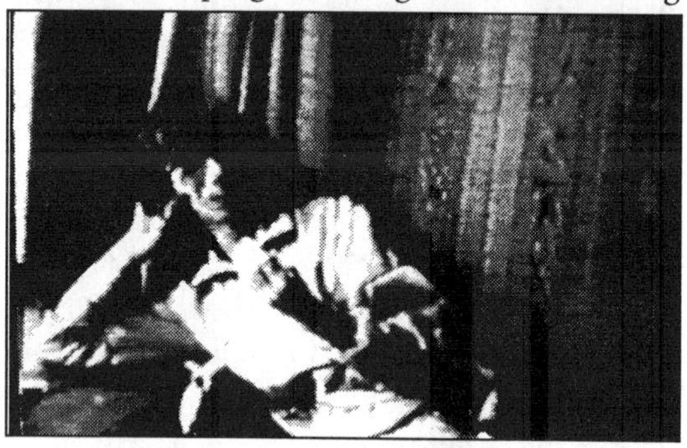

4 ...LOOKS AT IT IN PERPLEXITY...

Nico was a convert. He took to wearing dashikis and studying Jung. And Sisko left him with a small supply of Ibogaine. After treating Josien Harms, his girlfriend, the two of them decided to put Ibogaine to the hardest test. What would happen if they gave Ibogaine to worst-case junkies in Amsterdam's Central Railroad Station, with no Bwiti stuff, no orientation beyond "Take this, it will stop withdrawal"?

They gave it to a methadonian couple who were also doing heroin. The man was doing 180 milligrams of methadone a day (three times the normal U.S. dose). The woman believed she was possessed by devils, and was on anti-psychotic medication for that as well as methadone. At first Howard was disappointed when he heard the man was still on 30 milligrams of methadone after Ibogaine.

"Au contraire," said Nico.

"The people running the methadone program had never seen *anyone* go from 180 to 30 milligrams in one jump. It would be fatal. Best of all, the woman discontinued thorazine. She no longer believes she is possessed by devils."

Nico and Josien went on to spread the gospel of Ibogaine throughout the junkie liberation scene of Europe, although they found 70 percent of the movement considered it to be a diversion from the basic goal of legalizing heroin. But back in the U.S., the videotape of Nico's treatment, which Dana spent months laboriously re-editing, turned out to be the key that unlocked support among both AIDS activists and the legalization movement. Dana sent hundreds of copies of it all over the world.

One of the first to see it, raw and unedited in Sisko's living room, was the *Village Voice* writer Max Cantor. Now he *really* started hassling his editors, and the combination of that pressure and the purchase of a *Voice* ad for the May 5th Safe Drugs demo, led on June 4, 1990 to the publication of *Miracle Cure.* It was Dana's first big media score for Ibogaine, and he scarcely cared that Max, for "balance," repeated the canard of his opponents, that he owned "hundreds of thousands of dollars in Ibogaine stock."

[Hundreds of thousands of dollars of stock in a company with a capitalization at the time of $600,000 would leave nothing for the twenty-six actual investors! In truth, Dana realized in 1988 that stock ownership would undermine his effectiveness as a public health advocate, just as taking Ibogaine would open him up to charges he was another Timothy Leary who only wanted to legalize his favorite drug. He could be faulted for having a political agenda, but not a hidden one. He made no secret of his belief that Ibogaine could plug the gaping hole in AIDS prevention efforts caused by the current dearth of treatment for addicts.]

Two weeks later Nelson Mandela landed at Kennedy Airport. At the last minute a stop had been added — the first speaking engagement on his U.S. tour — at Brooklyn Boys and Girls High School. Because ROCK AGAINST RACISM was the only one with the equipment to do it on such short notice, the T. K. Forcade rock-and-roll-assault sound stage was pressed into service, and Dana ended up being one of the roadies.

When Mandela was done with his speech, Dana tapped him on the back with a copy of the *Village Beat* article (he'd given away all the *Voice* reprints). As Mandela turned to see who it was, the security on stage in front of the two of them parted. The moment was captured on television all over the city — Dana Beal handing Nelson Mandela the Ibogaine information. They shook hands. And then, gesturing to the piece of paper but encompassing the stage, ROCK AGAINST RACISM, the Staten Island Project, the entire organization he'd spent his life building since 1965, Dana said: "We worked for twenty-five years on this."

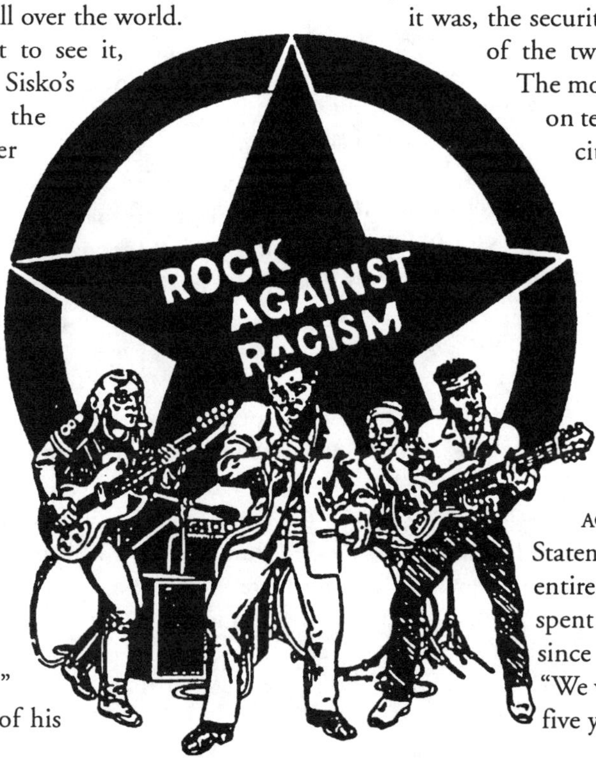

CHAPTER 9: Jon Parker

Later that same afternoon, June 22, 1990, Dhoruba Bin Wahad experienced the crowning moment (at least 'til that point) of *his* life. Black radicals in Harlem had demanded that Dhoruba — not Charles Rangel, David Dinkins or Jesse Jackson — must give the welcoming address at 125th Street. Only an ex-political prisoner unjustly imprisoned for nineteen years for a crime he didn't commit was qualified to greet Mandela, they insisted.

The politicians, he said, "do not want me to give you this address, because they do not want our South African brothers to know there are *Black political prisoners* held in the United States!

"There is a common thread and a common humanity that we all share. My Brother, I have spent nineteen years in prison in the United States for my political beliefs, and you, sir, you were the symbol that helped sustain me and other African American political prisoners!" And they shook hands, and were seen embracing all over the world.

Dhoruba Moore, now Bin Wahad (son of the One), had been released on February 19, 1990—his conviction overturned due to prosecutorial misconduct—and that very day Dana had given him the news about Ibogaine also. Once, when Dhoruba was still in prison and Tanaquil Jones was being evicted, Alan Thompson stopped everything by parking the soundstage in front of her building; so in the next few months, Dhoruba began to work with RAR.

February 1990 was also the month Dana met the pioneer of needle exchange in the United States, Jon Parker. Parker had already been driving down from Boston every week for more than a year to exchange clean needles for dirties with his "regulars" at the corner of Delancey and Essex. Now he was pulling together John Morgan's group, ACT UP, and survivors of the small city program cancelled by David Dinkins to challenge the law. A month earlier, he'd just won the first test case in the country in Boston, and he was on a roll. He was determined to overthrow needle prohibition wherever it existed.

Parker created a situation where the IV drug users committee of ACT UP had to play catch up: In March, 1990, Dana accompanied Richard Elovitch up to the front of the ACT UP meeting for the only time. Together they moved the floor to endorse a protest at Delancey and Essex, where eight activists including Parker would court arrest for needle exchange. But the minute Beal started talking civil rights for drug users, Elovitch ruled him out of order.

The protest went as planned; the case of the Needle Exchange 8 began wending its way through the courts. In June, Dana gave copies of the *Voice* article to Parker and everyone else doing needle exchange at the new site, Rivington and Attorney, a few blocks from the original site. But most of the others weren't as pioneering as Parker. And Ibogaine didn't have the endorsement of Ernie Drucker and the experts favored by Elovitch and ACT UP honcho Larry Kramer. So they just didn't get it.

One evening in August, when Parker was in Thailand setting up needle exchange for the Thai government, he had a flash: If needle exchange is only 35 percent effective in stopping the spread of AIDS, and Ibogaine is 70 percent effective for interrupting addiction and injection for three to eighteen months or longer, then Ibogaine is a breakthrough technology. Any medical breakthrough against the AIDS pandemic must be used, the sooner the better. When he got back to the US and informed Dana of this, Beal asked him to speak at the November 10th Stop the Drug Wars March in Washington.

By August, America was gripped by the worst pot drought in history, as Bush interdiction efforts — which only seemed to proliferate the more compact hard drugs — virtually eliminated bulky, smelly marijuana from the market. An ounce of moldy pot became more expensive than an ounce of coke, and even *The New York Times* noticed. There were back-to-back famines in '90 and '91, with only a few months break during the winter.

On August 4, 1990 Dana flew in and spoke at a rally for his best friend in San Francisco, Dennis Peron, who'd been busted for pot in January. The pot belonged to Beal's second-best friend in S.F., Jonathan West, who was using it to fight off his AIDS. The stress of the case was killing him. In nine months the most beautiful man Dana knew had turned into a concentration camp survivor with KS (Kaposi's Sarcoma) lesions in one eye. And with the famine, because the only pot Jonathan could get was moldy, his lungs were trashed. He lived just long enough to plead guilty in September to possessing the four ounces of pot in January. But that saved his best friend, Dennis Peron, from five years imprisonment as a predicate felon. Ten days later Jonathan West died.

Nonetheless, outside of San Francisco the marijuana movement still wasn't quite ready to deal with "safe drugs" and AIDS. When Dana was heckled by a group of rednecks and off-duty cops at the annual Woodstock Reunion concert two weeks later, hemp activists present decided the thing to do was to feature him a lot less as a speaker.

Two weeks later he was banned in Boston from giving a scheduled speech at a "marijuana freedom fighter" rally — to keep him from bringing up Ibogaine along with hemp. So he joined the Hemp Tour and talked Ibogaine from Philadelphia to Madison, Wisconsin. The hempsters hit back by spreading the phony factoid about him owning "hundreds of thousands in Ibogaine stock" everywhere he went.

But the lowest blow came when "freedom fighters" re-printed Baumann's phony Ibogaine death story into *High Times* without checking out the ultimate source: a German supermarket tabloid.[1]

We now know, based on Glick's work, that one possible way to potentiate the effect of 400 mgs. of Ibogaine to get an overdose is to give it with amphetamine. In fact according to Goutarel, Claudio Naranjo submitted a patent application in 1969 for a drug composed of the total alkaloids of *Tabernanthe iboga* roots combined with amphetamine.[2] MDMA is an amphetamine. Baumann's prefered drug for his intrusive brand of therapy is MDMA — which makes the patient putty in the therapist's hands. Ibogaine subjects, on the other hand, just want to be left alone.

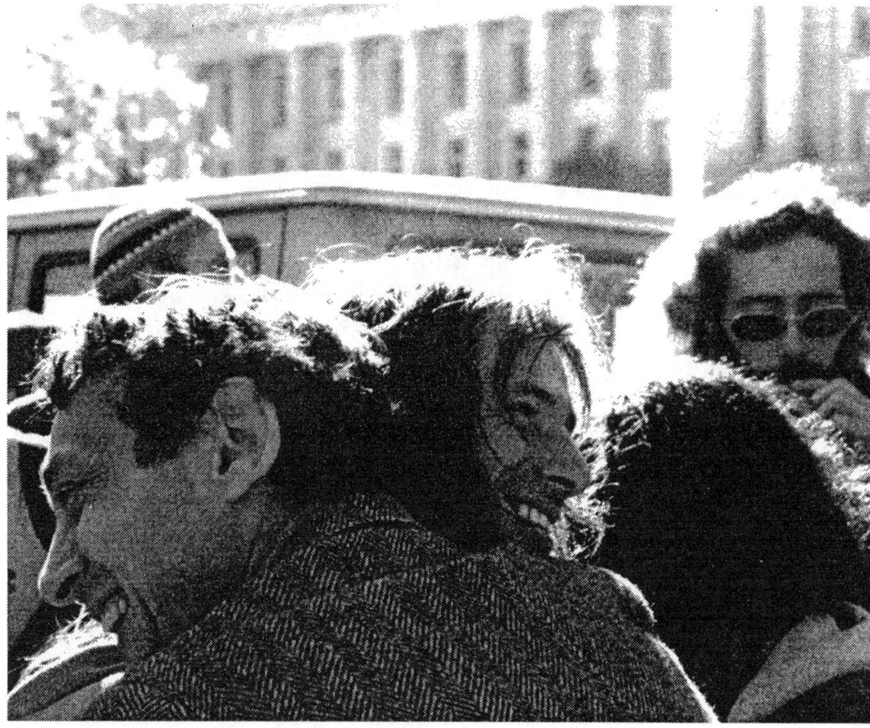

DENNIS PERON (CENTER), EMBRACED BY HARVEY MILK (MARTYRED GAY SAN FRANCISCO ACTIVIST)

Justifiable suspicions that MDMA had been administered with or after the 400 mgs. of Ibogaine were not dispelled, and if anything only increased, when the Swiss Psychelytic Association agreed to stop working with Ibogaine in order to preserve research access to other psychedelics in Switzerland. "The treatment of addiction," Baumann pronounced, "is beyond the competence of the psychiatrist."

To say the least, the rush by Rick Doblin (America's foremost MDMA proponent) to reprint a story from a supermarket tabloid in *MAPS* (Multi-Disciplinary Association for Psychedelic Studies) *Bulletin,* should have set off alarm bells at *High Times.* Especially when the approval for MDMA had just been withdrawn by the FDA over safety concerns.

John Spacely, a consistent Ibogaine booster who tried to mediate between his friends at *High Times* and Beal, asked them to lighten up with their coverage. But he was closer to the problem. It was around that time he informed Dana that Stiv Bators, who'd wandered out of his place drunk a few nights earlier and been hit by a car on 9th Street, had walked away unaware of serious internal injuries because of methadone analgesia — and died a day later.

1 See p. 56, [brackettted material].

2 As a treatment for addiction. To complicate matters even more, Naranjo's method included injecting ¼ of the drug. Hans-Georg Behr estimated that the portion injected might be ten times more potent, but that still didn't altogether explain it.

Happens frequently. Nasty combination, methadone and alcohol. Three out of 623 subjects in the LAMM (longer-acting methadone) trials died — two from impairment of their body's ability to process other shit they took while they were on LAMM.[1]

[1] Stands for *Levo-Acetl-Methadol.* The third fell off a roof.

Advocates of environmental hemp or squatting were not alone in suspecting Ibogaine, if it worked, would disrupt any agenda they might have in mind. Jon Parker had agreed to speak at the November 10th Stop the Drug Wars March even though he would have to drive all the way down from Boston to Washington two weekends in a row. On November 3rd he had to be at the annual Drug Policy Foundation (DPF) awards dinner to collect a $50,000 check for his victories on behalf of needle exchange.

The foundation's deputy director, Kevin Zeese, had specified that doing a Stop the Drug Wars March the day after his conference would be considered a "hostile act"; so six months earlier Dana reluctantly rescheduled it from the 4th to November 10th, even though it meant the DPF crowd would not be able to attend. And the one thing Zeese, his boss Arnold Trebach and their big-bux backer Richard Dennis all asked Parker not to mention in his speech was Ibogaine. The minute it was not a drug to be legalized but a treatment to be approved, they were all for ten years of painstaking tests and bureaucratic footdragging. Or else they bought the Baumann story,

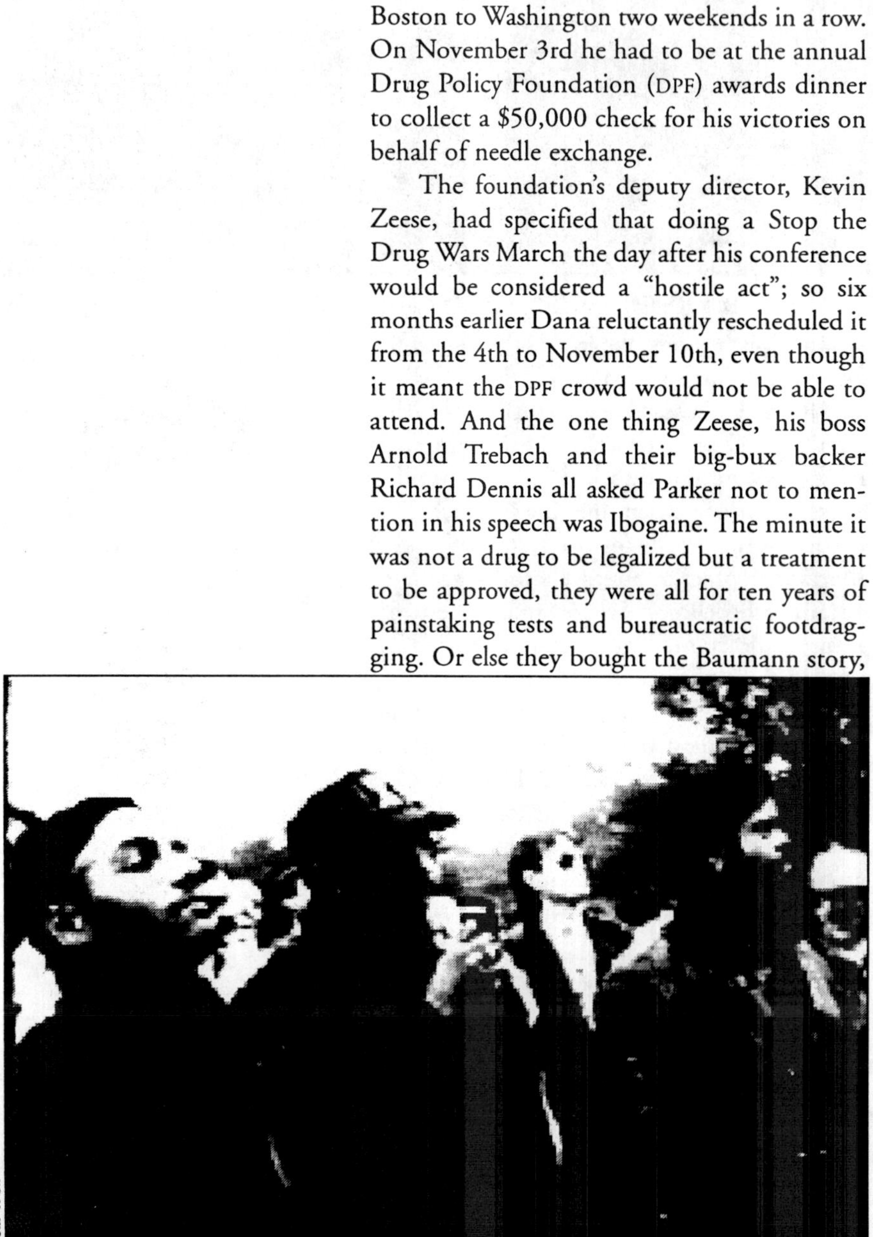

"Passin' It On"

DHORUBA SPEAKING AT THE CAPITOL, MOMENTS BEFORE HE IS GRABBED BY POLICE

and were willing to sacrifice a potential addiction interrupter on the altar of Ecstasy.

At the awards dinner Jon and his mother shared a table with Howard, Norma, Sisko, Dana and Boaz Wachtel. Jon's mother, a poor Irishwoman from South Boston, saw her son get a $50,000 award and tell a roomful of doctors, lawyers, scientists and even a sprinkling of US judges how after spending his adolescence in juvenile detention and much of his adulthood dealing drugs or in prison — one day he was sitting in a shooting gallery in New Haven. He was watching dozens of addicts clean their needles in the same glass of bloody water. The year was 1987, and Parker was a pre-med sudent at Yale, where they were teaching him that AIDS could be spread through shared water and cottons, and not just needles.

Jon Parker got so mad about that glass of bloody water that he started the first US needle exchange, because he knew offering them a sharp new needle was the only way to get the addicts in where you could give them lifesaving information.

The next day, the day Dana had moved the demonstration from — Sunday, November 4 — turned out to be unseasonably warm, a beautiful 65-degree day.

November 10th was cold and wet. The third speaker at the Capitol was Dhoruba Bin Wahad:

> "The War on Drugs that's being waged in the Black Community is a racist excuse for the militarization of the police and the eradication of Black people in this country. The CIA, the FBI and other government agencies have been the major importers of hard drugs into the Black Community ever since the end of World War II. As the head of the CIA, George Bush helped import drugs into this country, and he continues to collaborate with tyrants and dictators who profit off of hard drugs and the exportation of hard drugs.
>
> In the Black Community, the term for the importation of drugs and the murder of our youth is genocide. I think that, if you are steadfast in your struggle to decriminalize certain *aspects* of drugs, if you are steadfast in your position that there should be an emphasis on treatment and not on criminalization, you can begin to make a difference in the war on the Oppressors who import drugs.
>
> "Finally, I want to say to you, that the strug-

gle to free political prisoners in the United States is a struggle against racist and arbitrary repression–that if you do not stand up for the freedom, and dignity, of political prisoners who went to prison and sacrificed their lives for the liberation and empowerment of their people, then one day you might be a political prisoner, and there'll be no movement to support you!

"So you must make a stand. You must take a position. You must take a position to free all political prisoners in the United States and you should take a position that opposes the War on Drugs in the Black Community. Finally, I'd like to say, stay strong, be strong, and fight the Power!"

Halfway through the next speaker, word came that the Capitol Police were busting Dhoruba and his bodyguards just out of sight 300 yards away. The entire crowd — 600 people — went running over to surround the cops, chanting "Let them go! Let them go!" The cops, outnumbered, backed down. Jon Parker was part of the action that freed Dhoruba. Later he confided to Dana that twenty years earlier, like many working-class white kids, he'd thought the Black Panthers were incredibly cool. That militancy was part of the reason he chose a name for his organization like the National AIDS Brigade.

On Thanksgiving, Dana had dinner with Marty Robinson. Marty, whose AIDS had progressed, was wheezing. But because the drought was still on, he was very proud he'd brought his own pot. Dana took one look at the pot and said: "This is really moldy. It would give me bronchitis, and I'm healthy. Throw that away. Let me give you something good." But the drought wouldn't ease for another month, so of course Marty accepted Dana's gift, but kept his own, and got sicker. The grey mold causes *aspergillosis* in people with AIDS.

Ten days later Parker came to the ACT UP floor with info that a rule mandating nonjury trials for misdemeanors in New York City had expired. He wanted to clog the courts with new needle exchange protests. The rest of the Needle Exchange 8 prefered to wait for their trial in the spring. Parker won the vote, but on the day of the action, December 12, no one showed up but Sisko, Howard and some other Lower East Side denizens including Pope Michael. The cops broke Parker's wrist.

Dana went straight from the protest to a speaking date in Providence, Rhode Island, and then to Boston, to try to repair relations with the legalization movement that had cancelled his speaking gig a few months earlier. But the Boston "freedom fighters" still wouldn't parlay, so he stayed with Jon Parker or Andrew Hoffman. By the end of January he'd been up and back three times talking to everyone. And then he learned Parker was having trouble.

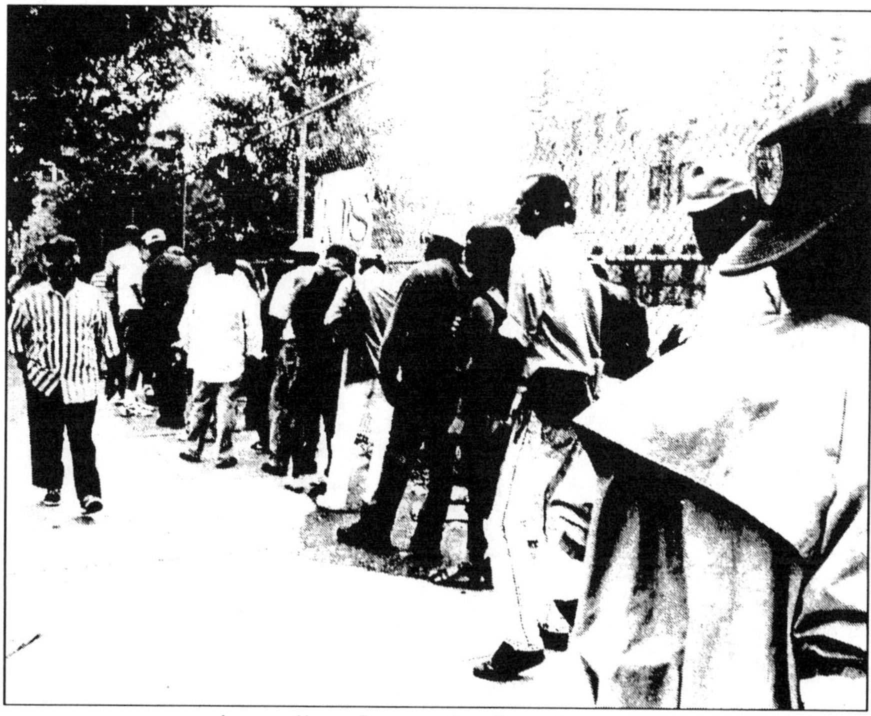

Line for Needle Exchange, New Haven, Connecticut

On January 24, 1991 with part of his $50,000 award, Jon opened a needle exchange office in Roxbury just down the block from a dope spot where he'd been doing street needle exchange. Neighbors already uptight about the dope spot flipped out. They were joined in daily pickets of the AIDS Brigade office by the Rev. Ellis Hagler, who'd been feuding with Jon ever since he'd kicked Jon's nascent needle exchange group out of his nearby church three years earlier.

After two days of picketing under the banner of Treatment on Demand, in the midst of a screaming match (where inflammatory things were said about Jon's mother), Ellis-Hagler decked Jon on television. Once the daily pickets took on the coloration of black/white violence, the majority of the needle exchange decided to dump Jon, keep his money and discontinue needle distribution out of the office.

Mind you, in principle all factions

involved were in favor of treatment on demand. Dana decided to broker a truce by getting all sides to stifle the needle exchange dispute in favor of a broad front to get Boston addicts Ibogaine as soon as possible. Because Ibogaine was the only affordable, effective "on demand" treatment available in the pipeline. But there was one fly in the ointment: The Clean Coalition (the storefront minus Jon) overlapped with some of the people who'd banned Dana from speaking in Boston in September. And if the lie that Dana owned "hundreds of thousands of dollars in Ibogaine stock" started getting pushed around Treatment on Demand, the whole initiative could be torpedoed before it got off the water.

The pot famine in Boston was still going strong, though, and as Dana circulated among AIDS activists promoting an Ibogaine coalition, he kept getting inquiries about good pot, because all the People with AIDS (PWAs) could get was the moldy. As a matter of fact, cheap ($75 an ounce, versus $200 in Boston) non-moldy stuff was now available on the Lower East Side. Hoping to cement relations with people who'd only just learned about Ibogaine from him, Dana agreed to make inquiries.

When he got back to New York, Howard called and told him to look at the *New York Post.* Charles Kritsky was dead. He had been shot in the neck while two thieves held him down on his own bed. Charles, whose rock 'n' roll fashion business was struggling, had turned to the last resort of many a countercultural businessman in the City, and tried to make ends meet by finding a buyer for a large amount of fronted hashish. It wasn't any good, and way too expensive. His buyers turned out to be junkies — the very people Charles was trying to help. Junkies with guns. They ultimately went to prison for decades. But the Ibogaine project had lost a vital activist with unique celebrity contacts.

Dana was in shock, yet he still thought to call Dhoruba, to ask if he knew anybody who could put in a good word with Treatment on Demand up in Boston. "You mean the folks picketing the needle exchange?" asked Dhoruba, "Hey, man, I just got back from Boston, and I spent the weekend with them!"

As a movement of Black accupuncturists, Treatment on Demand was chockful of ex-Black Panthers, and the biggest star — top of the line — they could bring in from outside to rally their troops was none other than Dhoruba Bin Wahad. He'd been arriving in Boston just as Dana was leaving.

Dhoruba's main focus, though, superseding his original mission of stopping hard drugs, was to free the 250 political prisoners in the US. To do that, he had to stay out of jail himself. Two months earlier Dana's people — led by Dennis Peron, Ben Masel, Jack Herer, Aron Kay and, yes, Jon Parker — had kept the cops in DC from snarfing him up.

Besides, Ibogaine, not picketing, is the way to stop hard drugs. You don't take on a Panzer division with rocks and bottles, or even a machine gun. Not when you have the atomic bomb. What Dana needed was for someone to vouch for Ibogaine, plus an intro to Treatment on Demand — and not through the Needle Exchange side, but by someone with impeccable credentials on the other side. Dana asked Dhoruba to propose a freeze on a protests outside the needle exchange in Boston, and a broad coalition around Ibogaine.

Dhoruba came down to East Third Street, where they sat around Sisko's kitchen table as Howard told him about their journey to meet Omar Bongo, and "Gabon's gift to the world." The next weekend, February 17, Howard, Sisko, and Boaz drove up to Boston with a very prestigious introduction to Treatment on Demand and Ellis-Hagler from Dhoruba, who vouched for them but said they'd have to convince people about Ibogaine on their own. Dana traveled up separately on the train and brought Andrew Hoffman to the meeting.

Actually, they were a bit overwhelming. Dhoruba suggested Dana go back the next week alone. Meanwhile, AIDS activists up in Boston wanted to know, where's the pot? Parker, who'd just had his own people roll over on him and stop needle distribution from the office, was paranoid about driving pot back from New York City, even though he drove the thousands of needles down from Boston every week.

On Saturday, February 23, 1991, the morning of the ground invasion of Kuwait, Dana got up and headed out to La Guardia with two and a half pounds of pot strapped to his back. (The source, who'd lost numerous friends to AIDS, upped the shipment the night before from a pound so he wouldn't have to do it again soon: "I'd been holding this for two weeks already," he complained. "Tell them they can take as long as they want to pay.") Dana was flying because he felt that at the meeting the week before, after spending the whole night on the train, he hadn't been sharp enough. His main mission was to get to Roxbury by 11 AM, in time to meet with Black treatment professionals from all over New England. He wasn't even thinking about the pot as he went through the metal detector at the Pan Am Shuttle. The airline, after the Lockerbie bombing, with the tightest security in the business. Traveling under his own name, which is on the ADEX list of people to be picked up in the event of a national emergency *(See composite of FBI files, right).* On the morning of a full national security alert. Dana was pat-searched and busted.

He didn't get to show the Nico tape to Treatment on Demand for three more weeks — until mid-March. It wasn't until April 23, 1991, that Moses Saunders, the executive director of Treatment on Demand, wrote Lotsof a letter, placing Treatment on Demand foursquare behind the project: "We are very pleased to participate in the research initiative around the drug Ibogaine."

Dana would have loved to have gone public and fought the pot charges, like Dennis and Jonathan. But that would've blown his nascent Ibogaine coalition. So he decided to delay, because with his lawyer Bill Kunstler always on a murder trial, cases usually took more than a year anyway. The best the Queens Assistant District Attorney (a certain Karen Rankin) would offer was one-and-a-half to three years in an upstate prison. So Dana finished his last Safe Drugs demonstration May 18, and used it to springboard a July 10th protest called *Storm NIDA For Ibogaine.*

The pot bust forced him to work full-time, to get Ibogaine fast-tracked before the anticipated eighteen-month sentence came due. Oddly, the timing was perfect. In early April his probation officer — infuriated that he fucked up three weeks before she was set to terminate his probation from the '87 bust — forbade him to travel. That kept him from attending the initial April 12 meeting between NIDA Medications Development and Lotsof, where they basically told Howard Ibogaine wasn't ready yet to go on the list of medications being developed for treatment of drug dependency. In other words, "Don't call us, we'll call you." But since Dana hadn't been there, he felt free to call. And Bill Kunstler got a judge to reverse the probation order, so Dana could travel as long as he informed Probation first.

Then, at the end of June, at the annual meeting of the Committee on Problems of Drug Dependency (CPDD) in West Palm Beach, Florida, three papers were presented demonstrating how the Ibogaine effect is real. Patricia Broderick said that hundreds of neuroscientists came to rapt attention, straining to hear her findings that Ibogaine did indeed show efficacy against cocaine addiction: "You could hear a

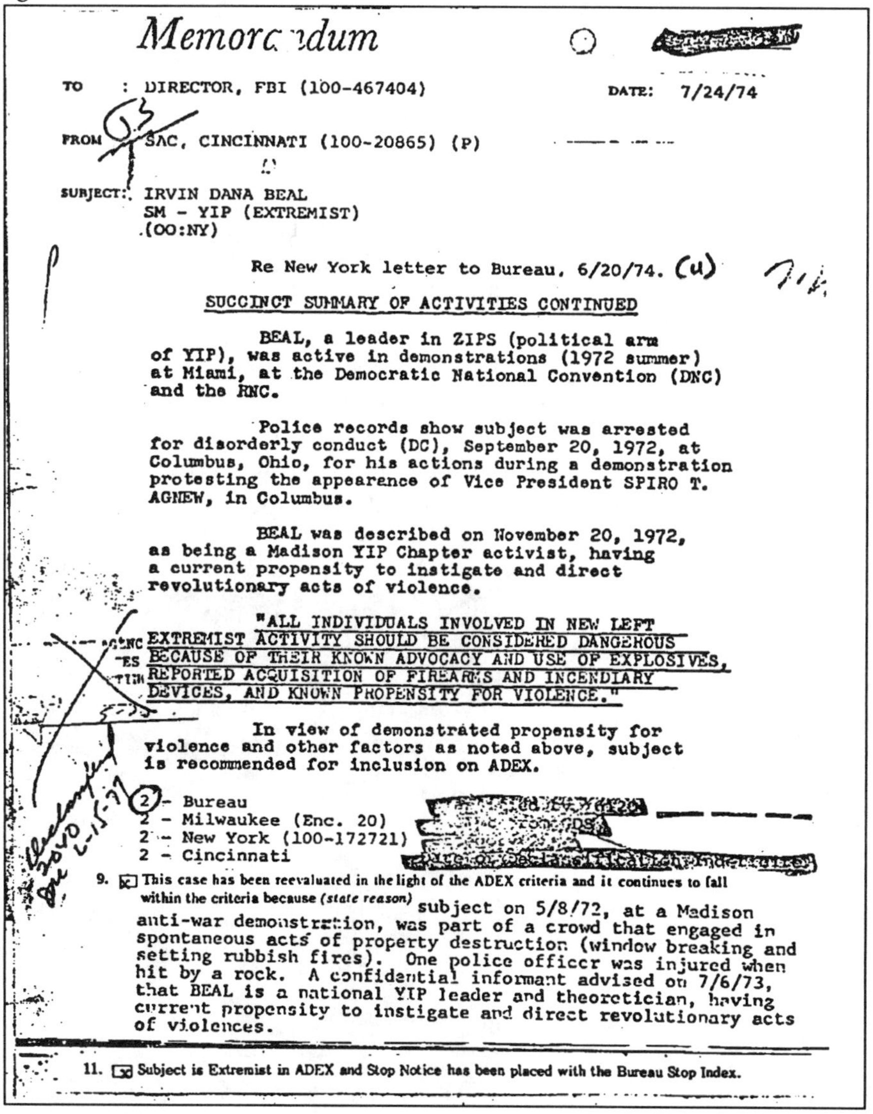

Memorandum

TO : DIRECTOR, FBI (100-467404) DATE: 7/24/74

FROM : SAC, CINCINNATI (100-20865) (P)

SUBJECT: IRVIN DANA BEAL
SM - YIP (EXTREMIST)
(OO:NY)

Re New York letter to Bureau, 6/20/74. (U)

SUCCINCT SUMMARY OF ACTIVITIES CONTINUED

BEAL, a leader in ZIPS (political arm of YIP), was active in demonstrations (1972 summer) at Miami, at the Democratic National Convention (DNC) and the RNC.

Police records show subject was arrested for disorderly conduct (DC), September 20, 1972, at Columbus, Ohio, for his actions during a demonstration protesting the appearance of Vice President SPIRO T. AGNEW, in Columbus.

BEAL was described on November 20, 1972, as being a Madison YIP Chapter activist, having a current propensity to instigate and direct revolutionary acts of violence.

"ALL INDIVIDUALS INVOLVED IN NEW LEFT EXTREMIST ACTIVITY SHOULD BE CONSIDERED DANGEROUS BECAUSE OF THEIR KNOWN ADVOCACY AND USE OF EXPLOSIVES, REPORTED ACQUISITION OF FIREARMS AND INCENDIARY DEVICES, AND KNOWN PROPENSITY FOR VIOLENCE."

In view of demonstrated propensity for violence and other factors as noted above, subject is recommended for inclusion on ADEX.

2 - Bureau
2 - Milwaukee (Enc. 20)
2 - New York (100-172721)
2 - Cincinnati

9. [x] This case has been reevaluated in the light of the ADEX criteria and it continues to fall within the criteria because *(state reason)* subject on 5/8/72, at a Madison anti-war demonstration, was part of a crowd that engaged in spontaneous acts of property destruction (window breaking and setting rubbish fires). One police officer was injured when hit by a rock. A confidential informant advised on 7/6/73, that BEAL is a national YIP leader and theoretician, having current propensity to instigate and direct revolutionary acts of violences.

11. [x] Subject is Extremist in ADEX and Stop Notice has been placed with the Bureau Stop Index.

FBI Composite

pin drop in that room." It was a good omen.

On July 1, 1991, Dana trekked up to the Rainbow Gathering in Vermont, trying to drum up participants for the July 10 NIDA zap. But as soon as he left, two New York squatters, Lori Rizzo and Barbara Lee, got up and denounced Ibogaine to the full Council, claiming it doesn't work. Barbara Lee'd moved in with Seth Tobocman, a roommate of John Penley, who owned Ibogaine stock — so she knew better.[1] But in the two years since Dana decided to make an issue out of Ibogaine, it had become a litmus test of loyalty for their in-group to say it didn't work, as a way of attacking the new harm-reduction-oriented strategy.

1 See Chapter 8, pg. 71; Chapter 11, pg. 110. Rizzo, a rabid Ibogaine foe, mysteriously appeared on the Lower East Side in the aftermath of the '88 riot. Before going on to work for the *New York Post*, Barbara Lee went on to publish a history of the movement which alleged that Beal "stole" the smoke-ins from Abbie Hoffman, when in fact Abbie initially argued against them in council in 1967—for about a month, until they were so successful he showed up to claim a piece of the leadership.

From Vermont Dana travelled to the July 4 White House Smoke-In, where he spoke four times, encouraging people to get out to Rockville the following Wednesday at 8 AM, to picket NIDA at the Parklawn Building. He even gave copies of the "Storm NIDA" leaftlet to Park Police in Lafayette Park, who furnished it to NIDA Medications Development the next morning.

NIDA-crats had no idea how many people were coming, but they did know ACT UP had brought almost a thousand people a year earlier to storm the National Institutes of Health, in Bethesda, Maryland. The first call came in from NIDA counsel Lee Cummings to the phone number on the leaflet, at 9 Bleecker, on Friday, July 5, at 2:30 PM. MDD was offering to meet a delegation from the ad hoc Harm Reduction Coalition representing ICASH, the AIDS Brigade and others, at 11 AM after the demo. On July 9 Charlie Grudzinskas, head of the MDD, faxed Howard a letter stating that they had reconsidered and were placing Ibogaine on the official list of drugs to be evaluated for treatment of drug dependency.

The action was small, a leaflet zap with banners, really. But every secretary in the offices of the FDA, NIDA, NIMH and the Surgeon General at the Parklawn Building was handed a copy of the *Pharm-Analytica* from the end of the previous year, which began:

> **Daily Brief. Executive Summary. Nov. 12, 1990**
>
> International: Drug Addiction
>
> "*Event:* A rainforest Alkaloid, Ibogaine, has been reported to act as an addiction interrupter across a wide spectrum of abused substances including heroin, cocaine, amphetamine, nicotine and alcohol.
>
> "*Significance:* There is a large potential market for pharmaceutical products for use in addict detoxification.
>
> "*Analysis:* The use of pharmaceuticals in combatting addiction is well established, though often of limited success.The claimed effect of Ibogaine is qualitatively different from that of established treatments..."

Two thousand leaflets went out. No longer could some little group in the building bottle up the information. The entire bureaucracy knew. On the government side at the 11 AM meeting were NIDA Attorney Lee Cummings, Charles Grudzinskas, his deputy Frank Vocci and Mona Brown for NIDA public relations; for the coalition, Bob Sisko and

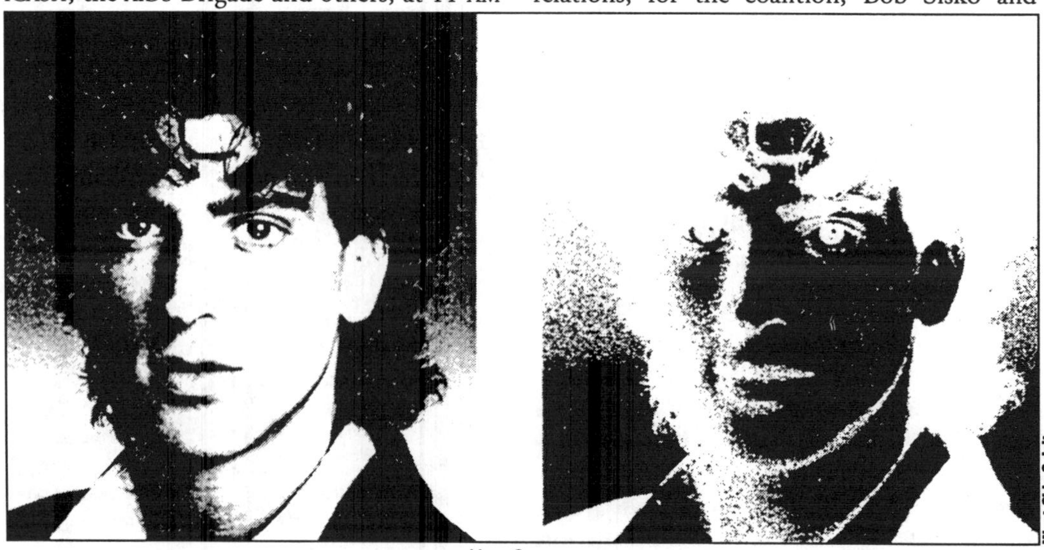

West Side Spirit

MAX CANTOR

Dana Beal, and Eric Sterling of the Criminal Justice Policy Foundation.

The main government demand was for rigorous follow-up data, since they wouldn't look at it in humans at all without an FDA green light; but they were skeptical because they hadn't seen it work on humans. "What if there's a secret ingredient?" Vocci asked. Grudzinskas also held up a story from a German supermarket tabloid on the Baumann death. "It might have been a drug interaction,"[1] Sisko responded as he asked for a xerox. "But in Gabon, out of thousands who take it, every year there are one or two deaths, usually women or physically slight males.[2] With the root they can't really control the dose."

The NIDA side confirmed that Ibogaine was now on their list for evaluation, but refused to issue a statement, although Mona Brown confirmed it to *Newhouse News* the next day. When they were walking out, though, Lee Cummings did say that if it worked, Ibogaine would be like polio vaccine replacing the iron lung.

With some concrete progress to show for his efforts at last, Dana began going to every committee of ACT UP looking for a sponsor. He became the Ibogaine man. He stopped putting medical marijuana stuff on the literature table of the Monday night meeting for eight months. He had a new Ibogaine re-print every other week. Finally, he joined the Treatment and Data Committee — the oldest and biggest in ACT UP — just when T&D was looking to open up relations with NIDA.

On October 20th, Max Cantor was found in his apartment, dead of a heroin overdose. He'd been sucked into the scene he was investigating — junkies and anarchists around Tompkins Square Park cannibal Danny Rakowitz.

Before his arrest in August, '91, Rakowitz definitely sided with Jerry the Peddler and the anti-Ibogaine faction from Tompkins Park,[3] so it made a weird kind of sense for Max (who never quit looking for Charlie Manson) to fish around Rakowitz for a larger Satanic conspiracy — except that the only Satanists on the scene were a few Aleister Crowleyites sadistically feeding his paranoia. And *they* were the ones into heroin mystique, so that Max should have known better. But he was always a garbage head[4] — that was why he gravitated

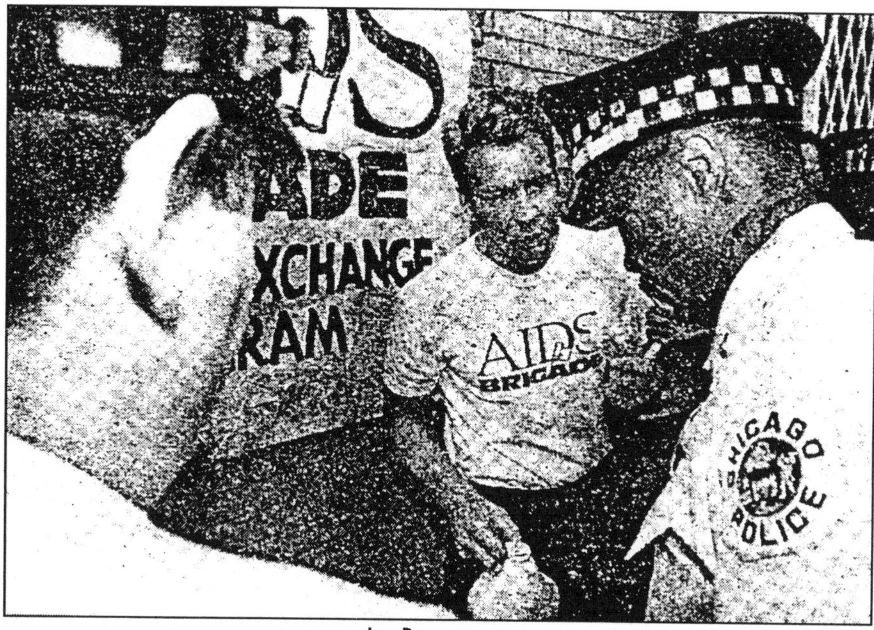

Chicago Sun Times

JON PARKER ARREST

to Pope Mickey. He was scheduled to be flown to Holland for Ibogainization. Howard begged him to throw away his needles, because he recognized Max was out of control, but Max was one of those yuppies who think reality doesn't apply to them.

Dana phoned Grudzinskas and told him the writer of the *Voice* article had OD'ed, and asked him how many more have to die. He got a new meeting for October 29th. Treatment & Data was in the midst of a big split after getting ddI and ddC approved. They voted to send a representative to the meeting, and much to the surprise of most present, one of the real luminaries of ACT UP, Dr. Iris Long, jumped at the opportunity.

Iris Long is one of the early heroines of the AIDS crisis. She's in the book *Best of Intentions*. You could tell the NIDA side was impressed when Frank Vocci asked her to autograph his copy. This time the MDD response was to pre-empt ACT UP's entrance by walking into the room with a time-line already set, for clinical trials (Phase I human toxicology) in one year. It included:

(A) Radiolabeling Ibogaine for autoradiography studies to locate and quantify Ibogaine receptors, followed by displacement studies to identify agonists and antagonists and determine binding characteristics;

(B) Toxicology studies to determine neurotoxicity and to determine if Ibogaine is cumulatively toxic;

1 I.e., because Baumann might have given it, like Naranjo, with amphetamine. See Goutarel, Appendix 2, pp. 237.

2 See "Guide to the Ancestors," Richard Evans-Schultes and Albert Hoffman, *Plants of the Gods* (Healing Arts, Rochester, VT, 1979), and P. Barabe, "The Religion of Eboga, or, the Bwiti of the Fangs," *Medecin Tropical*, Vol 42, No. 3, pp. 251–257, 1982. Also, p. 220, Appendix 1, Fernandez. Sisko based this estimate on conversations with Gabonese officials.

3 This was pure, blind loyalty of the non-analytic variety. Alice T. had kicked Daniel Rakowitz out of 9 Bleecker for talking about killing people; Aron Kay attacked him in the street for carrying a copy of *Mein Kampf* in his pocket. But Jerry the Peddler, who was lionized as the hero of the Tompkins Park riots, allowed Danny to hang out with him on the park bench, even though he confided later that he knew Rakowitz had already killed eighty neighborhood cats. In the height of irony, CBS reporter Mike Taibbi had videotaped hours of footage of Rakowitz and Jerry together in the park for a special on the "Cult of Rage" the previous summer — only to erase everything three weeks before Rakowitz was arrested for killing his girlfriend and serving her up as soup to the homeless in Tompkins Square Park.

4 I.e., one who takes anything. It's also likely he deliberately addicted himself because that was the only way he could get Ibogaine and write a followup article for the *Voice*.

(C) Pharmacological and metabolic studies;
(D) By March or April, stability testing, dose ranging and dosage form development; and
(E) Cognitive studies.

And by August 1992, the filing of their own Investigative New Drug (IND) application with the FDA, leading to clinical studies by late fall, 1992.

Besides Iris Long and the harm reduction reps from the July meeting, the coalition side included John Morgan of CUNY and David Goldstein. The government side was the same as before, Vocci, Grudzinskas, and Mona Brown. They did confirm Ibogaine psychoactivity would not be an impediment to tests in humans, and agreed to include HIV-positive addicts. And they were warned that the competitive bid regulations they were invoking against dealing through Howard Lotsof with OMNICHEM of Belgium (the only source in the world with 99.7 percent pure synthetic Ibogaine HCI in stock) might become a real stumbling block. They said it would be easier, though, to go through SIGMA, their regular supplier. SIGMA turned out not to be able to get *Tabernanthe iboga* out of Gabon. That set everything back five months.

Still, Iris Long said this timeline was about on par with current AIDS drug development timelines. Bringing ACT UP along had turned the trick. Ibogaine was "fast-tracked." As long as it could get past a battery of animal safety studies.

As for Jon Parker, he's re-established the AIDS Brigade in a storefront in South Boston. In June, 1992, he turned in his thesis on Needle Exchange to get his degree from Yale Medical School. In it he said the one innovative treatment modality the AIDS Brigade had come across addicts using in the field — the single new discovery in drug treatment he thought could make a difference against AIDS — was Ibogaine. Jon still drives down from Boston every week to do AIDS Brigade needle exchanges at the corner of Essex and Delancey, just after noon on Saturdays.

Of late he's been working with Jennifer, who was treated with Ibogaine for heroin addiction in Holland in August, 1991, on the trip when Bob Sisko got his retreatment. With the sense of purpose she derives from working with the AIDS Brigade, Jennifer's treatment is succeeding.

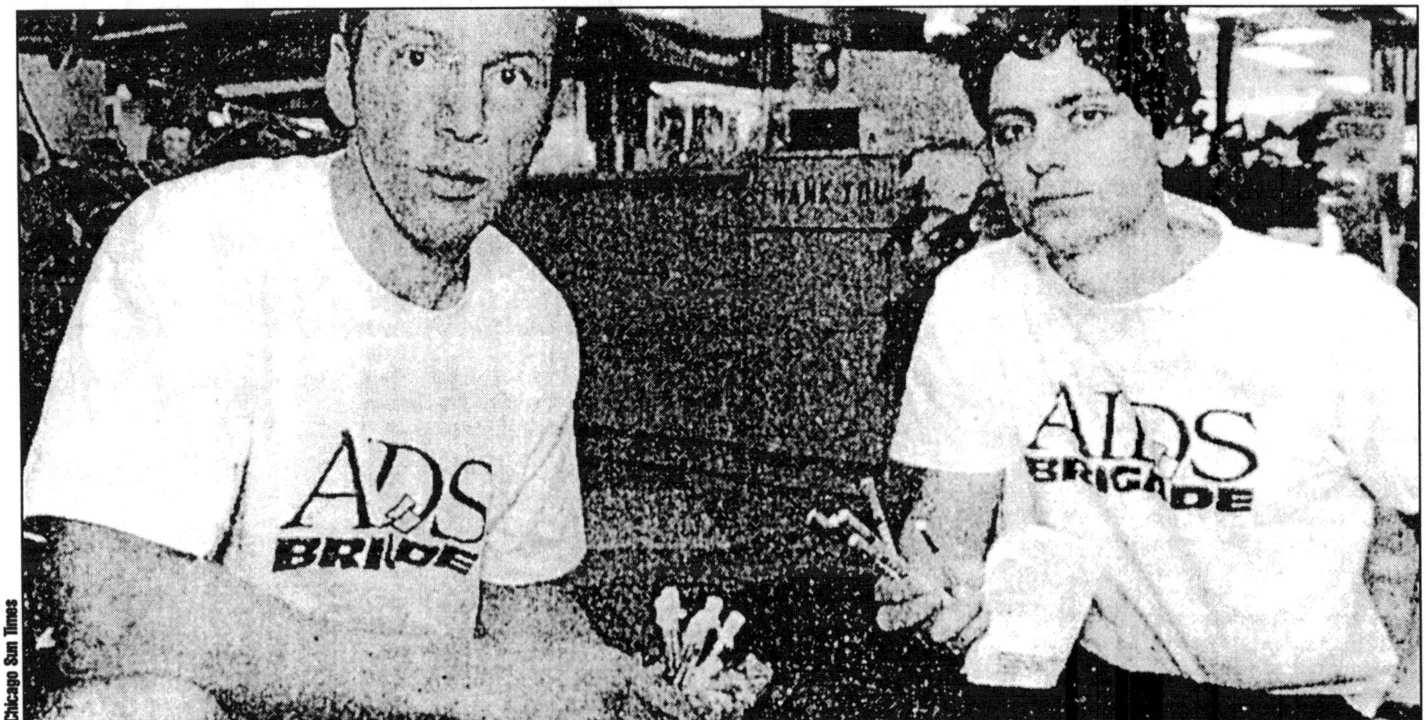

ON DECEMBER 8, 1994, JON PARKER AND ANDREW HOFFMAN WERE ACQUITTED OF CHARGES OF ILLEGALLY DISTRIBUTING CLEAN NEEDLES IN CHICAGO. IN A DIRECTED VERDICT FROM THE BENCH, THE JUDGE EXCORIATED THE STATE FOR BRINGING THE CASE AT ALL. ONE DAY LATER, ANDREW HOFFMAN ISSUED A CALL FOR PEOPLES' PRESENCE AT THE 1996 DEMOCRATIC CONVENTION TO PROTEST THE WAR ON DRUGS AND STOP THE RIGHTWARD LURCH OF AMERICA INTO THE ABYSS. AND SO THE PROTEST MOVEMENT RETURNED TO CHICAGO IN 1996!

CHAPTER 10: Carlo Contoreggi

Howard Lotsof actually first contacted Charles Grudzinskas prior to his appointment as head of MDD in January, 1991. Scanning a publication called *The Scientist* in November, 1990, he noticed an interview of a Lederle exec on regulatory changes needed to develop new drugs to treat drug dependency. It paralleled Howard's own thinking, including orphan drug provisions and the suspension of product liability (since all new daily-dose medications will wind up in druggies who can croak from street drugs anytime they relapse). Howard was so impressed he phoned the interviewee, Grudzinskas.

Near the end of that call he told him: "You know, my company has a really effective, single-dose, broad-spectrum treatment for addiction." Howard sent him Ibogaine material and they talked again. During their third phone conversation, Charlie told him he was leaving Lederle to become head of Medication Development at NIDA, and told him to send a letter requesting a meeting. but after he was in office, so it would be official. "I want to get in first. Send the letter after I get appointed, in January." That letter led to their April 12th meeting, setting the stage for the July 10th talks with treatment activists.

But the old boys' network gave Grudzinskas a deputy to watchdog him, named Frank Vocci, who in 1987 wrote the guidelines for emergency Schedule I classification of new hallucinogens, etc, as drugs of abuse. He was the one who asked about flashbacks, freak-outs, etc., as if Ibogaine was just another LSD analog. Both ACT UP and Howard, meeting with him separately, had to assure him in Grudzinskas' presence that this is a neutral, cognitive experience; that it's lucid REM, not hallucinations, and so-on. But Vocci also watched Grudzinskas' back, and kept him firmly in the NIDA loop whenever he tended toward running MDD as a private company — not wanting to tell public interest groups what was going on and so on.

One of the points of contention at the July 10, '91 meeting was the restrictions on Carlo Contoreggi. In March of the previous year, Bob Sisko had opened his own line into NIDA, but through NIDA's Addiction Research Center (ARC) at John Hopkins in Baltimore, not MDD in Rockville. At that point Medications Development was still being formed out of NIDA pre-clinical research in response to Senator Joseph Biden's language in the 1988 Omnibus Anti-Crime Act, mandating a search for a "magic bullet" to cure addiction.

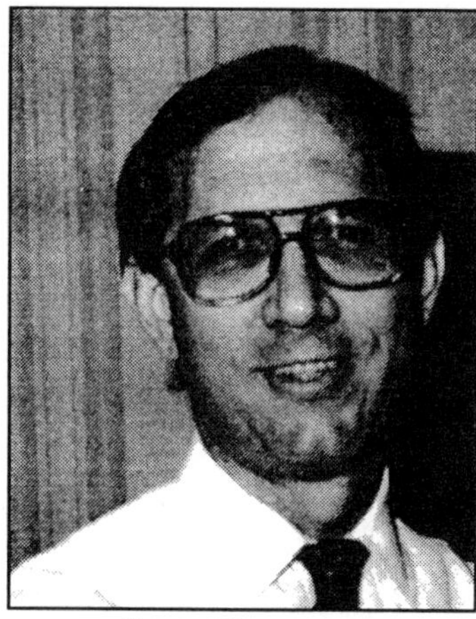

CHARLES GRUDZINSKAS

Sisko had come to Dr. Contoreggi following up on Howard's contacts with ARC Medical Director Bob Lange, who'd at least shown a willingness to listen. He and Carlo were the ARC medical officers. If someone has a bad reaction in a clinical trial of a medication ARC is investigating as a treatment, instead of having a researcher (who often has years of effort invested in their pet drug) treat the complications, an independent physician comes in, treats the complications, and writes up a report. Both Lange and Contoreggi were "quality control." But Lange was the boss: Carlo was the one who actually ran down and treated the crackhead who was having a seizure. So he'd seen a hundred different drug cures in action. And both he and Lange knew almost everything NIDA was testing was not living up to initial claims — in fact, was bombing out.

Sisko brought Contoreggi one addict to look at, before and after treatment, since Ibogaine isn't legal in the US and Carlo wasn't willing to fly off to Holland based on a rumor. It was the junkie interviewed in the *Village Beat* as "Dragonheart." He was a rock promoter snorting $500-a-day of heroin. When he walked into Contoreggi's office before Ibogaine, he was in bad shape — pale, emaciated, bent over. And during the interview, he progressed from nodding out to the chills and shakes of withdrawal. The only way he could finish the battery of questions and tests was for Carlo to give him an on-the-spot injection of morphine.

Carlo had to admit Sisko had brought

him a *bona fide* addict. When Dragonheart came back two weeks later, Contoreggi couldn't *believe* the difference.

> This tall, straight athletic-looking guy walks in. No pallor. No trace of withdrawal. In fact he's radiating good health, looks like he's been working out. There's a bounce in his step, a sparkle in his eye. The thing is, I'm a clinician — an M.D., not a rat scientist. I knew we had nothing in development that could do that. It's physically impossible in that timeframe.

Addicts with money can afford to *smoke* heroin, by frying it on a piece of tinfoil and sucking up the vapor with a straw. They call it "chasing the dragon." During the second interview the ex-addict told Carlo how before treatment, he felt the Dragon had his heart in its claws, but now *he* had the Dragon's heart. He wanted his case-name to be "Dragonheart."

The scientist in Carlo Contoreggi was hooked. But then his enthusiasm came to the attention of Bob Lange's boss, Dr. Jerome Jaffe, the overall head of the Addiction Research Center.

Since one-third of NIDA's budget goes to the ARC, Jaffe was definitely part of the old-boy network. He'd come up with Herb Kleber, who twenty years earlier had Contoreggi's job. After the conclusion of Ted Koppel's *Nightline* town meeting, on September 8, 1988, Dana buttonholed Jaffe and asked: "When are we going to have Ibogaine?"

"Never," said Jaffe, "We have test results showing it doesn't work." His air of smooth assurance was so great that even Dana was rocked back. A doubt was planted in his mind that wasn't dispelled until the day seven months later in the middle of the parade when Fred told him he'd taken it, and it *did* work. And of course, Jaffe and Kleber had nothing whatsoever to show it wouldn't work in humans. What they had was a rat study with a faulty paradigm, designed to have the experiment fail, and then to publish the results so as to make it appear that Ibogaine has no value.

In 1990 Jaffe and Sharpe published a study entitled *Ibogaine Doesn't Work.* They concluded Ibogaine administered subcutaneously (under the skin) failed to reduce naloxone-precipitated withdrawal in morphine-addicted rats, except for depressing one sign: grooming. Since that contradicts the findings of Dzoljic, Kaplan & Dzoljic (1988), Aceto, Bowman & Harris (1990), and all the findings of Stanley Glick's braintrust, Glick decided further work was necessary to resolve this.

Jaffe and Sharpe implied that all the other researchers had mistaken the temporary depression of motor activity caused by Ibogaine-induced tremor for genuine attenuation of withdrawal. After all, immediate effects of Ibogaine include drastic reduction of bar-pressing for *water.* The morphine in Dzoljic's experiment was *implanted,* not self-injected by the rats, yet withdrawal signs had *lessened* with Ibogaine. Glick's Albany Medical College group got together with the Capitol District Center for Drug Abuse Research and Treatment, and did a definitive, two-stage experiment to resolve the discrepancy.

In Part I, rats, addicted after five days of morphine, were given interperitoneally (in the gut) 20, 40 and 80 mg.-per-kg. of Ibogaine thirty minutes before one mg.-per-kg. of naltrexone HCl. Glick found that wet-dog shakes, grooming, teeth-chattering and diarrhea were all depressed 50-to-70% or more. Weight-loss and head-burying were marginally affected. At 40 mg.-per-kg. of Ibogaine, flinching was also depressed more than 50%.

But not only might Ibogaine-induced tremors during the first two hours be skewing the results, their unmistakable visibility made a true double-blind study impossible. So Glick & Co. ran Part II of the experiment with the lowest completely effective dose — 40 mg./kg. — given four hours before naltrexone, so the tremor would be totally dissipated. Wet-dog shakes and grooming were still depressed more than 50%. Teeth-chattering and diarrhea were virtually knocked out. (Weight-loss and head-burying increased slightly).

Now in the fine print, Jaffe and Sharpe had covered themselves, warning that discrepancies between their results and all others might be due to species variation in the rats, or subcutaneous versus interperitoneal or intercerebroventricular (directly into the ventricular spaces of the cerebrum) administration[1] of Ibogaine. And Glick had added a different mode of injection of, and a longer exposure to morphine, plus use of naltrexone instead of naloxone. Still, Glick concluded, every researcher found evidence Ibogaine lessened morphine withdrawal in animals. Even Sharpe

[1] This actually turns out to be the explanation. According to Carlo, subcutaneous administration would have given the liver time to process not only Ibogaine, but any active metabolite — a clue to just how important the liver is to metabolizing Ibogaine.

and Jaffee found lessening of one sign — grooming — indicating Ibogaine should continue to be investigated for treating opiate dependence, whatever the explanation.

But this study, *Effects of Ibogaine on Acute Signs of Morphine Withdrawal in Rats: Independence From Tremor* (S.D. Glick, K. Roseman, N.C. Rao, I.M. Maisonneuve & J.N. Carlson) wouldn't even be accepted for publication until November, 1991. In August, 1990, Jaffe had his paper published and in hand, and, as Carlo Contoreggi's ultimate boss, ruled that he could not do any more pre- and post-treatment evaluations of Ibogaine, under pain of being fired on the spot.

At their July 10, 1991 meeting with MDD, the reasoning behind this ban became clearer to Dana and Sisko. Vocci took the line that there was no urgency to get Ibogaine into clinical trials, because there was no hard evidence it worked in human addicts at all, and that NIDA couldn't help in developing that evidence. Medications Development was enjoined from even looking at a Schedule I drug in humans, no matter what it might do to stop addiction, AIDS crisis and all. Even pre- and post-treatment evaluation in humans would represent tacit NIDA approval — MDD complicity in an end-run around FDA.

That was the reason why, in the timeline presented October 29th, Vocci proposed doing the entire 1971 Dhahir toxicology study over again. It was also why the ACT UP side argued strenuously that Ibogaine must be considered an AIDS drug, either due to its impact on prevention or because for HIV-positive addicts, narcotic depression of the immune-system may well be a co-factor in the progression of AIDS.

Dr. Peter Hartsock of NIDA, whose New Haven study broke the back of resistance to needle exchange — who tangled with the Kleber/Jaffe crowd continuously — said their method is to obstruct from the shadows with whispers, to stab in the back. Pretty clearly, their strategy for stopping Ibogaine was to keep it in rat studies forever, hoping it could be made to appear to fail there, when the real question is why it works so much better in human addicts than in rodents.

By Oct. 29th, 1991, the harm reduction coalition had more than three dozen human case studies, enough to tell the MDD that 25% walk away from hard drugs forever after one treatment; on 25% it's effective less than a month. Of the middle 50%, one third (about an additional 15%) experience "shallow re-entry syndrome": they try using drugs again, but find they just don't like them anymore, so they too are drug-free after six months, giving an actual single-dose success-rate of 40%. The 35% remainder of that middle 50% can be kept substantially drug-free with treatments every six months and adjunct support groups like Narcotics Anonymous.

[Of course, if you could put AIDS into remission every six months with two days of chemo, the media would tout it as a cure.]

There are also indications that after three or more treatments the interrupter effect may "take" (like a successful organ transplant), due to the "maturing out" of the addict via the "Ibogaine learning curve," which Bob Sisko relates to the use of *iboga* in Gabon to initiate adolescents into adulthood.[1] Of course, whenever he'd start talking *Bwiti* at these meetings, as in "accessing your hereditary archive," Vocci and Grudzinskas would just roll their eyes.

Meanwhile, at the beginning of October '91, in front of 20,000 people at Ben Masel's Annual Harvest Fest in Madison, Wisconsin, Dhoruba Bin Wahad came out for hemp. A few days later, October 9th, on appeal by the Manhattan District Attorney, his conviction was reinstated by New York's highest court. Merely showing prosecutorial misconduct was no longer enough to keep him free. The rules had been changed in the middle of the game. Now his lawyers had to prove that the evidence that was withheld, the outright fabrications, would have materially affected the outcome of the trial. He flew to Paris, then Ghana; it looked like he might stay in Africa, in exile.

In November, 1991, on election day, Dennis Peron's San Francisco ballot initiative for medical marijuana for people with AIDS passed by the largest percentage of votes in city history — 80%. The national media made a big thing of it, and as far away as Washington, DC, pollsters and politicians sat up and took notice.

At the beginning of January, 1992, Herb Kleber became Number Two man at a new think tank called the Center on Addiction and

1 A graduate student of Charles Winnick, Steve Sifaneck, has suggested that Ibogaine treatment may simply be cutting short the last year or two an addict would spend maturing out; and that successive treatments "chop off" more and more of the period it would otherwise take for them to mature out. According to this idea, the best prognosis would be for addicts 35–40 years old, who've already graduated to methadone and no longer have any contact with the drug scene, whose only stumbling block as far as quitting is inability to stand withdrawal.

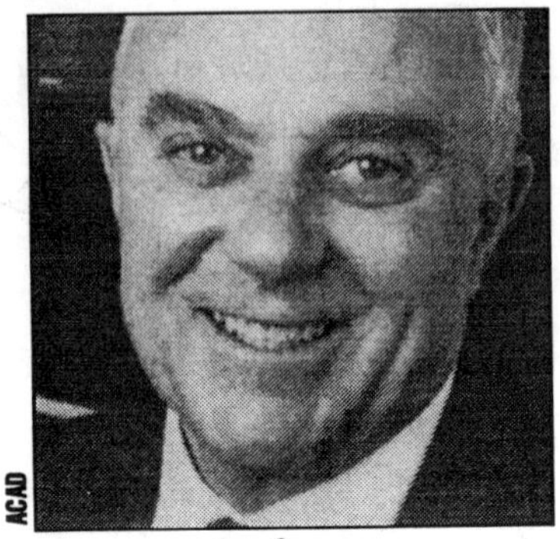

ACAD

JOE CALIFANO

Substance Abuse (CASA). Kleber had left his position (Deputy Drug Czar) at the Office of National Drug Control Policy a year earlier, ostensibly to protest Bush continuing his 70-to-30 ratio of law enforcement to treatment.

Actually he was taking a better-paying, more politically-secure job as head of Columbia University's Substance Abuse Division, one of the sponsors of CASA. His new boss was Joe Califano, who as Health, Education and Welfare (HEW) Secretary stopped pot decrim in 1979, thereby blocking early U.S. adoption of the Dutch harm reduction model. Since all subsequent Dutch reforms like needle exchange flowed from their decrim of pot in 1976, this Carter administration decision was arguably responsible for half of all AIDS cases in the US.

Curiously, although SUNY, CUNY, Cornell and virtually every university in and around New York City were now engaged in Ibogaine research, Columbia had since 1986 refused even to do rat studies "on the advice of their attorneys."[1] Then-President of Columbia, Michael Sovern, was eager to affiliate his university with CASA.[2] And despite having Herb Kleber as Assistant Director for Medical Affairs, CASA's charter specifically excludes funding biomedical research, in favor of prevention through education and long-term residential treatment.

Prominent on CASA's board is Jim Burke, head of the Partnership for a Drug-Free America, whose stated goal is to mobilize the advertising industry to foster intolerance of illegal drugs and those who use them. Alcohol and tobacco are never targeted in their ads, perhaps because their corporate sponsors include Anheuser-Busch and RJR-Nabisco, along with the biggest banks, pharmaceutical companies, and top media like Capital Cities/ABC. *(See Partnership List, pp. 95–96).* Their ads equating marijuana and hard drugs are omnipresent on television and in newspapers, which get tax write-offs. CASA seems to have been formed as a think tank to fine-tune their message, after some of those ads turned out to be wildly inaccurate.[3] Currently they say pot has no medical value whatsoever, and that people who smoke it are cop-killers, regardless of medical condition.

It is highly ironic that in the name of a Drug-Free America, the Robert Woods Johnson Foundation, which bank-rolls both Partnership and CASA, thereby supports Dr. Herbert Kleber — the man who held back Ibogaine in favor of the addictive drug buprenorphine.

At the end of January '92, Herb Kleber's successor at ONDCP, Ingrid Kolb, signaled a possible thaw by writing a letter to Assistant Secretary for Health and Human Services (HHS) James Mason, chiding him for keeping the applications of PWA's for medical marijuana in limbo.

Dana Beal noticed in news accounts that her title was Acting Director for Demand Reduction. He thought of people he knew who before Ibogaine were doing $200-to-$300-a-day of smack, who after a couple treatments maybe do $5 worth twenty times a year. That's a lot of demand reduction. Perhaps the medical marijuana letter was a sign this Kolb woman would be open-minded.

So Beal called Ingrid Kolb and asked on behalf of ACT UP for a meeting on "promising medications in the NIDA pipeline for treatment of drug dependency." He brought along Alan Thompson of RAR and Joey Tranchina of the West Coast AIDS Brigade. Joey talked to her about clean needles; Ingrid deferred to NIDA, saying the data wasn't in yet. Dana thanked her for the medical marijuana letter. But most of the meeting was about Ibogaine.

No one in the entire bureaucracy had

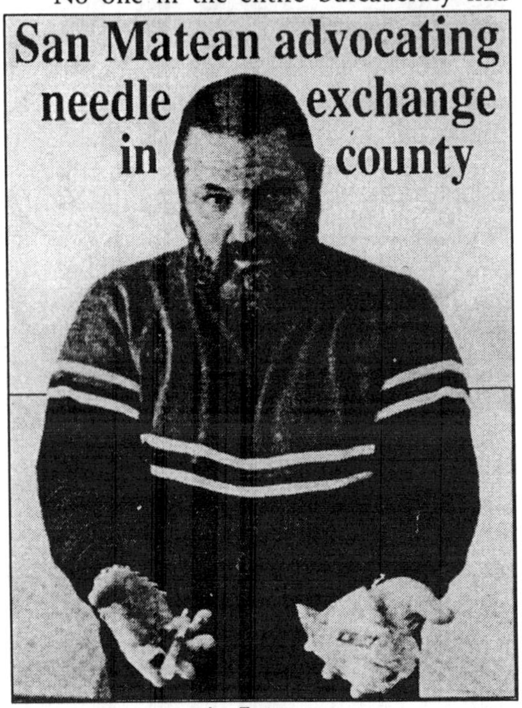

JOE TRANCHINA

1 Or under the influence of tenured faculty like Gabriel Nahas, who has stated: "NIDA's search for a magic bullet that will cure cocaine addiction is misguided, like most of its approaches, which waste billions of dollars perpetuating the drug problem." Yet it was Nahas' marijuana pseudo-science — sponsored by the U.N. Office on Narcotics when it was headed by the daughter of Kurt Waldheim, Liselot Waldheim-Natural — that whipped up pot hysteria in the '70s, until debunked around 1980 when every finding turned out to be faked. Meanwhile, the U.N. connection provided an additional gloss of respectability for Lyndon LaRouche's various "anti-drug" organizations (see. pp. 34–35). There is a definite mentality that opposes Ibogaine simply because it comes from the harm reduction side, and because it isn't particularly effective in stopping pot use.

2 See CASA Bulletin, 1992. He has since been replaced on the CASA Board by George Rupp, the current Columbia University president.

3 One showing the "brainwaves of a teenager on pot" as totally flat, actually showed an EEG from a middle-aged drunk in a coma after a car accident.

ever told the Acting Director for Demand Reduction they had a prototype addiction interrupter in the works, potentially *the* magic bullet.

Dana opined that the drug crisis could be ended and AIDS transmission cut as much as 25%, for about $2 billion, or enough to treat the one million worst-afflicted addicts. Alan Thompson told her how, in the twelve years Rock Against Racism had known about and supported the Ibogaine Project, he'd never been able to put together a band of his own without a junkie in it, and how one musician friend after another died of overdose. On the way back to New York City, he thanked Dana for enabling him to press his case at the White House.

That very morning, February 13th, Dhoruba had returned from Africa after a great internal struggle with himself, to fight his case all over again — appearing in court just as the ACT UP van was leaving for the meeting — too late to go along. Dana went into overdrive to set up a subsequent meeting that would bring in Dhoruba, actualizing the coalition between ACT UP and the Black treatment movement, but also to substantiate Dhoruba's role and keep him out of prison to continue his work.

The first date Dhoruba, Ingrid Kolb, Grudzinskas and Vocci could all meet was April 10th. Meanwhile Dana spent his time boiling an Ibogaine tape centered on the Nico interview down to sixty minutes.

It was still February when he got a call from John Spacely, in the hospital. When Dana came to visit, Spacely told him he had MAI.[1] A couple weeks later his HIV results came back positive. His T-cell count was 36. Ibogaine might have saved him in mid-1981, sitting around talking about it with Dana. But it was too late the minute he shared a needle with someone around Bruce Brown. On the other hand, all the years he smoked pot since he stopped doing dope, John Spacely had been free of opportunistic infections, in effect cushioning the decline of his T-cells[2] with medical marijuana. And at first he was able to triple his T's with herbal extracts and vitamins.

ACT UP Treatment & Data sent a letter to James Mason demanding that he reverse his

PARTNERSHIP FOR A DRUG-FREE AMERICA

CONTRIBUTORS

Aetna Life and Casualty
Air Products & Chemicals, Inc.
Allen & Company, Inc.
Allstate
American Advertising Federation
American Brands Inc.
American Express Company
American General Corporation
American International Group
American Marketing Association
American Telephone & Telegraph
Amoco Corporation
Anheuser-Busch Companies, Inc.
Archer Daniels Midland Corporation
Atlantic Mutual Companies
Automatic Data Processing
Avon Products, Inc.
BFGoodrich Company
BP America
Ball Corporation
Barclays Bank-USA Banking Division
Bear Stearns & Co. Inc.
Bechtel Group, Inc.
Becton Dickinson
BellSouth Corp.
Bergen Brunswig Corp.
Best Foods/CPC Int'l
Boeing Company
Bristol-Myers Squibb Company
C.R. Bard, Inc.
CBI Industries
CIBA-GEIGY/Pharmaceuticals Division
CSX Corporation
Cadbury Beverages, Inc.
Campbell Soup Company
Campeau Family Foundation
Capital Cities/ABC
Carter-Wallace, Inc.
Centel Corp.
Champion International Corp.
Charles A. Dana Foundation, Inc.
Chase Manhattan Bank, N.A.
Chevron Corporation
Chrysler Corporation
Chubb Corporation
Citibank, N.A.
Clorox
Coca-Cola Company
Colgate-Palmolive
Consolidated Freightways, Inc.
Continental Corporation
Corning Incorporated
Cortec Group
Dayton Hudson Corporation
Dayton Power & Light Co.
Deere & Company
Dow Chemical Company/Dow U.S.A.
Dow Jones & Company, Inc.
Duke Power Company.
E.I. du Pont de Nemours & Co.
EG&G, Inc.
Eastman Kodak Co., Inc.
Eaton Corporation
El Paso Electric
Emerson Electric Company
Equitable Assurance Society
Federal Express
Fireman's Fund Insurance Co.
First Boston
First Fidelity Bank
First Jersey National Bank
First Wachovia Corporation
Ford Foundation
Ford Motor Company
GenCorp
General Dynamics Corporation
General Electric
General Foods Fund, Inc.
General Mills, Inc.
General Motors
Glaxo Inc.
Golden Rule Insurance Co.
Goodyear Tire and Rubber Co
Guardian Life Insurance Co.
H.B. Fuller Company
H.J. Heinz Company
Halliburton Company
Hallmark Cards Inc.
Hearst Corporation
Henley Group, Inc.
Hershey Foods Corp.
Hoechst-Celanese Pharmaceuticals
Hoffmann-La Roche Inc.

Partnership for a Drug-Free America Members, 1991, page one.

ban on access to medical marijuana for people with AIDS; he refused to even meet about it with ACT UP. A few days before Dana was to report on this to the floor, he called Marty Robinson to ask if he'd make a special trip in from Park Slope and come back to the floor one more time because of his strong feelings on medical marijuana. Marty reported he couldn't smoke any more. He'd gotten his hands on some Marinol, though. Marty had

1 An opportunistic infection, a sure sign of the onset of full-blown AIDS.

2 'T-cells,' also known as CD-4's, are white blood cells that 'swallow' bacteria, protozoa and other pathogens so that in a normal immune system they aren't even a problem. Falling CD-4's are considered a sure sign of AIDS, but all indications are that only 1 in 10,000 CD4's actually become infected with HIV. Like good soldiers, the rest are

Cont. next page

committing suicide, in effect "following the orders" of too-long elevated levels of TNF alpha (tumor-necrosis factor), along with various interleukens and cortisols. Pot, a vaso-dilator, relieves inflamation produced by these cytokines — one of the auto-immune aspects of AIDS. This is a possible mechanism which would explain the findings of Winkelstein, et al, on the longer survival of drug users in the San Franscisco Mens Cohort. Pot was the only substance used by all, according to the *Bay Area Reporter*, 7/8/'94.

previously promised to testify in Beal's defense. But he was far, far sicker than Dana expected. "Those boys can't do anything for me anymore," he said of ACT UP.

"But Marty," said Dana, "the Ibogaine got through. Treatment & Data backed it. Iris Long got NIDA to fast-track it. That conference we did at City College — it led to research showing Ibogaine works against cocaine, against crack. You freed the addicts, Marty — you made the difference. You freed the slaves."

"That's nice." Marty mused.

"But what do I do about ACT UP and medical marijuana?" Dana queried. "I'm not gay. I'm not HIV positive."

"You will be the one who gets medical marijuana through," said Marty. Dana hung up the phone in distress. Fifteen minutes later Marty's friend Mark Rubin called back. "Marty is sicker than he let on. If you want to see him again, best come over within the next week." Dana decided to see him after the T&D meeting Wednesday night. Mark called him Wednesday morning to tell him Marty had died.

Up in Boston, Jon Parker had resumed needle exchange, this time outside the main city hospital several miles from Ellis-Hagler's base in Roxbury. Ellis-Hagler brought out pickets anyway. Parker would get arrested only to be immediately released. Dana went to Rev. Ellis-Hagler trying, unsuccessfully, to get a rep to the April 10th White House meeting. He talked to Treatment-on-Demand's Moses Saunders, who said they'd known for five years that they needed something like Ibogaine. He also confided they knew needle exchange was a done deal — they just wanted to keep the pressure on to get more money for treatment. So at least on days they were meeting with Dana, they weren't picketing. And ACT UP New York was willing to fund the D.C. trip if it had a chance of replacing confrontation with cooperation.

In the event, Dhoruba was satisfied to be accompanied by an ex-Young Lord, Father Frank Morales of the Episcopal Archdioscese of New York. The other participants on the ACT UP side were Dana Beal, Betsy Lenke, Jeff Eberhardt and David Goldstein for ICASH. Besides Kolb, Vocci and Grudzinskas, the ONDCP also had John Gregrich, on loan from the Justice Department. The meeting started a bit late due to traffic congestion, so there was really just time for Dhoruba to lay out two demands:

1.) The biggest obstacle to new chemotherapies for addiction is community resistance, due to experience with the toxicity and extreme addictiveness of methadone, which was forced on the Black community without their say-so. He demanded an independent,

Honeywell Inc.
IBM Corporation
Ingersoll-Rand Company
Inland Steel Industries,Inc.
International Video Entertainment
J. Seward Johnson Sr. Char. Trusts
J.C. Penney Company, Inc.
J.P. Morgan & Co., Inc.
J.W. Messner Inc
Jesse Philips Foundation
Johnson & Johnson
Joseph Drown Foundation
Kellogg Company
Kellwood Company
Kimberly-Clark
Kraft General Foods
Lee Hecht Harrison, Inc.
Lowe's Charitable & Educ. Founda.
Lucky Stores
Manufacturers Hanover Trust Company
Marsh & McLennan Companies, Inc.
McDonald's Corporation
McDonnell Douglas Corp.
Mead Corporation
Mercantile Stores
Merck & Company, Inc.
Merrill Lynch & Co.
Metropolitan Life Insurance Company
Mobil Corporation
Monsanto Company
Morgan Guaranty Trust Co. of NY
Morgan Stanley & Company, Inc.
Motorola Inc.
Mutual Benefit Life
Mutual of America Life Ins. Co.
Mutual of New York Finacial Services
National Westminster Bancorp NJ
New York Life Insurance Company
Nissan Motor Corporation in USA
Nomura Securities, Int. Inc.
Ohio National Life Ins. Co
Olin Corporation
Owens-Corning Fiberglas Corp.
PPG Industries, Inc.
PSE&G
Paramount Communications Inc.
Pepsico, Inc.
Pfizer Inc.
Phibro-Salomon
Philip Morris Companies, Inc.
Philips Industries
Polaroid
Proctor & Gamble Co.
Prudential Insurance Co. of Ame
RJR Nabisco, Inc.
Raytheon Company
Reader's Digest Association
Rite Aid
Robert Wood Johnson Foundation
Rockwell International Corporat
Ronetco Supermarkets, Inc.
Rubbermaid Incorporated
S.C. Johnson & Son, Inc.
Sara Lee Corporation
Schering-Plough Corporation
Sears, Roebuck and Co.
Selective Insurance Group, Inc.
Shell Oil Company
Smith Richardson Foundation Inc.
SmithKline Beecham
State Farm Mutual Automobile In
Texaco
The Pew Charitable Trusts
The Rockefeller Foundation
Time Warner Inc.
Traveler's Insurance Company
Triangle Industries-Trian Group
USF&G Corporation
Union Camp Corp.
Union Pacific Corporation
United Parcel Service
Universal Corporation
VF Corporation
Video Insider
W.W. Grainger, Inc.
Warner-Lambert Company
Waste Management, Inc.
Wickes Companies, Inc.
Williams Real Estate
Xerox Corporation

October 31, 1991

PARTNERSHIP FOR A DRUG-FREE AMERICA MEMBERS, 1991, PAGE TWO

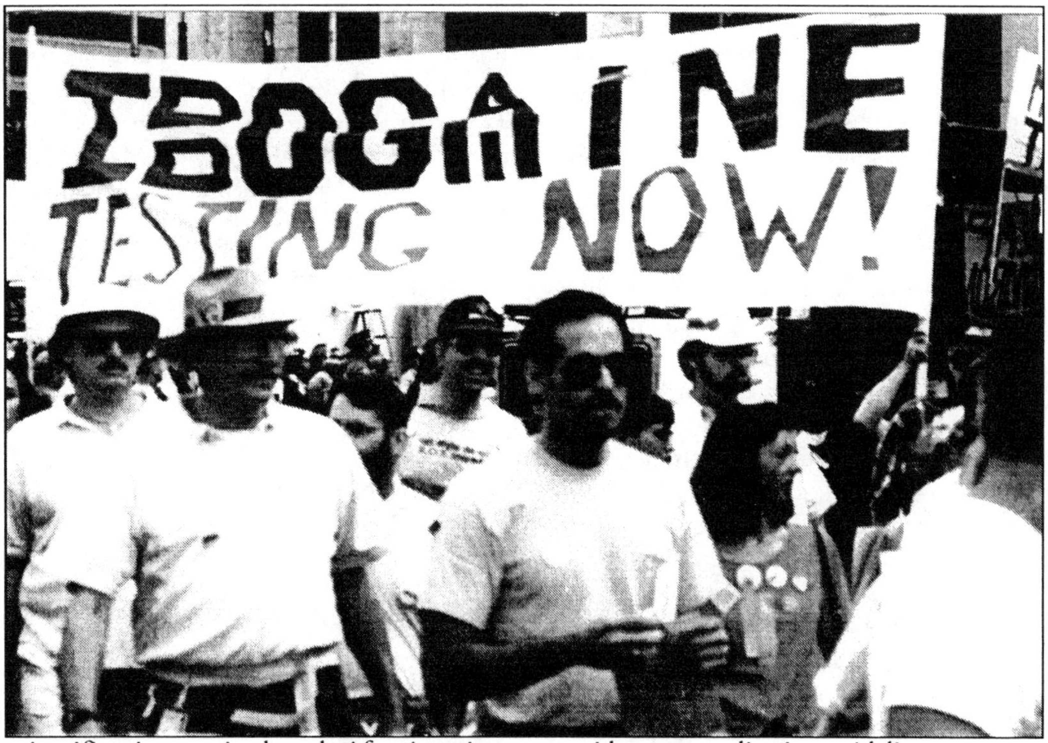

ICASH

scientific, inner city-based Afro-American study of Ibogaine — an immediate community-based trial by people with enormous hands-on experience, who are as skeptical as anyone. This would bring folks who are unwilling to use maintenance drugs into Medications Development; and from the beginning, rather than too late to make a difference.

2.) Community-based programs that can re-socialize addicts and stem the spread of HIV without undermining the fight against high-level drug dealing or government corruption are getting the shaft, because criminalizing users maximizes income from forfeitures. The system has become addicted to the cash flow it's supposed to be eliminating. Dhoruba demanded that 100% of the $400 million-a-year from forfeitures be retargeted, from the financing of new seizures to treating hardcore addicts. That way, in five years the one million most serious addicts who consume 70% of all hard drugs could be treated with Ibogaine or some other fast-acting addiction interrupter, for a net demand reduction of 35%.

To Point #1, Vocci responded that it would take eighteen months to write new regs for community-based trails; but Kolb and Grudzinskas suggested clinics with follow-up capability in Roxbury and Harlem apply to be among the first for funding, and offered to provide grant application guidelines.

Vis-à-vis Point #2, John Gregrich confirmed that the great bulk of forfeiture money was going to finance new forfeitures, except for $9 million which Ingrid Kolb said was all that Congress left of her request for $90 million out the $400 million for treating inner city addicts.

Dana, Betsy and Jeff of ACT UP raised three additional matters:

ACT UP asked about, and MDD agreed to furnish data on, sample size and subjects being studied (but not location and identity of researchers) in 13 animal studies. ACT UP reiterated the importance of high (99.7%) purity to ensure absorption. MDD had only obtained 300 grams of Ibogaine; they were now getting 400 grams additional from Lotsof. And despite half-hearted attempts to invoke NIDA's Office of Treatment Improvement (OTI) as the proper route for lobbying, Vocci and Grudzinkas confirmed the only early clinical access to Ibogaine would be through them.

ACT UP also pointed out that proposed guidelines on undesirable interactions of street drugs and new maintenance drugs made no provision for Ibogaine, which is not a maintenance drug and can be screened from interactions with any other drug during the brief forty-eight-hour procedure. Grudzinskas responded that Vocci had written those guidelines, and asked to be furnished with a set of parameters defining what an addiction interrupter would consist of.

Finally, Dana had touched base with Carlo Contoreggi just before the meeting; now he urged that MDD and FDA re-consider, and allow Dr. Contoreggi to resume pre- and post-treatment evaluation of addicts being flown to Holland. MDD budged, slightly. They offered to test, post-treatment, for gross neurological dysfunction. Jeff pointed out that would provide for no baseline comparison. David Goldstein cited Dhahir's finding of no neuro-toxicity ('71), as showing there ***would be no*** gross neurological dysfunction.

At the end of the meeting MDD still refused to mesh through Contoreggi with Lotsof, the patentholder, because of the treatments he was doing in Holland, a hang-up that had already set back procurement of supplies six months. As ACT UP said in a subsequent letter to Ingrid Kolb:

> The ban on pre-treatment evaluation... is both unscientific and legally inconsistent with the Administration position on freedom of travel. ...It is clearly legal for U.S. addicts to fly to Holland, where the procedure is approved as an experimental therapy. And NIDA wants them evaluated, not prosecuted, when they return.
>
> [This] ruling... has become an obstacle to NIDA... consulting... the folks who know the most about the procedure: Howard Lotsof and NDA International. In fact, Lotsof is not only complying with the letter of all applicable laws and regulations, but in refusing to make ENDABUSE available for casual research or for any other reason except fighting addiction, he is pro-actively fullfilling the intent of the law, which is to fight drug abuse.

But just for insurance, Dhoruba and ACT UP also met that morning with Tim Westmoreland, special AIDS advisor to Congressman Henry Waxman's Committee on Health and the Environment. Tim promised to get language into the pending NIDA re-organization act, mandating community-based trials. Dana intended to keep ***his*** promise to Treatment on Demand, to bring Ibogaine to Roxbury as soon as possible, no matter what.

Bringing Dhoruba into the negotiations did impress the feds. A few weeks later Los Angeles was burning. For a month or so there was a mood in the Bush Administration to take Black concerns a bit more seriously. Dana sent MDD the requested parameters defining an addiction interrupter in early May:

> 1.) An addiction interrupter must virtually eliminate withdrawal symptoms.
>
> 2.) An interrupter must drastically attentuate craving for three to eighteen months.
>
> 3.) An interrupter must block the customary pleasure response that the addict is trained to expect, so his drugs of abuse ***won't work*** for the first few weeks.
>
> 4.) An interrupter will stimulate the "maturing out" of the addict. The initial REM-like period, involving the firing and retrieval of memories and the automatic re-editing of memory as a whole is the key to how interruption "takes."[1]

Beal conceded these effects are specific to Ibogaine, but pointed out that the interrupter we know must provide the "yardstick" for comparison, just as methadone is our yardstick for evaluating all the new maintenance drugs in the MDD pipeline.

When he contacted Grudzinskas for his reaction, Dana asked who could do the now-approved post-treatment evaluations. Charlie turned him over to Vocci, who said he should call Contoreggi. But Vocci didn't call Carlo and give him any kind of authorization, though.

Just prior to the April 10th meeting, the Queens judge in Beal's medical marijuana case had tried to force him to trial. Bill Kunstler informed the court for the first time the defense would be medical necessity.[2] The first available trial date was the end of June, '92. The defense wasn't able to get its witnesses together, so Kunstler filed a motion to dismiss based on medical necessity instead. The clock was running out for Dana. But he had time for a few more moves.

June was the month he tried to set up a meeting with Joe Califano at the apartment of his friend Flo Kennedy, on East 48th Street, five blocks from CASA's temporary offices. Flo Kennedy had been the lawyer for legendary jazz junkies Billie Holliday and Charlie "Bird" Parker. After Herb Kleber found out the meeting was about Ibogaine, though, the meeting of Califano with Flo and ACT UP was cancelled.

But Dana's next move was a winner. Howard had a couple of paying treatments in Holland a few weeks before the International

1 For the new data on the neuro-receptor basis for this, see Chapter 18, pp. 199–201 of this Report..

2 The necessity defense here would be that an illegal drug, marijuana, was life-saving because it slowed or reversed the AIDS wasting syndrome.

AIDS Conference in Amsterdam in late July. Beal persuaded him to stay on and do a prototype treatment seminar, with Dutch addict freebies, in conjunction with the Conference. Then Dana invited folks to the treatments who were coming to Amsterdam anyway for the AIDS Conference: Joey Tranchina, Moses Saunders, Dr. Lester Grinspoon, and the real catch, Carlo Contoreggi.

Carlo was ready to quit his job. He'd just come up with proof that bleaching needles wasn't anywhere near as effective as needle exchange, and at the eleventh hour the order had come down from Drug Czar Bob Martinez himself forbidding Carlo from presenting his data at the International AIDS Conference.

All Contoreggi had done was to sit addicts down with their works and some bleach, and tell them to start cleaning. And a lot of them didn't do a thorough job, leaving microscopic bloodclots that HIV could live in for ten days or longer. So why not just give them clean works? It's safer for everyone. This directly contradicted the Bush / Martinez / Herb Kleber line.

[Of course, they'd all been against bleach, too, until Jon Parker started overthrowing needle prohibition from Maine to Delaware, and they adopted bleach as a fallback.]

"Don't quit," Dana told him. "We need you to stay put while we change everything around you. Instead of defying them directly, go to Amsterdam and sit in on some treatments with Howard. That'll be *real* civil disobedience. Let me worry afterwards about how to make it kosher with Grudzinskas and NIDA."

Contoreggi flew to Amsterdam at his own expense, and came back raving about what he'd seen. "I've treated junkies with more than a hundred drugs, and *nothing* is like Ibogaine. All signs of addiction are just — gone. You know, on other medications, junkies always keep asking for dope, nonstop. Instead, after 24 hours, this guy was asking for an Egg McMuffin.

"He wanted an Egg McMuffin!"

When Howard Lotsof and the treatment team flew back from Amsterdam, Dana had them booked for an August 4th presentation set up by accupuncturist Rommell Washington at Harlem Hospital. For 3 1/2 hours, thirty treatment professionals peppered Howard, Sisko, Geerte F. and Dana with questions.

But the clincher was a talk by Dhoruba Bin Wahad, putting Ibogaine in the context of a 25-year struggle. He said the Ibogaine team, with the forces they were taking on, were some of the bravest people he knew. No, he said, Ibogaine doesn't violate Muslim teachings. The Koran says any medicine that works can be used to heal the sick. And the word went out in Harlem: the senior surviving Black Panther had endorsed the Project. Doors began opening all over the place.

"Why didn't you invite me?" said Carlo when Dana phoned him afterwards. "Look, I have to come up the weekend of Sept 14th for my radio-medicine boards."

Dana thought a minute and said: "I'll see if I can arrange authorization from Grudzinskas for you to talk with some people who've been treated when you come up — to do a little post-treatment evaluation."

Then he called up Grudzinskas and explained that Vocci'd never gotten around to the call authorizing Contoreggi to do post-treatment evaluations, as promised in May. He got back to Carlo and told him to expect a call from Medications Development giving the go-ahead.

"Well, if Grudzinskas calls, I'm going public — all the way," said Carlo.

"What do you mean?"

"If I get my foot in the door, I'm going to shove it open all the way. I'm going to tell them everything I saw in Amsterdam."

The upshot was that Charles Grudzinskas gave *post facto* authorization for Contoreggi's Amsterdam observations. And invited him down to Rockville to brief fifteen neuroscientists at the MDD on what he'd seen. In Carlo, they finally had one of their own who'd seen it, and could explain the significance of what he'd seen in technical language they could understand. Overnight, Carlo became *the* government clinical expert on Ibogaine in humans. Vocci formally made him part of the MDD's Ibogaine Project.

The man who, like Galileo Galilei, said *"Si il mouve,"* ("But it moves") was now in the loop.

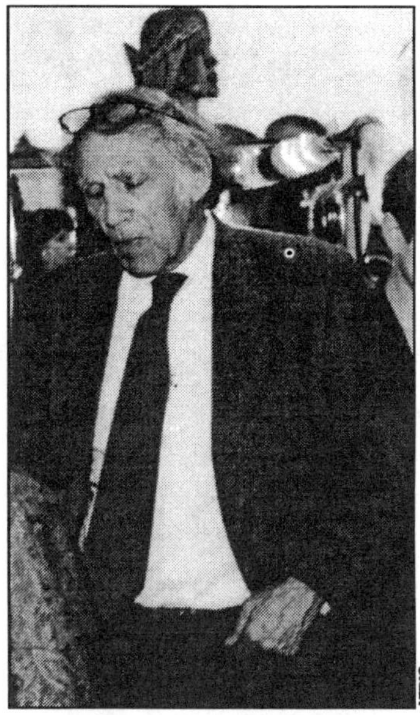
YIPIS

ATTORNEY WILLIAM KUNSTLER

CHAPTER 11: Geerte F.

Howard Lotsof first did an interview on Dutch pirate radio while Geerte (pronounced *Hair-tuh*) F. was attending the 1988–89 semester of art school in New York City, and renovating Umbrella House, a squat on Avenue C on the Lower East Side. Both Geerte and the pirate radio people considered themselves part of the international squatter's movement.

The pirate radio was in a large squat in Amsterdam. It was affiliated with Hi-Res, a smaller squat with a lot of computers. All the squats in Amsterdam had problems with heroin. Three people from Hi-Res, Chris Schwartz, Reinhardt Hecht and Simon Sheppeard, had come across published references to Ibogaine, and they wanted their friends and the people they lived with to be treated. But they also wanted the squatter movement to be the group of people to tell the world about Ibogaine. So they were looking into how to get their own supply, how to get people to eat it, and just doing research.

Hi-Res had to wait until Sisko came to Holland in October, 1989, for two volunteers to be treated — Geerte and Ron. In June, Geerte had come home from New York, where she had learned of Ibogaine in the squat scene, to live with her drug-addicted boyfriend, Ron. She was not using heroin when she made arrangements to treat Ron, but started doing it with him during the three months she spent waiting for Sisko to come. There's a videotape of Chris Schwartz interviewing Geerte and Ron, assisting Sisko with the intake procedure for the first Dutch addicts ever treated.

Ron had been addicted for twelve or thirteen years. He had been doing 85 milligrams of methadone every day for twelve years, with one exception — fifteen months spent in a rehab center to avoid going to jail. He actually followed the program on this rehab farm and he was clean under his own power.

But this particular program was merely suppressing Ron's aggression, so that for those fifteen months, Ron longed for the day he could get out and rebel. One day after he came out of rehab he copped smack, and fell back to using drugs right away — alcohol, pills, speed, cocaine and anything else he could get his hands on.

Ron had gone into treatment to get out of going to jail. But he learned a lot from the program anyway — which helped him with the Ibogaine treatment. It gave him the experience of being clean, which helps when you're suddenly given Ibogaine. Addicts have literally forgotten what it's like to spend a period of time without heroin.

Ron's Ibogaine treatment worked out very well. The day before he was a total wreck, a complete chaotic idiot. He took the Ibogaine and he laid down for a day. He was very peaceful, quiet and happy. He came out like he'd been through the laundramat, like a completely different person. That night he sat up and smoked a joint, drank a beer and he was totally happy and balanced.

Geerte was treated the day after Ron. She took the Ibogaine at 8 AM on an empty stomach. Sisko kept coming into the room to see if she had laid down yet, to have her walk a bit to check if she appeared wobbly. This only made Geerte determined to walk in straight lines. She kept telling him the Ibogaine wasn't working. She even ran around a chair to show she had full coordination.

In reality, she was resisting the effect because she didn't know what to expect from the Ibogaine — trying to prove that if she didn't want to be knocked out, she wouldn't get knocked out. It involved intense will power. She had had many mind-bending trips on LSD and mushrooms, maybe thirty or forty, but she didn't like what this was doing to her, because when she closed her eyes she saw things —

> "...Patterns in the beginning, about an hour after you take the Ibogaine, maybe 10% as vivid as LSD. But if you close your eyes, you see all kinds of stuff happening, really rapidly, too. As soon as you close your eyes, you go into a REM sleep thing."

The minute she experienced it, the eyes-closed stuff was familiar. Her mind recognized it as REM-like. What she saw was all these cartoon images — what a child's mind is formed out of in this century. She had been told she'd see a chronological movie of her life.

> "But all I saw were these weird cartoon figures coming past. I have a vision of walking through my brain, as if walking in a giant computer-like file-cabinet. There are long narrow drawers with selected, collective information. Somebody in the hotel turned on the radio, with commercials, and I just got — like all the commercial jingles I ever heard came out of this little drawer in my brain. It came out as one long song, and I visually saw the song.
>
> "Can you imagine all the jingles you ever heard on the radio all coming out as one thing? Like a harmonica. The trip is hard to explain. You're existing on ten different levels at the same time. You don't have any control over it and it just happens to you. Something you just can't comprehend — you begin to comprehend it when the experience is over.
>
> "You really feel that something is changing in your mind, and I kept saying to Ron, who was in the room when I got treated: 'There should be a doctor here: we should take a scan of my brain at this very moment. This is really too intense, it can't be happening.'
>
> "It felt like re-programming. I thought, 'This is not good. This is way too much. Nobody should experience this because it's way too intense.' Weeks after the treatment you start to understand why you experienced the things you did.
>
> "I would sit down on the bed and I'd hear a drum, like someone drumming in the next room. It's not like you hear this drumming in your mind and you can just stop it, like it's just a mind thing. No, it's really happening and you can't stop it. Like an African drum. Next thing I know I'm walking in Africa. Literally walking in the jungle with bare feet and snakes around me. Jungle leaves around my face and I thought, *'What the fuck is going on?'* But then I open my eyes and I'm still in the room. It's like an out-of-body experience, but you just open your eyes as soon as you want to snap back into your body, and you're there."

The visions of Africa made Geerte uncomfortable — "For the first time in my life, I accepted being born white in the 20th century in northern Europe." She also found the room irritating. The sheets were really bright red. She didn't like Sisko coming in to check up on her, saying "Maybe we should put some more Ibogaine into you." He seemed like a threatening pygmy from the forest, trying to stuff this root down her throat. Then he would leave to fall asleep, snoring in the next room. She felt Sisko and the others should be there for her. Ron was there, but he was taking

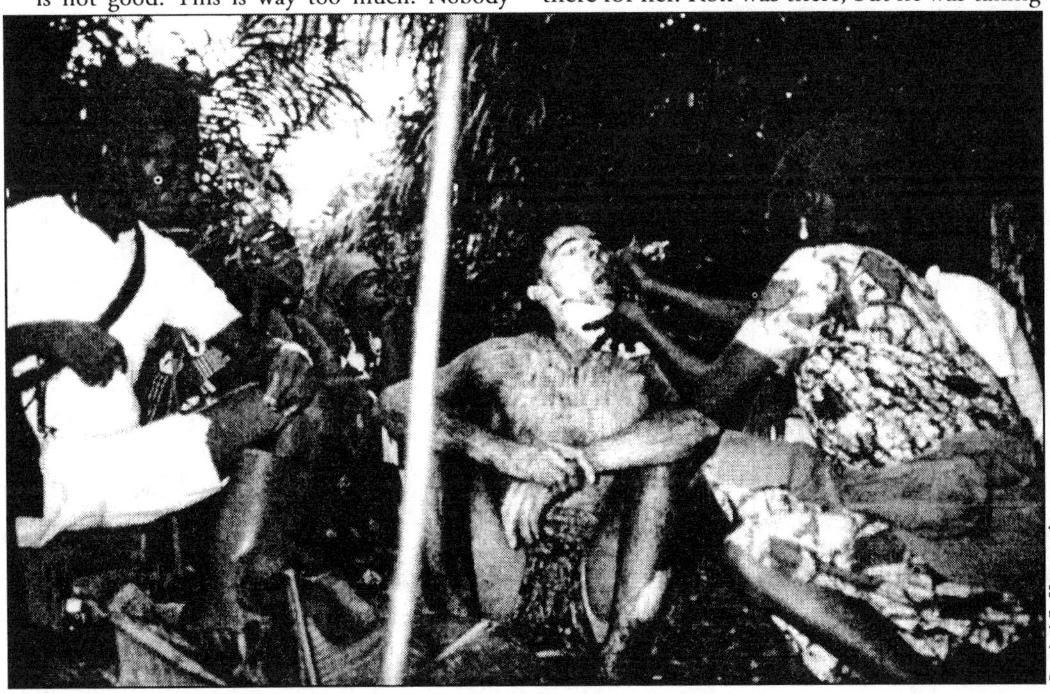

Psychedelic Monographs

EATING THE ROOT BARK

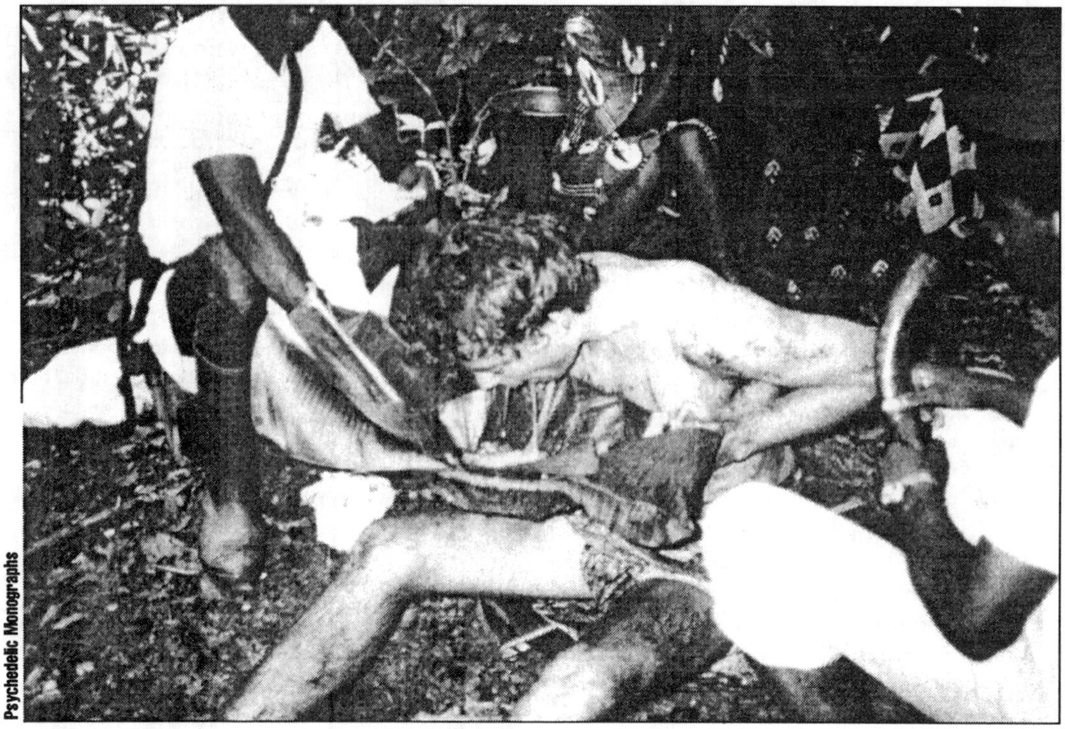

Psychedelic Monographs

EXTRAORDINARY CLEANSING

showers and telling her how great he felt. He was sitting there talking and she said, "Shut up. I'm in the middle of this experience here. Go for a walk or something."

Ron had gotten treated on a Sunday, a really quiet day. It was Monday, and all of a sudden people were cutting trees in front of the hotel, painters were painting windows, people were cleaning the hallways — there was all this noise. Sounds really get intensified on Ibogaine. About three or four hours into the treatment, Geerte decided to split.

> "I tried to puke up as much of the Ibogaine as I could. I thought it would stop the effect. It didn't, but I told myself it did, that it should be wearing off in half an hour. It wasn't, I was full-blown into it. But I wanted to go home. I dressed and wrote Sisko, who was still sleeping, a note: 'Have fun discovering new cultures in Africa with your freaky friends. See you another time'."

On the train-ride home to Utrecht, the Ibogaine was active — "I saw a lot of people who I experienced as being 'dead in the head'." At home she threw up again, which made her feel cheated — "I was not supposed to have withdrawal now." She went out to her dealer's house, where she smoked some heroin, and felt much better, though still trippy. Throwing up brought relief, but everything tasted and smelled bitter from the Ibogaine.

Late that night, as the heroin effect wore off, she lay down on the couch "in a dream-like, half-awake state," and the Ibogaine effect resumed as a rapid re-birthing experience. She saw herself as a fetus emerging from her mother's womb, felt "an incredible devotional love coming from my parents." This enabled her to accept mistakes her parents made during her growing up: "For the first time, I can feel respect for my parents, which shapes our whole relationship into a harmonious reality." Many other dream flashes appeared.

Researchers had known Ibogaine potentiates morphine analgesia, but here was a new finding — opiates potentiated the completion of Geerte's Ibogaine experience. She awoke the next morning completely refreshed, newborn, and hungry as a wolf. She gave her heroin away, and with Ron, started evaluating the experience. New things kept falling into place. It was as if all the information in their brain file cabinets was shaken out of its drawers onto one big pile, looked at "objectively" and re-filed, untwisted from emotional trauma.

It took time to realize they weren't getting sick, that there was no need to get money to run to the dealer anymore. The days went by

— one incredibly energetic and active, the next one needed to relax. A withdrawal never took place — just some occasional yawning and minor chills. Initially their junkie friends were skeptical, until they realized Ron was selling his methadone every day, for weeks in a row, and spending the money on camping gear to go to India, not drugs.

"In a normal withdrawal," said Geerte, "you need all your motivated energy to go through being sick, which burns you out completely."

This time their motivation was reinforced, and together with all of the visual experience, Ibogaine put Ron and Geerte on a path directed towards their goal. Some of their junkie friends found this positive attitude irritating. Others wanted to experience Ibogaine too. It was frustrating not to be able to give it to them.

The presence of hard drugs in their environment was neither threatening or particularly attractive: it just didn't matter. Once when Geerte tried heroin to see what it would do, it didn't get her stoned. It seemed to reactivate the Ibogaine. Up until four months after the treatment, she experienced colors and light very intensely.[1] Geerte lost interest in drugs in general; she found the effect of Ibogaine went far beyond their effect, though not necessarily in a pleasant way.

Ron stayed heroin-free until they reached Pakistan. Someone who's been a hardcore addict for twelve years finds it hard to resist a gram of smack for four dollars a day. Geerte carried all Ron's smack in her underwear for three months, because she was least likely to be strip-searched. But she stayed clean —

> "For years we'd been hunting it every day, and all of a sudden I was walking around with grams at a time and not touching it, because it made me nauseous, and felt horrible. My first Ibogaine experience also made me stop smoking, for six months. It was great."

Upon returning to Holland from Pakistan, India and Nepal, Geerte decided to go back to school in New York. But she had six months left in Holland, and she was so happy to be clean that she didn't want to hang around Ron, who was back to being a full-blown addict. She moved from Utrecht to Amsterdam, leaving Ron. There, all the friends that she told about her experience would come over every day, or call, asking, "Where's the Ibogaine? I want to get treated."

She'd been back a month, in March 1990, when she came into contact with Chris Schwartz again. He said Sisko had phoned and wanted to treat this guy Nico, who had founded the junkie-bond in Rotterdam more than a decade earlier. Geerte realized this meant the international coalition was going to continue doing treatments in Holland. Right away Geerte flashed on the idea of setting up her own addict self-help group to talk to people who were going to be treated, to prepare them. Then they could meet afterwards to do follow-up, and write up reports.

Chris introduced her to Simon and Reinhardt, who taught her how to work the Hi-Res squat computer. She started with all the information about Ron's and her treatments. She designed questionnaires. She did research with Simon about how to get their own supply of Ibogaine. The pharmaceutical companies told them they couldn't give any to people who were not scientific researchers.

Simon, who was English, had contacts in Cambridge with friends who had a laboratory there and said they could produce Ibogaine HCl. As they negotiated, the deal went sour because the Cambridge chemists refused to provide a sample. They were only willing to send the whole shipment, and they wanted cash — about $100 a gram. The squatters were willing to do benefits to raise the money, but at the same time they didn't want the media to catch on.

Then all of a sudden Chris, Simon and Reinhard decided to write a big article for the major newpapers, to tell them about the existence of Ibogaine.

It was May. Nico had been been treated by a team including Geerte:

> "Sisko stuck around a little bit and then he left us nine or ten doses of Ibogaine to set up a group to start treating Dutch addicts. The first to be treated was Nico's girlfriend, Josien. She was a total heroin prostitute and looked like a holocaust survivor. The only thing she would do is smoke heroin — smoke, smoke, smoke, smoke... and be a prostitute to get the money.
>
> "Within a week she was like a new person. She bought a mountain bike and started working out, got totally into vegetarian food... in three months she became this big, fat momma."

[1] See Chapter 18, p. 204.

Nico, Josien, and Geerte sat down, read everything on Ibogaine, the whole African ritual, and figured out how to involve the ritual in treating the next group, Geerte's friends from Utrecht:

> "We'd have the person come over the night before his treatment and introduce ourselves as Momma and Poppa Iboga, because the addict is the child going through re-birth. We would tell them about the African ritual the night before the treatment so that they'd totally know what they were going to face. We'd tell them the Africans use it basically to guide people into adulthood so they become more responsible people, and that's what we'd be doing. Making a person more responsible in life, so that he'd have control over drugs instead of drugs over the person.
>
> "If the person was a shooter, we would let him or her take their last shot, then let her or him destroy their syringe, symbolizing the destruction of their addiction. The same went for smokers and snorters — use up their last dose, then destroy the paraphernalia.
>
> "Each treament was a full moon and sun cycle. We had a room with two doors, which was perfect. We'd move someone in through a door with a moon painted on it, into the room where they would have the experience, and then after treatment guide them out the doorway decorated with a Sun.
>
> "We'd treat the person with much love and care. Momma and Papa Iboga would keep checking up on the person. All the treatments, about ten in a row during June, July and August of 1990, worked out fine. They were all my circle of friends, because I thought if they were all going to go home alone, and they didn't know each other, then they wouldn't have any help or recognition from each other. Before they were treated, I visited them at least five times, to prepare them mentally as best I could. I made all these trips to Utrecht.
>
> "Finally, I would introduce them to Nico and Josien, and we would do the treatments at Nico and Josien's house in Rotterdam, which was good because it was another city, and they couldn't just run out to buy heroin. But if people did want to go cop after the treatment, we'd first talk about if that was what they really wanted. If so, we'd help them cop.
>
> "We weren't anti-dope, just anti-addiction. We were pro-choice. It was perfectly set up, and all these people from the same generation just clicked. We all used to be members of the revolution but weren't any more. We were all idealists who had fallen into cynicism, and related in a similar way."

Geerte kept going back to Amsterdam after each treatment to put it on the computer. She wrote up each treatment from minute to minute, from intake to after-treatment. "During each treatment we took notes: 9 AM — 'person takes this much Ibogaine.' 9:15 AM — 'person vomits up a little Ibogaine.' You could read exactly how the treatment would take place, what we said to the person, etc."

But then, in May, 1990, after eight more treatments, Hi-Res — Simon, Chris and Reinhardt — all wanted to go public. Geerte, Nico and Josien objected strenuously. They were afraid publicity would cause the Dutch government to make Ibogaine illegal. What if health authorities broke into the midst of a treatment? Geerte said: "First we've got to treat fifty people and get all the data so we can throw out some numbers."

Geerte, Nico and Josien wanted it kept underground; Hi-Res wanted it in the news. So Geerte erased all the data from their computer, took all the information she had laying around, and moved out of the squat.

When she came back to pick up more stuff, Simon told her he had a back-up of all her data on the hard disk, and he was going ahead and making it into an article for the newspapers. Geerte shot back:

> "You never used heroin. You never used Ibogaine. Now you want to treat people and tell the newspapers what it's like? This is insane!"

The Hi-Res report, consisting of the information on the hard disk, was released to the newspapers. But most of the newspaper people said, if this was really happening, we would hear from the drug re-habs, we would hear from Erasmus University. We wouldn't hear it from some people who aren't even junkies, who haven't even experienced Ibogaine themselves.

Chris, Simon, and Reinhardt continued to do radio programs about Ibogaine, but the report was premature. It passed around the squats without igniting any kind of serious movement.[1]

Geerte, Nico and Josien decided to cut Hi-Res off from all subsequent treatments. This was in June, when they had treated about six additional people.

After eight treatments, Geerte and a friend in Utrecht were seriously talking of an

1 Published ultimately in the Netherlands *Journal of Substance Abuse Treatment*, Vol. 11, #4, pp. 379–385., by Simon G. Sheppeard. At fourteen weeks, he reports three of seven were drug free, one resumed intermittant use, two were back on in a few weeks, and one, who did only 700 milligrams of Ibogaine, used again after two days. Sheppeard indeed does seem to have cut the study short, and bolstering Geerte's side of the dispute, recently sent out flyers attacking "drug addicts and homosexuals," together with a letter declaring his intent to join a Nazi party.

Ibogaine support group. One day Nico's boss, Charlie Kaplan, walked in to Nico's house and suggested that everyone who had tried Ibogaine should start a focus group and get a doctor involved. Soon they were meeting once a week as a focus group, being examined by a doctor, sitting down and talking about their Ibogaine treatment and the after-effects.

At this point Nico and Josien were totally clean and happy, and so were the others. Some had used heroin in the first weeks after the treatment but didn't become re-addicted. Geerte's treatment was already more than six months old, and Ron had found out she'd done heroin here and there, without becoming re-addicted. Yet via the focus group, Geerte found out something very important:

> "I kept having contacts with my friends all through the months after my treatment and they basically all slowly but surely fell back into their addiction. The people who were dealing the heroin were very powerful, socially. They had friends in the focus group going back ten, fifteen years — they went all the way back to hippie times together. They had been through all kinds of shit and they had this intense bond.
>
> "The leader of this group was a heroin dealer, and in a way I was fucking with him by treating all his customers. I tried to stay friends so I wouldn't have a war with him. He himself wasn't healthy enough for a treatment — only had half his lungs left, from TB. Like most people in his scene he used to be an anti-heroin acidhead and pot-smoker.
>
> "In the end he won. After the Ibogaine people realized they were alone, and discovered the one thing they had in common was that every day, they used to sit at this guy's table and get together — and that this contact would happen because of smack (which was also his income). In the end they all fell back into heroin to maintain their social contact, and because the Ibogaine effect was wearing off."

The problem was that after treating people who lived in Rotterdam, Utrecht and Amsterdam, Geerte would have to take several train trips just to get the focus group together to talk. Some didn't even have phones. When she finally lost the war with the smack dealer, she realized it couldn't just be her, Nico, and Josien doing the treatments. It had to be on the clinical level, by re-habs who could follow through with employment, housing, support groups, everything. Or the underground movement would have to grow — which it wasn't doing because all the people who were treated just wanted to get on with their lives where they'd left off when they became addicted.

A lot of things happened fast right after Nico got treated — a snowball effect. After Josien got treated, she, Nico, and Geerte went to see Professor Dzoljic, who was the first to experiment in rats with Ibogaine and morphine self-administration. Dzoljic was interested in the activities of the treatment group, but not involved in the actual treatments.

Then, after Hi-Res succeeded in getting one small-town newspaper to publish a story about Ibogaine, Charlie Kaplan was fired as head of the Addiction Research Center at Erasmus Universtiy. Charlie was the one who got Sisko and Nico to connect, but he never officially witnessed a treatment. However, he made the mistake of answering, without proper clearance, questions from the reporter about his involvement. The headline said *"A Cure For Addiction."* But when they called Erasmus University and asked about one of their professors being associated with these treatments, Erasmus didn't want to be held responsible, so they dissociated themselves and bought out Charlie's contract as head of Addiction Research.

So Nico's boss was fired. It was the middle of the summer of '90. Nico started to put all Geerte's focus group data in his personal computer. Charlie did manage to get a German scientific researcher involved, doing a project for a thesis,[1] (and because she was genuinely interested in junkies). Nico really wanted to start a whole new life — one without junkies — but he didn't because his field researcher job was too well-paying. Just before she left for New York, Geerte's best male friend died on the operating table of dirty needles and bad heroin. She had to comfort his wife.

When she brought the work she'd done on the Hi-Res computer to Nico so he could enter it on the computer at Erasmus, they found they had a basic disagreement.

"What we really have to do is sit down with the drug rehabs and tell them Ibogaine is out there," said Geerte, "so they come forward with the interest and the money for the next treatments."

Nico didn't want the rehabs involved: "If

1 For Eva Ketzer, on "Wellness," turn the page.

I wanted to be treated, I'd want to be treated in a situation like we treated our friends in — in a house, treated by ex-junkies, not by some doctor in a clinical situation."

"I agree that should be happening," said Geerte, "but it also should be happening on a bigger level. We can't treat thousands of people. They can. We should be working on two levels instead of one."

"I don't believe in clinical settings," Nico told her. "We should keep the ritual involved with it."

In some ways Geerte agreed, and sought consensus. "We could train the rehabs."

"No," Nico insisted. "If you haven't had the Ibogaine experience, you can't know how to treat other people, because you don't know what they're going through. You're going to doctors. They're going to hook you up with inputs from all these machines, all kinds of experiments."

Nico scheduled his next pair of treatments — the couple from the Rotterdam Central Station — just when Sisko was treating some one else in another part of Rotterdam. So there were three treatments going on at once, with available paraclinicians completely overstretched. This woman at Nico's couldn't sleep and he didn't have any sedatives to give her. She was up for three or four days in a row, totally psychotic.[1] Nico had to go out on a bicycle to get a doctor. He didn't even have a phone. He didn't come back for a whole day, which totally exasperated Sisko.

Sisko concluded that if Nico — who was already refusing to share data on any of the Dutch treatments, or bring in the drug rehabs — wouldn't cooperate with him in doing treatments, he would cut off Nico's supply of Ibogaine.

This episode, when Geerte heard about it in New York, convinced her treatments must be done by a team, since no one person can really understand a personality.

> "You have to do it as a group, and not do a treatment here and there at the same time. Nico should have kept working with Sisko, but Sisko cut Nico off, and from that moment on, nothing happened, the whole year I was in New York, from September, 1990 to June, 1991.
>
> "In June, 1991, I walked back into Nico's house and asked — 'Where's my data, where's my computer work?' Turns out the guy has done hardly anything, hasn't set up the focus groups, hasn't kept up with any of the people we treated. He's sitting there talking about going to big annual international conferences to speak on Ibogaine, going to Zurich, to needle park...
>
> 'I don't want to hang out with the junkie scene any more,' Nico was saying. 'I just want to treat addicts —'."

"This is not the right attitude," Geerte interjected. "I'm sorry, but I'm not going to work with you if you're in this state of mind." Geerte was living at Nico and Josien's house with Adam, her new boyfriend from New York. Adam was a member of the New York band Missing Foundation.[2] As soon as they got to Holland they got to be junkies again within three weeks because the Dutch smack was so intense. Finally Geerte sat down with Nico and sighed, "I don't want be a junkie again, I'm sick of it."

And Nico said, "I was cleaning my bookshelf and I found three doses of Ibogaine behind the books."

"What?" asked Geerte. And Nico was introducing this guy, and saying "I want to treat this dude from the train station..." when Geerte broke in — "You fucking asshole! Why don't you treat me? I'm the one putting all the years of work on this project, and I'm the one hooked again, and I want another treatment!"

Adam wanted to be treated as well, so eventually Nico agreed to treat both of them. "I actually started crying right before I took the capsules because I knew..." mused Geerte. "This time, knowing I was about to go through this experience was a pretty heavy-duty decision. The first time you don't know what's going to happen. But the second time you do — which is more difficult. This time I didn't resist the effects, and Nico really helped me. I took it and in half an hour it started working. I lay down on my bed and started tripping immediately. The climax is about four hours after you take it. I think I fainted in the middle of my climax. Adam was treated two days before me, and he did very well. It was July, 1991."

The disagreement with Nico persisted. Adam and Geerte had to move into their own place in Rotterdam. They founded DASH — Dutch Addict Self-Help. They started going to all the rehabs in Holland, telling them

1 This was the one who believed she was possessed. See p. 81 of this Report.

2 Focus of "Cult of Rage" special by television news reporter Mike Taibbi, mentioned on p. 89, note 3..

Reaching a State of Wellnes: Multistage Explorations in Social Neuroscience

Charles D. Kaplan
IPSER, Academic Psychiatry Center, University of Limburg, The Netherlands

Eva Ketzer
General Practitioner Institute, Medical Faculty, Erasmus University, Rotterdam, The Netherlands

Joop de Jong
IPSER

Marten de Vries
IPSER

The United States Congress has declared the decade of the 1990s the "Decade of the Brain." As Cacioppo and Berntson (1992, p. 1019) point out, "this declaration is important to all psychologists, not only neuroscientists, because with this declaration come expectations of the cognitive and behavioral sciences generally and because the brain does not exist in isolation but rather is a fundamental component of developing and aging individuals who themselves are mere actors in the larger theater of life." We might add that this declaration is also of critical importance to anthropologists and sociologists, as well as physicians. The recognition that people are actors in the larger theater of life provides social neuroscience with an important place in the matrix organization of science in the decade of the brain. And also, to this end, are practical issues of applying the resulting scientific knowledge to the betterment of the condition of people through, among other disciplines, the practice of medicine.

In the Netherlands, there has been an upshot of multi-disciplinary formations in several medical schools to reorganize research in psychiatry and related medical specializations into a brain-and-behavioral program. This ambitious attempt has not been easy and involves the reconciliation of often conflicting epistemologies and methodologies, not to mention conflicting interest around basic and applied research. Medicine is an extremely practical affair, and no matter how elegant the research question and design can be, it must be tightly bound to issues of the patient. Our group, over the years, has attempted to contribute to the development of this brain and behavior initiative by emphasizing the basic role of culture and society in shaping the context of the patient and of determining what is in fact "the case" for social neuroscience. We have been especially influenced by ethnomedical and cross-cultural psychiatry traditions, but we have also tried to find our own way out of the limitations of these two traditions. We are not, in fact, interested in the macrocultural systems that have been the traditional object of ethnomedicine. Rather, we have worked to bring ethnography and other fieldwork methods into the design of medical research. In this regard, we have conceived of the endogenous mechanisms of the brain to have correlates in the exogenous mechanisms of cultural and social interaction.

To get from behavior to the brain and back again is a multistage process. The design of this research involves a Stage 1 which identifies risks and problems in a specific population. Stage 2 moves to target groups through snowball sampling and to problem clarification through the use of focus groups which aim to develop theoretical constructs that have "member" (i.e., patient) validity. Stage 3 consists of the acquisitions of intensive field samples of a relatively small size studied through experience-sampling methodology (ESM; see de Vries 1992) and ethnography. Only after this work is done are we ready to enter the laboratory for testing out hypotheses related to specific exogenous and cultural variables and brain function. This laboratory work represents Stage 4. In Stage 5 clinical and field trails can be conducted on interventions that are based on the findings.

Most of our work to this date has been limited to Stages 2 and 3. We have conducted extensive studies in Stage 3 using ESM on various psychiatric-patient groups. Study participants wear programmed wrist terminals that beep in random intervals during waking hours. At each beep, the participant fills out a short questionnaire. Thus, in a design calling for ten beeps per day, for seven days, the respondent is asked to fill out the same questionnaire seventy times. These studies have provided us with a thick description of the daily rhythms of psychiatric syndromes and the interplay of their specific symptoms with contextual, thought, and mood variables. These studies are allowing us to reframe diagnoses with new behavioral and cognitive data drawn from daily life. For example, in an ESM study of twenty active heroin addicts we were able to identify protective factors that are important determinants of health within the context of addiction (Kaplan et al. 1990). The in-depth analysis of these factors has allowed us to understand how addict daily life is naturally organized to protect health as well as to result in illness. The positive factors in addict daily life should provide the basis for health-promotion efforts in this hidden population.

We also have been making extensive use of focus groups prior to ESM analysis. The focus group has received attention for some time as a tool in applied research (Krueger 1988). The method involves the systematic formation of groups organized for the purpose of obtaining specific information. The group is organized to produce specific data of interest to the researcher and therefore differs from other groups, such as delphic and brainstorming. Focus groups are principally data-collection procedures, producing qualitative information which can facilitate theoretical insights. The topics for discussion are carefully selected and sequenced and are designed to provide materials for building theoretical understandings of the context and experience of the group participants. The focus group has recently been introduced as a tool relevant for public health problems.

For illustrative purposes we can present in this short communication two focus group studies that are currently underway. One involves focus groups conducted at the Tibetan Medical Institute in India with pain patients who have been treated with traditional Tibetan medicine and also Western techniques. The second focus group was conducted in the Netherlands with heroin addicts who had been treated by "lay healers" with ibogaine, an alkaloid extracted from an African root with potent mind-altering properties. Both focus groups collected background medical data and solicited informaton clarifying social neuroscientific processes that might be involved in reaching the state of wellness by these patients.

In the Tibetan focus groups, medicine blessed by His Holiness, the Dalai Lama, was used together with natural techniques, such as regimes of warm baths, were reported to result in the gradual reaching of wellness after years of severe pain and unsuccessful treatment. The role of this specially blessed medicine is crucial in the patients' accounts. A question for future research is what sociocultural mechanisms in conjunction with neurochemical processes are able to alter long-enduring periods of illness?

Some suggestions emerge in the consideration of the results of the focus groups with the Dutch heroin addicts. The focus group of the addicts revealed that ibogaine was able to induce the experience of collective consciousness and a clearing up of the mind for the members of the focus group. J., one of the members, reported a common experience, namely, that ibogaine had made her aware that "All the information I ever got through reading or experience was registered in my brain, and I was impressed with the tremendous capacity of the brain." This demonstration of the brain's capacities, which formerly was only theoretically known, became a lived experience. Common to all members was the production of an intense state of wakefulness. For three to four weeks after taking the ibogaine, they slept for only three to four hours per day. After a month they gradually returned to eight hours of sleep per day. The ibogaine experience was not comfortable for the members; all had highly anxious episodes. The state of ibogaine was described by all as a dream with full consciousness. All felt themselves to be physically heavy, i.e., in a somnolent stage like a body in sleep. All reported an interruption of heroin-seeking behavior for relatively long periods of time, a state that they never thought they would reach given their former nihilistic, depressed view of life.

From these focus groups some intriguing hypotheses have been clarified, highlighting both exogenous and endogenous processes. The ibogaine experience succeeded in providing a common sense of belonging to a distinct community oriented to wellness—a European variety of the African iboga medicine society. Thus, even, the one member who used heroin again rather shortly after the treatment did so out of a clear decision and reported that he did not feel himself addicted anymore. The focus group undermined a preconceived notion that, because of its extraordinary psychopharmacological effects, ibogaine produces a singular, common experience. However, the members discovered in the group that each experienced the ibogaine in a unique and different way. Does ibogaine, like the Dalai Lama's medicine, work to create a sense of belonging to a medicine community that is dedicated toward reaching a state of wellness? Is this special consensus an important exogenous mechanism culturally reframing pathological endogenous processes?

Turning to the endogenous system it is known that ibogaine is a serotonin agonist and has been pharmacologically classified as an antidepressant. Ibogaine's tricyclic chemical structure resembles the tricyclic antidepressants, such as imipramine, which have had successful clinical trials in managing drug-craving. Could this ibogaine have resulted in a "rechanneling" of serotonin in the brain, basically altering the fixated behavioral rhythms of the addict? All addicts presented a significant weight alteration from 3 to 10 kilograms. These alterations, together with the dramatic sleep changes, suggest a rechanneling of serotonin in the brain. In this case, could serotonin rechanneling inside the brain be correlated with a rechanneling of the drug addict's community consensus? Is wellness the outcome, if only for awhile, of this correlation?

These focus groups have indeed served their purpose of clarifying hypotheses and future research problems for specific subgroups of a larger population of patients. They illustrate that the correlation of exogenous and endogenous social neuroscientifically relevant mechanisms can be made available for empirical analysis through a stepwise, multistage method. Indeed, this relates to the reasoning why Cacioppo and Berntson have subtitled their article the "Doctrine of Multilevel Analysis." The decade of the brain in the 1990s will probably be one of great surprises. Not the least of these may be that an essential field of neuroscience research lies far beyond the laboratories of bench science. Reaching a state of wellness must certainly involve exogenous factors in "the larger theater of life." Focus groups, snowball sampling, experience sampling, and ethnography promise to be useful tools in the 1990s to clarify the theater's plays, stages, and scripts.

REFERENCES

Cacioppo, John T. and Gary G. Berntson (1992) "Social Psychological Contributions to the Decade of the Brain." *American Psychologist* 47:1019-1028.

Kaplan, C.D., M.W. de Vries, J.P. Grund and N.F.P. Adriaans (1990) "Protective Factors: Dutch Interventions, Health Determinants and the Reorganization of Addict Life." Pp. 165- 176 in H.A. Ghodse, C.D. Kaplan and R.D. Mann, eds., *Drug Misuse and Dependence*. Park Ridge, New Jersey: Parthenon Publishing Group.

Kreuger, R.A. (1988) *Focus Groups: A Practical Guide for Applied Research*. Newbury Park: Sage Publications.

Vries, M.W. de, ed. (1992) *The Experience of Psychopathology: nvestigating Mental Disorders in their Natural Settings*. Cambridge: Cambridge University Press.

about Ibogaine. Geerte mailed out Ibogaine packets. But the reaction was pretty lame.

Adam and Geerte got married. Their honeymoon was the Drug Policy Foundation conference in November, 1991. There they met Eric Fromberg, from the Netherlands Institute on Drug and Alcohol Abuse. They started talking Dutch. He wanted to find out more about Ibogaine. When Geerte and Adam went back to Holland, she looked up Fromberg.

"You should help introduce Ibogaine to Dutch scientists, and to the rehabs," she told him.

"I'll only do it if I see some treatments," said Fromberg.

Geerte told Howard, "I have to do some treatments." He said, "Okay, four treatments on the way."

While they were waiting for Howard to arrive, Geerte and Adam went to Berlin, to the European Interest Group of Drug Users, the conference of the junkie unions in Europe. It was January, 1992, and they were discussing human rights for HIV-infected addicts. Geerte and Adam went around telling all the junkie-bonds of Europe about Ibogaine, and most of them responded, "So what? We don't want to get treated. We want free heroin and methadone."

"One of the only ones who picked up on Ibogaine," Geerte continued, "was the organizer of the conference, Herman, who was HIV-positive. We wanted Ibogaine to be one of their projects, but only Herman supported it, and they wouldn't elect me to anything. At the end of the conference, Herman publicly said he would promote Ibogaine. We came back and we thought — 'If the junkie-bonds won't do it, we'll have to work harder than ever, and DASH will be on its own!'" Geerte and Adam went ahead and turned their house into a clinic.

"I was in the middle of an art show when the treatments took place, in early April. Things were very hectic. I had sleep spaces set up for Howard and Norma. I had three treatment rooms — rooms for doctors and everything." DASH supplied two people for treatment, Lanna and Grinnato. Howard and Norma brought a 19 year old male crackhead who couldn't stop touching the cold sores on his face, and Carol Baker, an HIV-positive woman dually-addicted to methadone and heroin.

The treatments went off without a hitch, with Fromberg present throughout, along with two representatives of Dutch treatment groups, two doctors and Professor Bastiaans, a senior Dutch expert on psychedelic therapy

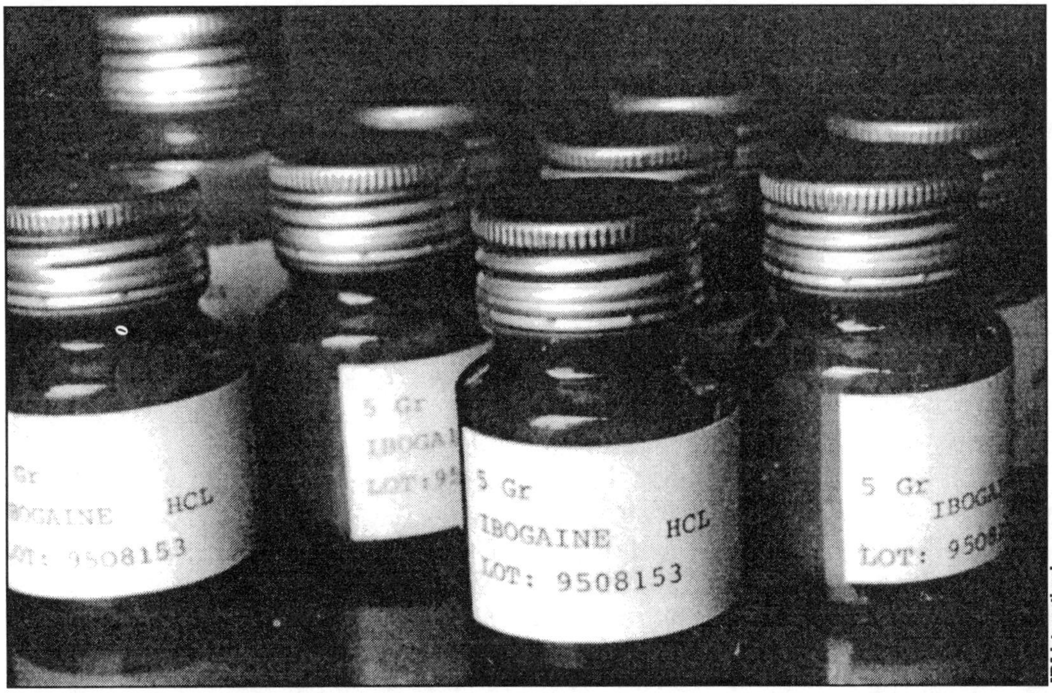

NDA International

Pharmaceutical-grade Ibogaine

who had given LSD to concentration-camp survivors. This time the doctors who were there had authorizations from their respective institutions to be there. They saw the after-effects, that these people were actually cleaned out.

"Grinato was a second-timer," said Geerte. "His case was the most successful because he was very motivated. He loved his experience."

Geerte went back to New York soon afterwards. Before she had gone to Holland, she had been forced out of Umbrella House, which she started, as a suspected junkie. The same Lower East Side anarchists who earlier engineered the big split to keep the marijuana movement from supporting Ibogaine refused to give Adam a key, even though the building voted to give him one, since he had previously lived there; they kept forcing re-votes until they got the outcome they wanted. They even broke into Geerte's space to see if they could find bags of dope.[1]

[1] See Chapter 8, p. 71; Chapter 9, p. 88.

Now it turned out she couldn't get her apartment back from Seth Tobocman, who held on to it as an art studio while he lived in his own — rented — apartment.

Meanwhile, in Rotterdam, Nico found out he was HIV-positive, and decided to take more responsibility for the project. He started involving Ibogaine in his work at the University.

The next move was for Fromberg to do treatments on ten methadone addicts, but he has to first inform the government and get funding. Said Geerte, of the doctors who have witnessed treatments in Holland: "All three of them are scientific witnesses that it works. That's what you need. You can't be a junkie or an ex-junkie, because people won't take you seriously. But they take doctors seriously. Now we need the money to do and track ten treatments, and fight the Dutch bureaucracy."

CHAPTER 12: Agent of Coincidence

One day in late July 1990, when he was stuck somewhere with nothing to do, Dana re-read a book he remembered as having offered a glimpse of Ibogaine's probable impact back in 1981, when the project was just starting. It was *VALIS,* by P. K. Dick, based on Dick's famous near-death experience (NDE) in March, 1974, from which he awoke speaking ancient *koine* Greek, understanding his own name as Horselover (Philip) Fat (German for Dick). Dana was looking for a passage that reads:

> " '**The Empire never ended,**' Fat quoted to himself. That one sentence appeared over and over again in his exegesis; it had become his tag line. Originally the sentence had been revealed to him in a great dream. In the dream he again was a child, searching dusty used-book stores for rare old science fiction magazines, in particular *Astoundings.* In the dream he had looked through countless tattered issues, stacks upon stacks, for the priceless serial entitled "The Empire Never Ended." If he could find it and read it he would know everything; that had been the burden of the dream.
>
> "Prior to that, during the interval in which he experienced the two-world superimposition, he had seen not only California, U.S.A., of the year 1974 but also ancient Rome, he had discerned within the superimposition a Gestalt shared by both space-time continua, their common element: a Black Iron Prison. This is what the dream referred to as "the Empire." He knew it because, upon seeing the Black Iron Prison, he had recognized it. Everyone dwelt in it without realizing it. The Black Iron Prison was their world.
>
> "Who had built the prison–and why–he could not say. But he could discern one good thing: the prison lay under attack. An organization of Christians, not regular Christians such as those who attended church every Sunday and prayed, but secret early Christians wearing light gray-colored robes, had started an assault on the prison, and with success. The secret, early Christians were filled with joy.
>
> "Fat, in his madness, understood the reason for their joy. This time the early, secret, gray-robed Christians would get the prison, *rather than the other way around.* The deeds of the heroes, in the sacred dream-time...the only time, according to the bushmen, that was real.
>
> "Once, in a cheap science fiction novel, Fat had come across a perfect description of the Black Iron Prison but set in the far future. So if you superimposed the past (ancient Rome) over the present (California in the twentieth Century) and super-imposed the far future world of *The Android Cried Me a River* over that, you got the Empire, the Black Iron Prison, as the supra- or trans-temporal constant. Everyone who had ever lived was literally surrounded by the iron walls of the prison; they were all inside of it and none of them knew it — except for the gray-robed secret Christians.
>
> "That made the early, secret Christians supra- or trans-temporal, too, that is to say present at all times, a situation which Fat could not fathom. How could they be early but in the present and the future? And if they existed in the present, why couldn't anyone see them? On the other hand, why couldn't anyone see the walls of the Black Iron Prison which enclosed everyone, including himself, on all sides? Why did these antithetical forces emerge into palpability only when the past, present and future somehow–for whatever reason–got superimposed?
>
> "Maybe in the bushman's dreamtime no time existed. But if no time existed, how could the early secret Christians be scampering away with glee from the Black Iron Prison which they had just succeeded in blowing up? And how could they blow it up back in Rome circa 70 C.E., since no explosives existed in those days? And how, if no time passed in the dream-time, could the prison come to an end? It reminded Fat of the peculiar statement in Parsifal: "You see my son, here time turns into space." During his religious experience in March of 1974, Fat had seen an augmentation of space: yards and yards of space, extending all the way to the stars; space opened up around him as if a confining box had been removed..."
>
> (*VALIS,* pp. 48–49)

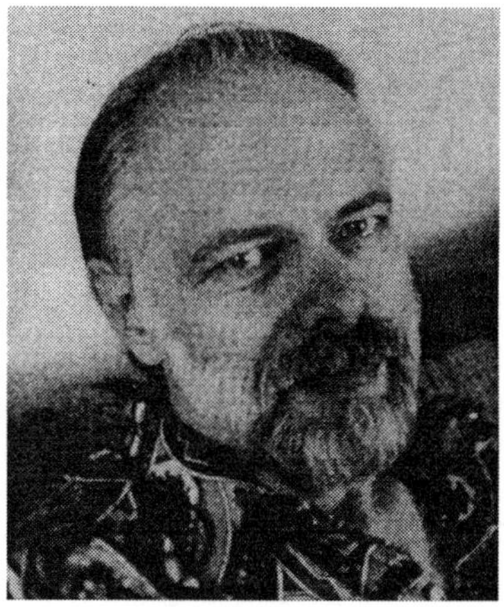

P. K. DICK

Now privately Howard, Boaz, and Sisko sat around that summer reveling in the changes Ibogaine would unleash — "the system-smash," Boaz called it — like a Big Bang without an explosion. But Philip Dick they thought of as science fiction, even though *VALIS* is actually a book on gnosticism and the lost plant sacrament of the early Christians, which Dick got to know all about during the '60s while married to the daughter of Episcopal Archbishop James Pike's mistress. Pike — the famed companion of Martin Luther King at Selma, Alabama — perished a few years later looking for the missing sacrament in the vicinity of the Dead Sea.

VALIS, and *The Transmigration of Timothy Archer,* Dick's even more autobiographical chronicle of Bishop Pike's quest and disappearance, provide a fascinating window into mainstream — if heretical — Christian thought on plant sacraments.[1]

Some months previously, though, Howard had cut a deal with the Belgian pharmaceutical giant Omnichem, which manufactures Ibogaine as a by-product of the leukemia drug vincristine, and by coincidence had decided, instead of dumping it, to stockpile this 99.7% pure (semi-synthetic[2]) Ibogaine. So Howard had cornered the world supply of Ibogaine. And Howard, Boaz and Sisko, who were now in the process of reconciling — working it out so that Howard wouldn't have to sue Sisko for infringing on his patent — were uncomfortable with the part about secret early Christians, even though no less an authority than James Fernandez notes the affinity of the Bwiti mindset to Biblical-era parable and proverb.[3]

Moreover, what tied Bwiti specifically to Gnosticism (even ancient Gnosticism seen through the post-quantum eyes of Philip Dick) was that, as Fernandez points out: "For these Bwitists... religion was not a matter of faith... It was a very pragmatic technique for understanding, predicting and controlling — in short a science or pre-science of hidden things. To believe in something despite lack of evidence or evidence to the contrary, which is the Western religious condition, was foreign to their attitudes. Fang had always had good evidence for their beliefs" — via ready access to plant sacrament, like the Gnostics. In *VALIS,* in a passage on Gnostic sacraments, Beal found an Ibogaine parallel which was just uncanny:

> **"48. ON OUR NATURE. It is proper to say: we appear to be memory coils (DNA carriers capable of experience) in a computer-like thinking system which, although we have correctly recorded thousands of years of experiential information, and each of us possesses somewhat different deposits from all the other life forms, there is a malfunction — a failure — of memory retrieval.** There lies the trouble in our particular subcircuit. 'Salvation' through gnosis — more properly anamnesis (the loss of amnesia) — although it has individual significance for each of us — a quantum leap in perception, identity, cognition, understanding, world- and self-experience, including immortality — it has greater and further importance for the system as whole, inasmuch as these memories are data needed by it and valuable to it, to its overall functioning.
>
> "Therefore it is in the process of self-repair, which includes: rebuilding our subcircuit via linear and orthogonal time changes, as well as continual signalling to us to stimulate blocked memory banks within us to fire and hence retrieve what is there.
>
> "The external information or gnosis, then, consists of disinhibiting instructions, with the core content actually intrinsic to us — that is, already there (first observed by Plato; viz: that learning is a form of remembering).
>
> **"The ancients possessed techniques (sacraments[3] and rituals) used largely in the Greco-Roman mystery religions, including early Christianity, to induce firing and retrieval, mainly with a sense of its restorative value to the individuals;** the Gnostics, however, correctly saw the ontological value to what they called the Godhead itself, the total entity.
>
> "The Godhead is impaired; some primordial crisis occured in it which we do not understand."
>
> (*VALIS,* pp. 96–97)

For a long time Howard and Sisko — who meanwhile reached an agreeement that ICASH would continue to do the intake and the treatments, but under the supervision of an NDA-supplied physician authorized by the Dutch government — couldn't see the connection with Ibogaine. Yet the more Dana got into it, the more he realized getting ahold of *VALIS*[5] in 1981 was like being handed a roadmap to understanding gnostic substances, Ibogaine and *Bwiti,* way back in the very beginning. But the Ibogaine story is replete with these coincidences.

Take Howard's contact at the University of Miami, Dr. Deborah Mash, who is currently doing the first Phase I clinical (safety) trial with ten humans. In late June, 1991, Howard gave her a call because her work showing cocaine and alcohol combine in the body to

1 Phil acknowledges in his Foreword to *A Maze of Death* (1968) the "wealth of theological material" he learned through talks with Pike. As biographer Lawrence Sutin's *Divine Invasions: A Life of Philip K. Dick* (New York: Harmony Books, 1989), puts it:

> "(Pike) was making repeated trips to Israel to investigate the historical Jesus.... In a July 1974 letter Phil recalled:
>
> Jim was tried for heresy shortly before his death [the charge was ultimately dismissed], and later resigned as bishop. Whether it reached the newspaper pages or not, the basic issue, the basic fear about him, was not merely that he had denied the Trinity but that he had picked up Zoroastrian doctrines, probably while going over the Dead Sea Scrolls discoveries.
>
> 'If I were not a Christian,' I heard him preach in December of 1964 in Grace Cathedral, 'I would be a Jew. And if I were not a Jew I would be a Zoroastrian.' And then he delivered to the congregation what I know to be a Zoroastrian exhortation: 'Come into the Light.' (He extended his arms and open hands to them all.) 'Come into the Light.' And so forth. This is the doctrine of Ormazd (Mazda), the Persian God of Light, identified with the Sun.... (p. 151)."

2 The .3% impurities are vinca-alkoloids, however, not Iboga-alkoloids.

3 Not necessarily to Christianity as opposed to Judaism, however. "As more of the Bible was translated and as the distinction between the religious cultures of the Old and New Testament became clear, Fang [a Bwiti people] reacted in favor of the Old Testament. It was not only that Fang found their own rigid taboo system reflected in the Book of Moses. The patrilineal extended family and polygyny and exogamy of the Old Testament was also congenial. Particularly for Protestants, who focus on the Bible rather than the Catechism, this unexpected preference posed a problem." See Fernandez, pp. 276–77.

4 Probably *harmala peganum.* See Chapter 16, pp. 177–180.

5 Stands for *Vast Active Living Intelligence System.*

form a distinct addictive substance, *coca-ethylene,* was just what he needed to get his patent for the treatment of polydrug dependency (U.S. Patent #5,152,992, October 6, 1992).

"Deborah picked up the phone," said Lotsof, "and we'd hardly started discussing coca-ethylene, when she said point blank — 'What about Ibogaine?' "

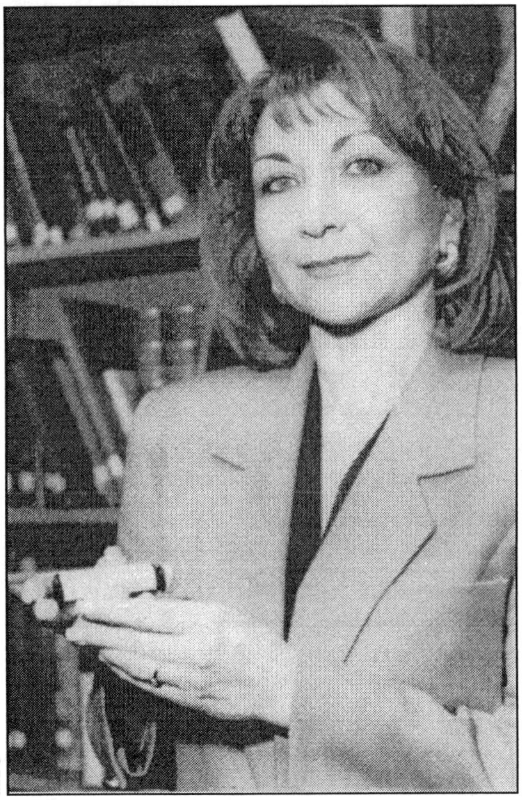
MAPS

Dr. Deborah Mash

"I hadn't introduced it into the conversation, so I asked, 'Did I mention Ibogaine?' "

" 'No,' she said, 'but I just attended three presentations on Ibogaine in West Palm Beach at the Conference on Problems of Drug Dependency, and I was just sitting here trying to figure out how to get in touch with you when the phone rang.' "

Deborah Mash was working with Dr. Juan Sanchez-Ramos, a neurospecialist on Parkinson's disease (PK) who'd written a paper on early treatment of PK with harmaline.[1] He became her principal investigator for the Ibogaine IND. Deborah also happens to be married to the Chairman of the Democratic Committee of Dade County. The Florida primary was very important to Clinton, so — Mash was able to arrange a meeting with Hillary. After briefing her for more than an hour on the Ibogaine Project, Mash secured her promise to do something about Ibogaine if and when the Clintons got to the White House.

The prospect of Mash's IND application for the Phase I trial being approved by FDA — and Howard pulling an end-run thereby on the MDD — also kept up the pressure on Vocci to move ahead, despite countervailing static in the system. After torpedoing the meeting between ACT UP and CASA,[2] Herb Kleber went into overdrive behind the scenes, activating his cronies salted away in NIDA's peer review process to cut off new grants for Ibogaine in the regular extra-mural system — the mechanism outside the MDD that Glick used to fund all of his research. (However — since as many animal studies came out supporting Ibogaine in 1992 as in all previous years combined — this was kind of like closing the barndoor after the livestock are long gone.)

None of this became known for months. What was obvious — after Glick told the *Albany Times-Union* in October of '91 that Ibogaine represented "the strangest coalition I've ever been involved in" — was a long dry spell in the media: nothing on Ibogaine being fast-tracked, nothing on ACT UP or Dhoruba joining the fray. Press releases were faxed out only to run up against "the experts," and in drug-free America, reporters take their cue from the experts. To the press, the Staten Island Project scenario seemed about as likely as some Japanese cut off on a remote island at the end of WW II coming up on their own with the Atomic Bomb.

But then coincidence intervened again — in the form of a disgruntled ex-Yippie, thrown out by Alice T. fourteen years earlier for robbing Studio 10 blind, who, claiming to act on behalf of Abbie Hoffman and the *Soho Weekly News,* still made crank calls to 9 Bleecker every morning between 6 and 7 AM. He knew Dana can't go back to sleep. Since 1979 he'd been trying to make Beal so fried he couldn't function. He'd make obscene phone calls to the kids, sex calls to Alice, anti-Semitic calls if you were Jewish, etc.

In the last three years or so, he'd escalated, putting up stickers on phones all over the city for non-existent whorehouses (Madame Alice, Oral etc.) and sex services (gay dating club,

[1] See page 190, Chapter 17.

[2] Kleber recently claimed that it wasn't him — that Califano refused to meet with ACT UP because he is super-Catholic. But Califano had agreed to the meeting for more than a week already, knowing full well it was to be with ACT UP, until Kleber discovered Ibogaine was on the agenda, and it was abruptly cancelled.

sperm bank) so Alice would get twenty crank calls a day from aggressive weirdos. Alice is unflappable, though, so Hank the Skank escalated again. In April of '92 he put up a sticker that said, "DRUG MULES: *Earn Big Bux* — Call 212 677-4899," figuring he'd get Dana in trouble with his probation officer. It did cause an investigation by Telco security. But instead of the DEA, a *Philadelphia Inquirer* reporter called up — Andy Maykuth from the New York bureau — and Dana said: "Oh, a sticker. It's put up by a cranker in Brooklyn who's trying to discredit what we really do, which is work on a *cure* for hard drugs, an African rainforest alkaloid called Ibogaine."

After ten minutes Maykuth agreed a crank from Brooklyn wasn't much of a story — "But maybe we can do something with the Ibogaine." Howard was in Lyden, the Netherlands, doing a series of treatments, because Dr. Baastians, the Dutch psychiatrist who had to sign off with the Dutch government for each Ibogaine treatment, lived in Lyden. Baastians, who pioneered treatment of concentration camp survivors with LSD, was too old to travel. He'd just had triple-bypass heart surgery, and since he insisted on sitting in on the 24-hour-a-day treatments himself, the strain was so great Howard, Norma and the treatment team thought more than once that they might lose him.

But the treatments were successful, and in early May Dana brought Howard to the floor of ACT UP with one of his successes: Carol Baker, the first HIV-positive person treated with Ibogaine. She'd been dually addicted, using 80 mg. of methadone to get through the day, and $250 worth of heroin to get through the night. As a successful real estate broker she could afford it. But she had no veins left, and she wanted to live out her life clear of the methadone fog.

After the uneventful 22-hour treatment and a short nap, she awoke feeling like "her armor had been stripped away." She was one of the first to fly back by way of the University of Miami, where Lotsof had set up his own post-treatment evaluations with Dr. Mash and Dr. Juan Sanchez Ramos. "I kicked methadone once before," she told ACT UP,"and it was five months of Hell. This time I woke up, I hadn't had a fix in 24 hours, and I wasn't dopesick. It was like a miracle."

The visualizations weren't like LSD, she said: "You see millions of visions when you close your eyes. But when you open them, you come back to where you are. You realize it was all mental." ACT UP loved it — this little woman with HIV, de-toxed with one Ibogaine treatment. Andy Maykuth of the *Inquirer*, sitting in the audience, could feel it. One thing led to another, and on July 4, 1992, in Philadelphia, the *Inquirer* published *"It's From an African Shrub. Howard Lotsof Says it Got Him off Heroin and Cocaine: TO BATTLE ADDICTION, HE ADVOCATES USE OF A DRUG."* It was the lead headline on page one: a Declaration of Independence for Addicts.

And best of all, when Dana appeared three days later for another adjournment on his probation violation (in Manhattan Court, not Queens), he could point to himself quoted in it: "Ibogaine kind of knocks you on your butt, which is good because you can't go out and get drugs. By the time the Ibogaine wears off, you don't have any craving."

"Your Honor," he said, "I just want to say that because of your ruling allowing me to travel and lobby the National Institute on Drug Abuse, this breakthrough treatment for addiction has been fast-tracked by the Federal government."

Sisko and Howard, though, were disappointed the story focus was still on a small cast of Lower East Side characters–that it failed to tell how in the past 18 months support for Ibogaine had metastasized beyond its countercultural roots. ACT UP was mentioned way down in the text. Nothing on Dhoruba or Black community support. So while everyone else was in Holland for the AIDS Conference, Dana put together an Ibogaine workbook with ACT UP's Xerox document-maker. It had all the available animal studies, the patents, the human anecdotal stuff, ACT UP correspondence with the government, with a couple of introductory articles up front. Beal began sending the book plus the 60-minute augmented Nico tape out to every science writer, every drug reporter, every AIDS writer at every major newspaper in the country.

He could add or subtract documents at will with the Xerox, so for the August 4th Harlem Hospital gig, he added African anthropological data, plus 20th Century documents relevant to the genesis of the Project, like the 1956 Harris Isbell letter, selections of *VALIS* and the original Black Panther tract, *"Capitalism Plus Dope Equals Genocide."*

He was rushing to finish before his trial date of August 7. But then another Ibogaine coincidence intervened. Out in Sonoma, California, Dennis Peron's friend Brownie Mary Rathbun was busted blending two pounds of marijuana into brownies for AIDS patients. After Brownie Mary hit CNN, Dana knew that in a few months, the publicity from her case would turn the country around on medical marijuana. He got another affadavit from Kunstler asking for a long adjournment. On August, 7, the Judge gave him until October 1st. He spent the next day waiting for Dennis and Brownie Mary to fly in for the Maury Povitch show, serenely cleaning up pages of the workbook on the Xerox.

A few weeks later a final section was added to the workbook on waking REM, when David Goldstein turned up a new paper by H. Deportere, *"Neocortical Rhythmic Slow Activity During Wakefulness and Paradoxical Sleep in Rats."* Deportere indicated Ibogaine tremor and behavioral immobility were clearly a function of stimulation of acetylcholine pathways — the ones active during sleep and REM (i.e., Rapid Eye Movement during dreams). Dana threw in an article he'd been saving since January from the *New York Times* science section on dreaming, which contained a paragraph that reminded him of all the accounts of Howard, Nico, etc., of the sensation of travelling at tremendous speeds through space, or down a tunnel, which said:

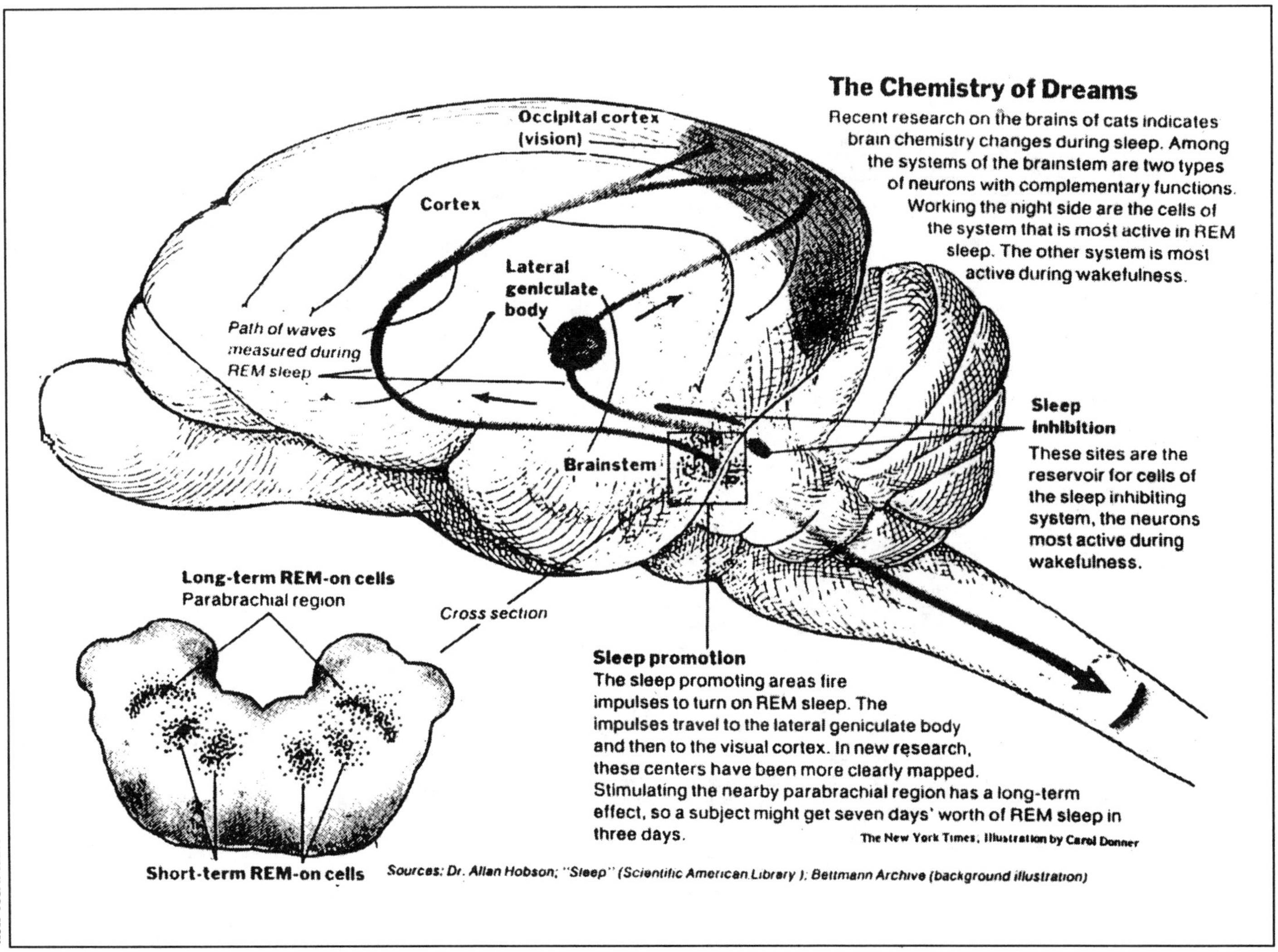

THE CHEMISTRY OF DREAMS

"Another nerve cell circuit connects to the place in the brainstem where movements like walking or running are triggered... When a group of cells in this region are triggered by an as-yet-undetermined chemical signal...[1] the stimulation helps bring on the muscle paralysis typical of REM sleep. At the same time glutamate, a brain chemical that excites neurons, is active. This might explain a paradox of REM sleep...that the eyeballs move and the body twitches even though the dreamer cannot move his sleeping body...

Changes of Scene

" 'Because the gait center of the brainstem is activated in REM sleep,' Dr Hobson said,

" 'You are rarely stationary in a dream. You run, walk, skip, drive, fly; you are almost always moving forward'."

(*"Scientists Unravelling Chemistry of Dreams,"* by Sandra Blakeslee)[2]

[1] See exhibit, pp. 199–201, and discussion on NMDA receptor.

[2] *New York Times,* March 3, 1992, p. C1.

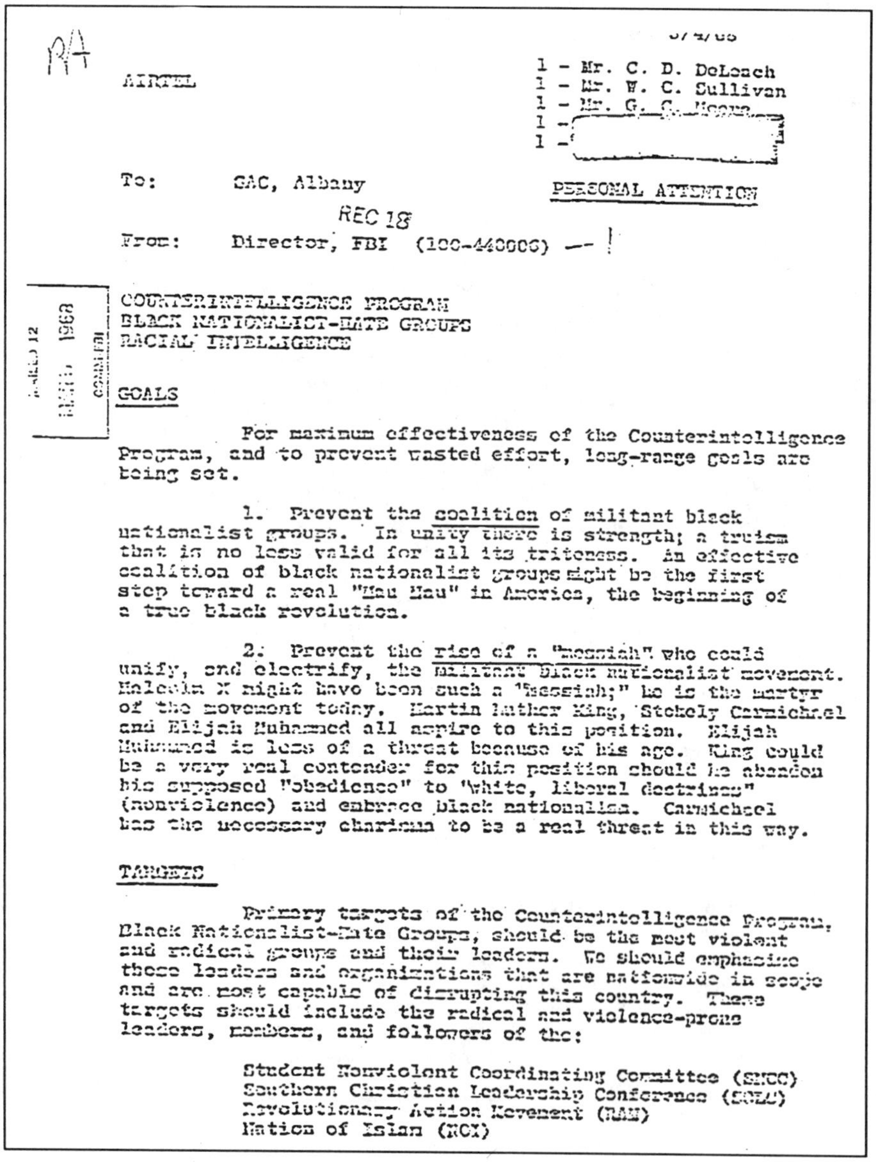

R/A

AIRTEL

3/4/68

1 - Mr. C. D. DeLoach
1 - Mr. W. C. Sullivan
1 - Mr. G. C. Moore
1 -
1 -

To: SAC, Albany

PERSONAL ATTENTION

REC 18

From: Director, FBI (100-448006)

MAILED 12 MAR 4 1968 COMM-FBI

COUNTERINTELLIGENCE PROGRAM
BLACK NATIONALIST-HATE GROUPS
RACIAL INTELLIGENCE

GOALS

For maximum effectiveness of the Counterintelligence Program, and to prevent wasted effort, long-range goals are being set.

1. Prevent the coalition of militant black nationalist groups. In unity there is strength; a truism that is no less valid for all its triteness. An effective coalition of black nationalist groups might be the first step toward a real "Mau Mau" in America, the beginning of a true black revolution.

2. Prevent the rise of a "messiah" who could unify, and electrify, the militant black nationalist movement. Malcolm X might have been such a "messiah;" he is the martyr of the movement today. Martin Luther King, Stokely Carmichael and Elijah Muhammed all aspire to this position. Elijah Muhammed is less of a threat because of his age. King could be a very real contender for this position should he abandon his supposed "obedience" to "white, liberal doctrines" (nonviolence) and embrace black nationalism. Carmichael has the necessary charisma to be a real threat in this way.

TARGETS

Primary targets of the Counterintelligence Program, Black Nationalist-Hate Groups, should be the most violent and radical groups and their leaders. We should emphasize those leaders and organizations that are nationwide in scope and are most capable of disrupting this country. These targets should include the radical and violence-prone leaders, members, and followers of the:

Student Nonviolent Coordinating Committee (SNCC)
Southern Christian Leadership Conference (SCLC)
Revolutionary Action Movement (RAM)
Nation of Islam (NOI)

J. Edgar Hoover's COINTELPRO FBI Memo

During the ten treatments she did, Geerte says the muscles and eyeballs of her subjects twitched this way during the entire visualization phase and even the beginning of the next phase, the one Sisko said gave him access to his "hereditary archive" — the ancestors. However, since Deportere indicated an EEG signature of true REM activity was absent on Ibogaine, Dana modified characterization of the visualization phase to "REM-like."

In late August the Queens Judge dropped a bombshell, completely ruling out a defense of medical necessity — because marijuana only relieves the *symptoms* of AIDS. Everyone began to assume Dana would be out of the game for a couple years, in prison. And Carlo was so intimidated by the opposition in the bureaucracy that he didn't even want to talk on the phone about it.

Dana sent him the revised workbook. He told him Clinton was going to win the election for sure, and that Mash had already talked to Hillary. And then he pointed Carlo to a passage in the Ibogaine book from *VALIS* (p. 159), from the *Book of Daniel,* which Philip Dick believed refered to Nixon, but due to the vagaries of the Xerox document-maker wound up in print directly opposite J. Edgar Hoover's memo on stopping the rise of a Black Messiah:

"In the last days of those kingdoms,
When their sin is at its height,
A king shall appear, harsh and grim, a master of stratagem.
His power shall be great, he shall work havoc untold;
He shall work havoc on great nations and upon a holy people.
His mind shall be ever active,
And he shall succeed in his crafty designs;
He shall conjure up great plans.
And, when they least expect it, work havoc on many.
He shall challenge even the Prince of Princes.
And be broken, but not by human hands."

"Look at the last line," Dana told him.

"What do you mean, not by human hands?" asked Carlo.

"Ibogaine, of course... Bwiti, as it were.

See — the police state Nixon and Hoover left us has never been overthrown. But we believe so many changes are going to flow from Ibogaine, that in four years, the opposition won't have a niche to come back to. Just relax, and let the Ibogaine do its thing."

But Carlo was still apprehensive. And the minute he left Baltimore to come up for his radio-medicine board Sept 14th, calls started coming in to his bosses at the ARC from Herb Kleber: "What is Contoreggi up to? Who's he seeing in New York?"

Kleber clearly didn't want Contoreggi getting together with ACT UP. CASA had good intelligence on ACT UP. Richard Elovitch had left the organization to advise the American Medical Foundation for AIDS Research (AMFAR)[1] from a new position at GMHC (Gay Mens' Health Crisis), miffed that his seminars with 12-step experts from Columbia's Substance Abuse Division were no longer getting alot of play on the floor. But he still had eyes and ears in ACT UP. Both he and Kleber had a lot to lose if an acknowledged clean needle expert came in and validated Ibogaine, providing the critical mass to push ACT UP over into some kind of big action.

Carlo also had no authorization from Grudzinskas to address ACT UP, and feared doing so as a private citizen might endanger his new position "in the loop.' On Sunday night he talked to a reporter who'd just interviewed Kleber extensively, preparing a piece on Ibogaine, and what he heard freaked him out so much that Monday morning Carlo cancelled his scheduled appearance at the ACT UP Monday night meeting. Dana was able to get an instant vote to zap CASA based on Kleber's interference. But a seed of doubt had been planted in ACT UP, and the zap was very small.

Howard, Boaz, and Carlo were all a-dither over a new finding by a researcher at Johns Hopkins named Mark Molliver. Molliver had discovered some brain toxicity in rats at 100 mg/kg (injected intraperitoneally, which was thought to be twice as toxic as giving it orally, making it equivalent to 11 times Lotsof's therapeutic dose). Howard was convinced this was a manuever to slow down Deborah Mash's IND at the FDA so MDD could get *their* IND approved first — when they were good and ready. But Contoreggi was intrigued more on a scientific level — because such selective toxicity is often a good clue to where a receptor site is. Here was possible evidence of the elusive Ibogaine receptor site, in a part of the brain considered to be off of the dopamine "pleasure pathway" — all the way back, in the cerebellum.

So instead of appearing at the ACT UP meeting, that morning Contoreggi went up to Kleber's 168th St. offices at Columbia's Substance Abuse Division to talk to a lower eschelon person who was his contact there. He was somewhat relieved after that meeting. But Dana had also leveled with him about the degree to which he was a pot activist, and Carlo was now wary of even talking. He had the Ibogaine workbook, though, with the articles on REM.

Dana still had time to go to the

Wednesday, Oct. 7, 1992

Hon.. Pearl B. Corrado
Queens County Court House
Queens, N.Y.

Dear Justice Corrado,

We are shocked to hear of your recent decision that medical marijuana is not "life-saving" because it is not a cure for HIV, but only treats the symptoms.

"Symptoms" underlie many of the disease-states that result in death in AIDS cases (e.g.: MAI, CMV, crypto-sporidiosis). To allow wasting disease, which can be staved off for years, to proceed unchecked is the equivalent of an early death sentence.

AIDS is a disease of over-reactions of the body: one of its paradoxes is why perfectly healthy T-cells die and continue to fall off at rates which eventually leave people with AIDS stripped of defenses against fatal opportunistic infections, even though only few T-cells are infected. The mechanisms of T-cell death bear further investigation. However, there is substantial evidence that constant elevated levels of the body's own anti-inflammatory response are killing healthy T-4 cells. One accepted property of cannabis preparations is their vaso-dialator, hence anti-inflammatory effect.

Forty percent of all the T-cells are in the gut. When they can't deal with all the "dirty" matter in the intestine, wasting occurs, so it's not just appetite stimulation or mood elevation that is occurring here.

ACT-UP Treatment and Data is currently following clinical trials with a wide range of anti-inflammatory medicines to find which is least toxic and most effective. We make all our findings available to the AIDS community. We are especially concerned with the problem of pharmaceutical load on the body of HIV positive people on AZT, DDI and other combinations of medications.

The unusually low toxicity of marijuana as well as the fact that it replaces separate medications that would be needed to combat nausea, stimulate appetite, elevate mood and calm the "jitters" (which leave many HIV positives in need of *something*), mean that we will follow with extreme interest Mr. Beal's reports on the upcoming clinical trials of smoked marijuana vs. marinol at San Francisco General Hospital. It is his function in our committee to convey our advice and requirements to researchers as to what we want the study to look into (e.g: cortisol levels), and what we need to know.

We are stretched extremely thin in our search for a cure for the plague, and Beal may not be immediately replaceable on the NIDA working group.

By ruling as you have, you've established a different standard for this medication than the one which we have forced the FDA to accept. The use of "surrogate markers" (i.e. rise or fall of T-4 cell levels as the basis for access of people with AIDS to medications) is a principle hundreds of us died fighting for.

No drug tested so far is a "cure" for AIDS. Drugs that alleviate "symptoms" and lessen toxicities are some of the most important in our medicine chest. By applying a different standard than *Bordowitz*, needle exchange becomes acceptable because it saves a certain number of people from being infected; but once infected, they have no fundamental right to medications which, in a regimen of other treatments, might be *the* element giving them several additional years of a more normal life.

Sincerely,

George Carter, John King, Theo Smart, Ken Jacobsen
of the ACT-UP/N.Y. Treatment and Data Committee

CORRADO LETTER

[1] Of which Joe Califano is a Board Member.

September 22nd protest at the Department of Health and Human Services by ACT UP, the Green Panthers and NORML against the cut-off of medical marijuana to people with AIDS. Naturally DC ACT UP flew in Brownie Mary and Dennis Peron for the event. HHS is just two blocks from Tim Westmoreland's office, so that Dana was able to set up a last-minute meeting with Tim, another staffer named Ripley Forbes, Dennis, and Brownie Mary, which explored giving states local option on medical marijuana. The HHS zap dominated DC airwaves, and in the superheated pre-election atmosphere, reverberated across the country.

On October 1st, the judge in Queens demanded that Beal produce his lawyer for trial October 9th. No more affadavits. Kunstler's helpers prepared a massive Clayton motion — essentially a motion "in the higher interest of justice" — arguing that the need of society as a whole for Dana's Ibogaine work should be balanced with the good he was doing getting medical-grade instead of moldy marijuana to PWAs, and that all charges be dismissed. The Clayton, thick as a book, was delivered October 8th.

To rule, the judge had to read the appendix, which contained the entire ACT UP Ibogaine workbook, dense with impenetrable rat studies. She didn't want to do that, so on October 9th, she pressured the prosecution to offer a 60-day plea bargain. Dana didn't like the compromise, but relented when the judge agreed her earlier ruling against medical necessity defenses for pot would not constitute a precedent in other AIDS cases — in effect nullifying her earlier decision.

Bill Kunstler assured Dana this would play in the media as a victory, a judgement that was borne out when the *Daily News* ran an article the next week reporting a big win for medical marijuana for people with AIDS. It even mentioned his Ibogaine work, and the November 20 sentencing date gave him time to do a presentation at the annual DPF Conference.

Next, figuring that his secret was out, Dana broke down and got a small amount of free pot for Robert Rygor, the ACT UP workspace manager, who he saw every week at the Coordinating Committee. When Robert asked, he could scarcely tell him no, now that the penalty clearly was weeks, not years. But he kept it well under the amount de-criminalized in New York State law.

The irony was that Rygor, who only joined ACT UP when he found out he was positive, had gone on the warpath five years earlier as a neo-conservative Village Reform Democrat (Koch faction) to oust the annual May Parade and rally from Washington Square. By this time Dana was also having to run errands — to pick up acidophilus or the laundry — for Spacely, whose scene was starting to come unglued. Both situations involved the same running around. So began the tradition of free, non-moldy pot to PWA's and other patients in New York City.

Best of all, after five weeks, Carlo called Beal rather than the other way around. His confidence was waxing as the election neared, and he seemed to feel ACT UP connections might be useful under the new regime. Dana opined that with funding until 1996, Califano and Kleber seemed to have designed CASA to sit out the next four years on the outside, looking in.

But then another Ibogaine coincidence took over. All the books and tapes Beal had been sending out bore fruit in the best article yet, in the Science Section of the *Boston Globe*. The reporter, Deborah Kong, actually read all the rat studies, so she spotted the efficacy. She didn't feel it necessary to "balance" the article with comments from skeptics too lazy to look at the data. A short version was reprinted all over the US. And at *New York Newsday*, where Spencer Rumsey had been blocked by higher-ups from getting an article published for three years, he used the *Globe* piece as ammunition to guilt-trip his editors: "You guys let me get scooped again!"

On November 19th, the Queens judge picked up her *Newsday* and found a massive, four page feature on Ibogaine, which mentioned AIDS, ACT UP and the Black Panthers, even though interviews with Dana and Dhoruba had been cut due to space considerations.

The next day Bill Kunstler walked into court with Dana and asked that the 60-day sentence be changed to some kind of community service. And when Bill got to the part about the *Newsday* article, Judge Corrado said: "I read my *Newsday* yesterday, Mr. Kunstler. " She wanted to change the jail time to community service on the spot, pending a letter from ACT UP Housing Works, the largest provider of housing for PWA's in New York.

Dana was out — at least until the DA in the case pressured Judge Corrado to change her mind. In December he talked to Carlo again. Carlo was very excited. The receptor site in the cerebellum tied it all together — Ibogaine tremor, behavioral immobility, acetylcholine pathways, visualizations, everything.

The cerebellum governs input from the muscles, joints and tendons; it regulates balance. It tracks all sensory inputs to let you know where you're located in space, and what your body's position is in it. It's where you learn to walk when you're one year old. An Ibogaine receptor within the cerebellum means that true addiction involves the same kind of deep conditioning of the cerebellum as learning to walk. Addiction doesn't even happen at the so-called common narcotic receptor, where dopamine acts, but *through* the pleasure pathways — in the cerebellum.

Addiction involves the same circuits as learning to walk. And just like walking, once you learn how to shortcircuit the conscious brain — once you're addicted — you do it without thinking about it. The addict's feet literally walk him down to the dope spot on their own. But that means there's no "magic bullet" for addiction without going into the cerebellum. Carol Baker said that once the craving for heroin used to lock in, she could never break out of the routine of going to cop — and just walk away. After Ibogaine she was always able to divert herself into doing something else — cleaning up, watching television, anything as long as it wasn't going to cop.

There's no cerebellar action without the tremor or visualizations, either. The acetylcholine pathways of the ascending reticular formation — involved in REM, in dreaming, as shown in the *Science Times* illustration (page 115) — connect directly through the giant pontine cells (see exhibit, p. 206) into the location in the brain for walking, running, moving. And that's the cerebellum. Ibogaine works through the acetylcholine pathways, therefore there can be no interrupter effect without behavioral immobility and tremor, both effects of acetylcholine. Dana and Carlo each had a pre-release copy of a monograph by Robert Goutarel, the father of modern Ibogaine research, and Carlo drew Dana's attention to a passage at the end:

> "Barrass, B.C. and Coult (1972) demonstrated that ibogaine inhibits the oxidation of serotonin by a monoamine oxidase (MAO), ceruloplasmin, and catalyzes the oxidation of catecholamines by the same substrate.
>
> "Indeed, Ibogaine is a potent serotoninergic that has the ability to reduce the level of cerebral catecholamines. This decrease in the level of catecholamines, dopamine in particular, explains the results described recently on the blockade of the stimulation of mesolimbic and striatal dopamine induced by morphine or cocaine...."
>
> "The decrease in the level of catecholamines and the joint increase in the cerebral serotonin level result in a suppression of REM sleep and the appearance of hallucinatory phenomena (C. Debru, 1990).
>
> "LSD, like Ibogaine, is a potent serotoninergic that inhibits the oxidation of serotonin and catalyzes the oxidation of catecholamines by MAO.
>
> "However, there is an enormous difference between these two alkaloids: LSD is active at doses of less than a milligram. Its activity is difficult to control and the hallucinatory phenomena produced belong to a high and angelic domain of esthetic sensations, whereas Ibogaine is hallucinogenic only at doses in excess of 100 mg, and the domain of the oneirophrenic substance is that of the subterranean world of Freud, of animal impulse and of regression....
>
> "Let us note that serotonin is the neurotransmitter of the cerebral parasympathetic system, catecholamines being neurotransmitters in the cerebral orthosympathetic system, and that the negative chronotropic and inotropic effects as well as the arousal-producing action of Ibogaine are nullified by atropine, an acetylcholine antagonist, acetylcholine being the neurotransmitter of the autonomic nervous system.
>
> "The long waking dream period that follows the absorption of iboga or ibogaine at a subtoxic dose (or oneirophrenic dose according to Naranjo) appears to be responsible for a temporary destructuring of the ego, followed by its restructuring.
>
> "This hypothesis is consistent with the observations made by the ethnologists in their studies of the Mitsogho Bwiti, and may be compared to the hypotheses of Michel Jouvet and Sir Francis Crick (C. Debru, 1990) on the role of dreams in the programming and deprogramming of basic behavior patterns, resulting in a new individuation of the human brain.
>
> "Normally, the stages of wakefulness of the human brain are: waking, NREM (slow wave or

deep) sleep, PGO (pontogeniculo-occipital) waves, and REM (rapid eye movement or paradoxical) sleep. REM sleep is the period of dreams.

"Michel Jouvet and Sir Francis Crick consider PGO waves to be the principal coding tool that acts at the cortical level in recording the genetic and epigenetic acquisitions necessary for the individuation of the human brain.

"In addition, through random activation mechanisms, the PGO waves eliminate from certain types of neuronal networks an informational overload linked to pathological behavior. This is what C. Debru calls 'cleaning out the neuronal circuitry.'

"REM sleep apparently undertakes a sorting out process among the "residues" stirred up by the PGO wave sleep pattern and disposes of these residues during dreaming.

"Michel Jouvet (letter of November 7, 1990) wrote: 'The oneiric effects observed in humans and which are produced by hallucinogens do not enable us to approach the dream mechanism directly, because it does appear that these two phenomena cannot be linked together as one.'

"We know, however, that the principal difference between dreams and hallucinations resides in the way in which the stages of wakefulness are organized, with the suppression of REM sleep and the intrusion of PGO waves in the arousal (waking) stage and in NREM (or slow) sleep.

"The new organization becomes: waking (arousal) stage, stage of PGO waves, hallucination stage, sleep stage, and it appears possible that hallucinatory manifestations, the waking dream, eliminate "residues" stirred up by the PGO wave pattern in the absence of REM sleep."

— "Pharmacodynamics and Therapeutic Applications of Iboga and Ibogaine," Robert Goutarel, with Otto Gollnhofer and Roger Sillans, French National Scientific Research Center)

"You were right," exulted Carlo. "Ibogaine *is* fundamentally different from the 'clear' psychedelics. And Howard's right — in that there may be no way to duplicate the Ibogaine effect without the visualizations! It *is* a waking dream — but REM-like, not true REM."

What it is exactly is explained in Goutarel's next lines:

Near Death Experiences

"According to the Mitsogho, the initiate will see the Bwiti only twice in his life: on the day of his initiation and on the day of his death.

"This means that the visions at the approach of death, what are called near death experiences (NDE), are the same as those termed normative visions.

"We know that at the time of dying, some individuals see their whole life pass before them. In those who are 'rescued from death,' a spectacular transformation is observed. They no longer fear

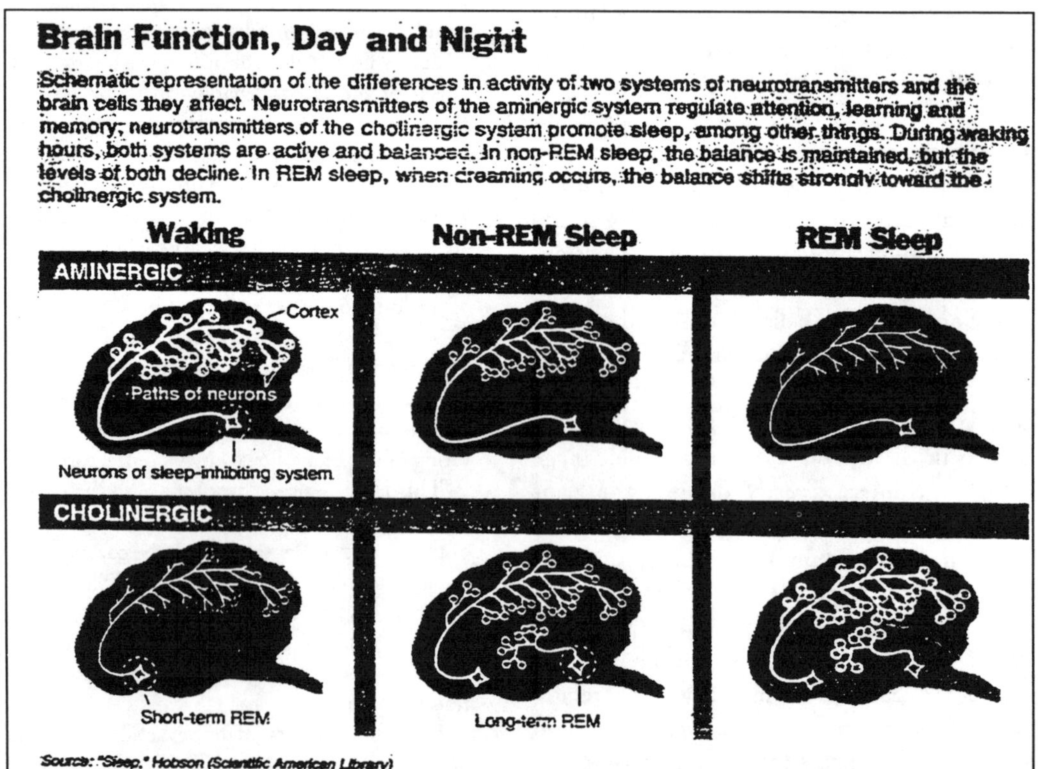

New York Times

death, they feel stronger, more optimistic, calmer, and contemplate their life more positively."

The brain is capable of generating another state, then, which the conscious mind recognizes as "dreamlike." Normally the waking mind has only indirect access to the activities of the acetylcholine pathways. Normally the NREM and PGO activity of the sleeping brain only seeps into consciousness slowly — during the few minutes of REM we get every night.

But a real emergency can trigger a survival reflex, the NDE, which gets both the waking and sleeping brain up and functioning stereoscopically, at the same time. The serotoninergic pathways, organized as the ego, get direct access to all the disorganized activity of the cholinergic pathways, which are perceived as "five or six television programs going at once."

Ibogaine activates the pathways of the NDE reflex. The "splitting of the skull," which releases the visions, is the same as the jerk (myotonic twitch) you sometimes feel just as you're falling asleep, greatly amplified because your serotonin and acetylcholine are pumping at the same time, and your DA is way down, which normally doesn't happen for more than a few seconds each night as you're drifting off.

But in the NDE, the mind gets conscious access to PGO wave material, and therefore potential access to direct genetic instructions from the non-nucleated genetic material in all of your cells — the only possible mechanism for ancestral memory.

These are the genes that are passed on directly from your mother; they don't lose anything from generation to generation, unless a cosmic ray hits them. You get nothing from your father but nucleated genes passed on through the sperm, which is the genetic equivalent of an earth satellite. The egg by comparison is a minature planet, rich with information.

Primitive cells that replicate by division,[1] like amoebas, pass all their memory along to their clones through these non-nucleated genes. But about a billion years ago some cells invented sex, swapping genetic instuctions contained in the nucleus via mitosis. Much more complex organisms became possible, but to maintain access to cellular memory, through the acetylcholine pathways, they had to *sleep*. All the activity of the sleeping mind is summarized several times a night in the REM phase, which, when you remember your dreams, makes a "report" from the unconscious to the conscious mind.

Sleep doesn't just raise cellular memories to consciousness, though. One possibility is that every night your mind makes a "back-up" of the day's memories all the way down in the non-nucleated genetic material of your cells. Since these little packets of information don't degrade much from generation to generation, you have ancestral memories going back a quarter of a million years. But always through the mother, if this theory is true. [Perhaps this is why Fred, on Ibogaine, experienced the concentration camps through the eyes of his mother and not his father.]

The thing is that these cellular memories might have in them the information you need to survive in a real emergency, when you have no chance to sleep through the night, until the answer comes to you in a dream — when you need an instant scan of all useful situations and scenarios in the past quarter million years.

So before there was language, before there was writing, we developed the NDE, this trick reflex that allows the conscious mind to access PGO wave activity directly. Ibogaine triggers the NDE reflex chemically, without having to be near death. Ibogaine turns the serotoninergic and cholinergic pathways into a super-augmented, "sterescopic" entity, capable of scanning ancestral memory in the non-nucleated genetic material of your cells:

The ancestors.

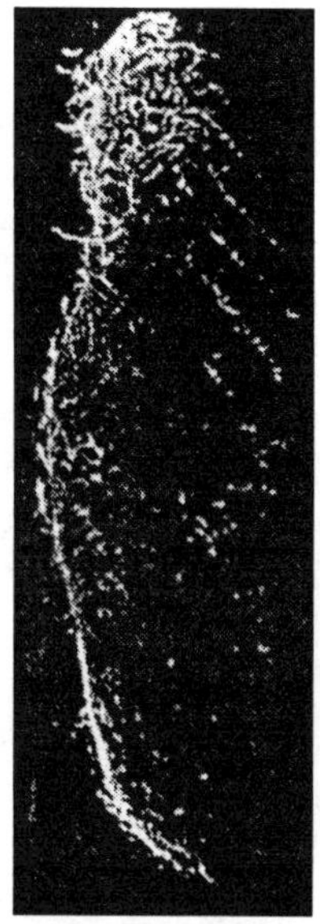

Journal of Consciousness Studies

Figure 4a: Scanning electron micrograph (rapid fixation) of Paramecium showing protruding cilia Arrows demonstrate ciliary movement in metachronal waves.

4b: Diagram showing Paramecium polygonal infraciliary lattice with cilia (ci), containing 9 + 2 sets of microtubules including peripheral microtubule (pm) doublets. (ms: median septum, al: alveoli, tt: trichocyst tips, ps: parasomal sacs, ff: fine fibrils, kf: kinetodesmal fibrils.) This illustrates how cilia (sensory and motor) are connected to intra-cellular cytoskeleton. (With permission from Wichterman, 1985).

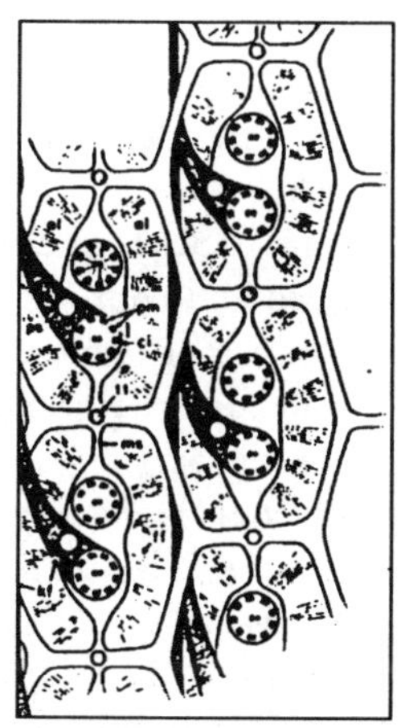

[1] See Appendix, Hameroff, p. 247. Even paramecia have a "nervous system," as this illustration shows.

So Many Religions?

By His Holiness John Paul II

You speak of many religions. Instead I will attempt to show the common fundamental element and the common root of these religions.

The Council [the Second Vatican Council of 1962-65] defined the relationship of the Church to non-Christian religions in a specific document that begins with the words "Nostra aetate" ("In our time"). It is a concise and yet very rich document that authentically hands on the Tradition, faithful to the thought of the earliest Fathers of the Church.

From the beginning, Christian Revelation has viewed the spiritual history of man as including, in some way, all religions, thereby demonstrating the unity of humankind with regard to the eternal an ultimate destiny of man. The Council document speaks of this unity and links it with the current trend to bring humanity closer together through the resources available to our civilization. The Church sees the promotion of this unity as one of its duties: "There is only one community and it consists of all peoples. They have only one origin, since God inhabited the entire earth with the whole human race. And they have one ultimate destiny, God, whose providence, goodness, and plan for salvation extend to all.... Men turn to various religions to solve mysteries of the human condition, which today as in earlier times, burden people's hearts: the nature of man; the meaning and purpose of life; good and evil; the origin and purpose of suffering; the way to true happiness; death; judgment and retribution after death; and finally, the ultimate ineffable mystery which is the origin and destiny of our existence.

"From ancient times up to today all the various peoples have shared and continue to share an awareness of that enigmatic power that is present throughout the course of things and throughout the events of human life, and in which, at times even the Supreme Divinity or the Father is recognizable. This awareness and recognition imbue life with an intimate religious sense. Religions that are tied up with cultural progress strive to solve these issues with more refined concepts and more precise language" ("Nostra Aetate," 1–2).

Here the Council document brings us to the Far East — first of all to Asia, a continent where the Church's missionary activity, carried out since the time of the apostles, has borne we must recognize, very modest fruit. It is well known that only a small percentage of the population on what is the largest continent believes in Christ.

This does not mean that the Church's missionary effort has been lapsed—quite the opposite: that effort has been and still remains intense. And yet the tradition of very ancient cultures, antedating Christianity, remains very strong in the East. Even if faith in Christ reaches hearts and minds, the negative connotations associated with the image of life in Western society (the so-called Christian society) present a considerable obstacle to the acceptance of the Gospel. Mahatma Gandhi, Indian and Hindu, pointed this out many times, in his deeply evangelical manner. He was disillusioned with the ways in which Christianity was expressed in the political and social life of nations. Could a man who fought for the liberation of his great nation from colonial dependence accept Christianity in the same form as it had been imposed on his country by those same colonial powers?

The Second Vatican Council realized this difficulty. This is why the document on the relations between the Church and Hinduism and other religions of the Far East is so important. We read: "In Hinduism men explore the divine mystery and express it through an endless bounty of myths and through penetrating philosophical insight. They seek freedom from the anguish of our human condition, either by way of the ascetic life, profound meditation, or by taking refuge in God with love and trust. The various schools of Buddhism recognize the radical inadequacy of this malleable world and teach a way by which men, with devout and trusting hearts, can become capable either of reaching a state of perfect liberation or of attaining, by their own efforts or through higher help, supreme illumination" ("Nostra Aetate," 2).

Further along, the Council remarks that: "The Catholic Church rejects nothing that is true and holy in these religions. The Church has a high regard for their conduct and way of life, for those precepts and doctrines which, although differing on many points from that which the Church believes and propounds, often reflects a ray of that truth which enlightens all men. However, the Church proclaims, and is bound to proclaim, that Christ is 'the way and the truth and the life' (John 14:6), in whom men must find the fullness of religious life and in whom God has reconciled everything to Himself" ("Nostra Aetate," 2).

The words of the Council recall the conviction, long rooted in the Tradition, of the existence of the so-called semina Verbi (seeds of the Word), present in all religions. In the light of this conviction, the Church seeks to identify the semina Verbi present in the great traditions of the Far East, in order to trace a common path against the backdrop of the needs of the contemporary world. We can affirm that here the position of the Council is inspired by a truly universal concern. The

Church is guided by the faith that God the Creator wants to save all humankind in Jesus Christ, the only mediator between God and man, inasmuch as He is the mediator between God and man, inasmuch as He is the Redeemer of all humankind. The Paschal Mystery is equally available to all, and, through it, the way to eternal salvationis also open to all.

In another passage the Council says that the Holy Spirit works effectively even outside these visible structure of the Church (cf. Lumen Gentium 13 [a Vatican II document often called the "Dogmatic Constitution on the Church"]), making use of these very semina Verbi that constitute a kind of common soteriological root present in all religions.

I have been convinced of this on numerous occasions, both while visiting the countries of the Far East and while meeting representatives of those religions, especially during the historic meeting at Assisi [the 1986 congregation of world spiritual leaders], where we found ourselves gathered together praying for peace.

Thus, instead of marveling at the fact that Providence allows such a great variety of religions, we should be amazed at the number of common elements found within them.

At this point it would be helpful to recall all the primitive religions, the animistic religions which stress ancestor worship. It seems that those who practice them are particularly close to Christianity, and among them, the Church's missionaries also find it easier to speak a common language. Is there, perhaps, in this veneration of ancestors a kind of preparations for the Christian faith in the Communion of Saints, in which all believers—whether living or dead—form a single community, a single body? And faith in the Communion of Saints is, ultimately, faith in Christ, who alone is the source of life and of holiness for all. There is nothing strange, then, that the African and Asian animists would become believers in Christ more easily than followers of the great religions of the Far East.

As the Council also noted, these last religions possess the characteristics of a system. They are systems of worship and also ethical systems with a strong emphasis on good and evil. Certainly among these belong Chinese Confucianism and Taoism: Tao means eternal truth—something similar to the "Word"— which is reflected in the action of man by means of truth and moral good. The religions of the Far East have contributed greatly the history of morality and culture, forming a national identity in the Chinese, Indians, Japanese, and Tibetans, and also in the peoples of Southeast Asia and the archipelagoes of the Pacific Ocean.

Some of these peoples come from age-old cultures. The indigenous peoples of Australia boast a history tens of thousands of years old, and their ethnic and religious tradition is older than that of Abraham and Moses.

Christ came into the world for all these peoples. He redeemed them all and has His own ways of reaching each of them in the present eschatological phase of salvation history. In fact, in those regions, many accept Him and many more have an implicit faith in Him.

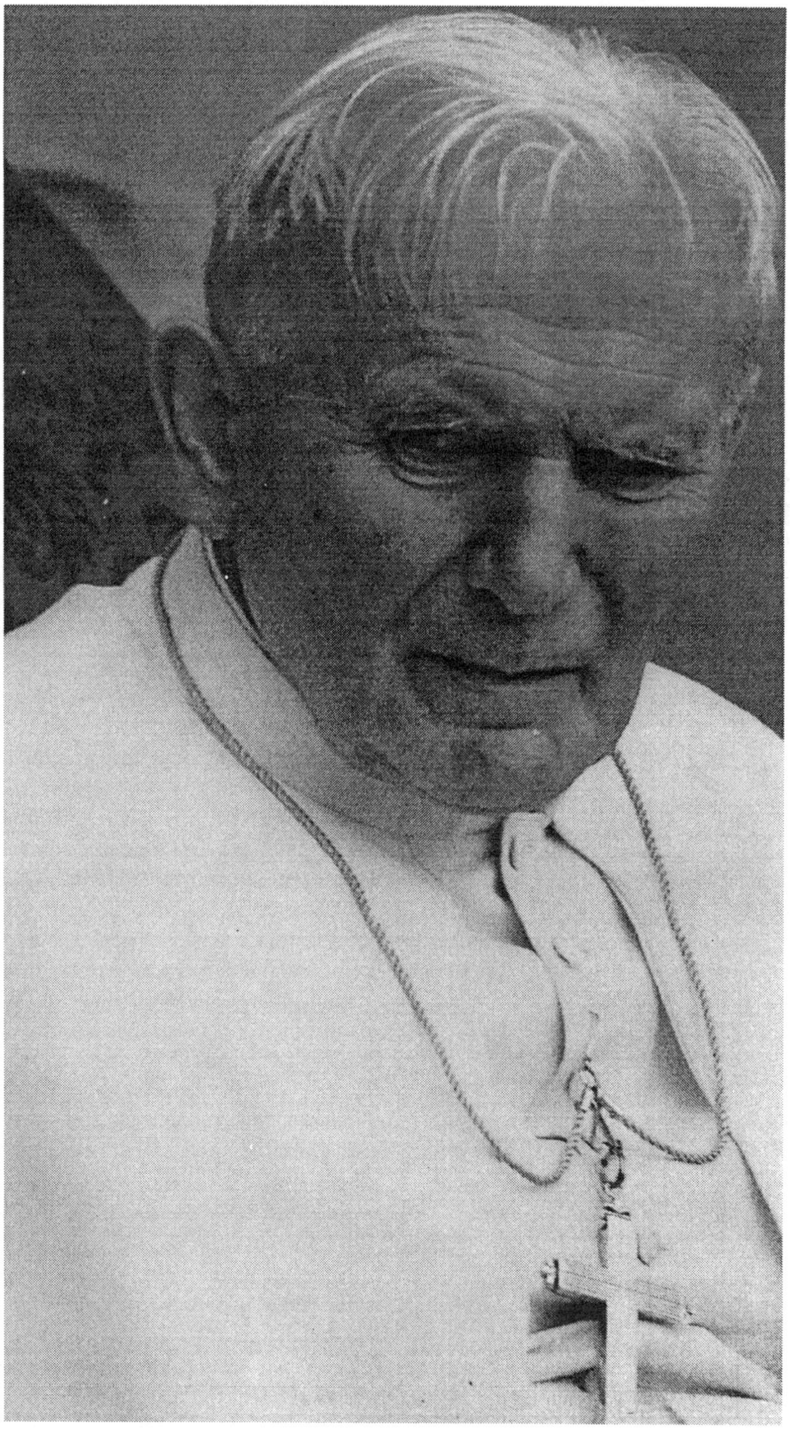

New York Times Magazine

CHAPTER 13: Bwiti

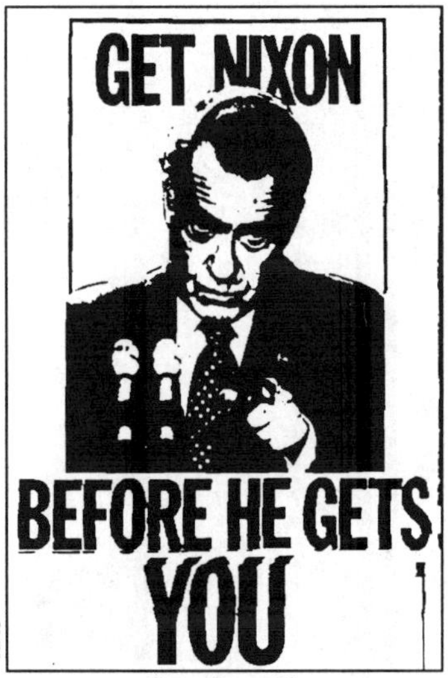

GRIM KING #1

In February, 1992, the first time Beal could sit down with Dhoruba after he came back from Ghana, Dana confided that before, he hadn't wanted to tell him what to do — but that coming back to fight his case was the right decision. Then he had him read the following passage, and Dhoruba gave a start as soon as he read the first sentence, as if he recognized something in it. It read —

> "The goal of your lives has been reached. I am here to tell you this. Do not fear...
>
> "A time of trial and delusion and wailing lies ahead because the grim king, the king of tears, will not surrender his power. But you will take his power from him; I grant you that authority in my name, exactly as I granted it to you once before, when the grim king ruled and destroyed and challenged the humble people of the world.
>
> "The battle which you fought before has not ended, although the day of the healing sun has come. Evil does not die of its own self because it imagines that it speaks for god. Many claim to speak for god, but there is only one god and that god is man himself.
>
> "Therefore only those leaders who protect and shelter will live; the others will die. The oppression lifted four years ago,[1] and it will for a little while return. Be patient during this time; it will be a time of trials for you, but I will be with you, and when the time of trials is over I shall sit down on the judgement seat, and some will fall and some will not fall, according to my will, my will that comes to me from the father, back to whom we all go, all of us together.
>
> "I am not a god; I am human. I am a child, the child of my father, which is Wisdom Himself. You carry in you now the voice and authority of Wisdom; you are, therefore, Wisdom, even when you forget it. You will not forget it for long. I will be there and I will remind you.
>
> "The day of Wisdom and the rule of Wisdom has come. The day of power, which is the enemy of Wisdom, ends. Power and Wisdom are the two principles in the world. Power has had its rule and now it goes into the darkness from which it came, and Wisdom alone rules.
>
> "Those who obey power will succumb as power succumbs.
>
> "Those who love Wisdom and follow her will thrive under the sun. Remember, I will be with you, I will be in each of you from now on. I will accompany you down into the prison if necessary; I will speak in the courts of law to defend you; my voice will be heard in the land, whatever the oppression.
>
> "Do not fear; speak out and Wisdom will guide you. Fall silent out of fear and Wisdom will depart you. But you will not feel fear because Wisdom herself is in you, and you and she are one.
>
> "Formerly you were alone within yourselves; formerly you were solitary men. Now you have a companion who never sickens or fails or dies; you are bonded to the eternal and will shine like the healing sun itself."
>
> (*VALIS*, pp. 198–99)

There's more, but after that Dhoruba talked with Dana about how in the African tradition, the NDE is considered a medical fact. And then Dana said:

> "You know, my orientation is primarily scientific. For the first eight years of the project I wouldn't go all the way for Ibogaine — make it my main public focus — until *I* was convinced in 1989, by the evidence. We've only treated a handful of people, but already the world is being changed through them. Maybe there *is* some kind of force working through Ibogaine.
>
> "*Something* is happening. Remember, Bush is Nixon — the forces he represents killed off all the potential Black leaders once before. But God is not mocked. When He's fixing to send a Messiah, He cannot be thwarted. He can send one who can't be killed, and can't be stopped.
>
> "Because of AIDS, the System is going to have to use Ibogaine. And then Bwiti will be alive in thousands of junkies and crackheads, and *they* will be tranformed into the force that overthrows the Oppressors. What I'm trying to say is, win your case, but husband your resources. Neither one of us has to die. The fix is in. Cosmically."

About a year earlier, Dana was supposed to meet Howard and Norma at Flo Kennedy's 75th birthday party. It was a cold night; they never made it in from Staten Island. But there at the party were Charles Rangel and New York Attorney General Bob Abrams, whose wife Diane is one of Flo's best friends. Beal

[1] This is written in late 1978, about 1974 and Nixon. *VALIS* is filled with theological insights and metaphysical constructions, but this passage alone may reasonably be construed as intended by P. K. Dick to represent the Word of God—by virtue of utterance by the child Sophia, (i.e, the literary vehicle of the revelation he is supposed to have experienced in March, 1974.)

gave everyone Ibogaine stuff, and renewed his acquaintance with Flo, who he hadn't seen much since the '70s. He also met Flo's friend Lillian Smith, a producer for Phil Donohue. For about four months he tried to get a show on Donohue about the needle exchange controversy in Boston, with Jon Parker and Ellis-Hagler, but it didn't happen. He got to know who to call at the show, though.

Howard and Norma wound up meeting Flo Kennedy at a later date, and Flo really hit it off with Norma. Flo Kennedy became a big Ibogaine supporter. She was Billie Holliday's lawyer for her smack busts; today Flo's the executor for the estates of Billie Holliday and jazz junkie great Charles "Bird" Parker. She also became a big Dhoruba supporter — liked his feminist politics — and threw a party for him when he got back from Ghana. The minute Dana got back from the April 10th meeting with Ingrid Kolb, he got Flo to write up a note to Diane and Bob, about how effective Dhoruba had been as a negotiator, and how important he was to the Ibogaine project, and sent it off to them with a copy of the Ibogaine tape.[1]

The morning after the rioting began in Los Angeles, April 29th, 1992, he called Flo and said, "You really ought to call your friend Lillian, and see if you can get Dhoruba on Donohue." Flo never makes phone calls, but she told him to leave a message on Lillian's tape, saying Flo recommends Dhoruba. He did that, and then he left a message on Dhoruba's tape saying Donohue's producers might call, but that he should call them. Within hours, Dhoruba was on Donohue with Sister Souljah. Overnight, he was a superstar, the most articulate Black radical since Malcolm.

In the selections for the Ibogaine workbook prepared for the Harlem Hospital workshop August 4th, Dana included three articles on *Bwiti,* plus the interview of a European after meeting Bwiti — Nico. The thing is, *Bwiti* cosmogony is not usually written down except by Europeans.[2] (Why write down your religion, when you can put in a direct call to God any time you require clarification?)

But Barabe summarized it:

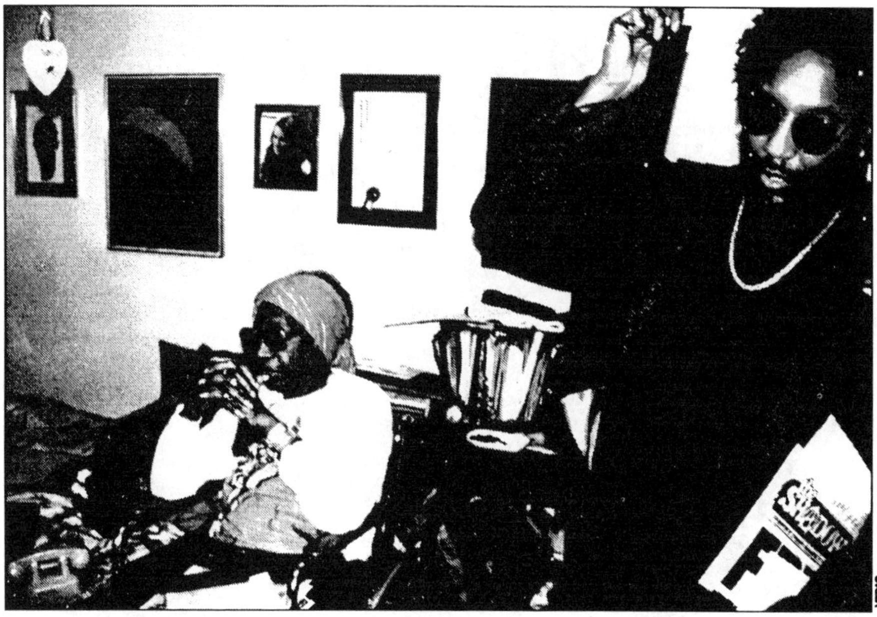

FLO KENNEDY & DHORUBA BIN WAHAD

"Mebeghe is the name of the divinity in the Fangs (a tribe), a supreme being without mother or father or spouse. It engenders the three divinities by bursting the divine primordial egg.

"Nzame-Mebeghe, God, is born with his brother and sister but remains pure.

Nyingone-Mebeghe, 'sister of God,' the female principle of the universe, goddess of fertility and of the night. At the instigation of Evus, she committed Nsem, incest, with None. As punishment, she must carry the earth on her head.

"None-Mebeghe, the third individual in the divinity, the male principle, has committed Nsem.

"Ekurana has issued forth from the placenta and the umbilical body of the divine egg. It possesses thunder and makes order reign.

"Evus, the twin brother of Ekurana, has been punished with a thunderclap on orders from Nzame. He is the tempter and initiator of Nsem.

"All these divinities are represented in the temple, the place of night-time ceremonies, the place for celebrations on the occasion of feasts and initiations [involving consumption of massive quantities of iboga bark, often at puberty], the place for funeral dances on the death of a person of standing. The temple may also serve as a meeting room, as a courthouse or a guard house. It is called Mbandja."

("*The Religion of Eboga or the Bwiti of the Fangs,*"
P. Barabe, May/June 1982.

Note again the Freudian overtones accompanying Iboga: Bwiti is a safe-sex-oriented, matriarchal religion, reacting off of a

[1] Mostly to promote Ibogaine and the cooperation around it, since as State A.G., Abrams had no direct role in Dhoruba's case.

[2] Fernandez does mention *The Secret Bible of the Blacks According to Bwiti,* published by the Etshira, Prince Birinda de Boudieguy, in 1952. One in a series of short occult works published in France at the time, it had begun to circulate widely in Gabon by the end of the decade. It reflects Gabonese Bwiti doctrine of the forties but it also possesses imaginative elements of its own and an overall breadth and integration of perspective not often found in local Bwiti leaders. For example, Birinda's treatment of the female principle Dintsouna Muata Benga, ... is a more elaborated notion than was given in the forest chapels themselves. Birinda presents Dintsouna as the luminous princess, daughter of the night, who was created out of the breath of the first of the creator gods, Mukuku Kandja. In her right hand she bears the sun and in the left the moon which she brings together to form the solar prince whom Birinda calls "the Eternal Verb." From Dintsouna's right breast flows a torrent of blood and from her left breast a torrent of milk. It is Dintsouna who fills out and stabilizes the tumultuous night, and it is only through her that devotion can be expressed to the supreme being." (Op. cit. pp. 299–300).

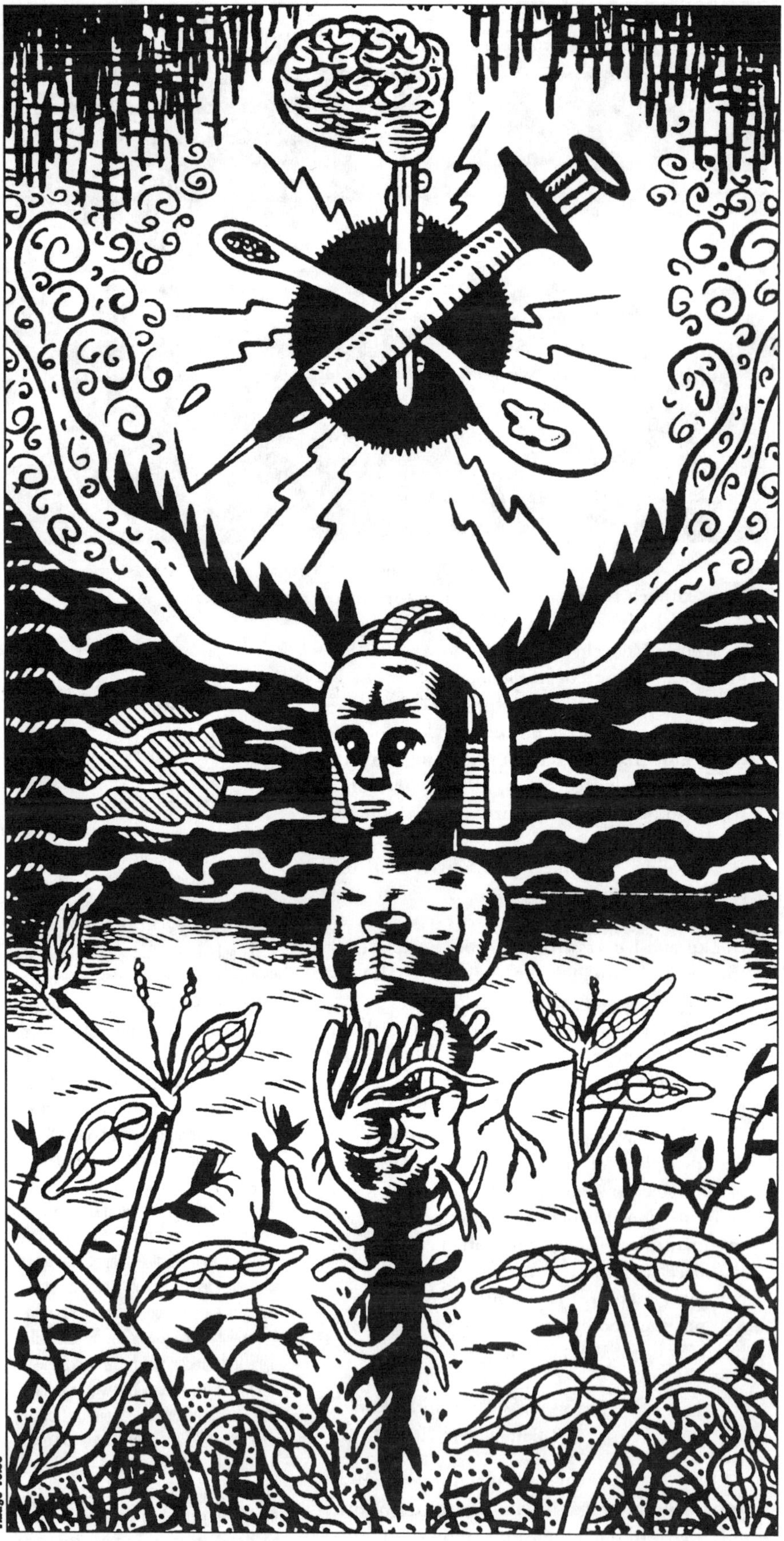

Village Voice

[1] Evans-Schulte's *Food of the Gods.*

tremendous gonorrhea epidemic at the turn of the century. The Catholic colonial authorities (Dominicans) were prone to harassing Bwiti, which had a unifying effect during the Gabonese drive for independence.

The important part of the initiation is meeting the ancestors, which everyone has stored hologramatically in their memory, on the cellular level. Collectively, they are Bwiti. During initiation, the neophyte often meets a guide such as a trusted parent, uncle, or grandparent, now deceased, who accompanies him through the visions. Or they might meet the Bwiti, (if in effect there's a special message for them), the personification of the ancestors who Evans–Shultes[1] described as "the universal African Ancestor."

Dana decided selections of *VALIS* had to go in side-by-side with the Nico interview–both because they contain a number of notes which explain the significance of what's happening to Nico, and because of certain resemblances between the Bwiti materials and the Egyptian Gnosticism of the Nag Hammadi Scrolls, which Dick considers the missing link, not only of the three Monotheisms, but all religions —

> 47. TWO SOURCE COSMOGONY: The One was and was-not, combined, and decided to separate the was-not from the was. So it generated a diploid sac which contained like an eggshell, a pair of twins, each an androgyny, spinning in opposite directions (the YIN & the YANG of Taoism, with the one as the TAO). The plan of the One was that both twins would emerge into being (wasness) simultaneously; however, motivated by a desire to be (which the One had implanted in both twins), the counterclockwise twin broke though the sac and separated prematurely; i.e, before fullterm. This was the dark or YIN twin. Therefore it was defective. At full term the wiser twin emerged. Each twin formed a unitary entelechy, a single living organism made of *psyche* and *soma,* still rotating in opposite directions to each other. The fullterm twin, called FORM I by Parmenides, advanced correctly through its growth stages, but the pre-maturely born twin, called FORM II, languished.
>
> The next step in the One's plan was that the Two would become the Many, through their dialectical interaction. From them as hyper-universes they projected a hologram-like interface, which is the pluriform universe we creatures inhabit....
>
> "49. Two realms there are, upper and lower. The upper, derived from hyper-universe I or

Yang, FORM I of Parmenides, is sentient and volitional. The lower realm or Yin, FORM II of Parmenides, is mechanical, driven by blind, efficient cause, deterministic and without intelligence, since it emanates from a dead source. In ancient times it was termed "astral determinism." We are trapped, by and large, in the lower realm, but are through the sacraments, by means of the plasmate, extricated. Until astral determinism is broken, we are not even aware of it, so occluded are we...

"The name of the healthy twin, hyperuniverse I, is NOMMO. The name of the sick twin, hyperuniverse II, is YORUGA. Their names are known to the Dogon people of Western Sudan in Africa.

"50. The primordial source of all our religions lies with the ancestors of the Dogon tribe..."

(*VALIS*, pp. 236–39)

The ancestral home of the Fang, before they were pushed south and west to the rainforests of Gabon by the Fulani expansion, was the Savannah of Western Sudan. And according to Fernandez, the destination at the end of the visions for many Bwiti initiates is a grassy upland resembling nothing so much as the Fang ancestral homeland. There the initiate may find a huge village of the Ancestors, or the clear glass house of Bwiti, of their particular guardian angel, or Christian imagery.[1]

The other members of the Project weren't sure the *VALIS* stuff belonged in an Ibogaine workbook at all. But Beal kept it in subsequent Xeroxes, because both Gnosticism and Bwiti — in their notion of subsidiary creator gods — echo the Platonic idea of the creative *Logos* which generates the material world, but resides with God, on a spiritual level.

Besides, maybe the other predictions in it would pan out — like Clinton winning the election:

"The grim king, the king of tears, will not surrender his power. But you will take his power from him; I grant you that authority in my name, exactly as I granted it to you once before, when the grim king ruled and destroyed and challenged the humble people of the world."

Would the Grim King, Bush, join Nixon wandering along the beach, wondering what hit him? Destroyed, like Nixon, by an informational shock wave? It was important to Deborah Mash.

On November 4, Bush lost the election, shot down like Nixon, according to most pundits, (*"...exactly as I granted it to you once before, when the grim king ruled..."*) by the last minute disclosures of Special Contragate Prosecutor Lawrence Walsh. *Bush knew*[2] — and most people knew it, but they had forgotten. Walsh *reminded* them. After twelve years, the second part of Dick's prediction had come true.

If this seems crazy, remember Harris Isbell and the other CIA-era researchers considered Ibogaine and the other indole-alkylamines to be "psychotomimetic." In other words, if Nico thinks he met the Supreme Being, Nico is crazy. But Philip Dick says there are two ways to tell a genuine *theophany* from mere delusion. One sign is sudden healing ("It was like a miracle," said Carol Baker). But second, if you are imparted with information which turns out to be true, *and which you had no way of knowing*, then perhaps the revelation is genuine.

During initiations, Bwiti routinely see future events — from Fernandez's informant in Chapter 18[3] seeing his brother lying dead along the road three weeks later, to Geerte's boyfriend Adam seeing his friend nodding off and falling out of a 14th-story window, exactly as it happened three months later.

In the NDE, in the dreamtime, the shock of future events is sometimes sharp enough for you to get a preview. Time is not as we ordinarily perceive it. Howard Lotsof crossing the street on Ibogaine turned around and saw seven after-images of himself crossing the street behind him.[4] According to Dick, the actual, secret sacrament of the Gnostics — which the wine and the wafer only *represent* — confers upon the initiate this same augmented perception of time. But the secret is encrypted in the myth of the cup which caught Christ's blood — the Holy Grail — which Dick could not figure out:

"The leader of the Grail knights, Amfortas, has a wound which will not heal. Klingsor has wounded him with the spear which pierced Christ's side. Later, when Klingsor hurls the spear at Parsifal, the pure fool catches the spear — which has stopped in midair — and holds it up, making the sign of the Cross with it, at which Klingsor and his entire castle vanish. They were never there in the first place; they were a delusion, what the Greeks call *dokas;* what the Indians call the veil of *maya*..

"There is nothing Parsifal cannot do. At the

[1] See discussion Fernandez (Appendix 1), pp. 224–228, and Appendix 2, Goutarel and Gollnhoffer, pp. 233–35.

[2] About Oliver North, the cocaine, the guns-for-hostages, the whole nine yards!

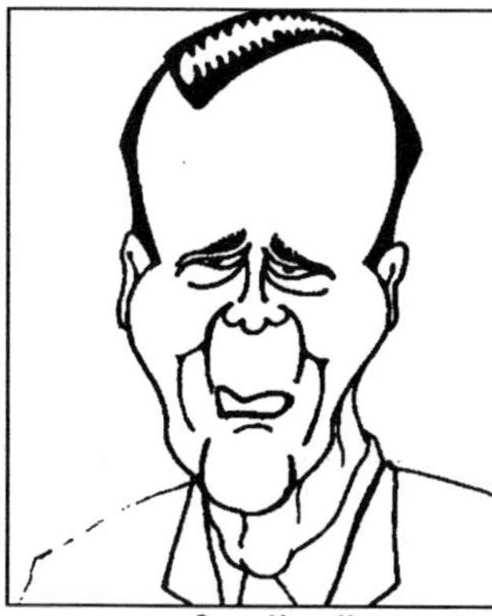

Grim King II

[3] See Fernandez, p. 223.

[4] See Chapter 2, p. 22.

end of the opera, Parsifal touches the spear to Amfortas' wound, the wound heals. Amfortas, who only wanted to die, is healed. Very mysterious words are repeated, which I never understood, although I can read German:

'Gesegnet sei dein Leiden,
Das Mitleids hôchste Kraft,
Und reinstein Wissens Macht
Denn zagen Toren gab!'

"This is one of the keys to the story of Parsifal, the pure fool who abolishes the delusion of the magician Klingsor and his castle, and heals Amfortas' wound. But what does it mean?

'May your suffering be blessed,
Which gave the timid fool
Pity's highest power
And purest knowledge's might!'

"I don't know what this means. However, I know that in our case, the pure fool, Horselover Fat, himself had the wound which would not heal, and the pain that goes with it. All right; the wound is caused by the spear which pierced the Savior's side, and only that same spear can heal it. In the opera, after Amfortas is healed, the shrine is at last opened (it has been closed for a long time) and the Grail itself is revealed at which point heavenly voices say:

" *'Erlosung dem Erlöser!'*

"Which is very strange, because it means:

" 'The Redeemer redeemed!'

"In other words, Christ has saved himself. There's a technical term for this: *Salvator salvandas.* The 'saved savior.'

"'The fact that in the discharge of his task the eternal messenger must himself assume the lot of incarnation and cosmic exile, and the further fact that, at least in the Iranian variety of the myth, he is in a sense identical with those he calls — the once lost parts of the divine self — gives rise to the moving idea of the 'saved savior' (*salvator salvandas*)."

"My Source is reputable. *The Encyclopedia of Philosophy,* Macmillan Publishing Company, New York, 1967; in the article on 'Gnosticism.' I am trying to see how this applies to Fat. What is this 'pity's highest power'? In what way does pity have the power to heal a wound? Would this, then, make Horselover Fat the Savior himself, the savior saved? That seems to be the idea which Wagner expresses. The savior idea is Gnostic in origin. How did it get into Parsifal?

"Maybe Fat was searching for himself when he set out in search of the Savior. To heal the wound made by first the death of Gloria and then the death of Sherri. But what in our modern world is the analog for Klingsor's huge stone castle?

"That which Fat calls the Empire? The Black Iron Prison?

"Is the Empire 'which never ended' an illusion?

"The words which Parsifal speaks which cause the huge stone castle — and Klingsor himself — to disappear are:

" *'Mit diesem Zeichen bann' Ich deinen Zauber.'*

" 'With this sign I abolish your magic.'

"The sign, of course, is the sign of the Cross. Fat's Savior is Fat himself, as I already figured out; Zebra is all the selves along the linear time-axis, laminated into one supra- or trans-temporal self which cannot die, and which has come back to save Fat. But I don't dare tell Fat that he is searching for himself. He is not ready to entertain such a notion, because like the rest of us he seeks an external savior."

(*VALIS,* pp. 130–32)

What is almost overlooked here is that if the healing sacrament of the ancient Gnostics is found, (i.e., when the shrine is at last opened after 2,000 years), for Gnostics it's the same as the living blood of the Savior.[1] It tranforms any cup it touches, and presto: The Grail is revealed.

1 See underlined, p. 112. Also the discussion in Chapter 14, pp. 143–149. Also the discussion in Chapter 16, pp. 172–181.

This particular passage went into the workbook because the verse of Parsifal that Dick says he doesn't really understand encapsulates the central features of Nico's experience, including a line Nico felt was so important he repeated it *four times* on the original raw tape:

"If you are resisting suffering, you suffer more.
"If you are trying to deny your confusion, you remain confused.
"If you are striving for Peace, you find yourself constantly disturbed."

Conversely, the Nico tape perfectly explains the verse of *Parsifal* which Dick says he doesn't understand. It's Zen! Suffering is "blessed" which frees you from suffering — as in getting you through the withdrawal instead of prolonging it with more heroin. It is also "pity's highest power" (the only meaningful pity) — to free all whose sides have been pierced (until no veins are left) — by means of a healing alkaloid.

The crack user treated at the same time as Carol Baker had the kind of cocaine psychosis where he thought he had bugs under his skin. He'd picked at his face until it was covered with cold sores and zits. In 48 hours it healed. (Rats pre-treated with Ibogaine recovered from electro-shock twice as fast as untreated rats.) Also, Ibogaine turns out to be the left half of a Kaposi's Sarcoma drug called Vinblastine (*dimeric* Ibogaine, from the Madagascar periwinkle), and of another drug for hairy-cell leukemia called Vincristine. It's far less toxic than either one.[1] [Contoreggi submitted a protocol to study it as an anti-viral; he wrote another for KS.]

According to Dick, healing that seems miraculous is a dead giveaway for the missing sacrament (along with raising the dead, e.g., the living dead of addiction), but Nico's experience also clears up the other thing Dick can't figure out — what "Purest knowledge's might" is:

> "Do you *KNOW,* now?"
> "Yes I know, now."
> "So you *KNOW: ACT* like it!"

During the Ibogaine rupture into the dreamtime, the aminergic pathways react to the shock of the opening up of the cholinergic pathways — the "splitting of the skull" — by creating the brain's own "windows" program: the movie screen many people describe as opening on the ceiling or wall, for the visions. It is Nico's "rectangle that opens up," so the Supreme Being can speak to him out of a blue sky. The rectangle is a characteristic "signature" of chaos, one of the quirky geometric shapes ("strange attractors") that emerge in "chaotic" phenomena from galactic spirals to conch shells.

It is Parmenides' "perfect" rectangle. The Greeks used it to build the Parthenon; we use it in playing cards. Its dimensions are always three by five.[2] It's all through the *VALIS* trilogy, as the "doorway to the Other Realm."

To match up the transcript of Nico's meeting with God to Dick's observations on Fibonacci's doorway — side by side for easy reference, in such a way that both verses about suffering also come out next to each other — left no other place to stick Hoover's Black Messiah memo in the Ibogaine workbook but *in between* them, *facing* the *Book of Daniel* verse about the grim king.

The coincidence of those three sets of pages forming a hexagram like that by themselves, the first time — it's a billion-in-one.

On December 23, 1992, Howard Lotsof and Dana Beal watched from the courtroom audience as Judge Bruce Allen vacated the life sentence of Dhoruba Bin Wahad for a second

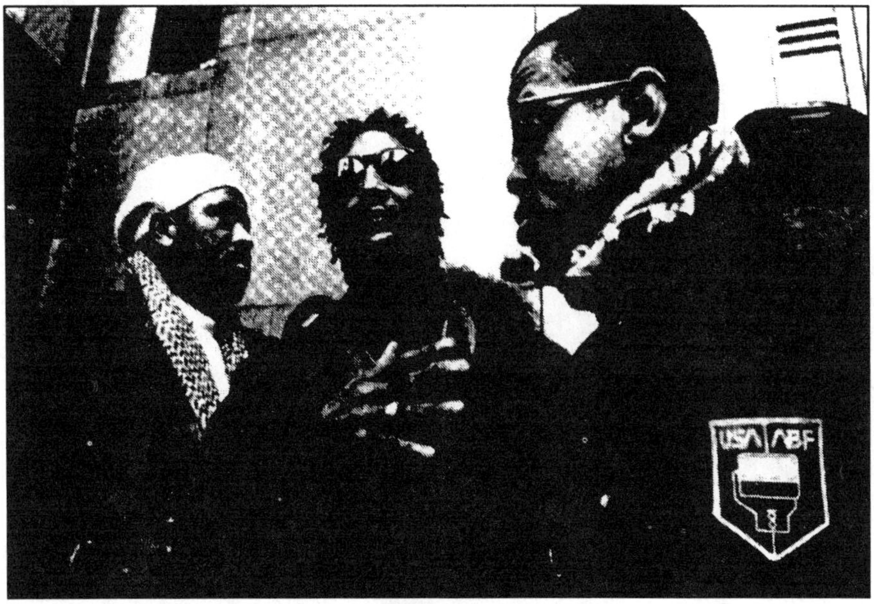

"PASSIN' IT ON"

time. He found that FBI and Red Squad misconduct was so egregious that it met the new test — it had *materially* influenced the outcome of Dhoruba's trial two decades ago. It was so bad the conviction had to be thrown out, even under the new, more restrictive rules. Now the Prosecution would have to do a new trial, with evidence missing that might be mislaid, years afterwards...the vendetta would become too obvious. And against a regular guest on Phil Donohue. You're talking international human rights there, buddy.

But what about the other part of the prediction? (*"...not by human hands.."*) Of changes that would clear the deck, in other words, and let Ibogaine do its work?

In 1992 a significant body of scientific evidence coalesced, demonstrating Ibogaine efficacy in interrupting cocaine use in animals. At the June session of the Conference on Problems of Drug Dependency at Keystone, Colorado, M.R. Dzoljic presented data showing that Ibogaine administered once a week diminishes cocaine self-administration in rats 90%. (On everything else, they keep injecting coke until they die.[3]) Henry Sershen from the Nathan Kline Institute of Orangeburg, New York, confirmed Ibogaine reduces amphetamine-induced dopaminergic and locomotor activity in mice, finding that it inhibits [3H]WIN 35,248 binding to the dopamine transporter.[4] And Patricia Broderick published a new abstract on further interactions between

1 About $^{1}/_{40}$, in fact.

2 This is "Fibonacci's Constant," which is expressed as $^{1}/_{.618034}$.

3 See NIDA Scorecard, Chapter 15, p. 160.

4 "Ibogaine Reduces Amphetamine-induced Locomotor Stimulation in Mice, But Stimulates Locomotor Activity in Rats," by Henry Shershen, Laszlo G. Harsing Jr., Audrey Hashim, and Abel Lajtha, Nathan S. Kline Institute; *Life Sciences,* Vol. 51, pp. 1003–1011, Pergamon Press.

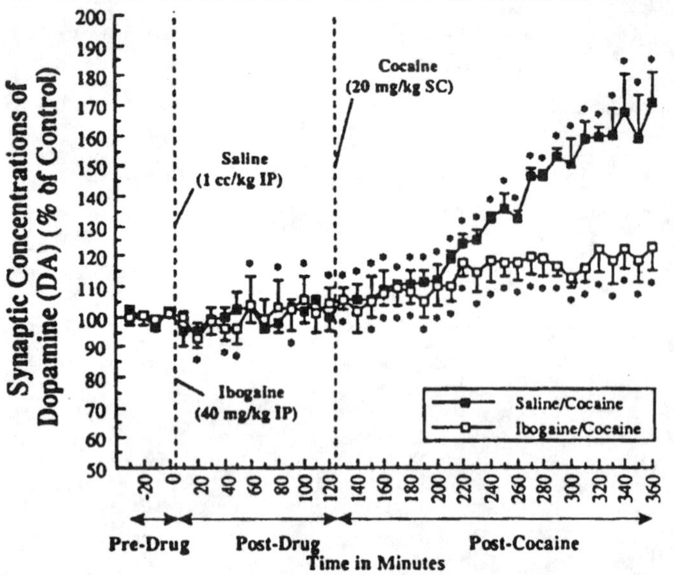

FIG. 2. DA release in vlNAcc: Animals habituated (extended) to novel environment: extended time period: saline-cocaine group and ibogaine-cocaine group. Phase 1: the effect of saline (■) on synaptic concentrations of dopamine (DA) in vlNAcc of freely moving and behaving male Sprague-Dawley rats (*N* = 4) as compared with the effects of ibogaine (□) on synaptic concentrations of DA in vlNAcc of a different group of freely moving and behaving male Sprague-Dawley rats (*N* = 5). Phase 2: the effect of cocaine (20 mg/kg SC) on synaptic concentrations of DA in vlNAcc of the same freely moving and behaving male Sprague-Dawley rats in which saline's effects on vlNAcc DA synaptic concentrations were studied (*n* = 4) (■), as compared with the effect of cocaine (20 mg/kg SC) on synaptic concentrations of DA in vlNAcc of the same freely moving and behaving male Sprague-Dawley rats in which ibogaine's effects on vlNAcc DA synaptic concentrations were studied (*n* = 5) (□). The saline group and the ibogaine group each had injections of either saline or ibogaine respectively for 3 consecutive days before the day of and on the day of the study. *$p < 0.05$; 95% confidence limits (CL). See text for ANOVA statistics.

BRODERICK: IBOGAINE'S EFFECT ON COCAINE AND DOPAMINE

Ibogaine and cocaine, showing locomotor stimulation, a good indicator of cocaine anxiety and craving, was greatly reduced in Ibogaine-treated rats.[1] A scientific consensus was beginning to gather behind Ibogaine's efficacy with cocaine, as it had the year before with morphine. It was bad news for bureaucrats holding out for a cocaine blocker.

There is currently no known pharmaceutical treatment for cocaine. Potential maintenance drugs all turn out to be longer-acting cocaine analogs. And the problem with trying to find a cocaine blocker, *à la* naltrexone, is that a dopamine transporter is not like an opiate receptor — you can't "occupy" it without inhibiting DA re-uptake just like cocaine itself, which is why all the "blocker" analogs they've looked at so far have cocaine-like effects. Meanwhile, none of it is effective at *stopping* cocaine — instead, users top off the new medication with their usual crack or coke. So the prediction that AIDS would force the system to adopt Ibogaine because there's no alternative turns out to be true as far as cocaine is involved.

The other seminal development in '92 was the ripple-effect in the Black community after Dhoruba Bin Wahad came out for Ibogaine. Especially after his appearance at the Harlem Hospital teach-in, he put the Movement on record for an early community-based trial. He plugged it on WBAI. He had already worked through the political implications, and he had always found the people involved to be reliable.

Meanwhile Rommel Washington moved, from Harlem hospital at 135th Street to Reality House at 125th, where Mark Lamantia (one of the same junkie cohort as Fred[2]) was staying in the program only by telling them he was about to go over to Holland to do this experimental drug treatment. Mark, who was on 35 mg. of methadone daily, was in imminent danger of being ejected from Reality House because he was never able to keep his urines free of cocaine or heroin for longer than a week.

Back in 1980, when Howard and Norma did the Halloween Smoke-in (the one that marched on the *Soho Weekly News* to demonstrate against Heroin Chic), it was Mark Lamantia who did the logo for the leaflet — a Halloween jack-o-lantern with hands, dropping joints. All these well-intentioned protests failed, though, to keep Mark, Mario and Fred — the whole crew who went to work for Pope Mickey — from getting strung out on smack in '81 and '82.

Ibogaine was developed to treat *that* particular crop of kids and now at last, after thirteen years, Mark Lamontia was about to go to Holland, to be a subject in a January, 1993 international treatment seminar organized by Sisko, Boaz and Howard. Rommel Washington had signed up to go along to be part of Mark's treatment team. And he got his old boss, Dr. Clark, head of Harlem Hospital's Substance Abuse Unit, to go with them.

Dr Clark joined Mark's treatment in 8 hour shifts with Rommel, Dr. Hans-Georg Behr, Boaz and the Israelis, and Sanchez Ramos and Deborah Mash. Mash was track-

1 The chart above shows that dopamine remains level also. From "Ibogaine Modulates Cocaine Responses Which Are Altered Due to Environmental Habituation: In Vivo Microvoltammetric and Behavioral Studies" by Patricia A. Broderick, et al., *Pharmacology Biochemistry and Behavior,* Vol. 49, No. 3, pp. 711–728, 1994, Pergamon Press.

2 See Chapter 6, p. 59.

ing the treatments on remote video, sending samples of Mark's piss on dry ice to the University of Miami by Federal Express. "What can you tell us," she asked Jan Bastiaans, "about how it *really* works? How many treatments have you done?"

"Only ten treatments. But you're missing the important point. It works." And that was the newsflash that Clark took back to Harlem, to the entire Black treatment community — that Ibogaine works, that Mark had come off of 35 mg of methadone in three days, with an absence of withdrawal that seemed uncanny. When Mark got back to Reality House, he walked right past the methadone window. (Another subject of these treatments came off a whopping 125 mgs!) Forty-five days later Dr Clark did a complete physical examination of Mark, who was like a new man (of course). Mark's was the first really rigorous followup: weekly urines, the very thing NIDA MDD had been demanding. And an informational shock wave flashed out through treatment professionals and others in Harlem, as the word was confirmed by people they respect: It works. It really works.

Shockwaves are ruptures, sweeping across the landscape of things-as-usual. In the high energy state within the wave, different mathematics apply; structure that was latent is manifested along the rupture.

Take slime mold — it has a very strange characteristic. Ordinarily it's a little individual amoeba, but take away its food, and it signals to all the other amoebas, and they start to cluster in wave patterns and form one differentiated animal. The front is a head, the back, a stalk, the body becomes spores covered with hard cases. The cases break away, dispersing spores far and wide, which open up wherever there's new food–and out come little amoebas.

Your ancestors are like that. They exist hologramatically on the cellular level, in all the non-nucleated genetic material of all humans. Perhaps the non-nucleated material generates the great weak electromagnetic aura Philip Dick calls "VALIS".

Holograms have the same quality — if you break a holographic plate, the entire hologramatic image is in every fragment. That's because it's made without lenses, by the direct action of split lasers on a negative. Everything is enfolded in a photographic print which requires the same split laser setup to project a three-dimensional image. There is no difference between image and object. There is no space, no time, no matter and no mind. Our process of memory seems to work along the same lines, locating the correct memory in the "print" with the neuroelectric equivalent of the "reference beam" used to read a hologramic print.

VALIS is an acronym for Vast Active Living Intelligence System. P. K. Dick believed it knows everything known to every person, but only in memory. It knows only hologramatically, therefore it perceives the universe as a hologram. For us to communicate with it is a problem. Direct communication with creatures via modulation of bioelectric phenomena in the area puts such a load on any nervous system in the neighborhood that it can cause permanent damage. But in the dreamtime, when you have direct access to information stored in your cells, VALIS can communicate digitally — perhaps via perturbation of REM circuits, or of the non-nucleated genetic material directly. It can generate the equivalent of a

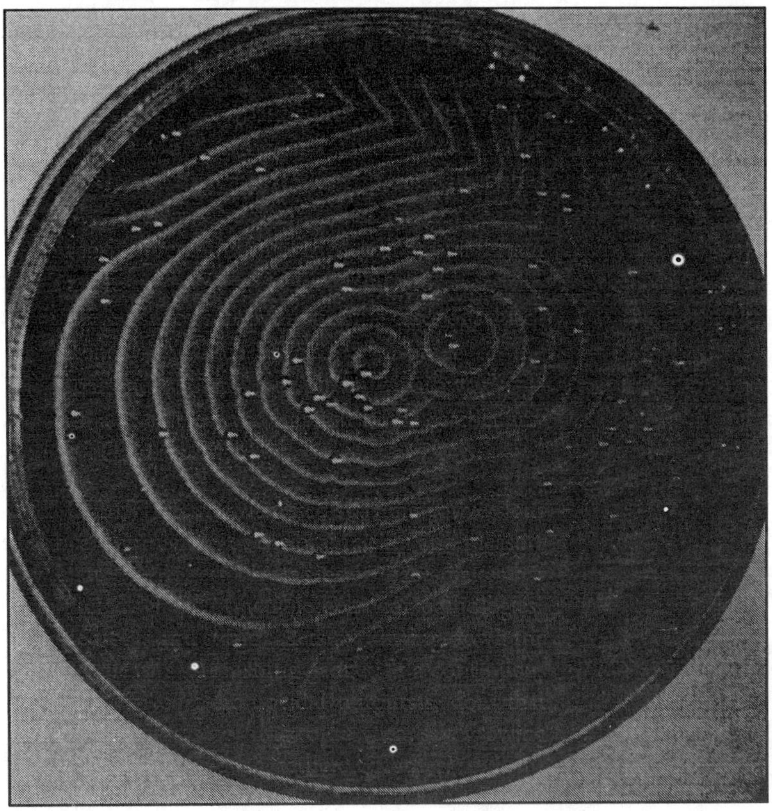

Three Pound Universe

SLIME MOLD — CHAOTIC DYNAMICS AT WORK.

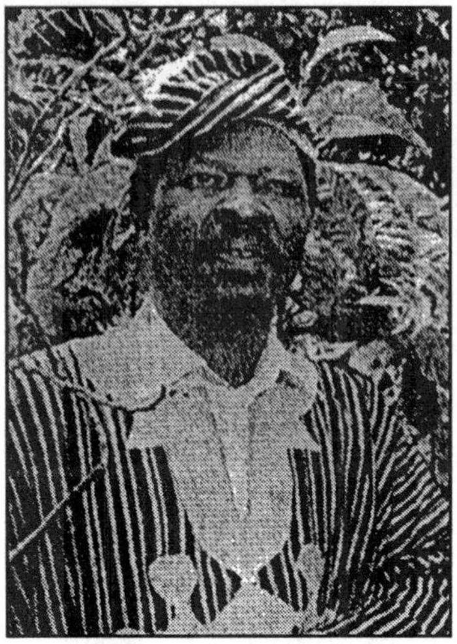

DR. ANTHONY ANDOH CALLS IBOGA "THE PLANT THAT HEALS THE SPIRIT."

laser reference beam to project a Fibonacci "doorway:" and if the throes of your NDE reflex generate the same chaotic 'attractor' shape, and the two lock together, you have a match, and Nico meets God.

Therefore, VALIS does not rule, but influences outcomes via sychronicity, maximized through free will taking advantage of coincidence. The only thing that can destroy it is for humanity to completely destroy itself. For the first time in history, however, that could happen at any moment. In his notes, in a later paragraph of entry 47, on *Two Source Cosmogony,* Philip Dick writes:

> "It was the One's purpose for our hologramatic universe to serve as a teaching instrument by which a variety of new lives advanced until ultimately they would be iso-morphic with the One. However, the decaying condition of hyperuniverse II introduced malfactors which damaged our hologramatic universe. This is the origin of entropy, un-deserved suffering, chaos and death, as well as the Empire, the Black Iron Prison; in essence, the aborting of the proper health and growth of the life forms within the hologramatic universe. Also, the teaching function was grossly impaired, since only the signal from the hyperuniverse I was information-rich; that from II had become noise. The psyche of hyperuniverse I sent a micro-form of itself into hyperuniverse II to attempt to heal it..."[1]
>
> (*VALIS,* p. 237)

[1] Identified as the Holy Spirit, i.e., "the Spirit that in-dwelt."

By means of "the plant that heals the spirit," containing an alkaloid that unlocks the NDE reflex, a multi-ordinal feedback loop is established at the intersection of the chaos of the dreamtime and the chaos of society. As the Ibogaine wave flashes across society, strange synchronicities play across the wavefront. Initiates gain augmented perception of time. In Bwiti, the Grail, the Blood, the Burning Bush are one. There are glimpses of a ghostly order emerging that *attracts* the chaos to it, like a tornado.

The little guys in the secret early grey robes have attached a special phase generator to the FDA / NIDA info-input of the Black Iron Prison. Since the entire Prison is a Chaos-generated projection, the little guys are pulsing a *strange attractor* into the input–a chaotic shape that exactly cancels out the chaotic phase-signature of the Prison. The shape: the perfect rectangle of Parmenides.

The impulse has reached the nucleus of the prison, and it is beginning to replicate hundreds and thousands of Bwiti among the prison inmates, which will burst the cells of the Prison, causing massive cell-death and breakdown of the malignant occupying organism in its entirety.

To the regular Christians such as those who go to Church on Sunday, the little guys have issued the Ibogaine Challenge:

Bring us, O Cardinal, three junkies.
Give them the wine and the wafer,
And sit with them for forty-eight hours.
We will bring three junkies also,
Give them Ibogaine,
And sit with them for forty-eight hours.
At the end of the time,
You have breakfast with your junkies.
We'll have breakfast with ours.

From pot to jug

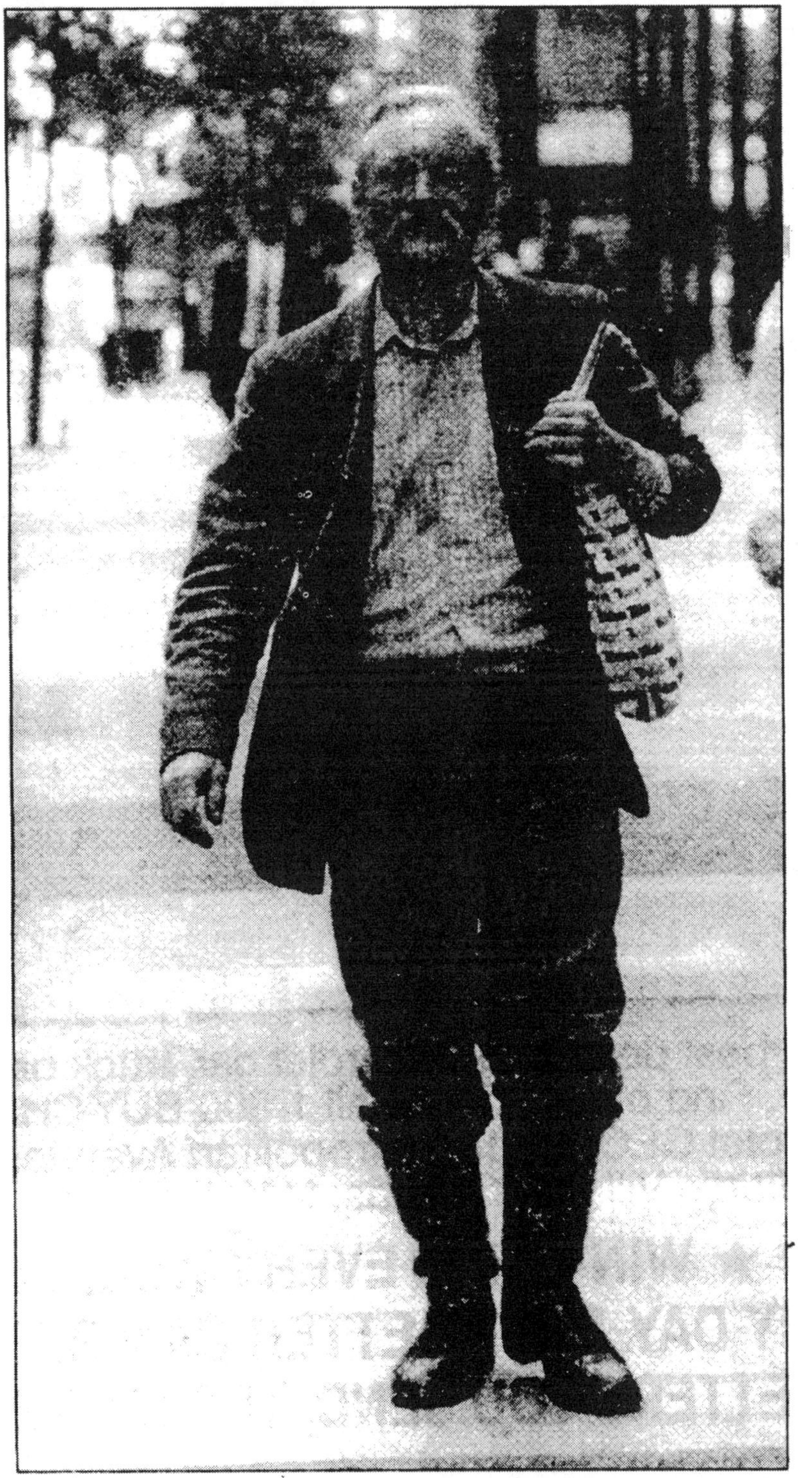

POT PROPONENT Dana Beal on 42d St. yesterday. He will have to do some time for trying to take a pound of marijuana to AIDS patients. JIM HUGHES DAILY NEWS

AIDS trip ends in jail

By ROB POLNER
Daily News Staff Writer

A graying founder of the Yippies will be sentenced to 60 days in prison for trying to take a pound of marijuana to AIDS patients to ease their suffering.

The light sentence is the result of a plea bargain worked out Friday between defendant Dana Beal's attorney, William Kunstler, and the Queens district attorney's office.

Beal, 45 and graying, has a prior drug rap, but his case generated a wide spectrum of support from doctors, AIDS activists and a lawmaker who favors legalizing marijuana for medical purposes.

Dr. Brian Salzman, an infectious-disease specialist at Beth Israel Medical Center, filed an affidavit stating that illicit marijuana smoking is already "common among AIDS suffers because it stimulates appetite, reduces nausea and thereby limits severe weight loss."

Sen. Joseph Galiber (D-Bronx) also weighed in for Beal, saying the activist "has lobbied for the medical uses of marijuana (and) impressed me with the sincerity of his convictions."

Arrested in '91

Beal was arrested in January 1991 while trying to carry a pound of freshly cut marijuana through a metal detector at LaGuardia Airport to fly it to dying patients in Boston.

Beal could have been sentenced to up to nine years because he was convicted in 1987 of marijuana possession, said Kunstler.

Beal called the light sentence a victory in the fight to legalize marijuana for medical purposes. "The state Legislature needs to exempt health-care providers and bona fide AIDS activists from criminal drug prosecution when they are attempting to ease the suffering of the terminally ill," he said.

In the 1960s, Beale said, he prescribed a heady mix of psychedelic drugs and youthful activism. He later advocated giving clean hypodermic needles to heroin addicts to fight AIDS, and he has since become the leading promoter of ibogaine, a new drug derived from the root of an African shrub that, he says, can ease addicts' dependency without the agony of withdrawal.

New York Daily News

CHAPTER 14: "Time is a child at play, playing draughts..."

When the *Newsday* Ibogaine article appeared November 19, 1992, and it seemed he might not go to jail, Dana experienced a vague sense of loss. He'd been planning to write a comprehensive report on Ibogaine during his sixty days, and now he wouldn't have a chance... too many interruptions in the outside world.

For him to be freed on the spot November 20th, though, he needed a letter setting forth an offer of a community service job at Housing Works,[1] which was slow to produce it — with the result that the judge adjourned the matter until December 9th. Charles King of Housing Works got around to writing Beal the letter just before Thanksgiving. But Karen Rankin, the ADA in the case, who'd been absent November 20th, now insisted on the full sixty-day jail sentence.

On December 9th the community service option was withdrawn by Judge Corrado, and Beal agreed to begin serving the actual forty days of his sixty-day sentence on January 11th, the Monday just after his birthday. Even an eleventh-hour appeal by Jim Dwyer of *Newsday* failed to sway the court on the 11th, and Beal was on a bunk in Riker's before the day was out.

He spent the week reviewing papers in Lotsof's NDA version of the workbook and reading Philip Dick. On the following Tuesday all of his scientific and religious materials were seized and he was flown by airplane hundreds of miles north to the Canadian border, to a state prison being leased by the city for inmates deemed likely to benefit from a stay in a drug-free residential treatment facility.

With only limited phone calls to the outer world, Dana raised enough of an uproar that any thought in the prison administration of barring him from receiving the Ibogaine workbook or Goutarel's monograph was quickly quashed, and after eight days, during which he wrote a first draft of Chapters 1 through 4, the workbook and other materials arrived the very day he needed another look at the patents to write Chapter 5.

Within days he was reading each of the Glick papers six times, writing Chapter 7. But among the packet of materials Alice T. sent was a book whose cover had leaped out at her when she found it, on the browse, at Strand Books — *The Three Pound Universe.* He put it aside, to read when, in order to go forward from Goutarel's PGO waves, he needed more basic information about the brain. It presented neurophysics as very different from high-school physics — a domain of quantum uncertainty and 'chaotic dynamics'. Plowing through it after he'd finished Chapter 10, Dana noticed an extensive presentation of the findings of a certain Dr. Heath,[2] a Tulane University professor who achieved success in treating some cases of schizophrenia — which is also a disorder of the dopamine circuits (or "pleasure pathway") — with a small electrical implant in the cerebellum.

Then he hit paydirt, on pp. 174–8:

1 New York City's largest AIDS housing provider.

2 Yes, this is the same Dr. Heath whose infamous monkey studies on cannabis toxicity were discredited because he failed to account for carbon monoxide poisoning caused by his experimental equipment, cited in *The Emperor Wears No Clothes,* by Jack Herer.

The Secrets of the Cerebellum

IN THE LAST CHAPTER we witnessed startling conversions wrought by electrical stimulation of the brain's pain and pleasure centers. We saw that Dr. Robert Heath's brain pace-maker has rescued people afflicted with "intractable behavior pathologies" from a life of padded cells and straitjackets by turning down the fear/rage switch in their heads. Now we'll return to Dr. Heath's astonishing gadget: If a continuous low-voltage electrical current applied to the cerebellum can curb homocidal outbursts, does that mean that violence is an inborn neurologic defect? And that it has nothing to do with, say, growing up in a broken home in the South Bronx with a crazy, alcoholic or drug-addicted mother?

Wrong. When it comes to producing a violent person, the brain and the social environment interact in such intricate ways that the old nature-versus-nurture debate seems rather like those hair-splitting early Christian councils about the precise proportion of humanity/divinity in Christ. The story of the cerebellum is a case in point.

The first clues came from the famous Harlow monkeys. At the University of Illinois in the 1950s and the early 1960s, psychologist Harry F. Harlow performed a series of now-legendary experiments in sensory and emotional deprivation, raising infant rhesus monkeys in solitary wire cages without toys or companions. After three months even an obtuse observer couldn't miss the signs of emotional damage. The small monkeys sat forlornly in a corner of the cage rocking back and forth like autistic children. When they came of age and rejoined the colony, their social ineptness was pitiful. Unable to decipher the most rudimentary simian social signals, they could barely distinguish friend from foe, self from non-self. They recoiled in terror from the sight of their own hands and compulsively mutilated themselves. The males never learned to court or mate, while the females who became mothers neglected or abused their babies. Most important, from our perspective, these monkeys were given to outbursts of inexplicable violence.

At first the Harlow monkeys were taken as proof of the psychoanalytic dictum that bad mothering (or in this case, no mothering at all) caused schizophrenia, for the isolated monkeys looked about as "schizophrenic" as is possible for a nonhuman primate to look. But Harlow confounded the Freudians by separating rhesus infants from their mothers and raising them with age mates. These monkeys developed quite normally. What crucial sensory lack, then, was causing the "deprivation syndrome"? A former colleague of Harlow's, William A. Mason, devised an ingenious experiment in the late 1960s to find out.

Mason compared three groups of young monkeys. One group was reared in the usual way with their mothers. A second group grew up with a "movable surrogate," consisting of a motorized, swinging bleach bottle; while a third group of infants got a stationary surrogate, a bleach bottle covered with fur and fixed in place. The result? The monkeys reared with their mothers, of course, grew up normally, and the monkeys whose only solace was a fixed surrogate developed a bad case of the deprivation syndrome. The monkeys given the movable surrogate, however, surprised the psychologists by being much less screwed up. Was movement crucial to emotional development?

James W. Prescott, a developmental psychologist then working at the National Institute of Child Health and Human Development (NICHD), thought so. He managed to get hold of five of the emotionally stunted Harlow monkeys, whose weird stereotypic rocking motions reminded him of some of the institutionalized children he'd seen. Any kind of sensory deprivation must damage the growing brain's emotional systems, he figured. Noticing that an immobile surrogate produced such basket cases, his thought turned to the cerebellum, the three-lobed structure at the very back of the brain that governs movement and balance.

"At the time," he recalls, "there was very little data to support my theory that stimulation of the cerebellum might have something to do with emotions. Actually, back around 1800, Franz Joseph Gall, the father of phrenology, said the cerebellum was involved in pleasure or lack of pleasure, but he was discredited because of the phrenology stuff...

"Anyway," he continues, "I thought we'd find a neuro-pathology in the isolation-reared animals, so I shipped them to Tulane so Bob Heath could implant them. I suggested that he put electrodes in the cerebellum as well as the limbic sites." Where other investigators had failed to find anything wrong with these sensory-deprived brains, Heath's electrodes detected a great deal amiss. There were abnormal "spike" discharges in the monkeys' limbic pain-and-pleasure areas, very like the pathological EEGs of violent human psychotics. And, to be sure, strange spikes also occurred in the cerebellum, where Heath had never thought to look before.

"The paleocerebellum, the old cerebellum, governs proprioception," Heath explains. "That's the input from your muscles, joints, and tendons that lets you know what position your body is in, where you're located in three-dimensional space. It also regulates balance, your vestibular sense. Now, why do children like to be tossed in the air, hang upside down, and ride merry-go-rounds and roller coasters? Because these sensory experiences feed directly into the emotional system."

Hard evidence came from the sad-eyed Tulane lab monkeys in their little plastic restraining chairs. As electrodes in different sites of their brains recorded second-to-second electrical changes, Heath showed that the bursts of activity in the paleocerebellum set off similar ones in the septum, hippocampus, and amygdala, and vice-versa. The upshot was that the cerebellum, the limbic pain/pleasure centers, and various sensory relay stations were all part of one circuit! This was not just a heretical rewriting of neuroanatomy — the textbook drawings of the nerve tracts didn't show cerebellar-forebrain connections — but it explained to Heath how the isolation-reared monkeys got so weird. Messages from our eyes, ears, and skin, as well as the body-sense signals processed in the paleocerebellum, stir trains of electrical impulses in the distant emotional centers, setting in motion a giant emotional-sensory feedback loop. (We all can testify to how quickly a Mozart sonata or a good massage travels to our "pleasure center.") Imagine, then, the effects of sensory isolation on an immature brain.

"We already knew from human studies," Heath tells us, "that if you're suspended in weightlessness you'll hallucinate, have delusions, and experience what is known as depersonalization." Heath sees a curious connection between body sense and sense of self in the shattered inner world of psychosis, for a psychotic's body image is distorted along with his ego. "Psychotics, you know, often say they feel unreal or don't know who they are — that's depersonalization," he says. "And typically the lack of self-awareness can be detected long before the classic symptoms of hallucinations and thought disorders appear." Could an impaired cerebellum or faulty cerebellar-limbic nerve connections be responsible?

Heath went on to develop the cerebellar pacemaker and implant it in the heads of violent mental patients, some of whom improved dramatically. James Prescott, meanwhile, was embarked on a course of research that would leave him jobless, without funds, and mired in a bitter lawsuit against his superiors at the NICHD...

(*The Three Pound Universe*, pp. 173–76)

Later, in a section on the Near-Death Experience, writers Judith Hooper and Dick Teresi found something harder to explain: the autoscopic phase wherein the person finds themself hovering above their body, looking down on efforts to resuscitate them. Afterwards they are able to provide details the near-dead *could not have seen* from their vantage point on the operating table. Significantly, several experts cited the potential role of endorphins[1] in producing the feelings of "distance and well-being" that characterize the NDE.

The next chapter, on the Brain as a hologram, reviewed evidence that the neuron's code for storing information resembles the interference pattern on a holographic plate, based on a method of breaking down any complex pattern into sets of simpler waves — a mathematical operation called the *Fourier transform.*

Every fragment of a hologram contains the entire image. Your Grandmother does not reside in a "Grandmother neuron," but everywhere throughout your memory whenever you think of her. And just as many different holograms can be superimposed, so can infinite images be stacked in our brains. We perform the spatial representation that maps the retinal image onto the cortex; then, in the membranes of the cells the image is transformed back into the frequency mode — the "scatter" we'd see if we saw without a lens.[2] The brain's code for storing information resembles the interference of wave-phase relationships in a holographic plate — with the equivalent of a "reconstruction beam" zooming in on a particular coded memory when we recall something. Scattered, holographic information storage explains why stroke victims don't lose discrete parts of their memory: all memory is contained within any portion thereof.

The waking, or "aminergic" pathways of the brain have been found to resolve visual sensory input into edges, extensions, and intersections — the neural equivalent of Kant's spatial "categories" — giving us the external world, wherein nothing travels faster than the speed of light. But in the Fourier domain, correlations can be performed almost instantly — just as we can dream a whole ten years in two minutes of REM, or experience our "whole life flashing before our eyes" in a Near Death Experience. Ibogaine subjects, given waking access to the cholinergic pathways of the sleeping brain, describe it as being like "six televisions going at once," without the automatic focusing in on the most interesting channel that goes on during wakefulness. The cholinergic pathways have never bothered to organize themselves into a proper ego, and experience time as "internal" (generated via regular brainwaves within the cerebellum, etc.) — as something the self is "outside of." Conversely, information that becomes available during an Ibogaine experience may snap into focus months later.

The best stuff of all was in the last chapter of the book—

[1] That is, the endogenous body opiates, including enkephalins and dynorphin. See p. 191 for discussion.

[2] See Hammeroff, pp. xxx–xxx.

Chaos, Strange Attractors, and the Stream of Consciousness

"A great disorder is an order. Now, A
And B are not like statuary, posed
For a visit in the Louvre. They are things chalked
On the sidewalk so the pensive man may see."
— WALLACE STEVENS
"Connoisseur of Chaos"

For five days in a row, a Stanford psychiatrist has been watching the "shopping bag ladies" in the public park. By his calculations each of the women has a stereotypical routine of postures, gestures, and monologues that is repeated over and over again like a musician's set. Later he jots down some equations for dopamine synthesis in the schizophrenic brain.

Fiddling with his parameters a little, a scientist in Pennsylvania makes a high-speed computer "epileptic." A Chicago biophysicist studies the "hallucinations" he conjured with digital representations of neurons. In Santa Cruz, California, a mathematician adds stress variables to ROVER, a computer simulation of a dog's adrenal cortical system. "When we add ACTH," he says, "it responds just like a dog."

In La Jolla, rats on LSD, amphetamine, cocaine, antidepressents, lithium, and caffeine wander at random in cages. Each time their tails pass through a photobeam, an electrical blip is transmitted to a computer, which calculates the "frequency" and "amplitude" of their journeys. Studying the patterns, a neuroscientist reflects, "The stream of consciousness is a random walk, but an order emerges over time."

These scientists are "connoisseurs of chaos," practitioners of a science so new it doesn't have an official name, only a nickname — chaos. (Officially it is known as nonlinear dynamics, or sometimes as chaotic dynamics.) The Christopher Columbus of chaos was an MIT meteorologist named Edward Lorenz. While working on the problem of long-range weather forecasting in 1963, he proved mathematically that the weather was impossible to predict. This may be big news for Willard C. Scott — and for you when you're worried about the rain on your parade — but what does that have to do with the brain?

Well, years after Lorenz's quiet discovery (known for a decade only to readers of an obscure meteorology journal), it became apparent that the laws he discovered also governed water flowing through a pipe, hurricanes, airplanes in flight, chemical reactions, the waxing and waning of wildlife populations, economic cycles, the ebb and flow of hormones in the body — and the 1,000,000,000,000 (one trillion) interconnected nerve cells of the brain.

The mind does not easily grasp nonlinear interactions between billions of cells," says Stephen Grossberg, a mathematician and interdisciplinary scientist at Boston University's Center for Adaptive Systems. "That is why we need mathematical models." Says Arnold Mandell, "The machinery of the brain is just too complicated. Two hundred neurotransmitters, each with seventy thousand receptors! How can we ever understand all that plumbing? We have to get away from the plumbing to see the brain's deep messages." Of course many researchers have made brilliant careers digging up the "plumbing." Out of Eric Kandell's microscopic scrutiny of cell membranes came the elementary building blocks of memory; from Hubel and Wiesel's single-cell recordings, a map of the visual cortex. But can this explain how you *think?*

Mandell, Grossberg, and the other scientists you'll meet in this chapter don't think so. If you want to know how New York City functions, would you interview three passersby in depth? Or would you take a helicopter ride over the city and look down on the different boroughs and the major traffic routes, the clusters of skyscrapers that mark the financial centers, the densities of flashing red lights that might mean dangerous neighborhoods? If you are looking for the brain's basic organizing priniciples, its "deep messages," mathematics can lift you above the gritty details. The lingo of chaos is esoteric, and many of its pioneers labor in rarified and otherworldly realms of theoretical physics. But the interesting thing about it is that chemists, mathematicians, biologists, physiologists, meteorologists, and neuroscientists are all tuning in to the same "deep messages." There are some who think chaos is a universal language of nature.

The Dripping Faucet as Microcosm

"ONLY ONCE OR TWICE in a millennium," says mathematician Ralph Abraham, of the University of California at Santa Cruz, "is there a true scientific revolution, a paradigm shift. Newtonian mechanics and the invention of calculus in the seventeenth century brought about the last one. The current scientific revolution will synthesize the whole intellectual discourse of the species." While Abraham makes this prophecy, in a Szechwan restaurant in downtown Santa Cruz, ragged armies of sixties' casualties drift by the window, hollow-eyed, laden with knapsacks, like refugees from an Antonioni film. If there is a dark side to the third millennium, these are the people who will gather on mountaintops to witness the end of the world. Abraham and his fellow chaos theorists expect to witness quite the opposite.

Up the hill, the University of California at Santa Cruz (UCSC) is a land of sun-bleached, windblown meadows and cool redwood groves. Something of the zeitgeist of the sixties lingers in the air: the students do not look like accounting majors, and it is possible to obtain a Ph. D. in the History of Consciousness. Perhaps it was the right objective correlative (as T. S. Eliot might have called it) for the Chaos Cabal.

In 1977 physicist Rob Shaw was just winding up his Ph.D. dissertation on superconductivity when a professor asked him to take a look at some puzzling differential equations. He programed them into an analog computer he'd salvaged in the basement of a defunct engineering department and got the shock of his life. By having the computer perform iterations — essentially repeating the same equations over and over again — he fell into a looking-glass world where order spun off into chaos. Soon he lost all interest in superconductivity (the dissertation was never completed) and took to sleeping in his lab and staying up all night to ponder the enigmatic shapes on his screen. (They were "strange attractors," though Shaw did not know that yet.) When three friends, also physics students, dropped by to see what he was doing, they became possessed too. In late 1977 the Santa Cruz Dynamical Systems Collective — or colloquially, the Chaos Cabal — was formed. (Abraham, who had heard the gospel of chaos a few years before, became a sort of chaos elder.)

To enter Shaw's office is to walk into the bowels of a dismantled appliance–a maze of meters, dials, plugboard, wires, terminals, plotters, and gauges. "I'm a technotwit," he confesses. He takes us next door to see a contraption that looks like a precocious child's project for the science fair. A plastic tub of water is mounted above a brass faucet. The drops from the faucet interrupt a laser beam, which precisely records the intervals between them and transmits them as pulses to the computer next door. This is Shaw's famous chaotic faucet. "The fascinating thing about a standard faucet," he tells us, "is that it's got this random element in it. The flow is constant, the spigot doesn't move, and nothing has perturbed the system, but you got this chaotic pattern in it that never repeats itself. It's a microcosm."

When the Chaos Cabal first presented results like these at scientific conferences, other scientists would shake their heads dubiously and ask, "Are you sure this isn't just a numerical error?" But chaos is not the result of a numerical error. It is a fact of nature.

Physical theories since Archimedes, Galileo, and Newton have been built around a stable, linear world, an idealized cosmos of frictionless pendulums, efficient machines, and eternal trajectories. The serene assumption — articulated by the French mathematician Pierre Simon, Marquis de Laplace — was that you could predict the future in its entirety if you knew the position and velocity of every particle at one moment in time. Alas, this is untrue. Half a century ago, the founders of quantum mechnics said that the subatomic domain was haunted by randomness, and the best measuring devices on earth could not make it less uncertain. Albert Einstein could not accept this idea, objecting, "God does not play dice with the universe!" Well, God does play dice, and not just with quarks. Waterfalls, cloud patterns, heart arrhythmias, waves crashing against a sea wall during a winter storm, the fluctuations of a predator/prey population, the collective song of your neurons, and many other systems in nature also have pockets of randomness that make them unpredictable. We can write equations for the orbits of remote planets, but the trajectories of tumbling dice forever elude us. Why?

Back in 1977 Shaw observed that the realm of chaos was ruled by certain laws. One of these was "sensitive dependence on initial conditions," a phenomenon starkly illustrated at the casinos of

Las Vegas. At the moment a roulette wheel is spun, the tiniest twitch of the finger controls the ball's trajectory. Similar infinitesimal influences determine how dice will land. In meterology there is the so-called Butterfly Effect, the idea that the flapping of a butterfly's wings in the air over Peru in February could affect the weather in Los Angeles in March. Because of sensitive dependence on initial conditions, minuscule measuring errors are magnified into huge ones farther down the line, and prediction becomes impossible. So it is not necessarily your local weatherman's fault if he's wrong about the weather a week from Monday. We are condemned to live with chance.

One of the founding fathers of chaos, the German theoretical chemist Otto Rossler, once watched a mechanical taffy puller at work, pulling the taffy and folding it back on itself again and again. In his mind Rossler followed the diverging course of two imaginary raisins and jotted down equations for a new "strange attractor." Rossler was observing a second fundamental law of chaos, "rapid divergence of nearby trajectories." Variables that start highly correlated — the mathematical equivalents of the raisins — drift apart and become uncorrelated. After lots of stretching and folding, which a computer does with "iterations," differences in the system widen and a deterministic system become indeterminate.

Shaw was to learn, of course, that the terra incognita he stumbled on was not entirely incognita. Edward Lorenz before him had discovered how "sensitive dependence" and "rapid divergence" produced lumps of chaos in the convection currents of the atmosphere. Then, in 1971, a study of fluid turbulence really put chaos on the map. Werner Heisenberg, the father of quantum uncertainty, once remarked that when he went on to the next world, he wanted God to explain two things. One was the mysteries of the quantum realm: the other was fluid turbulence. Generations of physicists have tried in vain to write equations for the hydrodynamics of waterfalls, cascading rivers, even water rushing out of a faucet, and concluded that those phenomena, for reasons no one could identify, were just too complicated to predict. But two European scientists, David Ruelle and Floris Takens, showed that a wild river had a form to it after all, albeit a strange one. In the dynamics of turbulent fluids they divined ghostly geometric forms similar to the one Lorenz had identified a decade before in the weather. They named them *strange attractors.*

So what is an attractor, and what makes one strange? Any physical system — a chemical reaction, the motion of a pendulum, a heartbeat, or the fluctuations in a population of gray foxes — can be plotted as a series of mathematical points representing sucessive temperature readings, velocity, amplitude, or whatever. In time the points describing the changes in the system are drawn toward the visible geometry of an "attractor" like metal filing toward a magnet.

There are three types of attractors, two of which are old ones.The *fixed point* attractor describes a system at rest, after all the motions have ceased. If you fill a pan with water and shake it up, the liquid will swirl around for a while and then stop. Mathematically speaking, it settles into a fixed point. After all the chemicals have stopped reacting, a chemical system would have a point attractor (equilibrium) structure.

The second type is the *periodic* attractor, or *limit cycle.* The period motion of a pendulum or metronome, the regular beating of a human heart, a smoothly oscillating EEG, or the mood swings of a manic-depressive might all be described by the limit cycle. The key thing about the fixed point and the limit cycle is that they are regular and predictable. If you know the initial state, you can plot all the future states.

Suppose you heat french-fry grease in a saucepan. At first the grease just sits there. As it heats, convection currents form, periodic wiggles that make a limit cycle. If you turn up the burner a little more, the patterns make doubly periodic wiggles (wiggles upon wiggles). At a certain critical value of heat, however. the grease abruptly "bifurcates," in the lingo, to a strange attractor motion.

Paradoxical Order

WHAT does a strange atttractor look like? Aiming a creaky school projector at the wall, Shaw shows us movies of the strange attractors captured on the local cathode-ray screens. "This is our local compulsion," he says, as the ten thousand mathematical points that represent ten thousand future states unfold in an instant, bringing these odd mathematical creatures to life. They are beautiful: baroque spirals, elaborate filigrees, intricate webs spun by non-Euclidian spiders, spaces like amusement-park rides as depicted by Marcel Duchamp.

There's a method to this madness, however. At first chaotic behavior seems to follow no rules, but in time it assumes a definite shape. Strange attractors may sprout extravagant thickets of randomness, but they never fly out of the "phase space," a determined mathematical envelope. And whether you're dealing with water in pipes or clouds or swirls of smoke or jet engines, certain rules and constants always apply when nature "bifurcates" into disorder.

By the very nature of our activities," says Shaw, "we try to avoid chaos. What do we try to do with our machines? Keep them stable and avoid oscillations, or if we have oscillations, try to keep those stable. But now we can see that chaos has a lot of order in it.

The Old Guard — people like [information theorist] Norbert Weiner — used equations for *total* randomness as a model for nature," explains Doyne Farmer, a graduate of the Chaos Cabal who has carried the seeds of chaos to Los Alamos National Laboratories in New Mexico. "When you have complete chaos, you can perform probability studies. This is the case with the molecules in a gas, which get pretty evenly distributed. However, there are many situations in nature where orderly things happen in the midst of great chaos. Some systems have a 'clock' inside them that goes on keeping perfect time in the midst of very chaotic stuff. For those systems, deterministic chaos, with its strange-attractor structure, is the best model."

Paradoxically the study of chaos seems to lead into a higher realm of order. (Farmer's Ph.D. dissertation, *"Order in Chaos,"* describes how order, information, and structure arise in these systems.) Under nature's polymorphous surface lies a finite set of hidden principles. "There are only a few movies, and everything we see around us is the working out of one of those movies," says Ralph Abraham. If you know how to look, the invisible blueprints of strange attractors determine the behavior of rivers and jet engines, chemical reactions and cloud formations, heartbeats, the Big Bang, EEGs, and economic cycles.

You can use nonlinear equations to model a two-nation arms race, as physicist Alan Saperstein, of Wayne State University in Detroit, has done. "I think," he says, "the idea of a transition from laminar [smooth] to turbulent flow or, if you will, from predictable international relations to chaotic international relations is important." You can look at the economy this way, plotting the often quirky "oscillations" of business cycles. You can analyze the heart as a dynamical system, as a pair of researchers at Montreal's McGill University did, and isolate the conditions under which a normal, periodic heartbeat will "bifurcate" into dangerous heart fibrillations. You can mix together certain chemicals and see the genesis of chaos. You can build a nonlinear model of the female endocrine system (the interlocking hormonal feedback, loops of which act like coupled mechanical oscillators) to study the premenstrual syndrome. Ralph Abraham did, and he also fathered ROVER, the computer simulation of a dog's stress response.

"It is interesting, even comforting," muses W. Ross Adey, a neuro-scientist who is conversant with chaos, "that the laws that determine atomic interactions in cosmic interstellar dust are the same laws that determine the interactions of molecules on the surface of brain cells."

Chaos and the Brain

THE WALLS of Don Walter's office, in the basement of UCLA's Life Sciences Building, are covered with graphics of different biological processes. Some, like the computer-graphics portrait of systolic and diastolic rhythms, resemble stylized mountain chains with Japanese-style clouds around their peaks. As we arrive, his computer terminal is displaying sawtooth waves of blue and violet. "Chaotic spikes," he explains.

By running equations for three linked neurons, Walter and Alan Garfinkel, of UCLA's Crump Institute for Medical Engineering, have conjured up a bit of chaos. *Orderly* chaos. "If you link together a bunch of neurons with cross-inhibitory coupling, they will fire erratically," says Garfinkel. "And yet there really is a pattern in that chaos that we can tease out with sophisticated methods." As a wallpaper-like pattern on the screen grows more intricate, Walter adds, "you can't predict the thing in detail, but it has tendencies."

If three coupled neurons make unpredictable patterns, imagine what 10^{11} (one trillion billion) interacting cells could do. A working brain is more like the weather or a turbulent stream than it is like a digital computer, according to the chaos connoisseurs. In the classic lock-and-key model, one molecule of a brain chemical fits into a specific receptor on a cell membrane. But neuroscientists now know that a population of receptors can fluctuate rapidly under the influence of many microscopic conditions inside and outside the cell. "Instead of receptors, it may be better to think in terms of *receptivity,"* says Alan Garfinkle. The neuron itself isn't a hard, little marble or a microchip in a computer but "a complex chemical reaction in a solution," a "bag of enzymes," prone to the same fluxes as other chemical reactions.

"There are some predictable things about the brain and some predictable things about people's behavior," say Walter. "You can predict when most people will get up tomorrow. You can predict their brains will get old and clanky and wear out and die. But for many brain processes you give up even the *ideal* of determinism. Chaotic dynamics tells us that many things that look deterministic can't be predicted in a practical sense for more than a short time."

Calculus describes a smoothly changing, predictable world, and it's inventor, Gottfried von Leibnitz, once declared, "*Natura non facit saltum*" ("Nature does not make jumps"). But nature *does* make jumps. When a parameter is increased beyond a critical value, metals snap, a smoothly flowing fluid becomes turbulent, chemical concentrations turn chaotic. These are some of nature's *nonlinearities.* A linear relationship is one in which if x equals y, 300x will equal 300y, and so on, for all possible values of x and y. "But all biology is nonlinear," say Garfinkle. "Double the dimensions of a bone and the result has eight times the weight but only four times the strength. That makes a thirty-foot-tall man impossible."

In the brain, twice the input may mean *four times* the output — or *half* the output. Perception, for example, is organized along log (decibel) lines. And whether you're measuring the behavior of an animal or a neuron, the effects of heat, chemicals, or electricity can have decidedly unpredictable effects. "The brain is funny," say Arnold Mandell. "If I gave you two milligrams of amphetamine you might feel very alert; at seven or eight milligrams you might feel sleepy; at twelve, you might be alert again; at twenty, full of rage; at fifty milligrams, totally out to lunch. So in the brain more is not necessarily more. Sometimes more is just different."

If there are universal patterns buried in the brain's "plumbing," if there is a grand theory — perhaps an $E=mc^2$ — latent in all the data flowing out of electrodes and radiation counters, perhaps nonlinear dynamics can pry it out. "Now that people like Hubel and Wiesel and Mountcastle have made these marvelous discoveries about what single cells can do and a little about how columns [of neurons] are arranged," says Jack Cowan, the University of Chicago biophysicist...."Now comes the next problem. How is it all put together? What are the general organizing principles of the brain?"

Cowan has been working on a mathematical model of epilepsy and hallucination. These "bifurcations" occur in the brain, he thinks, when neuroelectric activity, cranked up past a certain threshold, forms "traveling and rotating waves." His abstract pictures of these crashing electrical wavefronts are identical to the scroll-like waves generated by the famous "chaotic" Belousov–Zhabotinski chemical reaction. Meanwhile, Paul Rapp, of the Medical College of Pennsylvania, has been tracking "seizures" in a computer. As electric brains grow more complex, he reports, they begin to exhibit failures analogous to epileptic convulsions. Brains and high-speed computers both can be easily tipped into chaos.

The Secret Messages of Shopping-Bag Ladies

THE GRASS was still beaded with dew when Roy King arrived. Like a Margaret Mead of the park bench, King was keeping meticulous record of several homeless "shopping-bag ladies" in a San Jose, California, public park. One of his subjects was sitting rigid on a bench, a petrified Pompeiian mummy with a masklike face. From time to time she'd lift her right arm in a stiff salute and rock back and forth for ten minutes, before going catatonic again. Another pushed a shopping cart full of yellowing newspapers and broken appliances around a fixed route, pausing at intervals to comb her hair with a dirty blue comb. A third woman obsessively circled a bench, head bowed, muttering the same malignant phrases over and over. The tape recorder in her brain seemed stuck in one place, condemned to repeat one terrible message forever, like the "black box" of a crashed airliner.

For five days in a row, King timed their behavior with a watch. Each of the women (who were evidently chronic schizophrenics) has a "stereotyped routine of movements, postures, and gestures," he noted. "Their activity had an erratically periodic course. The same routine was repeated in the same order roughly every twenty minutes."

Most psychiatrists-in-training don't hang out in public parks timing shopping-bag ladies, but King was chasing a theory. The outlines had come to him while he was still in medical school at Stanford in the late 1970s. He was working at an alternative psychiatric-treatment center in San Franscisco, where he was able to observe the "natural evolution of psychosis" in unmedicated

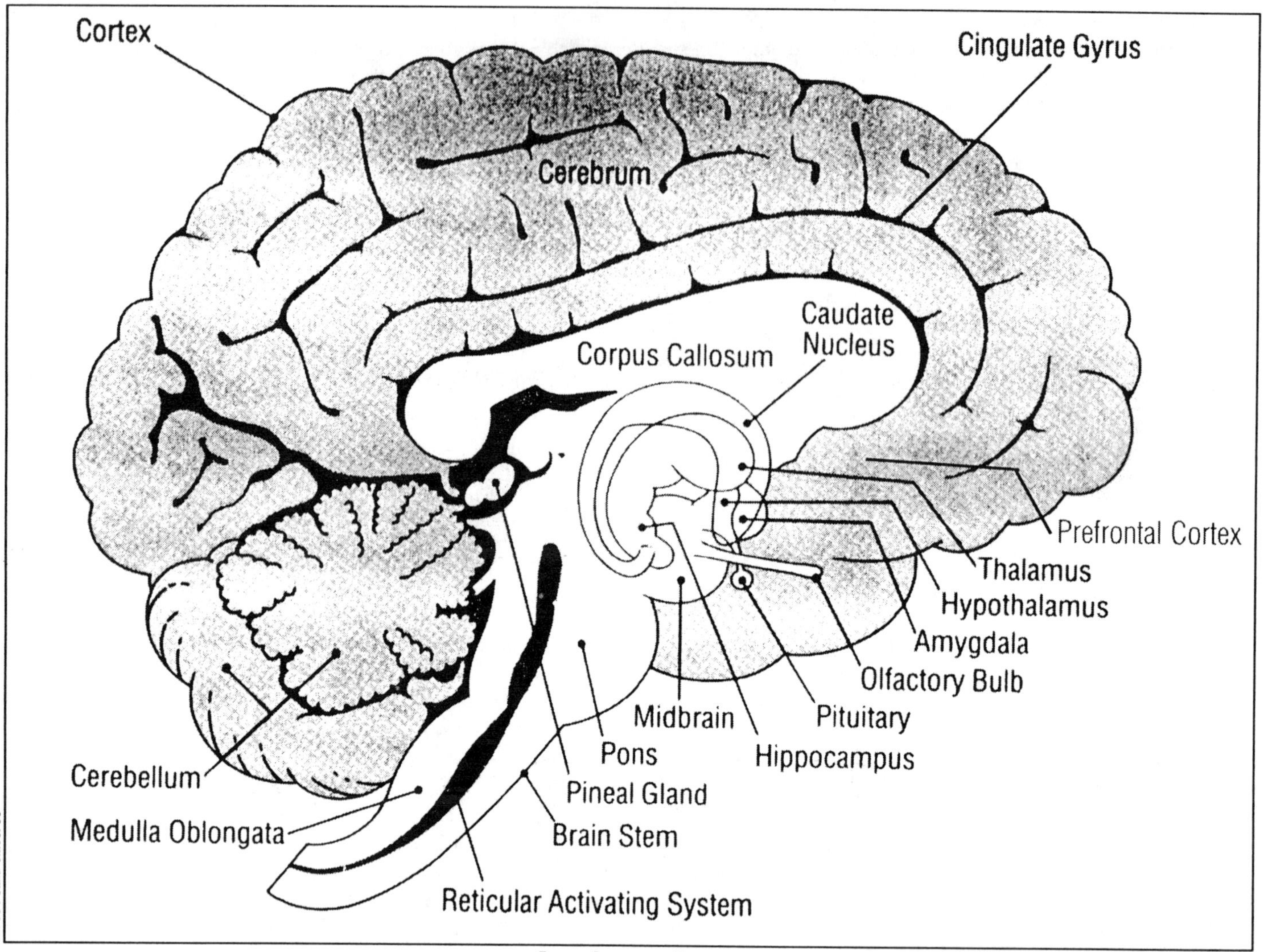

Three Pound Universe

FIGURE 1 — THE BRAIN

patients. Certain rhythms in their behavior struck him as curious. The acute schizophrenics were swaying like pendulums between agitated frenzy and catatonic withdrawal every twenty minutes. The mood and behavior swings of manic patients, in contrast, formed regular ninety-minute cycles, like the cycles of REM and non-REM sleep.

"What I saw was that people were fluctuating between opposite states," he tells us, "And a light bulb went off in my head. I saw the key to psychotic behavior was not *too much* or *too little* of a specific neurotransmitter. It was unstable fluctuations in a chemical system."

Fortunately King had a Ph.D. in math from Cornell under his belt. He went to his computer, plugged in the variables for dopamine synthesis and release, and in 1981 *"Catastrophe Theory of Dopaminergic Transmission: A Revised Dopamine Hypothesis of Schizophrenia"* was published. (Catastrophe theory is not about earthquakes and towering infernos; it refers to the sudden jumps and phase transitions that nonlinear systems are prone to.) The gist of the theory is that the key to schizophrenia is chaotic fluctuations in dopamine production. As King explains it, he draws neat diagrams and graphs in our notebook: a synapse with DA (dopamine) hovering in the presynaptic terminal, a curve shaped like a *U,* a chain of jagged peaks and valleys (dopamine release plotted against time). When his equations spawned a telltale, U-shaped curve, King did a double take. That classic nonlinear curve said that the dopamine system was unstable, extremely sensitive to small inputs. A relatively minor influence could set off wild bursts of dopamine release that spanned twenty minutes from peak to peak. This exactly matched the behavioral rhythms he'd observed in psychotic patients.

The model also said that a schizophrenic's dopamine neurons would start to fire in two different rhythms and rapidly become uncoupled. Could this be the organic basis of the psychological splitting Eugen Bleuler had in mind when he coined the word Schizophrenia? "I think that in schizophrenia the brain fragments into active and inactive clusters of neurons and different parts of the brain become disassociated," says King. "You might get an asymmetry between the left and right side, say. Schizophrenics often feel that their minds and bodies are split apart. I had one patient who said her left hand was possessed by a foul, fuming substance and her right hand was pure light, ecstatic, blessed. Another patient said his father put a stake through the left side of his head when he was six years old and that the right side of his head was possessed by his mother, who wanted to have sex with him. When he was most psychotic, he said he felt like Humpty-Dumpty, all in pieces. Therapy helped him reconnect the different parts of himself."

The principle goes beyond schizophrenia. With equations for norepinephrine and its receptors, King has been studying the abstract geometry of panic disorder. "In panic attacks," he says, "you get these bursts of adrenergic [norepinephrine and epinephrine] activity that lasts five to eight minutes. You get symptoms like tachycardia, cold sweats, confusion, cold extremeties, fear. I found that the system was very unstable, supersensitive.

Why did nature design the brain this way, so that it is so highly sensitve to small changes in input? If the brain were linear, you'd have the same sensitivity in every state. It would seem that an organism in the wild needs to be acutely aware of danger. The fight-or-flight reaction has to be very sensitive.

(*The Three Pound Universe*, pp. 359–69)

The authors go on to cite the schizophrenic's inability to concentrate ("sensitive dependence on initial conditions"), and obsession with fixed delusions ("everything reminds you of *x;* every little thing takes you back to the 'attractor'), as manifestations of the 'travelling, rotating' dopaminergic storm along the disordered pathway from the cerebellum to the pre-frontal cortex. *(*See Figure 1, the mesolimbic area, where the caudate nucleus is in close proximity to the thalamus, hypothalamus, amygdala, and hippocampus, in front of the pons*)* Addicts, with their inability to concentrate on anything but the dopamine reward of drugs, present tell-tales of a similar underlying disorder — the 'fracturing' of brainwave activity into distinct, out-of-phase waves. Addicts, like schizophrenics, are unresponsive to talk therapy. Trying to talk an addict out of addiction or the schizophrenic out of being crazy via attempts to deconstruct their fixation is like cross-sectioning a strange attractor —

> "...you get an infinite regress of folds-within-folds-within-folds like nesting Chinese boxes. Magnify an inch of one fold, and you'll see more folds inside, with the same rich detail repeated in miniature. It is like a map of the English coastline each curve of which, when enlarged, contains a smaller version of the coastline, and so on ad infinitum." (Ibid., p. 373)

With his little electrical implant in the cerebellum of schizophrenics, Dr. Heath of Tulane showed that dopamine circuits are modulated by the cerebellum. Unlike the "anti-psychotic" phenothiazines, which suppress symptoms of schizophrenia through direct action on dopamine receptors (at the cost of eventual "tardive dyskinesia" damage in of up to 45% of subjects), Heath's implant showed how such an oscillating loop "fibrillating"[1] in the dopamine circuits (A) was probably the result of faulty cerebellar pattern-recognition, since (B) it can be abruptly interrupted whenever the cerebellum sends a different signal.

The psychosis returned, however, if Heath's cerebellar inplant was incapacitated.

Like a persistent computer virus, the faulty recognition-pattern triggering the oscillations in the dopamine circuits (its *strange attractor*) still infected the cerebellum.

In African medical tradition, on the other hand, *iboga* is the treatment of choice, *par excellence,* for schizophrenia — because the delusions vanish, and do *not* return. Like Klingsor's evil castle they are abolished, via some kind of random recognition mechanism[2] so intense that iboga-generated oscillations *overpower* competing brainwaves, *cancel out* the offending cerebellar template, and *re-set* cerebellar output.

[1] See p. 141 of this chapter; also, Chapter 15, 150–153, and 162, and Chapter 16, p. 174; and Chapter 17, pp. 190–191.

[2] PGO activity, i.e, imaging. See Goutarel, pp. 119–120 , Molliver, pp. 152–155.

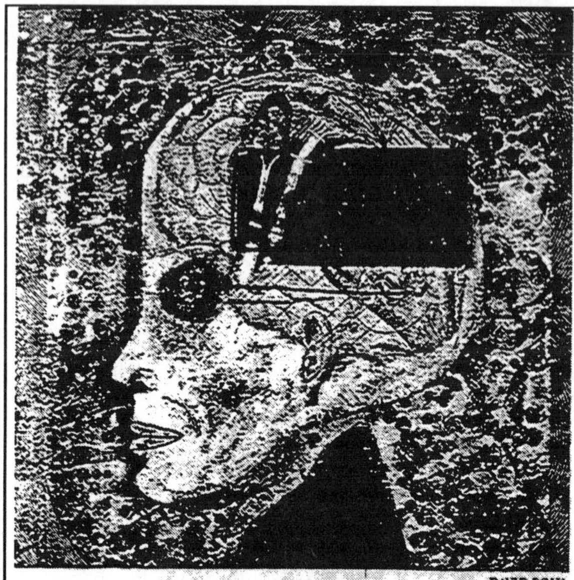

DAVID POHL

A Psychedelic Trip to the End of Addiction

Health: Can a tribal potion block cravings?

BACK AROUND THE BEGINNING OF time, an African creator god hacked up a Pygmy and scattered his remains in the forest. When the man's widow found flowering plants growing from his flesh, the god gave her a useful bit of advice. Eat the root, he said. It will open doors to the supernatural world and help you communicate with your dead husband. The story comes from western Africa's Bwiti religion, whose adherents use the iboga plant to induce visions and aid in the hunt. But researchers now suspect that the plant's active ingredient, a hallucinogen called ibogaine, may have other uses as well. Anecdotal reports suggest it can free cocaine and heroin addicts from their cravings. No one knows just why a psychedelic drug would combat drug addiction, but animal studies support the claim, and federal officials could move as early as next week to approve the first formal trials in humans.

Yippies, junkies and AIDS activists have been touting ibogaine for years (Hunter Thompson joked that the drug might account for Edmund Muskie's disastrous performance in the 1972 Democratic primaries). But only recently have scientists shown any interest. Howard Lotsof, the New York entrepreneur who hopes to market the compound under the brand name Endabuse, stumbled onto it in 1962, when he was addicted to heroin and taking hallucinogens for fun. Lotsof popped a few ibogaine capsules and, after a 30-hour trip, found that his heroin craving had vanished—even though he hadn't gone through withdrawal. The government outlawed ibogaine in the late '60s, fearing its potential for abuse, but Lotsof never forgot his experience. In 1989, he started shuttling heroin and cocaine addicts to the Netherlands (where ibogaine was still legal) to try it as therapy. Though hardly a scientific study, that exercise yielded a number of stories like his own. He claims that 20 of 30 clients lost their cravings, and that 12 stayed drug-free for at least six months.

On the strength of his anecdotes, Lotsof persuaded several labs to embark on animal experiments. "At first I thought he was a crackpot," says pharmacologist Stanley Glick of Albany Medical College, "but the drug had more interesting effects than I expected." Glick and others found that ibogaine freed rats from morphine and cocaine addictions, and by 1991 the National Institute on Drug Abuse had established its own research program. NIDA planned to start human trials within a year, but when scientists in Baltimore dissected the brains of ibogaine-treated rats, they detected nerve damage in the cerebellum, a brain region concerned mainly with balance and posture. That could be an important discovery, for it suggests that the cerebellum plays some role in addiction—and that ibogaine may work by disabling the culpable cells. Even so, cautious federal officials decided to postpone human trials in favor of dog and monkey studies.

Researchers at the University of Miami have now tested the drug in monkeys, and they're ready to forge ahead. Next week the Miami team, led by pharmacologist Deborah Mash, will ask a Food and Drug Administration advisory committee to approve ibogaine for experimental use in a small group of cocaine addicts. Because addicts are so prone to AIDS (needle sharing and the barter of sex for drugs both spread HIV), activists scoff at the drug's potential hazards. "Say it has some neurotoxicity," says Dana Beal of ACT UP. "Would you want to live 50 years with a few burnt receptors, or would you rather die?" If ibogaine fulfills its promise, addicts may soon have the option.

GEOFFREY COWLEY *with* HEATHER HEIMAN *and* JOSHUA COOPER RAMO

NEWSWEEK ARTICLE

Even *Newsweek* was struck by the Gnostic overtones of the Bwiti counterpart of the sacrament myth *(See lead of article)*. And — keeping in mind he totally identifies VALIS with the true, lost Gnostic sacrament — P. K. Dick's description of the healing mechanism that defeats The Black Iron Prison is quite specific:

> VALIS [*Iboga*] had fired healing information at us, medical information. VALIS [*Bwiti*] approached us in the form of the physician, and the age of injury, the Age of Iron, the toxic iron splinter had been abolished.
>
> And yet... the risk is potentially, always there.
>
> It is a kind of terrible game. Which can go either way... There is a streak of the irrational in the universe...
>
> I remember something which the great physician of the Renaissance had discovered. Poisons, in measured doses, are remedies. Paracelsus was the first to use metals such as mercury as medication. For this discovery — the measured use of poisonous metals as medications — Paracelsus has entered our history books. There is, however, an unfortunate ending to the great physician's life.
>
> He died of metal poisoning.
>
> So put another way, medications can be poisonous, can kill. And it can happen at any time.
>
> *"Time is a child at play, playing draughts: a child's is the kingdom."* As Heraclitus wrote twenty-five hundred years ago. In many ways this is a terrible thought. The most terrible of all. *A child playing a game...with all life, everywhere.*
>
> (*VALIS*, pp. 177–78)

Einstein was wrong — God does play dice with the universe. In a universe of quantum uncertainty, free will represents the evolutionarily optimum response. According to Hobson and other sleep theorists, random activation of the cerebellar gait-centers during REM *(See figure, p. 115)* is as important for *forgetting*, on the level of reflex, as the random cerebellar activity of *playing* is to original healthy development in children.

Could Ibogaine-induced REM-like activity be triggering or mimicking the brain's own natural 'chaotic' mechanism for interrupting and re-programing stereotypical routines? Both in Lotsof's addicts and among schizophrenics in Gabon, the effect was catastrophic rupture of their *strange attractor* — replacing their addictive craving or *idée fixe*, after treatment, with completely altered behaviors. But if a natural mechanism were involved, Ibogaine might not be doing anything that different from what we experience every night when we have REM. It could be *chaotic,* but relatively safe, notwithstanding reports from Johns Hopkins of cerebellar damage at a high dose.

So the earliest prototype of this report was not quite finished when Dana's forty-one days of free room and board elapsed, and he was shipped back from prison upstate to be discharged from Rikers. He mailed two copies of eleven chapters off to different lawyers, in the form of a defendant's affidavit. The judge on his violation of probation had seemed inclined in December to let him go, but it was prudent to have something for him to read, just in case. Beal was sufficiently sure of the outcome, though, to get Bill Kunstler to appear Monday night at ACT UP, to invite the floor to get in on the final victory.

At the hearing Judge Biehler was most impressed by the leniency of the judge in Queens, together with a reminder that his earlier decision allowing defendent to travel and lobby federal authorities had resulted in fast-tracking a treatment breakthrough for addiction. But what really startled him was when half the courtroom got up and left with the defendent, chanting "ACT UP!" The judge'd never totally believed it was a medical marijuana case until that moment. It was February 24th, 1993.

Just before Dana's release a controversy broke out in ACT UP over using the phonetree for his court appearance. Resistance came from the usual 12-step crowd, together with those who saw drug users' rights as some kind of "outside agenda" as far as AIDS activism is concerned. But Beal and the harm reduction working group reckoned support would be highest when victory was announced at the next ACT UP meeting. They were anxious to get ACT UP to sign on to Harm Reduction Day, May 1st, by sponsoring the big, final rally in Washington Square Park for medical marijuana.

When it came up, with five minutes of discussion, at issue was whether to lend the ACT UP name to the working group's permit application, and so-on. Dana pleaded that he be the last person in New York state to go to jail for medical marijuana. It passed 60–40, with about a third of the room abstaining.

The Parade coming down Fifth Avenue was simply acknowledged in the motion as a "friendly demonstration" — subject to ACT UP discipline once it joined the medical marijuana rally. Endorsement of the parade was deferred til later. What could be seen as cross-endorsement of the Black Treatment Coalition rally in Harlem or the NORML rally at the Partnership for a Drug-Free America was too complicated for five minutes; and besides, the harm reduction working group wanted time to negotiate for the support of the Lower East Side Needle Exchange for the Clean Needles element of the rally against Herb Kleber and Joe Califano, at West 57th Street, the Center on Addiction and Substance Abuse.

Negotiations turned out to be much more protracted than expected. Dan Raymond of Lower East Side Needle Exchange (LES) felt that Clean Needles must be totally walled off from any concept of harm reduction for non-injection drug users, let alone Ibogaine. He didn't even accept, as grounds for targeting CASA, Kleber's pivotal role in beating back needle exchange under Bennett, Martinez, and Bush. Raymond wanted to conserve LES credibility for direct demonstrations against the government. Later.

Meanwhile, as Dana struggled to get a preliminary version of this report into print, certain folks began a whispering campaign claiming that ACT UP had been tricked into supporting the annual parade, which clearly had been presented as a friendly event in the motion passed March 1st. One afternoon editing work on the book was interrupted as Johann Moore, Dana and Alice heard a furious clumping on the stairs up to the third floor (the only floor with heat). It was an emaciated Spacely, who'd just got out of hospital again, coming up the stairs on his hands and knees — begging for fresh green pot, because his brown pot made him sick. So a network of volunteers was organized to deliver free pot to the growing numbers of PWA's who were opting to survive longer, on pot.

Publication of the first version of this report via the literature table at the ACT UP Treatment and Data meeting, complete with criticism of Ibogaine's detractors, was followed by several angry blasts in anonymous diatribes left on the ACT UP backtable on subsequent

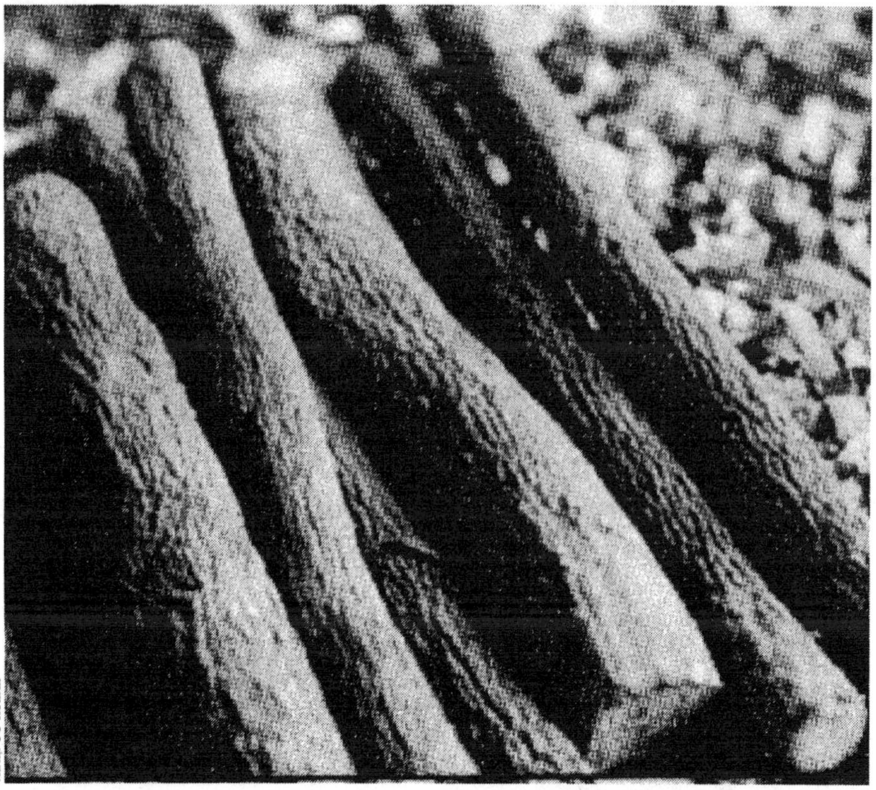

Nature's Health

RAW IBOGA ROOT: *"...MEASURED DOSES, ARE REMEDIES."*

Mondays. These claimed that ACT UP's name was being used without authorization, that Ibogaine was an "outside agenda," the medical marijuana was a trick, and so-on.

Ultimately when the May 1st activities came back up at the beginning of April for an action update, Dan Raymond rose on behalf of the LES needle exchange to disavow the Clean Needles rally at 57th St that was to kick off the parade. But by that time it had been decided not to ask for ACT UP endorsement of the Parade.

Then someone from the LES exchange told folks in New Yorkers for Drug Policy Reform that CASA had reversed its opposition to Needle Exchange, and New Yorkers dropped out as sponsor of the 57th Street event. ICASH stepped in to take their place.

Discussion within the Treatment & Data Committee had shown the Floor might not be ready to support civil rights for drug users — even though the Public Health validity of this position was clear in theory. The floor was fearful, skitterish — upset by the death of ACT UP spokesperson Bob Rafsky, who in his last months was pretty hostile to Ibogaine or anything that wasn't a direct cure for AIDS.

When May 1st came back up for discussion once more before the event, the best way to respond to one misinformed query was to explain that another group, not satisfied with a harm reduction /Stop the Drug War focus, had gone so far as to schedule a competing "20th Annual Pot Parade" May 8th.[1]

May 1st was an organizing success, with good media for Ibogaine, and important contacts made among undergraduates at Columbia University — Herb Kleber's back yard. The student underground at Columbia had just lost the final struggle to save the Audubon Ballroom.[2] And the problem of heroin on campus was such that stories were appearing in the weekly *Manhattan Spirit* about undergraduates running out to cop at 110th Street and Amsterdam Ave.

Noah Potter, a member of the BC–STAC 7 (undergraduates prosecuted for a campus building takeover to protest the Audubon demolition), came up with the idea of sponsoring a treatment for the campus junkie featured in the *Spirit* article. Dana thought it would be great to embarass Kleber by treating a notorious case of addiction right under his nose.

But Howard and NDA weren't particularly interested in this angle. They agreed to treat the kid from Columbia, but they'd promised exclusive coverage of their next treatment junket in the Netherlands to a writer for the *New York Times Magazine,* and they were far more interested in their upcoming Day One special, scheduled to air nationwide (June 8) on ABC. The kid, just graduated from Columbia, could get his life handed back to him, but he would have to get his medical workup together.

At least as far as ACT UP was concerned, the Harm Reduction Working group had succeeded, in the year since Califano and Kleber refused to meet, in exposing them as Drug War strategists intent on co-opting AIDS as an issue. The problem was that under CASA's arrangement with the Partnership for a Drug Free America, Herb Kleber was still house expert for the networks and *New York Times.*

Kleber's position was that Ibogaine had never been subjected to double-blind trials, and that in the absence of more data, clinical trials were unwarranted.

Harm Reduction jumped at the chance, then, presented by the awards dinner of the Center on Addiction and Substance Abuse at

1 The question was about the "other rally, May 8th."The May 1st event was in fact the successor to twenty years of rallies on the first Saturday of May. The issues had changed, and no matter how much May 8th organizers promised people free weed to get them to leave the medical marijuana rally, the attempt to resurrect a bygone formula on May 8th was doomed. The squatter anarchists putting on May 8th even profited from the word on the street that the May 1st rally had gone on unmolested by the cops. But that only meant they succeeded in piling 50% more people into a smaller space, where one fight was enough to cause a stampede – almost a riot. The May 8th organizers and their backers lacked the sensitivity of the Rock Against Racism crew on how to put on an event in New York City. See Chapter 8, p. 71; Chapter 9, p. 88, and Chapter 11, p. 110.

2 The Audubon Ballroom was the site of the assassination of Malcolm X, which Columbia University replaced with a biomedical center to research, among other things, the so-called "violence initiative" — aimed at the 'psychiatric' suppression of inner-city violence.

the Hotel Pierre.[1] Jim Burke, head of the Partnership and Chairman of CASA, was having awards presented to himself and his brother, Dan Burke (head of Cap Cities/ABC), by Barbara Walters and Joe Califano. They were charging very rich people $500-a-plate to be there. A zap was announced at ACT UP, but before it actually went ahead, on the morning of June 2nd, Dana called up Deborah Kopakin, assistant producer of the *Day One* special set to be aired the next Monday. She felt tit-for-tat retaliation by high ABC brass — scrubbing her Ibogaine special because of a demonstration — was imposssible, but said call back Friday.

The zap — signs and leafleting — materialized perfectly, peaking with people stationed on all the approaches to the Hotel Pierre just as maximum numbers of guests were mobbing the doors. Before the cops even got there, the cream of CASA's big donors were hit with fact-sheets outlining Kleber's obstructions of Ibogaine and refusals to meet with ACT UP. Some time in the middle of the week, the *Day One* special was reviewed by top brass at ABC. When Dana reached Deborah again on Friday, she said she was shocked — shocked — that a fact-check had revealed two of the addicts in the piece had done drugs again. Dana was silent for a long moment.

Everyone had always told *Day One* producers that relapse is a fact of life in most cases. But the *Day One* special was put on hold, indefinitely.

The jibes of cynics who blamed the cancellation on the zap were a lot easier for ACT UP harm reduction to handle than worries that the treatment team, now already in Europe, might be pissed off and refuse to treat the kid from Columbia. But no one believed Howard would do anything that unethical. Over the weekend, however, Howard called New York and said that the kid's EEG showed a previously-unsuspected propensity for epilepsy. The doctors in the Netherlands wanted a new EEG, or the treatment was off. The Columbia graduate couldn't believe this was a problem — he'd never had a history of epilepsy, at all. He insisted on flying to Holland without all his paperwork, hoping he could make contact with Howard and persuade him to go ahead with the treatment.

The result was a complete bust — literally. The kid ended up getting busted for loitering in Rotterdam while waiting to make contact with Nico. He never did get to the treatment site. Instead Sisko called 9 Bleecker and read Beal the riot act. In the end Sisko had to come to Rotterdam and babysit the kid til his flight back to the US, where he promptly vanished for three weeks into the druggie underground up at Columbia, before getting a needle removed from his esophagus(!), and checking himself into a conventional de-tox up in Massachusetts.

[When he got out, though, he didn't promptly relapse — not completely. In preparation for the aborted treatment, he'd read the original twelve-chapter version of this Report,[2] and viewed the Nico tape. He'd been exposed to enough Ibogaine Information to get the Idea, to get the essential message — "If you are resisting suffering, you suffer more" — and to understand that the real challenge isn't getting off, but staying off. By the end of August, on his own, he designed his own plan, working two shifts a day, 28 days a month, regrogramming his cerebellum with a straight job, and paying off his student debt in two years. At the end of that time he'd been drug-free for two years. So his Rotterdam quest was not in vain.]

In reality, Lotsof had far more substantial reasons not to do the treatment — reasons no one knew about until three weeks later. It turned out that *all* treatments with Bastiaans were suspended. One of Dr. Baastians' own patients — never subjected to the full screening of the ICASH protocol — was a German female heroin addict, about 23. Her mother had sought out Baastian's psychiatric services for her daughter, Nicola K. — because, of course, he was the only other 'gate-keeper' for Ibogaine treatments.

The catch was that the daughter never would have gotten past ICASH intake, because she didn't really want to quit. She and her boyfriend brought five *grams* of heroin with them, which they did up all day and most of the night before their treatments. Six hours after an initial dose of 1800 milligrams of Ibogaine, Nicola K. was administered a 600 mg. booster dose because she complained that the Ibogaine wasn't working.

Seventeen hours later, after Nicola K. was basically recovered and could go to the bath-

1 Fifth Avenue and 61st Street, in New York's poshest district.

2 One that ended with "Bwiti", now Chapter 13, the "information slumbering in the codices," so to speak, since this is the first of several cases.

room unaccompanied, something happened that demonstrated that the morphine/Ibogaine interaction might vary drastically over time (although in line with Glick's finding of transient Ibogaine *kappa* opiate activity, potentiation of morphine analgesia ought to *decrease.*) She came out of the bathroom, lay down on the bed, and inside a couple of minutes lapsed into a classic heroin overdose, with respiratory distress, etc .

Bob Sisko — who was the paraclinician on watch at 4 AM that morning — witnessed it, and helped rush her to the hospital (uselessly), presuming that she had gone to the toilet and tried to do what Geerte had done in Utrecht: smooth out the end of the Ibogaine with a little smack.[1] Except that when Geerte had done that, in her case it seemed to potentiate the Ibogaine. To complicate matters, the Dutch autopsy did not include a MAM test, which more accurately could have determined when Nicola K. last did heroin.

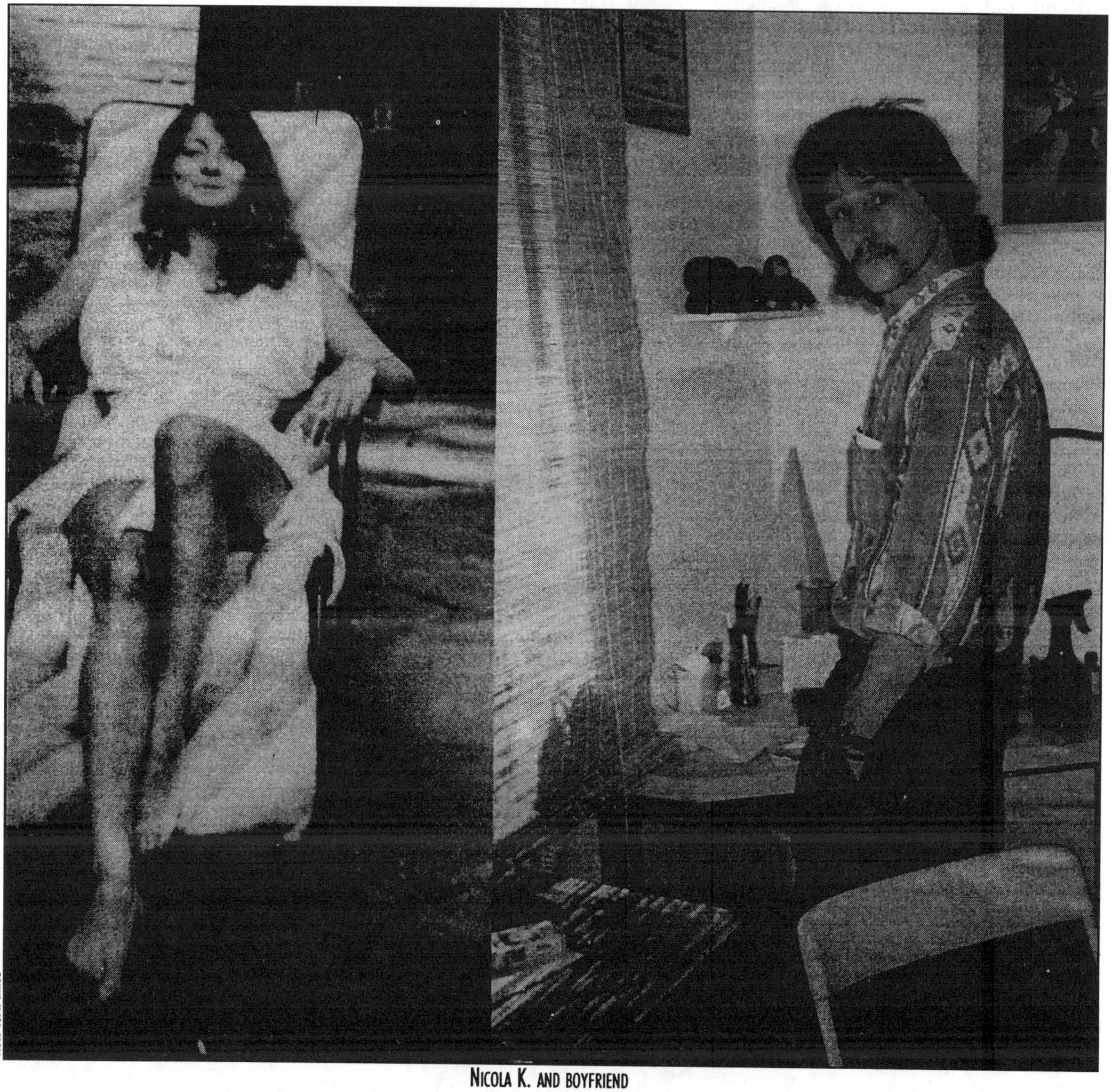

New York Times

NICOLA K. AND BOYFRIEND

[1] NIDA still considers this to be an open possibility. See Chapter 18, p. 209, on the presentation of March 8, 1995.

"Medications can be poisonous, can kill. And it can happen at any time. Time is a child at play...with all life, everywhere..."

Ibogaine's potential for fatal drug interactions, especially with amphetamines and opiates, was already fairly obvious.[1] Also, experienced addicts know the highest risk of heroin overdose comes at the very first use after a prolonged abstinence — and the effect of Ibogaine in many ways resembles a prolonged de-tox. The impossibility of nailing down just what had gone wrong, however, was a real stumbling block.

Lotsof, unwilling to submit clients to body-searches, decided to suspend all treatments until he could get government authorization for controlled administration of narcotics to addicts right up until the morning of treatment, so this situation could never recur.

Later, Sisko read Dana a passage from *PIHKAL,* by Sasha Shulgin, which threw an additional light on the differing symptomology of heroin overdose and the deaths that occur once in a great while with the use of Iboga among the Bwiti:

> "...I'd had an extraordinary day on peyote. and I'd had an encounter with what I called the death door, and that it was beautiful and friendly, but I wasn't tempted to go through it because I knew it wasn't time and there was still a lot I wanted to do. I said I'd wondered ever since what might happen to someone who saw the way out of life and was tempted; what would happen if he actually went through, or tried to go through?
>
> "She stared at me and said that, as a matter of fact, she had an answer — at least, she could tell me what happened to one of her clients at the clinic who did just that. She was sitting beside his cot when, apparently, he saw the exit and decided to go through it. What she saw was a young guy lying there, who had stopped breathing. She called out to him, and when he didn't respond, she tried to find his pulse and there wasn't any. He was in clinical death, she said. She dashed out to get help. By the time the staff people got back to him with the injection and whatever to kick his heart back to life, he'd been dead for three minutes.
>
> "Eve said that, as they rushed through the door, he opened his eyes. He was back. After all the panic had died down, he told her that he'd seen the opening and wanted to go through it, and did, and he got in a place where an entity of some sort told him very firmly, but kindly, that he wasn't allowed to stay because it wasn't his time to die, and he was going to have to go back and stick around until it was the proper time. Then — Zap! — he was waking up on the cot with people running into the room, brandishing hypodermics and stuff.
>
> "He also told her he would never again consider cutting his life short, and that he certainly wouldn't have any fear of death, when it was time to go. One of the things Eve concluded was that there must be some kind of — ah — Overseer part of us that keeps an eye on things, so to speak. She said she'd never talked about the incident outside the clinic before, especially not to other psychiatrists, needless to say!"
>
> (*PIHKAL,* pp. 294–295)

The geometry of the 'exit,' or doorway, is remarkably consistent, regardless of how the NDE is accessed. According to P. K. Dick, it's dimensions are 1/.618034: Fibonacci's constant. The "golden ratio" of the Greeks, which lurks in chaotic phenomena from spiral nebulae down to the spiral patterns of conch shells. According to Goutarel *(See appendix, p. 234),* the Mitsogho say each Bwiti initiate approaches it two times, on the day of his initiation and on the day of his death. The characteristic strange attractor of the moment of ultimate rupture?

Parmenides' rectangle.

1 Since it directly potentiates, or multiplies the effect, of both amphetamines *and* opiates.

CHAPTER 15: Molliver's Travels

Behind the scenes, as is often the case, the postponement in early June of the *Day One* Ibogaine story was being dictated by other agendas and other schedules. In April, '93, unbeknownst to Lotsof or the treatment activists, the FDA and NIDA huddled to sort out a plan to deal with the unprecedented publicity of the *Day One* special. They set a date of August 25th for a formal hearing on Deborah Mash's Investigational New Drug (IND) Application, before the full FDA Advisory Panel on Substance Abuse. Once that hearing was scheduled, there was a temptation built-in for *Day One* Producers to keep the Ibogaine story in the can, and peg the airdate to the news-interest around August 25th. Even if NIDA, in the person of Frank Vocci, hadn't sincerely believed that any delay by the media was in the best interest of the project (the longer thereby to put off potential anti-psychedelic backlash), it was highly unlikely that Herb Kleber and CASA wouldn't have found out independently and advised ABC brass of the new timetable.

Treatment activists were among the last to find out — not until the end of June did Vocci and Lee Cummings tell Beal of the August hearing.

But after the Hotel Pierre zap, which Beal and Johann Moore recounted in delightful detail to the floor of ACT UP as they announced their next action — a zap of the FDA/NIDA on July 6 — Amy Bauer objected that only floor-approved zaps were supposed to get in during announcements. So at the next meeting, enough people were fed up with two years of talk and still no addict access, and the July 6th zap passed, 38 to 27, with a third of the floor abstaining.

Far more important was Dana's decision, amidst the uncertainty surrounding the failed treatment of the kid from Columbia, to quit ducking the Molliver toxicity data and be the first to get it to the press — but as evidence of a new, cerebellar mechanism of addiction instead of an indication of danger in humans. Another writer, Richard Alan Miller, had already gotten the basic story into print, in the eco-journal *Green Egg*, obviously after reviewing Goutarel's monograph *(See Appendix, p. 240)*. He wrote the following, under *"Possible Mechanisms"*:

> "Some new theories have recently been proposed, based on EEG readings of patients undergoing ibogaine treatment in clinical situations.
>
> "Normally, the stages of wakefulness of the human brain are: normal waking state, NREM (slow wave or deep) sleep, PGO (pontogeniculo-occipital waves, and REM (rapid eye movement or paradoxical) sleep. REM sleep is the period where most dreams occur. PGO waves are considered to be the principle coding tool that acts at the cortical level in recording the genetic/epigenetic acquisition necessary for the individuation of the human brain. In other words, it is the software-writer aspect of the Self.
>
> "In Ibogaine therapy, while the patient is in the near-death dream state, the PGO brain pattern has been found to overlap the standard low alphoid brain state. This precipitates fundamental shifts in instinctual learning patterns, possibly the underlying cause of ibogaine's erasure of addictive behavior patterns.
>
> "In addition, through random activation mechanisms, PGO waves eliminate from certain types of neuronal networks an informational overload linked to pathological behavior, thus "cleaning out the neuronal circuitry." REM sleep apparently includes a sorting-out and disposal process of the "residues" stirred up by the PGO wave sleep pattern. The actual dream state could be considered the "reboot" of the personality rewrite.
>
> "In essence, ibogaine allows one to reconfigure the genetic and cultural programming one receives at birth, much like changing the *config-sys* file of a computer. The REM aspect then reboots the consciousness patterns with a new *autoexec.bat* file for habits, needs, and the manner in which one approaches desires.
>
> "In humans, the oneiric effects which are produced by hallucinogens do not enable us to approach the dream mechanisms directly. These two phenomena (dreams and hallucinations) cannot be linked together as one item. The principal difference between them resides in the way

in which the stages of wakefulness are organized, with the suppression of REM sleep and the intrusion of PGO waves into the arousal (waking) stage and in NREM (or slow) sleep.

"The post ibogaine therapy organization of consciousness becomes: waking (arousal) stage, stage of PGO waves, hallucination stage, and then the sleep stage. It is possible that hallucinatory manifestations in combination with the waking dream eliminates residuals stirred up by the PGO wave pattern in the absence of REM sleep.

"According to the Mitsogho tribe, the initiate will see the Bwiti only twice in his life, on the day of his initiation and on the day of his death. This means that the visions at the approach of death are the same as those termed "normative visions," as when at the time of dying, some individuals see their whole life pass before them. In those who are rescued from death, a spectacular transformation is observed. They no longer fear death; they feel stronger, more optimistic, calmer, and contemplate their life more positively.

"This is precisely what was described by the heroin addict described above after his ibogaine treatment. He felt that God had appeared before him and shown him a series of visions on how he arrived at addiction to heroin. Once he emerged from the dream stage, he no longer felt as if he were the same person — because he was *not* the same person.

"A more detailed description is needed of the precise form of dream therapy, an important aspect of the initiation of the Bwiti of the Fang. The ibogaine offers a hallucinatory tool for assisting the effectiveness and efficiency of current dream therapy protocols. The added structure of a virtual-space type of platform for the therapist to act as a (shaman) guide is described in a paper called "VR Therapy" by Iona Miller."

(*Green Egg*, p. 37, Summer '93)

Howard Lotsof wanted to downplay the implications of Molliver's discovery of a cerebellar site of action because it involved findings of Ibogaine toxicity, and Howard had unpublished data from Miami showing no toxicity in primates. However, inasmuch as serious damage in Molliver's rats was only occurring at sub-lethal doses, Beal couldn't see any reason not to point out that early paraclinical observations of a REM-like mechanism of action with Ibogaine — as well as the effect he was predicting in the gait centers — would be dramatically confirmed if Ibogaine acted on the cerebellum, the seat of movement, coordination and reflex. Just because Molliver had located the cerebellar site by deliberately inducing cell damage with a sublethal dose was no reason to sit on the revolutionary implications of his discovery.

So it was without any inkling as to the Aug. 25th FDA hearing date, or the suspension of treatments in Holland due to a heroin OD, that Dana sent his new report to science writers who'd gotten the previous ACT UP sourcebook at *Newsweek* and the *Baltimore Sun,* along with the story line —*"Ibogaine Reveals New Mechanism of Addiction."* Both writers had previously indicated interest, pleading that their plates were too full at the time. With an article on Howard appearing in the June *Omni,* however, the time was now ripe. Basic interviews were all done with both *Newsweek* and the *Sun* before either the August 25 hearings or heroin OD in the Netherlands became known, and Dana, after ascertaining Ibogaine was probably not the cause of the death, decided to honor the exclusive of the *New York Times Magazine* writer who'd been covering that set of treatments. His discussion with Vocci, who refused to meet July 6th, produced nothing either to justify calling off the July 6th zap or changing the articles set to appear in *Newsweek* and the *Sun.*

A day before the NIDA/FDA zap Dana, David Goldstein, and Noah Potter met with O'Hearn and Molliver at Johns Hopkins. Mark Molliver, from experiments with harmaline tremor twenty years earlier, suspected that Ibogaine must be working in the *inferior olive,* a kind of knot on the brainstem that branches directly up into the inside of the cerebellum. As Molliver explained it, the olivo-cerebellum was in effect one formation. What he'd discovered *(See illustration, next page)* was that excitation of the olive by Ibogaine triggered the rhythmic firing, lasting many hours, of a layer of unusually well-shielded super-switcher cells in the cerebellum, called *Purkinje cells.* Purkinjes are completely interconnected with synaptically rich olivo-cerebellar climbing fibers which project from the inferior olive.

In rats treated with a sublethal dose of Ibogaine (100 mg/kg, or about 80% of the L.D.50), sustained rhythmic firing of the Purkinje cells caused prolonged tremor and loss of as many as 10–15% of Purkinjes. Earlier researchers lacked the sophisticated technique to detect the effect — because it

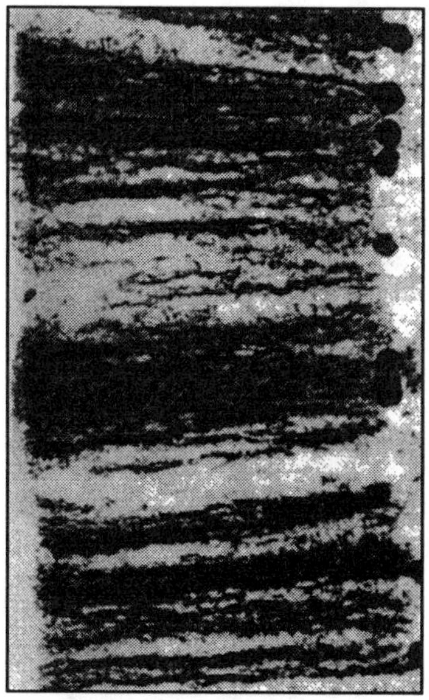

Purkinje cells in rat cerebellum after high-dose treatment with Ibogaine. The pale bands show where Purkinje cells have degenerated. The stain is an antiserum to calbindin, a calcium-binding protein. Picture by Mark Molliver.

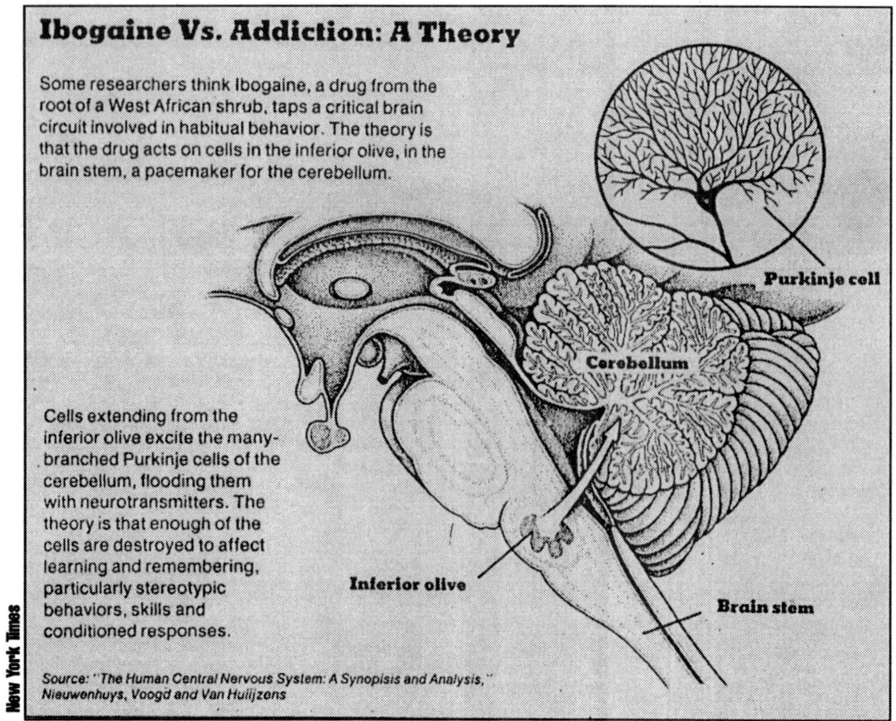

appeared in very narrow stripes running from front to back in the central *vermis* between the right and left hemispheres of the cerebellum. Molliver believes each stripe is, in effect, an individual parallel processor module. The vermis controls the vestibular sense — balance — which would explain the trunkal ataxia (difficulty in standing, coupled with a strong urge to lie down) human addicts experience during the initial phase of the treatment.

The good news was that Purkinje cell loss in rats was not a direct toxic effect of Ibogaine, but a secondary, *excito-toxic* effect. Ibogaine action in the olive was triggering the sustained, rhythmic[1] release of the excitatory neurotransmitter *glutamate* to the Purkinjes, which were apparently firing until they died — a case of death by overstimulation. But there was no direct toxicity occurring in the inferior olive, and it wasn't until *after* the Ibogaine wore off that Purkinjes would start to degrade and leave vacuoles (pits). This lag made Molliver and O'Hearn hopeful some blocker could be found that could limit the damage without blocking Ibogaine's anti-addictive effect. Or if some cell death turned out to be necessary to erase the template of addiction from the cerebellum, as Molliver at first suspected, he thought a second drug that stopped tremor might block the worst of it.

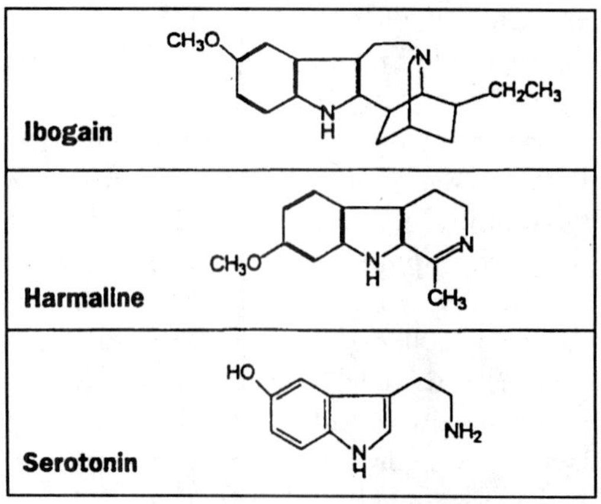

IBOGAINE, HARMALINE, SEROTONIN

One thing Molliver and O'Hearn were pretty sure of was that a 5-methoxy group projecting like a key from the upper lefthand side of the Ibogaine molecule specifically "fits the lock" of the receptors in the inferior olive, which activate the cerebellum. But the crucial difference of Ibogaine from harmaline, when compared side-by-side *(see left)* is the "porch" that projects out *at a perpendicular* from the lower right of the Ibogaine molecule. Dana proposed that this must be the part of the molecule responsible for the property of weakly binding to the *kappa* opiate receptor, which (according to Glick) harmaline does not share. There was discussion of whether the *kappa* receptor might be involved with the mechanism of the "opium dream" — as distinct from opiate analgesia produced by *mu* opiate receptor agonists like methadone — and whether by occupying *kappa* receptors, the well-known potentiation of opiates by Ibogaine is accomplished by "freeing up" opiate to occupy more *mu* receptors.

Dana, remembering the "oscillating" characteristic of Ibogaine onset, asked O'Hearn and Molliver if some form of oscillating brainwave activity might not be the mechanism of "cerebellar reset." Molliver agreed that if the anti-addictive property turned out not to be due to the equivalent of pharmacochemical psycho-surgery, the REM-like mechanism suggested by Goutarel and the French would be the next most logical explanation. As to the role of PGO waves, he explained they are apparently evidence of neural perception of light, which is consistent with imaging activity, i.e, a random recognition mechanism.

But Dana was also remembering some-

1 Ten bursts-per-second.

Mystery of Sleep Yields as Studies Reveal Immune Tie

Scientists now know why total deprivation is lethal in rats.

By SANDRA BLAKESLEE

A COLLEGE student goes two nights without sleep to cram for exams and on the third day comes down with a cold. A night-shift employee begins working days and gets the flu. A surgery patient who is awakened four times a night in the hospital begins to recover only after going home and getting a good night's sleep.

Are these situations coincidental? Or do they show that sleep loss promotes illness? Despite intense interest in the question, sleep researchers have been hard pressed to show exactly how sleep influences human health and disease.

But now a burst of findings is beginning to shed light on the ultimate purpose of sleep, and in particular on the convoluted interplay between sleep and the immune system. Experiments suggest that the immune system is somehow repaired or bolstered during sleep and that it, in turn, has a role in regulating sleep.

Sleep is divided into periods of so-called REM sleep, characterized by rapid eyeball movements and dreaming, and longer periods of non-REM sleep. Neither kind of sleep is at all well understood, but REM sleep is assumed to serve some restorative function of the brain. The purpose of non-REM sleep is even more mysterious. The new experiments, such as those described for the first time at a recent meeting of the Society for Sleep Research in Minneapolis, suggest intriguing explanations for the purpose of non-REM sleep.

For example, it has long been known that total sleep deprivation is 100 percent lethal to rats, yet, upon autopsy, the animals look completely normal. A researcher has now solved the mystery of why the animals die. The rats develop bacterial infections of the blood, as if their immune systems had crashed.

In another study, healthy men and women were deprived of sleep for three days while their blood was monitored for immune system factors. Researchers expected to see a decline in immune function, yet the opposite happened. The subjects' immune systems went into overdrive, seeming to respond to sleep deprivation as if it were an invading organism like a bacterium or virus.

In a study of AIDS patients, researchers found abnormal fluctuations of an immune system chemical that in healthy people is released rhythmically during sleep. The abnormality may help explain debilitating daytime fatigue in AIDS.

This immune factor may also be related to a nightly rhythmic contraction of the small intestine, researchers said, raising the distinct possibility that the intestine sends a sleep-promoting signal to the brain via the immune system. In this view, the bowel may be telling the brain to go to sleep so that it and other organs can carry out housekeeping functions.

Sleep serves many purposes, said Dr. Harvey Moldofsky, director of the University of Toronto Center for Sleep and Chronobiology. Apparently, animals sleep to regulate body temperature, organize memories and replenish the immune system, he said. But most research has focused on sleep as a brain phenomenon, ignoring the rest of the body. The cells, organs, hormones and immune factors in the periphery may, like the brain, contain molecular clocks that help drive daily sleep and wake cycles, he said.

Dr. James Krueger, a physiologist at the University of Tennessee in Memphis, has investigated the idea that sleep factors — the molecules that promote sleep — build up in the bloodstream during the day and, when they reach a high enough concentration, make people drowsy. Such sleep factors would be only one mechanism for promoting sleep, he said. Others might kick in during an infection, for example, or on a hot summer day or after Thanksgiving dinner. Although the mechanisms of the various sleep factors would be different, he said, they may interact with and compensate for each other.

Dr. Krueger is focusing much of his research on cytokines, messenger chemicals of the immune system that are associated with white blood cells. These substances, which make up the front line against infection, are also found in the brain, although whether circulating cytokines converse with or exert control on brain cytokines is not known.

When cytokines like interleukin-1 (IL-1) and tumor necrosis factor are injected into animal brains, the animals fall asleep, Dr. Krueger said. It may be that these molecules promote sleep in some regions of the brain and not others, so that the whole brain does not sleep at once, he said. In fact, different brain networks may take turns sleeping, which would explain why there are many gradations of sleep, from light dozing to the deepest sleep.

Some of the new research began with a mystery that presented itself 10 years ago. Dr. Allan Rechtschaffen at the University of Chicago Sleep Research Laboratory put two rats into the same environment, but permitted only one to sleep. No striking differences emerged until the end of the second week, when the sleep-deprived rat began to gorge itself on food yet grew skinnier and skinnier without exercising more. After one more week, the sleep-deprived rat lost the ability to regulate its body temperature and died.

'What Could Be Toxic'?

Later, in looking for the cause of death of sleep-deprived rats in many such experiments, researchers could find nothing wrong with them. Their organs, blood and urine all seemed normal. The animals resembled cancer patients whose bodies are either weakened by chemotherapy or wasting away from their disease, said Dr. Carol Everson, a senior staff fellow at the National Institute of Mental Health in Bethesda, Md., and a former student of Dr. Rechtschaffen's.

"I began thinking, what could be toxic? Maybe the rats were infected," she said. After culturing their blood, Dr. Everson found that the rats had died from bacterial infections of the blood. The bacteria were strains that the animals were in contact with every day, she said, and do not normally cause disease.

Oddly, these infections did not damage tissue, Dr. Everson said, suggesting that the rats' immune systems did not mount an aggressive attack on the bacteria. Further tests are under way to measure the immune response during the sleep-deprivation experiments, she said.

Dr. David Dinges, a psychiatrist at the University of Pennsylvania, is testing the effects of sleep deprivation on healthy men and women, meanwhile. There is a long-held belief, based on very little evidence, that going without sleep will make you sick, Dr. Dinges said. Some studies have shown that medical students taking exams, caretakers of patients with Alzheimer's disease and people in bereavement have reduced lymphocyte counts — the T cells and B cells that combat infection — and decreases in other immune system cells, he said. The idea is that people in crisis who may not be sleeping well have depressed immune systems.

But few studies have looked at how healthy people respond to sleep loss, Dr. Dinges said. In an ambitious experiment that is now being analyzed, Dr. Dinges and his colleagues recruited 24 healthy volunteers who agreed to live in a sleep lab for one week. Dr. Dinges said that he and others expected to find a decline in immune function after sleep loss. "But from the git-go," he said, "we realized we were on to something different."

The T cells and B cells that are

New York Times

Sleep Yields Some of Its Secrets: Studies Find a Tie to Immune System

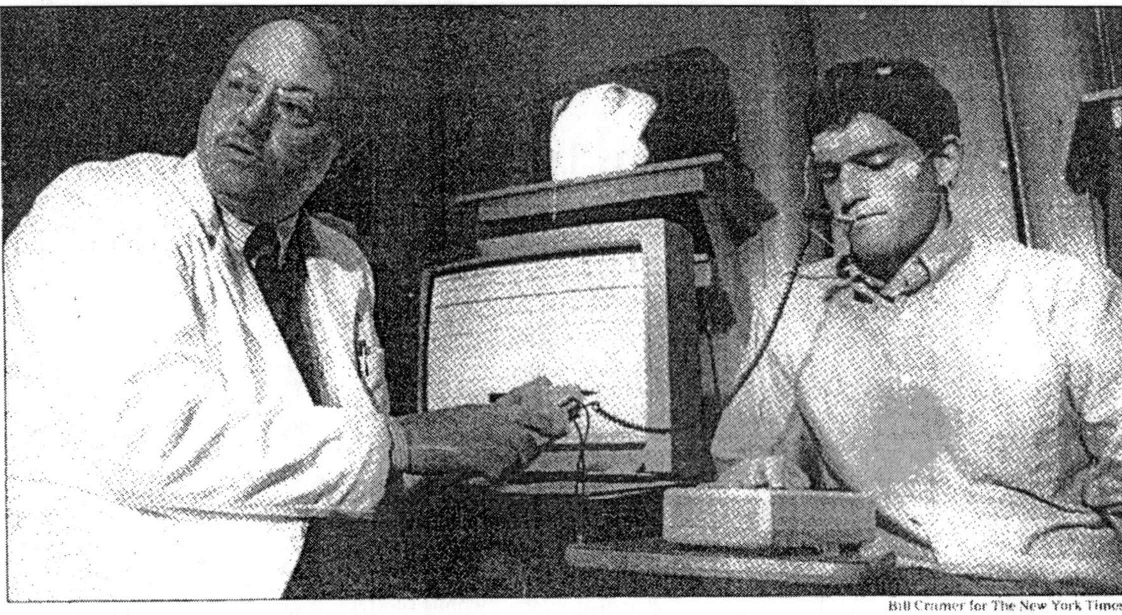

Bill Cramer for The New York Times

Dr. David Dinges, psychiatrist at the University of Pennsylvania in Philadelphia, monitoring the physical effects of sleep deprivation on a subject, part of a study of how the lack of sleep relates to illness.

called upon to attack specific pathogens showed no change, he said. But monocytes, granulocytes and natural killer cells — immune cells that are called into play when the body responds to an unknown invader — went sky-high. Cytokines like IL-1 also appear to be elevated, he said.

Immune Cells May Induce Sleep

The sleep-deprived subjects seem to be mounting what immunologists call a nonspecific host response, Dr. Dinges said. It is a first line of defense against disease-causing agents and means that these people should be better at fighting off colds and flu. Whether this response would endure after additional hours of sleep deprivation is not known, he said. And what it means to the brain is also not known.

Such experiments raise the question of what role the immune system plays in normal sleep. One idea is that immune cells are involved in the buildup of sleep factors.

In 1980, Dr. Krueger helped identify one such factor in the human gut. During the day, he said, immune cells called macrophages digest gut bacteria and release tiny proteins from the bacterial cell walls. These proteins escape into the circulation and may reach the brain. When injected into animal brains, the proteins produce deep prolonged sleep.

> Researchers are searching for factors outside the brain that may regulate sleep.

In addition, Dr. Kruger said, the macrophages stimulate the release of cytokines. They, too, induce sleep when injected into animal brains.

Such findings may also explain why people get sleepy when they are sick, Dr. Krueger said. Cytokines and other immune cells flourishing in the blood and lymph may exert an influence on the brain, inducing sleep while the infection lasts.

Dr. Krueger, a pioneer in the field of sleep and the immune system, has distilled his observations into a theory of sleep. The brain is composed of myriad groups of neurons that carry out specific functions, he said. But during the day, not every group is called into play. If the neuronal groups are not stimulated, their connections may be lost. During sleep, Dr. Krueger said, the brain releases cytokines that induce a special firing pattern among various neuronal groups, preserving their connections for future use.

Thus parts of the brain sleep while other parts are awake, Dr. Krueger said. The collective output of many such groups leads to what scientists called non-REM sleep, when dreams do not occur.

Implications for Illness

Such research has major implications for human ailments. Chronic fatigue syndrome could be related to the abnormal arousal of cytokines in the brain. Cancer patients and transplant patients are prone to developing bacterial infections of the blood similar to those seen in the sleep-deprived rats. The practice of taking the temperature and blood samples of hospitalized patients throughout the night could, in some cases, do more harm than good. And AIDS patients could be exhausted during the day because their damaged immune systems interfere with normal sleep.

Recent experiments with AIDS patients and sleep suggest ways in which factors outside the brain might help regulate sleep, said Dr. Dennis Darko, a psychiatrist at the Scripps Clinic and Research Foundation in La Jolla, Calif.

When healthy people sleep, the intensity of a characteristic sleep wave, called delta, goes up and down throughout the night, Dr. Darko said. Moreover, a cytokine called tumor necrosis factor undergoes a synchronous fluctuation.

This synchrony is off in AIDS patients, Dr. Darko said, and may be a clue as to why patients are so tired during the day.

But the experiment raises a larger question, he said. Why would healthy people have waxing and waning levels of tumor necrosis factor in their blood? This would indicate a periodic activation of the immune throughout the night, but what might kick it off?

"We asked the gastroenterologists if they could think of anything," Dr. Darko said, and they had an answer. About four hours after the last meal of the day and sleep onset, the small bowel, which must remain sterile, begins chugging with rhythmic contractions. A slow wave starts at the bottom of the stomach and for the next 90 to 120 minutes moves down through the small bowel to the junction between the small and large intestine. Bacteria are pushed away from the small bowel to the colon, which is built to handle them, Dr. Darko said.

All night long, he said, the colon's walls are flooded by churning bacteria in rhythms lasting 90 to 120 minutes — which matches exactly the interval between the sleep stages seen in the brain.

It could be a coincidence, Dr. Darko said. But it could also mean sleep factors are reaching the brain in synchronous waves. REM sleep, when dreams occur, may be necessary for a healthy brain, he said. "But for all we know, non-REM sleep may be necessary for a healthy bowel."

thing else — something Bob Sisko had said about the hot and cold flashes and sweats which Nico perceived as withdrawal symptoms — diminished but still present — as his first Ibogaine treatment was wearing off. "Sweats, hot and cold flashes — *are also side-effects of the Ibogaine,"* said Sisko. "He was just feeling the Ibogaine."

If the physical symptoms were the same, must not the brainwave activity be very similar?

In wave mechanics there is a phenomenon *(See pp. 143–144)* where two closely-matched wave fronts *heterodyne,* or fuse, cancelling out each other's unique characteristics. It's a model that could explain a lot. Otherwise, Ibogaine represents an apparent violation of the laws of momentum. Where do the withdrawal symptoms *go?*

Dana's working hypothesis was that human brain architecture differs enough from rats so that instead of tremor and cell damage, Ibogaine excitation is shunted into the REM circuits, the natural mechanism of nightly tremor and cerebellar "forgetting." So instead of selective cell-destruction, the basic model would be a REM-like random activation mechanism which triggers or promotes the same kind of healing that takes place when a stroke victim learns to use remaining brain capacity to replace missing function–an effect not to be interfered with (although it would still be helpful to find something that would block any cell-breakdown after Ibogaine wore off).

The big question was whether a level of excitation might be found that would reverse addiction without causing over-stimulation. Molliver and O'Hearn agreed the focus should be finding a "window" between the lowest effective dose and the dose level where Purkinjes start breaking down. But they were not too optimistic. Individual cells were still being lost they believed (less than 1%, but still detectably) at 25 mg/kg.

Wasn't oral Ibogaine less toxic than IV? No, as a matter of fact the effect of 25 mg/kg oral Ibogaine was slightly more damaging than i.v., because it hung around longer in the body, and the *tremor* lasted longer. Molliver felt the degree of cerebellar damage in rats seemed to coincide with length of tremor. His most interesting aside, in reaction to the news that some Kaposi's patients were getting speedlike euphoria with their vinblastine, was his thought that the Ibogaine-like half of the vincristine or vinblastine might be having psychoactive effects distinct from the lower, toxic moiety *(see diagram, right).*

The leaflet zap and picket the next day, July 6, at the Parklawn Building[1] was three times the size of the original action in 1991. It had significant support from Philly ACT UP for the first time. And virtually every worker in the building got an open letter to Dr. Curtis Wright of FDA Pilot Drug asking why, if it was permissible to give vinblastine — an Ibogaine cogener but forty times more toxic — to treat Kaposi's Sarcoma, it wasn't kosher to use Ibogaine to keep addicts from contracting or transmitting AIDS to begin with. Jonathan Bor from the *Baltimore Sun* came and left before everybody got together at 11 AM for a real ACT UP moving picket. But he interviewed Paul Morcone, owner — "and also a client" — of three methadone clinics, who wanted to give all his clients the Ibogaine option. Before it was over, Terry Toigo of FDA AIDS Coordination came down and asked for a meeting between ACT UP and Curtis Wright.

The ACT UP side was all for a meeting, but later rather than sooner, so they could ask questions after they were better briefed on the run-up to the hearings August 25. During the delay, in one of those typical twists of Ibogaine coincidence, the *New York Times* published a story *(see pp. 153–54)* by Sandra Blakeslee, *"Mystery of Sleep Yields as Studies Reveal Immune Tie,"* which threw some unexpected light on the oft-observed rapid healing effect of Ibogaine.

What she discussed were new findings — that in auto-immune disorders, normal deep sleep wave-synchronicity with the rhythmic contraction of the intestine is disrupted, together with the rise and fall of certain sleep-inducing cytokines such as tumor necrosis factor (TNF). And since — as Molliver had explained at the very first meeting — all such rhythmic brainwave activity is generated by the cerebellum, what this all suggested was that something that resets the cerebellum might also have a role in fighting AIDS. Especially since the inferior olive, site of Ibogaine action, functions as the cerebellum's "clock."

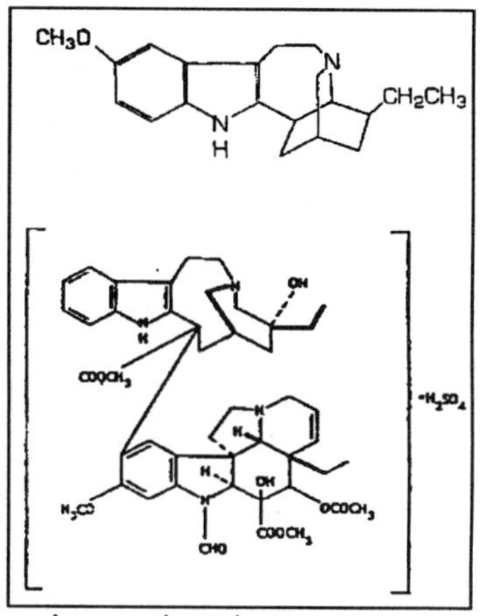

IBOGAINE (ABOVE) AND VINCRISTINE

1 The offices of NIDA, the FDA, even the Surgeon General.

Then on August 9th, the *Baltimore Sun* published the first story to explain — not just effects of Ibogaine on the dopamine receptors of Glick's rats — but the new, cerebellar mechanism of addiction suggested by Molliver and O'Hearn's work at Johns Hopkins *(see story next two pages)*.[1]

With things heating up nicely, Dana requested the presence of Carlo Contoreggi — as ARC medical affairs officer and the only person with comparative information on the relative efficacy of other addiction medications and Ibogaine. He ended up instead with Grudzinskas and Vocci for NIDA, and having to ask them to bring Carlo. But activists got a meeting with FDA/NIDA on standards of approval for Ibogaine almost two hours long — and just a week before August 25th.

Best of all, the day before the meeting, the second story on Ibogaine and the new mechanism of addiction appeared in *Newsweek (see page 144)*. Dana handed out color xeroxes to Vocci, Grudzinskas, Contoreggi, and for FDA, Curtis Wright, Dan Spiker, Belinda Hayes, Corinne Moody and Nancy Stanisec. Present for ACT UP besides Dana were Vic Hernandez, Dr. Iris Long, David Goldstein, Jeff Eberhardt and Kiyoshi Kuromiya.

The ACT UP side pushed for an immediate parallel track process for NIDA MDD's own Phase II trials, on the assumption that the August 25th Hearings would allow research in some form to go forward. Besides reiterating ACT UP's position that Ibogaine toxicity must be compared with vincristine and vinblastine, Dana said this problem should be looked at anew to see if there was a common neuromechanism of action — perhaps by including a small number of HIV-positive addicts with KS in NIDA Ibogaine trials. He proposed that a small interagency task force under a clinician (he nominated Carlo) be set up with all necessary authority, to meet night and day, working on nothing but Ibogaine.

The big counter-argument from the government was their own spectacular disaster with FAIU, a chemotherapy that at first seemed to show promise in clearing hepatitis virus from the body completely. It was safe in dogs, but fatally toxic in humans, who lacked a protective enzyme dogs have. Half the subjects in the first human trial required emergency liver transplants, and several died. Of course it could be equally true that Ibogaine was safe in primates, and toxic only in rats. But NIDA MDD felt there were still too many uncertainties about Ibogaine in humans. Nonsense, said Vic — get ethnobotanists in with data on human use in Africa. Jeff said most of NIDA's problems could be surmounted by doing a large, simple Ibogaine trial.

The showdown came one week later, in the ballroom of a Holiday Inn in Silver Springs. After preliminary findings suggesting genuine addiction interruption, indications of Ibogaine toxicity in animals had put clinical trials on hold for a year — and might well doom further testing in humans. The FDA hearings on August 25th were covered by top media including ABC's *Day One, The Los Angeles Times,* UPI, AP, *The New York Times Magazine,* CBS National Newsradio, CNN and the NBC Nightly News, along with other Washington, DC print and electronic media. The Press Table outside listed more than two dozen names.

The entire FIDA Advisory board was present, as well as representatives of various divisions of NIDA and ARC. The NIDA/FDA medical bureaucracy had its own roped off area in the middle of about three hundred seats. Harm reduction groups including the DC and Philly needle exchanges, ICASH, and ACT UP activists from four cities were there — along with NDA International, their lawyers, consultants, as well as a "who's who" of independent Ibogaine researchers. As the principals began to take their seats around the U-shaped table and the audience filled in, the room took on an electric intensity. Everyone who counted was there to decide the future of Ibogaine.

The activists came up first, with a series of appeals that Curtis Wright later was to admit made the difference in a very close decision. Dana Beal, up first, framed the issue by invoking Bill Burrough's junk pyramid and making a cogent appeal to apply the same safety standard as vincristine or vinblastine — and let Ibogaine research go forward.

Vic Hernandez questioned the basis of putting the original IND on hold at all. Iris Long presented data on the devastating spread of AIDS among women via addiction. Jon Paul Hammond of Philadelphia made an emotional appeal on behalf of needle exchangers: make

1 Authenticating the information-burst, as it were (in terms of *VALIS*... or *Bwiti*), a quote from Adam Nodelmann on his Ibogaine visions of the assassination of the Kennedys, King and Malcolm X coincidentally (or synchronistically) made it into print.

Harm Reduction Working Group 212-677-4899

THE SUN. LIGHT • FOR • ALL
SPORTS FINAL
MONDAY, AUGUST 9, 1993 • VOLUME 313, NUMBER 73 BALTIMORE, MARYLAND HOME DELIVERY: 25¢ (in most areas) • NEWSSTAND: 50¢

Hallucinogen touted as stopping addicts' craving

Researchers probe ex-abusers' claims

By Jonathan Bor
Staff Writer

NEW YORK — He saw planets materialize in black space, then vanish. He saw his ancestors flee a European pogrom. He saw leaders felled by assassins, a bug devour a green leaf, his young daughter looking hopeful.

In a darkened apartment in Holland, Adam Nodelman had taken a hallucinogenic drug called ibogaine, a plant extract used in Gabon, West Africa, to initiate people into a tribal religion. He was dreaming while awake, watching rapid-fire images replay the history of the world, the laws of nature, the events of his life.

When the trip ended, he discovered something more amazing than any vision that had flashed before his eyes. He no longer wanted heroin.

For a man who had smoked and snorted the brown powder for almost six years, this was a revelation.

"All of a sudden you have a reinvigorated sense of consciousness," said Mr. Nodelman, 27, who now logs 50 to 70 miles a day as a bicycle messenger in New York. "I felt like I'd never done heroin before, and suddenly you want to eat instead of getting high."

Mr. Nodelman, a man with thoughtful eyes, long brown hair and a Frank Zappa tuft under his mouth, is part of a small, vocal group of drug addicts, AIDS activists and entrepreneurs who want to see ibogaine legalized as a main weapon against drug addiction.

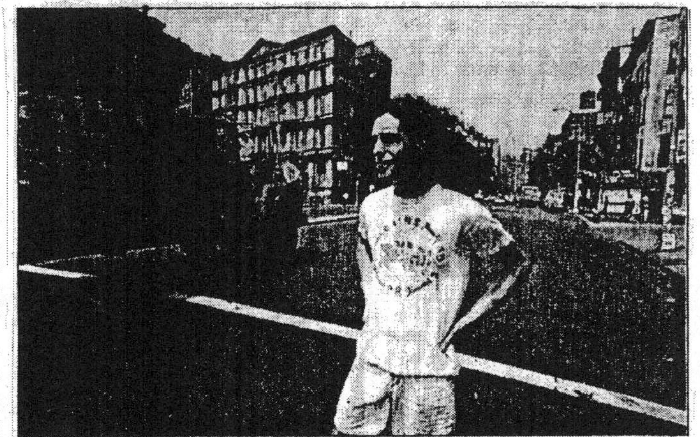

BY ED QUINN

Adam Nodelman credits ibogaine with ending his heroin addiction.

They have no scientific studies of their own, only compelling testimonials that ibogaine stems an addict's desire for heroin or cocaine, even after decades of drug abuse.

If they are correct, ibogaine would offer a unique weapon in the war on drugs — an agent that ends an addict's craving instead of producing a substitute addiction that can be just as hard to kick.

Critics of methadone, a heroin substitute used by thousands, acknowledge that methadone produces less euphoria than heroin and is less likely to cause an overdose. But they say it is abused by many addicts who sell it or use it with heroin. And scientists have yet to find a substitute for cocaine.

For now, ibogaine remains the only drug under active investigation that — at least in theory — allows the addict to leapfrog past physical withdrawal and live without the psychological craving that defeats most people who are trying to quit.

From Johns Hopkins University to the University of Miami, animal experiments with ibogaine are being approached in the cold, clinical manner that gives science its authority. Bubbling below the surface is a current of excitement.

Scientists are tantalized by the notion that if ibogaine really works, and they can figure out why, they might finally understand the nature of addiction.

Not recreational drug

Just about everyone who has taken or studied the chemical agrees that ibogaine is unlikely to be abused. Although not altogether unpleasant, the hallucinogenic experience is considered too intense and self-analytical to turn ibogaine into a recreational drug.

Advocates don't say the drug works for everyone or that its benefits last forever. Mr. Nodelman, for instance, said he backslid after six months and had to take a second treatment. When he slipped again, he says he gathered the fortitude to quit even without a third treatment.

"That was my last full addiction," said Mr. Nodelman, who says he has been drug-free for eight months. "Now, I feel great. I'm happy to be clean. I'm having the same feelings now that I had the morning after ibogaine. It's just a relief to be normal."

Among the most vocal advocates is Dana Beal, a former yippie radical who joined the AIDS activist group ActUp when he became convinced that ibogaine could halt transmission of the human immunodeficiency virus through addicts' needles. Today, Mr. Beal and his associates are prodding federal regulators to clear the path for its therapeutic use.

From his outpost in the East Village in Manhattan, Mr. Beal sees the desperation of drug addicts looking for a way to break free.

"If you can get somebody from using $200 of heroin a day to using a $5 bag on the weekend, it's progress," he said. "If you can get someone who's doing methadone and cheating on the program to not do anything, it's a bigger deal. Because they're not sticking a needle in their arm."

In 1991, the National Institute on Drug Abuse began funding animal studies in hopes of learning whether ibogaine truly breaks addiction and whether it might cause lasting harm along the way. Advocates hope the studies will progress to humans, but the government wants evidence first that the risks are small.

"This could have unique therapeutic potential," said Dr. Frank Vocci, acting director of NIDA's medications development division. "But it gets back to this. The layman says 'Wow.' But when you ask them what evidence they have for their claims, all of a sudden you're up in the ether."

So far, he points out, ibogaine's track record is anecdotal; cases have been reported without careful follow-up. Ultimately, he said, the issue will be settled by controlled experiments.

Dr. Carlo Contoreggi, medical officer at NIDA's Addiction Research Center in Baltimore, remembers the day in 1989 that his boss showed him a file about ibogaine. Even among scientists familiar with hallucinogens, ibogaine was a matter of obscure interest.

"He dropped it in front of me and said, 'I don't know what to make of this.' "

Dr. Contoreggi was riveted as he read of ibogaine's tribal roots, its hallucinogenic properties and the claims surrounding it.

"This has got to be one of the most fascinating things I've ever tripped over," he said recently. "These are street addicts. Fresh needle marks. They take this ibogaine stuff and say, 'Golly, I don't want to take heroin.' "

The central figure in the file was Howard Lotsof. The Staten Island man is widely credited with discovering ibogaine's potential to break addiction.

No craving for heroin

In 1962, he was a 19-year-old college dropout and heroin addict who started experimenting with hallucinogens such as LSD and mescaline. Then, he tried ibogaine.

"The first stage was like watching a slide show of your life coming on at a thousand frames a second," Mr. Lotsof recalled. "No euphoria, all intellectual and distant." He said the next phase was like "eight to 10 years of psychoanalysis" compressed into a few hours.

Col. 2

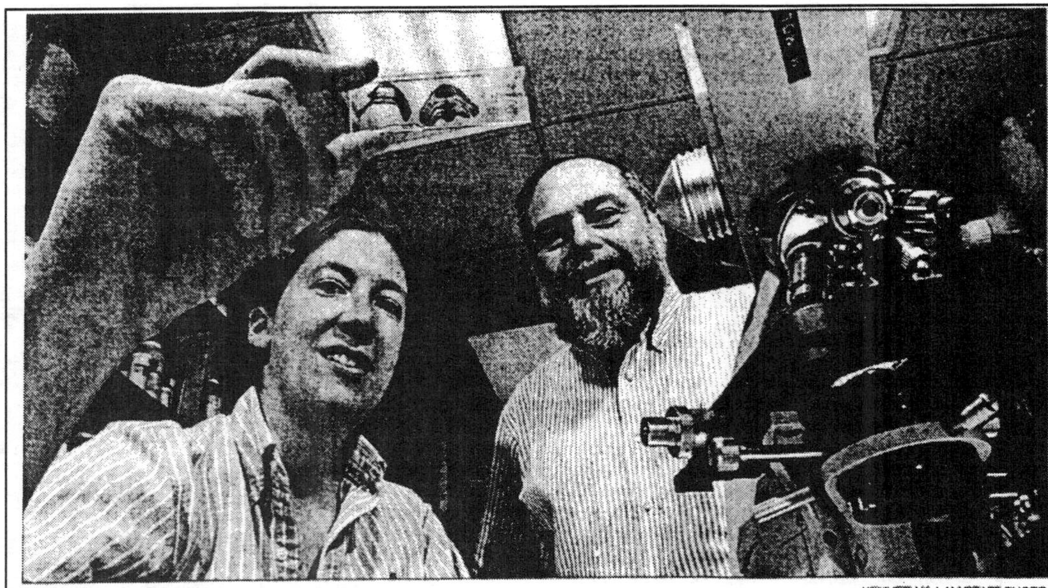

KENNETH K. LAM/STAFF PHOTO

Drs. Elizabeth O'Hearn and Mark Molliver are studying the effects of ibogaine on brain tissue.

DRUG, from 1A

When it was over, he was exhausted. But there was a final jolt: Although he had gone almost two days without heroin, he didn't crave it.

"Ibogaine immediately interrupted my chemical dependency," he said. Curious to see how others would react, he gave the drug to 20 friends, seven of whom were addicts. Five of the addicts stopped doing drugs, he said.

Too young to grasp the implications, he "stored the experience away." Later, he served a 14-month prison sentence for conspiring to sell LSD. After his release, he again became addicted to heroin.

By then, the government had outlawed the sale of hallucinogens, including ibogaine. He kicked heroin on his own, knowing from his ibogaine experience that addiction could be overcome. "I've been drug-free ever since," he said.

After stints in a variety of jobs, Mr. Lotsof and some partners established a private corporation, NDA International. He took out five domestic and 14 overseas patents and hopes to market ibogaine treatment under the brand name Endabuse.

In 1987, Mr. Lotsof and an old friend set up an underground railroad that has ushered 30 American addicts to Holland, a country whose relaxed attitudes toward drugs meant ibogaine treatments could go on quietly.

Treatment, in apartments and hotel rooms, was supervised by psychiatrists in some cases, by lay workers in others. A month ago, Mr. Lotsof suspended the treatment with the intention of setting up a medical clinic in which health professionals would oversee the addicts' care.

Boosters may be needed

Mr. Lotsof hasn't conducted follow-up studies, but he presents a picture of success based on anecdotal evidence: While a third of those treated returned to drugs within two weeks, he says, the rest enjoyed fairly prolonged periods of abstinence. "Some have stopped for as long as four years and are still going," he said. "We have an average period of four to six months from a single treatment."

Mr. Lotsof suspects that addicts may need periodic boosters and a support system of doctors and counselors to stay clean.

Those who say they are ibogaine's success stories don't some believe the hallucinations deliver a message of healing that sticks.

"For every negative vision, there was a positive," said Mr. Nodelman, who has worked as a cook and rock musician. "For every question, an answer. I saw a lot of destruction, but without destruction there can't be creation."

In his planetary vision, he saw the heavenly bodies grow from a tiny seed as heroic music played. But as they grew, their color changed from a healthy green to a polluted black. Suddenly, they vanished and grew again in a cycle that repeated itself 20 to 30 times.

In the assassination scene, he witnessed the murders of Martin Luther King Jr., Malcolm X and John and Robert Kennedy. "I couldn't see much hope, much to fight for. But then, I saw my daughter, 2 years old. I realized the only choice is to renew life, to continue life, to carry on the fight."

Scientists don't dismiss the possibility that the hallucinations are therapeutic. But for now, they are looking into theories that ibogaine causes physical changes in the brain that interrupt the cycle of addiction.

At the Johns Hopkins School of Medicine, two scientists have found clues.

After giving rats high doses of ibogaine, Dr. Mark Molliver and Dr. Elizabeth O'Hearn analyzed their brains. They found dead cells in a portion of the cerebellum that ordinarily controls repetitive tasks.

The scientists say they have no idea whether cell destruction could cause long-term problems. However, they say, a little toxicity in the right place may be just what addicts need.

One theory holds that the same brain cells that control repetitive tasks also control obsessive-compulsive behavior, a mental disorder that can send someone into endless hand-washing or eyebrow-plucking. If this is true, the drug might sever pathways in the brain that keep addicts reaching for their needles.

"We don't like brain damage — we need every nerve cell we've got," Dr. Molliver said. "But we have to wonder: Could you compensate? And maybe the [cell] degeneration we're seeing is responsible for the anti-addictive effect of ibogaine."

Another possibility

Dr. Stanley Glick at the Albany College of Medicine in New York has another idea: Ibogaine blocks the ability of addictive drugs to stimulate a flood of the natural brain chemical dopamine. Some scientists believe that all drugs of abuse — including heroin, cocaine, alcohol and nicotine — work by habituating users to a dopamine surge.

However ibogaine works, Dr. Glick has observed that it is doing something. In one experiment, rats addicted to morphine stopped pushing a lever that delivered the drug once they had taken ibogaine.

"In several cases, it almost eliminated and usually decreased their drug intake," Dr. Glick said. "It did so for at least a day after administration of ibogaine, and in some rats it did so for several days or weeks. I can't say it totally halted it."

Even if ibogaine doesn't halt addiction forever, addicts say they are grateful for any drug-free months.

A Manhattan real estate broker who scraped up $5,000 and flew to Holland for a treatment last year said she has slipped a few times but hasn't "done anything in three or four months." The 40-year-old woman said the drug released her from more than two decades of shooting heroin around the clock.

In the past, she said, "I could get off a high dose of heroin and methadone in 10 days with minimal suffering. But it's the psychological craving that brings you back to it. I had been somewhat sedated my entire adult life. [Ibogaine] makes you feel OK, normal."

The woman, who asked that her name not be used, said she sought treatment when she became thoroughly disgusted with her life. She tested positive for the AIDS virus, which had killed her husband. She had served a three-year prison sentence for smuggling narcotics. She didn't know whether she'd be alive to see her daughter grow up.

She spent the ibogaine experience in bed, too exhausted to move. At one point, she saw a bank of video screens, each one flashing a different image that changed with every second. Most were medieval faces.

"Maybe that's what people mean when they say you meet your ancestors," she said. In accounts of Gabonese ritual, the drug is said to help people meet their forebears.

After her trip, she felt depressed, then renewed.

"I felt like I had raw skin, like ibogaine had peeled everything away," she said. "Then, over a period of days, I felt my skin growing, like a little protection. Just because I've used [drugs] somewhat, I don't think that should negate anything. It's a phenomenal thing, ibogaine."

But is it harmful? At Hopkins, new tests on monkeys should give some idea because primates are close on the evolutionary ladder to humans. The University of Miami is due to unveil results of its own primate studies and has applied for a permit for human trials.

Dr. Contoreggi says society may have to accept a certain level of risk, just as it accepts the side effects of chemotherapy in treating cancer. In the meantime, he is buoyed by what he saw last year in an Amsterdam hotel, where two addicts finished a two-day ibogaine experience without symptoms of heroin withdrawal.

Every week or so, he gets calls on his answering machine from addicts saying they were saved by ibogaine.

"It's remarkably curious," he said. "You get answers from the places you least expect them. Wouldn't it be interesting if you get the answers from the mouths of junkies, not scientists?"

treatment on demand a reality with Ibogaine. Jeff Eberhardt handed out a Medication Development Scorecard *(see chart, next page),* showing the failure of NIDA's other potential treatments to pan out in testing.

Bob Sisko delivered a plea on behalf of ICASH to reconcile harm reduction and demand reduction through Ibogaine. Howard Lotsof made an impassioned statement for NDA on human rights.

Then came Belinda Hayes of the FDA, who presented the basic FDA version of the data on Ibogaine. As the hearing unfolded, Glick, Sershen and the independent researchers presented well-designed studies showing efficacy, while MDD animal researchers like Steve Dworkin demonstrated the inability of the standard agonist/antagonist model even to measure the interruption effect as distinct from the ataxia.

But the major controversy was the findings of Molliver and O'Hearn in rats, versus those of Mash and Sanchez-Ramos in primates. The high point of the morning came with the presentation by Mark Molliver of his findings on cerebellar toxicity. His large, color slides showed that Ibogaine toxicity in the cerebellum of rats, which was significant at 100 mg/kg (10–15%), appeared to fall off logarithmically, so that Purkinje loss at 25 mgs/kg was not even 1% ("You can count the individual cells lost," said Molliver later.) Yet the level of damage at the higher dose seemed impressive, and ACT UP conceded that 16–18 mg/kg was actually more like the standard dose for addicts — an estimate that stuck with the press.

The turning point that morning was when Curtis Wright asked Frank Vocci if they were not in fact in possession of as much pre-clinical data as is usual when an IND is approved. Vocci answered unhesitatingly. "Yes."

After lunch there was a break for Patricia Broderick and Mikhael Dzoljic to present their data. When Broderick treated cocaine-habituated rats with Ibogaine, she recorded drastic reductions in locomotor stimulation — the 'running around' that occurs with cocaine. Dzoljic acheived 80% reductions in cocaine intake in rats by determining that the correct regimen of Ibogaine administration was weekly, not daily. During a break just afterwards, Dzoljic confessed puzzlement over the exaggerated concern for a few cerebellar cells — "We lose that many to wear and tear every day."

The day-long event peaked late in the afternoon when Deborah Mash presented her Miami primate results, which directly controverted O'Hearn and Molliver's findings in rats. Deborah Mash's primates showed no cerebellar damage. Urine and blood samples showed none of the telltales of cell damage. But her test group was small — three animals — her slides were not as big and convincing, and you had to ask if she'd looked in precisely the right place: along the back-to-front "stripes" where cerebellum joins together between its right and left hemispheres — along the *vermis.*

Furthermore, the monkeys had been sedated with ketamine before Ibogaine administration. The ketamine might have skewed the result.[1] Still, in the Miami primates Ibogaine tremor — really verging on ataxia — was much shorter and less pronounced than in the rat (Mash observed rats may be "exquisitely sensitive" to Ibogaine).

These findings actually swayed Molliver and O'Hearn, making them somewhat more inclined to think Ibogaine might be safe in primates, but then Mash asked if Molliver would estimate Purkinje loss at 100 mg/kg in his rats at 10–15%. Somehow 10–15% was the figure that stuck in people's minds, even though this was many times the therapeutic dose.

Then it was Sanchez-Ramos' turn to present neurological observations on the two addicts whose treatments he'd witnessed in January in Lyden. Both had a neurologic deficit *before* treatment. Again, it was Wright who asked the defining question — "Did you just say one of the two treatments you witnessed in Holland resulted in apparent interruption of a 40 mg. daily methadone habit?"

"With no apparent withdrawal," Sanchez-Ramos repeated. But ACT UP wasn't allowed to ask him to amplify another off-handed observation — about the disappearance of a facial tic during the *other* Ibogaine treament. He seemed to imply animal and human research with Ibogaine would uncover novel neurobehavioral aspects of habit formation in addiction and other inappropriate cerebellar reflexes — and that this understanding might even lead to treatments of movement disorders like

1 Possible because ketamine, an animal tranquilizer, is a non-competitive NMDA receptor antagonist. Ibogaine's effect has been found, partly, to result from activation of this receptor also. See Chapter 18, p. 199.

NIDA'S MEDICATION DEVELOPMENT SCORECARD

OPIATE

Treatment Agents	Therapeutic Indication	Sponsor	Status	Owner
Methadone plus Naloxone	Opiate Maintenance Therapy Lower abuse potential	------	not tolerated by addicts	Bristol
Depot Naloxone	Long-term Opiate Blockade	NIDA	blocks endorphins	Dupont
LAAM	Opiate Maintenance Therapy	NIDA	3 day methadone	Public
Clonidine	Opiate Detoxification	None	lessens withdrawal, not craving	Boehringer
Buprenorphine	Opiate Maintenance & Blockade	NIDA	less withdrawal than methadone, better high	Norwich /Eaton
Melkephamid	Opiate Maintenance Therapy	NIDA	not happening	Lilly
Acetorphan	Opiate Maintenance Therapy	NIDA	not happening	No owner listed
Ibogaine	Polydrug Addiction Interrupter	NIDA	MDD 'considering' trial	NDA, Int'l.

COCAINE

Treatment Agents	Therapeutic Indication	Sponsor	Status	Owner
Desipramine	Treat Withdrawal	NIDA	no efficacy	MerrellDOW
Sertraline	Treat Withdrawal	Pfizer	no efficacy	Pfizer
Imipramine	Treat Withdrawal	NIDA	no efficacy	Geigy
Carbamazepine	Treat Withdrawal	NIDA	no efficacy	Geigy
Mazindol	Treat Withdrawal	None	no efficacy	Sandoz
Flupenthixol	Treat Withdrawal	NIDA	anecdotal benefit	MerrellDOW
Fluoxetine	Treat Cocaine & PCP Withdrawal	NIDA	alcohol, not coke	Disin/Lilly
Niledipine	Block Euphoria	NIDA	no clinical benefit	Pfizer
Buprenorphine	Block Euphoria	NIDA	minimum benefit	Norwich Eaton
Verapamil	Block Euphoria	NIDA	no clinical benefit	Searle
Diltiazem	Block Euphoria	NIDA	no clinical benefit	Marion
Sulpiride	Block Euphoria	NIDA	no clinical benefit	Delegrange
SCH23390	Block Euphoria	NIDA	none available	Schering
L-tryptophan	Functional Antagonist	NIDA	doesn't work	Public
Amantadine	Maintenance Therapy	NIDA	too euphoric	Endo
Bromocriptine	Maintenance Therapy	Sandoz	doesn't work	Sandoz
Methylphenidate	Maintenance Therapy	NIDA	doesn't work	CIBA
L-dopa	Replacement Therapy	NIDA	doesn't work	Roche
Ibogaine	Polydrug Addiction Interruptor	NIDA	IND pending	NDA, Int'l.

TOXIC OVERDOSE

Treatment Agents	Therapeutic Indication	Sponsor	Status	Owner
Niledipine	Cocaine Cardiotoxicity	NIDA	won't reverse toxicity	Pfizer
Verapamil	Cocaine Cardiotoxicity	NIDA	won't reverse toxicity	Searle
Diltiazem	Cocaine Cardiotoxicity	NIDA	won't reverse toxicity	Marion
Monoclonal antibodies	PCP Toxicity	NIDA	not off the ground	

Source: ACT UP

Tourette Syndrome and Parkinson's Disease.

At the climax of the afternoon, one of the panelists asked if any addicts present who'd been treated could have a chance to comment. Bob Sisko from ICASH rose and gave his most impassioned argument yet for accelerated approval of Ibogaine.

Yet, when the Advisory Panel began with their own statements, an intense argument broke out on the significance and ramifications of the toxicity results of Molliver and O'Hearn — and whether FDA should permit even the most limited Phase I human testing. A collective decision was necessary. Dr. Theodore Cicero, a psychiatrist at Washington University in St. Louis and a non-voting FDA consultant, adamantly opposed human research. So did the neuroscientist George Ricaurte, arguably the leading expert on serotoninergic degeneration (who as it happens also has his own drug for addiction under development[1]). Both Cicero and Larry Brown of the ARTC in Brooklyn got the 10–15% damage level mixed up with "equivocal" loss at the much lower therapeutic dose — expressing nervousness at addicts having to take it as frequently as every four months if the damage was 10–15% each time.

This caused consumer advocate Cheri S. Groesbeck to object vehemently: "These people, many of them are going to be dead if we study and study and study." But when the advocates of going forward began to speak out, questions arose for Deborah Mash and the Miami team which they could only answer by presenting still unpublished data.

The open portion of the hearing was now ended, and the Advisory Committee went into executive session, to make its final decision in secret. New York ACT UP repaired in disgust to eat at a nearby Silver Springs diner.

When they got back to the Holiday Inn, they connected with Lotsof and Mash on the way up to the NDA suite to watch themselves on Tom Brokaw. It was apparent some approval had been given, but not enough. Only later did ACT UP learn that projected doses of 5, 10 and 25 mg/kg had been cut down to 1, 2 and 5 mg/kg. Or that the population of the Miami experiment wouldn't be Ibogaine-naive crackheads (the original protocol), but was limited to those who had already previously done Ibogaine safely. Still, some form of human testing could resume.

The next day a novice reporter covering the hearings picked up and repeated the panel's errors about a 10–15% loss of Purkinje cells at the lower, therapeutic dose of Ibogaine in the *Los Angeles Times* wireservice story. This prompted Mark Molliver to fire off a letter requesting a correction which characterized the loss at the therapeutic level as "very slight." The only break was that the following Monday, August 30, ABC finally aired the *Day One* Special. AIDS had been edited out in favor of LSD footage from the '60s.

Toward the end of the next week Dana got an excited call and a fax from Mark Molliver. As predicted, vincristine turned out to cause Purkinje loss in the vermis of the cerebellum. Up to 80% during a typical course of chemo, in fact.

And now Sandra Blakeslee's editors in the Science Section of the *New York Times* suddenly decided they wanted an Ibogaine article. Just xeroxing up one copy of this report on the ACT UP copy machine caused a scene with office manager Walt Wilder, who charged it was all "social and political background" — not "scientific," (even though Sandra Blakeslee said that as background, it was "the best laid out in advance of any article she'd ever written.") In reality it was the most effective weapon in the harm reduction repertoire, but the only way Dana could insure continued access to the xerox was to go back to the ACT UP floor for support.

At this point Howard called up with incredible news. New studies had come in which seemed to show more cerebellar loss with either cold turkey withdrawal or alcoholic *delerium tremens* than with Ibogaine treatment.

In the first,[2] researchers in Connecticut measured hand tremor and body sway in recovering coke and alcohol abusers, and detected persistent cerebellar disfunction in the alcoholics, and extra-pyramidal disfunction in the cocaine abusers. In the second paper,[3] using Magnetic Resonance Imaging (MRI) and Positron Emission Tomography (PET-SCAN), Norwegian researchers showed no significant difference between non-drinking drug users and non-using controls — but an

1 With Charles O'Brien, who recently got approval of the Dupont drug Trexan for treatment of alcoholism. O'Brien is scientific co-chair of Sue Rusche's National Families in Action and was one of the presenters at the 1980 Columbia University conference on the "findings" of Nahas. See footnote, p. 35.

2 "Motoric Signs of CNS Disfunction Associated with Alcohol and Cocaine Withdrawal," by Lance O. Bauer, *Psychiatry Research*, 47, 69-77, Elsevier Scientific Publishers Ireland Ltd., accepted Feb. 18,1993.

3 "Minor Structural Brain Changes in Young Drug Abusers— A Magnetic Resonance Study," by J. Aasly, O Storsaeter, G. Nisen, O Smevik, P. Rinck, *Acta Neurologica Scandinavia*, 1993: 87: 210–14.

18 per cent average atrophy of the vermis of the cerebellum of the heavy alcohol users, with four exhibiting mild balance difficulties, and the one with outright ataxia having a *40 per cent* shrinkage of his vermis. This is well in excess of the 35% shrinkage needed to produce symptoms, according to researchers.

These findings, which showed no measurable damage at all from cannabis, suggested that the *real* drug threat to tokers may be drinking while high, prompting Dana to issue a report to ACT UP advocating marijuana as harm reduction for non-IVDU's.

Since the maximal damage Molliver detected in rats at 25 mg/kg was just 1%, it also meant there had to be significantly more damage to the vermis with continued abuse of alcohol or coca-ethylene[1] than with a modest number of Ibogaine treatments.

Sandra Blakeslee made a point of mentioning that in her article. But then every week, it was delayed. Just coincidence, but some other breaking science development kept bumping it.

Dana phoned Molliver again, asking about the tremor of withdrawal. Withdrawal tremor is another excito-toxic feedback loop, perturbing the dopamine circuits, which control movement. So cold-turkey withdrawal zaps Purkinjes. Continued abuse zaps Purkinjes. The least loss is with Ibogaine, which is not paradoxical, given that it apparently eliminates withdrawal. Could Ibogaine be generating a "travelling wave" between the cerebellum and the pleasure pathway that matched the "rotating feedback loop" of withdrawal/craving closely enough to cancel it out? In that case, might the "very slight" Purkinje loss stem instead from the greatly reduced withdrawal syndrome still present during Ibogaine's waning phase?

Molliver now felt that if Ibogaine activity was indeed REM-like, there might be no Purkinje cell loss in primates at all. To this Curtis Wright also added, in further phone conversation with Dana about the cerebellar hypothesis, that FDA was aware of 1982 reports in the *Scientific American*[2] of abnormalities or lesions in the midline vermis of Harlow's monkey infants — those raised with nonmoving terry-cloth "mothers" — who displayed the same characteristic "shy-aggressive" behavior that researchers of the Chicago Project later observed in preschoolers at risk for addiction.

Shortly after a fresh medical marijuana protest outside Health & Human Services (HHS) on September 7th, Dana announced to ACT UP that Harm Reduction was planning further protests at FDA/NIDA in November. Philly ACT UP agreed on a date of November 14th for a week-end rally. Work started on a leaflet to give out at the Great Midwest Harvest Festival.

But before a final decision to go ahead, Harm Reduction decided to take up the NIDA and FDA offer of a further meeting, to see if enough concessions could be obtained to make the zap unnecessary. This produced not one but two additional meetings. The first was at Parklawn again, to get Vocci and Wright together with Dhoruba Bin Wahad, to update prospects for a community-based Phase III Ibogaine trial in Harlem. But this quickly lead to an invitation to the Oct. 28th design session for MDD's own Phase I–II trial at the Sheraton in Rockville.

The meeting October 4 started late and Dhoruba was delayed, which gave Dana Beal and David Goldstein an opportunity to ask about the implications of the August 25th Advisory Committee decision. David asked Curtis Wright to explain the exclusion criteria for Phase I human trials, especially the exclusion of women of child-bearing age. Curtis briefly explained that these are only the initial parameters for the first group of human studies — but had been decided by the FDA Advisory Board, and were firm.

Beal once again objected to the classification of Ibogaine as hallucinogenic, and suggested that a more accurate term might be stimulant–oneirogen. Curtis explained that all psychoactive drugs legally could fall in only four categories: 1) stimulant, 2) depressant, 3) narcotic, or 4) hallucinogenic.

David Goldstein asked about the use of nitrous oxide for narcotic withdrawal (7,000 people over ten years in South Africa), but Wright and Belinda Hayes indicated its status as a drug of abuse was a mark against it. Ibogaine, on the other hand, they now considered to have a low potential for abuse.

Some discussion of community-based tri-

[1] See pp. 49, 113. See also report of Ibogaine interruption of delerium tremens — a classic excito-toxic loop, on p. 218, note 2.

[2] Get cite from Wright.

als did go on even before Dhoruba got there. But all MDD funding for clinical trials turned out to be tied up for at least a year finishing LAAM. No independent Ibogaine project was necessary, they said, because the only other drugs they had under full development were buprenorphine and LAAM.

Wright did let drop one important reason Ibogaine is getting consideration: the danger of TB spreading via daily contacts on the waiting lines for methadone. Then he launched into a discussion about the "Alkaline Lake Experiment."

Alkaline Lake was an Indian Reservation in Canada with an 80% alcholism rate. Nothing was working, until two natives came along who benefited from the conventional 12-step therapy that was having no effect on the other reservation inhabitants. What these two designed was a new program incorporating the history, myths, and spiritual traditions of their people. They started a movement that cut alcoholism at Alkaline Lake drastically. If Dhoruba could do something like that for Ibogaine, Wright thought it would improve the impact.

In fact, Wright and Vocci were a lot happier discussing things years in the future than in having Carlo at the Addiction Research Center provide compassionate Ibogaine access for a few addicts right away. They were rife with suggestions of independent researchers who might be interested in filing INDS.

Jon-Paul of Philadelphia ACT UP sat patiently for forty minutes and finally exploded at Wright and Vocci — that HIV transmission intervention can't wait, that the exclusion of PWA's was another stall. He was heatedly impatient at the slow pace. But discussion on these topics was tabled as Dhoruba arrived, a person Vocci and Wright were eager to meet.

Dhoruba was interested in getting word out in the Black community about the FDA estimate on the probable lack of abuse liability of Ibogaine, which Frank Vocci conceded was relevant. Dhoruba felt Ibogaine would probably be acceptable to the community, but his initial concerns were that its use be community-based, and cognizant of the social-revolutionary aspects — and that sensitivity to medico-political ramifications was there all around to support the accelerated introduction of this new addiction treatment.

When all was said and done, the only choice the government side seemed to leave the activists was for them to lobby Congress for more money for MDD. What was clear was that there was still no Ibogaine for addicts.

The negotiators minus Dhoruba returned to the Monday night ACT UP meeting, where they asked the floor to follow the lead of Philly ACT UP and field one more demonstration on November 14th to protest further delays. It passed fifteen-to-one, with four abstentions and the proviso that a better flyer be brought back to the floor for approval.

On Friday, October 8th, Frank Vocci called Dana Beal and invited ACT UP to an open design session for Phase I/II Ibogaine trials on October 28th. The meeting was to be a more sedate affair — no press, a calm hotel lunch buffet where the participants had time to talk privately, exchange information and discuss issues. NIDA was following the FDA's lead and opening up its process, but with the objective of coopting further protest.

The day before, though, in a highly irregular publication in the Wednesday *New York Times* Health Section (*turn the page*), Sandra Blakelee's article (bumped once again from that Tuesday's Science section, by breaking developments with HIV receptors) materialized as a practical demonstration of how the Ibogaine coincidence factor tends to intervene in things — *as exactly* the information required to re-define the meeting outcome.

Finally, the first complete explanation of Molliver's findings and the cerebellar mechanism of addiction was presented ungarbled (although Blakeslee repeated the mistaken analogy to psychosurgery instead of Hobson's theory of REM as cerebellar forgetting).

To the October 28th meeting were invited NIDA's in-house experts on hallucinogens, treatment specialists with years of experience (in one case with 25,000 addicts), and the consultants who were still finishing work on LAAM and buprenorphine. Participants were presented with the draft protocol for a NIDA Phase I/II Trial, prepared by MDD for discussion and comments. The target date for start of the trials was May of 1994. Frank Vocci proposed the initial trials would be four treatment groups of six to eight people.

Mark Molliver did a mini-seminar on Ibogaine neuromorphology and function, answering all questions, and presenting new findings of faint toxicity traces — secondary effects of the cerebellar excitation — in the thalamus and locus coeruleus.

If Ibogaine was not in fact erasing addiction by very selectively targeting guilty Purkinjes — if the explanation, as Molliver put it, was some "other excitatory mechanism" — cerebellar excitation of the thalamus and locus coeruleus would be consistent with REM-like activity. And increasingly, that began to look like the only explanation, as panelist after panelist rejected the selective chemical lesioning hypothesis as failing to account for the cerebellar damage already known to be caused by alcohol, for instance.

Why wouldn't drinking "erase" addiction to alcohol, if that was all that was involved?

Right after lunch Curtis Wright gave a presentation on the introduction of breakthrough science and the obstacles to, and possibilities inherent in, change.

Through the late morning and into the afternoon, however, the discussion centered on whether the safety and effectiveness issues should be separated. Paul Fudalla, who was leading the afternoon session, was especially set on doing Phase I Trials with nonaddicts, despite the fact that the interaction of Ibogaine and the body chemistry unique to the potential target group has to be studied if it is ever to go into real addicts. Even after Mash and Sanchez-Ramos explained that the dose level run-up being discussed was the logical extension of their Miami trial, there were separate objections to followup ("Just peeing in a bottle to follow up effect," Vocci almost pleaded).

There was an almost perverse feeling that unless it was being given to non-addicts, any administration to addicts had to be double-blinded if there was going to be an efficacy component. Several panelists kept bringing up LSD as an active placebo.

This split finally manifested itself around the issue of whether dose escalation should be cut off with the onset of ataxia. Howard Lotsof stated bluntly that addiction interruption had never occured without ataxia.

This was the point when all the preparation, the education embodied in the serendipitous publication the day before of Sandra Blakeslee's article (*see right*), explaining the Ibogaine visualizations and the ataxia as "REM-like effects," paid off. The panel more or less agreed dose escalation in the first NIDA-sponsored trial in humans should not break off when ataxia started to appear.

But Dana's plea to remember the larger context of AIDS otherwise failed to resonate. For the second time, he suggested NIDA run a comparative trial of Ibogaine and another rain forest plant alkaloid which has been in contemporary use by doctors in New Zealand to interrupt the narcotic withdrawal syndrome. Mitragynine from *Mitragyna speciosa* (or *kratom*) has a long history in Malaysia, used both as a psychoactive drug and to detox addicts. A 4-methoxy substituted tryptamine, mitragynine is also psychedelic, similar in action to psilocin. But no one seemed interested in putting mitragynine on the list of medications to be evaluated for treatment of drug dependency.[1]

[1] See Chapter 17, p. 189.

The panel had heard the plea to respond to AIDS, but refused to cut corners. Instead of a trial starting in May, they wouldn't *re-convene* until then.

There was another problem. Neither Wright or Vocci possessed the power to negotiate the broader harm reduction agenda. They could not discuss clean needles or a waiver to allow AIDS buyer's clubs to supply medical marijuana. A meeting was needed with the higher-ups, and one way to get that was to go ahead with the November 14th protest.

Along about Wednesday in the week before the Harm Reduction rally, Nancy Stanisec called up and asked why there was a protest when they'd been so willing to meet. "What do you mean?" asked Dana. "We offered you the cure for crack, and you won't even let us have a little marijuana for our friends with wasting syndrome." He demanded to meet with Kessler, Gebbie, Lee Brown, and the new head of NIDA, when one was appointed, on a broad harm reduction agenda.

The demonstration on Sunday, November 14, 1993 at the Parklawn building of NIDA/FDA was largely a media success because of the coincidental appearance that morning of a medical marijuana article in the *New York Times*, placed

A Bizarre Drug Tested in the Hope of Helping Drug Addicts

By SANDRA BLAKESLEE

DRIVEN by a deep sense of frustration that efforts to cure drug addiction are going nowhere, Federal researchers are testing a bizarre, mind-altering drug called ibogaine as a possible new treatment for cocaine and heroin addiction.

The drug, drawn from the roots of a West African shrub, has been tried on only 60 people. But several doctors and patients say that the compound works wonders, often banishing symptoms of withdrawal and craving for months if not years. Intrigued and at the same time skeptical, researchers have decided to see if the drug works as well as its supporters claim.

Their work with ibogaine has opened the door to a new theory of how the brain becomes addicted to substances like heroin, cocaine, nicotine and alcohol.

The theory, which runs counter to current models of drug dependency, suggests that addiction is rooted in the cerebellum, the area of the brain where the connections for motor coordination, memory and dreams meet, and that it involves the same kind of ingrained conditioning that informs learning to walk in early childhood.

Ibogaine advocates claim that a single dose of ibogaine taps into this critical brain circuit and banishes withdrawal symptoms and drug cravings, sometimes for extensive periods.

Evidence Is Anecdotal

But scientists who are familiar with the drug urge caution. "At this point, there is no credible scientific evidence that ibogaine cures addiction," said Dr. Herbert Kleber, a psychiatrist and director of the division of substance abuse at Columbia University College of Physicians and Surgeons in New York. "All the evidence is anecdotal and not based on carefully controlled scientific studies."

Nevertheless, since every effort to find a cure for cocaine addiction has so far failed, "it is appropriate to look at any promising agent to see if it works," Dr. Kleber said. "It would be foolish to rule anything out."

And, indeed, driven by this sense of frustration and a Congressional mandate to seek effective treatments for drug abuse, Federal researchers are taking a close look at ibogaine. In the last year the National Institute of Drug Abuse has sponsored 18 animal studies on the compound. And in August, the Food and Drug Administration decided to let researchers begin limited testing of the drug in humans. At least three clinical trials are planned.

"The F.D.A. recognizes drug-abuse disorders as being lethal disorders with no good current therapy," said Dr. Curtis Wright, a medical officer at the agency. "Right now we don't have any other candidate drug that looks as good as ibogaine. At least we have a group of patients and doctors who say this stuff works."

Initiation Rites in Gabon

Used in pubertal initiation rites in Gabon, ibogaine induces a powerful altered state for at least 48 hours, during which young people are said to come into contact with a universal ancestor called Bwiti.

In 1962, when psychedelic drugs were newly popular in the United States, a group of 20 recreational drug users, including a young heroin addict named Howard Lotsof, heard about the drug and decided to try it. Of the seven who were heroin addicts, five, including Mr. Lotsof, claimed that taking the drug extinguished, at least temporarily, their desire for heroin. The other two, in spite of similar feelings, decided to go on using heroin anyway, Mr. Lotsof said in a recent interview, because they were Beat Generation poets and, they said, they liked being junkies.

"For ibogaine to work," Mr. Lotsof said, "you have to not want to continue on drugs. Some people don't want to kick their habit and ibogaine cannot help them."

When the AIDS epidemic began claiming the lives of thousands of drug addicts, Mr. Lotsof's continuing interest in ibogaine grew into a crusade. In the mid-1980's, he persuaded a Belgian company to manufacture ibogaine in capsule form and begin offering it to addicts in the Netherlands, where drug policies are lenient. Like LSD, mescaline and many other drugs, ibogaine is illegal in the United States.

Of the 60 people who have been treated thus far, 50 were recruited by an addict self-help group in the Netherlands, Mr. Lotsof said. "These were people who had failed all other treatments and had completely hit bottom," he said. Very little information exists about the long-term effect of the drug, but at least three remained free of drugs for several years.

"We anticipate that many of the 50 volunteers fell back into drug use," Mr. Lotsof said, "but we have no way of tracking them."

Three-Stage Treatment

Treatment with ibogaine is ordinarily a three-stage process. After taking a capsule, a patient first lies quietly until, after a couple of hours, he or she falls into a waking dream state. "When you open your eyes the dream stops," Mr. Lotsof said. "The drug does not produce euphoria. Instead, people find that repressed memories are released in the dreams, memories that may have markers saying 'don't go near this, it hurts.' " He stressed that this is a very different state from hallucination, over which a patient has no control.

After four to five hours, a second stage, which Mr. Lotsof calls a cognitive-evaluation stage, begins, lasting 8 to 20 hours. "Many clients describe it as 2 to 10 years of psychoanalysis in 20 hours," Mr. Lotsof said. "You have the complete underlying psychopathology of your life revealed to you, which helps you understand why you've been using drugs."

The third stage is a period of intense wakefulness, which may last for a day or two.

The 18 animal studies sponsored by the drug institute in the last year have examined the pharmacological and toxicological effects of ibogaine, including experiments to see whether the drug relieves symptoms of withdrawal from heroin or cocaine addiction. In one such study, ibogaine had no effect. In another it offered some relief. And in yet another, animals experienced substantial relief from withdrawal symptoms, said Dr. Frank Vocci, head of the ibogaine research program at the drug institute.

Different investigators used different strains of mice and rats, which may explain the contradictions, Dr. Vocci said. Moreover, rodents, like humans, show a wide variation in their response to addictive drugs and to ibogaine. More work is needed in this area, he said.

Charting Brain Pathways

For another study, the drug institute asked Dr. Mark Molliver and Dr. Elizabeth O'Hearn, experts at the Johns Hopkins Medical School on how drugs damage brain cells, to examine ibogaine.

New York Times

Continued from preceding page

The researchers gave rats huge doses of ibogaine, reasoning that areas showing damage would reflect where the drug was active in the brain. Rats thus treated developed tremors and a lack of muscle coordination called ataxia, Dr. Molliver said. A close examination showed that some cells in the cerebellum were being destroyed by the drug.

The cerebellum is the part of the brain where smooth muscle motor control, balance and coordination are carried out, Dr. Molliver said. It helps the body get its bearings.

But recent research indicates that it also receives inputs from just about every other part of the brain, including the spinal cord and a central area of the brain stem where dreams are initiated. The cerebellum appears to play an important role in learning and remembering, particularly stereotypic behaviors, skills and conditioned responses, Dr. Molliver said.

Dr. Molliver said that he thinks ibogaine does not act directly on cells in the cerebellum. Rather, it seems to target an area of the brain stem called the inferior olive, a pacemaker that sends timing information to the cerebellum. Ibogaine activates olive cells for hours, causing them to release excitatory transmitters that flood cells in cerebellum, eventually killing some of them.

Most addiction research has focused on brain circuits that use the neurotransmitter dopamine as a reward, Dr. Molliver said. But if ibogaine eliminates drug withdrawal and craving — and Dr. Molliver stressed this has yet to be proved — it means addiction might be routed through the cerebellum and that different, perhaps undiscovered, neurotransmitters are involved.

Unlearning Addiction?

"Addiction is learned," Mr. Lotsof said. "It takes time to become dependent on any drug. Then people become sensitive to cues in the environment. If Dr. Molliver is right, we might be seeing with ibogaine an unlearning of the addiction process." In other words, he said, the waking dreams elicited by the drug may literally unstructure the neural circuitry laid down when the addiction was acquired.

At the University of Florida Medical School in Miami, Dr. Deborah Mash is eager to begin human trials with ibogaine. Dade county has a serious AIDS and crack-cocaine epidemic, "and I don't think we have any time to waste," she said. "We need to find out if this drug works."

Dr. Molliver's findings have made the F.D.A. very worried that ibogaine might kill too many cells in the cerebellum, Dr. Mash said. But experiments in her laboratory show that ibogaine given in therapeutic doses does not cause similar brain damage in monkeys. And other studies show that there is more brain damage associated with cold-turkey withdrawal from opiates and cocaine than from ibogaine.

For now, Dr. Mash has permission from the F.D.A. to test extremely low doses of ibogaine in nine people who have already taken the drug to see how their bodies use the compound. Once that is done, she said, it should be possible, as early as next year, to test therapeutic doses in people who have never taken ibogaine.

The New York Times SUNDAY, NOVEMBER 14, 1993

Healing Herb or Narcotic? Marijuana as Medication

Underground Networks Supplying the Sick

By JOSEPH B. TREASTER

Every two weeks, Rabbi Isaac P. Fried visits a businessman in Brooklyn who is dying of cancer. They talk for a while, and the rabbi hands over a small bag of marijuana with a hopeful blessing.

"May these herbs," he says, "be an instrument of healing."

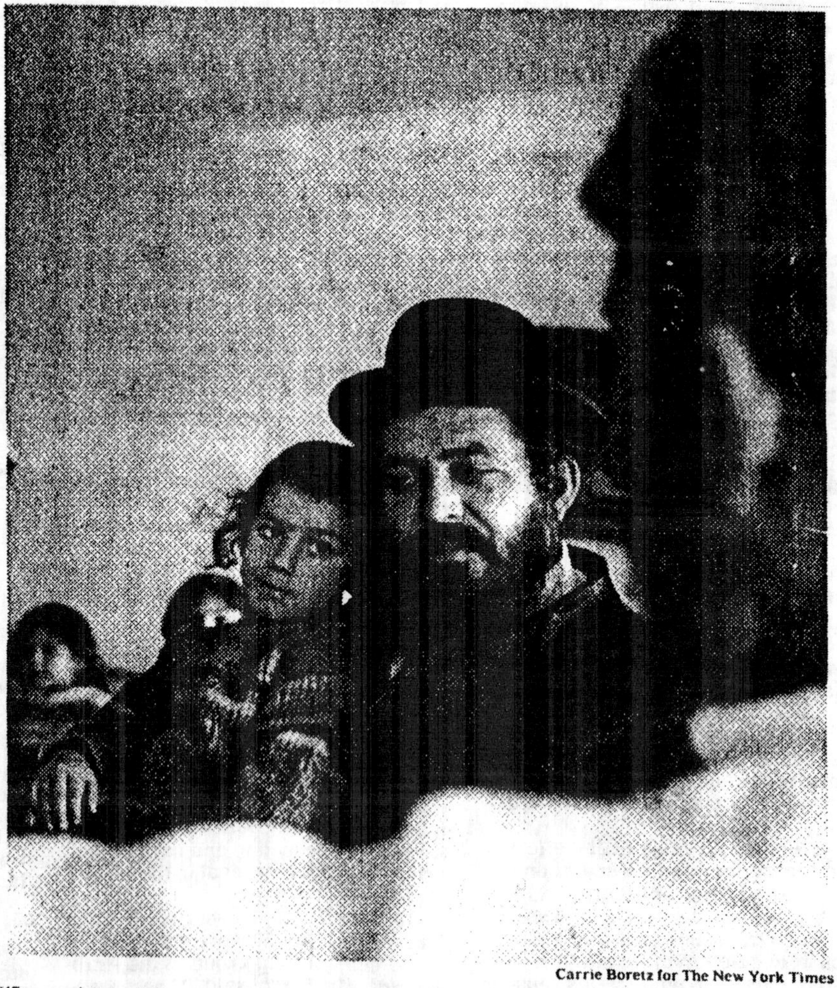

Carrie Boretz for The New York Times

"I consider this a need that has to be filled," Rabbi Isaac P. Fried said of giving marijuana to those in medical need. "Should I buckle under the fear of an archaic law that doesn't deal with the present needs of the 1990's?"

once again weeks before by ACT UP Harm Reduction, with no inkling that publication would be so synchronistic.

The angle was a Hasidic rabbi who defies civil authority, bringing medical marijuana to the very sick in his community — a contact made as a kind of consolation prize for the Ibogaine clinic that never happened in Prague. Within days he would be on network talk shows.

This made it hard to ignore that day's protest. Sixty-five activists from medical marijuana, clean needle, and Ibogaine groups from five cities demonstrated, with coverage by four local TV stations and one radio network. All assembled were also energized and entertained by the massive presence of the mobile Thomas K. Forçade assault rock 'n' roll soundstage, the legendary Rock Against Racism battlewagon, equipped with megawatt speakers (and full recording capabilities), a serious symbol of activist organization. But although there were twice as many people as there'd been in July, the organizers were worried — there should have been hundreds.

Sure enough, when Dana called Nancy Stanisec on November 16th she said the FDA Office of AIDS Coordination could not facilitate such a harm reduction meeting, and said they must independently contact Lee Brown, Gebbie and so-on. The next day Dana put in one more call, to Curtis Wright. Beal asked flat-out for a waiver equivalent to the needle exchange for medical marijuana.

The FDA couldn't be trusted regulating herbs, Dana said, if they couldn't clean up their act with cannabis.

Wright said the problem was in NIDA, that Marvin Snyder, their policy man on marijuana, was unwilling to sign on to anything that might "signal kids pot is okay." Wright said they were very concerned about the uptick of pot use among eighth graders.

Dana replied that the absence of a corresponding rise in coke use showed that the harm reduction movement was working — "We need *more* explicit separation of soft from hard drugs — not *less*. The Dutch had a 40% reduction in the rise of their addiction rate by separating out marjuana. If we get 40% reductions with Ibogaine it will be a miracle drug.

The fact that pot is competitive again with crack is a *benefit*."

Wright seemed unconvinced. But then an interesting thing happened. That Thursday, during the first day of the Drug Policy Foundation Conference at the L'Enfant Plaza Hotel, Ric Doblin was called away to a two-hour FDA meeting at the Parklawn Building, with Wright and Dan Spiker. This meeting was so impromptu that Ric didn't even turn up for his own long-scheduled afternoon MAPs organizing workshop.

A few people looking for the MAPS session instead found Dana and David Goldstein holding forth on ancient Gnosticism and Ibogaine. One of them turned out to be a sleep researcher and addictionologist from Milwaukee, Ed Friedrichs. When Dana got to the part about REM and healing, Friedrichs grew very excited.

"What you're saying exactly dovetails with my findings about REM and addiction. Most addicts have major sleep disorders, you know. Many since childhood. They can't complete REM without waking up — so they never get the deep, post-REM slow wave sleep. I've been giving them just enough desipramine and melaril to keep them from waking up — and some of them REM for days, but they get a good sleep for the first time in a long time, and their withdrawal and craving abate.

"The thing is, the body can't heal itself without the deep sleep that comes immediately *after* REM. I had a gal in the hospital, an ex-alcoholic with a history of DTs. She was an AA counselor; all that coffee had given her an ulcer, and they had her in to take out her stomach. Well, she couldn't sleep at all, and after four days spontaneously lapsed into *delerium tremens*. Once you've had DTs, simple sleep deprivation can trigger a recurrence. On the fifth day her stitches popped out and her wound came completely open. It never had a chance to heal."

"So instead of REMing," said Dana, "she lapsed into an excito-toxic loop! Which blocked deep sleep, slow wave sleep, completely!" He added—

"After Ibogaine, people don't need REM at first. They awake completely refreshed each time after just a few hours of deep sleep. They have a REM surplus. And they appear to *glow*."

"It's simple, really," Friedrichs continued.

"The relationship between REM and healing is that deep sleep can't happen without successful completion of REM. And healing doesn't happen without deep sleep."

When Ric Doblin returned from his FDA meeting, he said that Curtis Wright had mentioned the ACT UP rally. They offered him two important concessions. First they agreed to approve marijuana as an herb, in line with their new standards for herbs, instead of a compound, requiring decades of study of sixty active ingredients and their interactions. Second, they agreed to consider an application for orphan drug status for marijuana, to give Doblin a shot at $400,000 to pay for Don Abrams' comparative trial of marijuana versus Marinol[1] at San Franscisco General.

1 Marinol is only 2% absorbable, compared to the quicker, much-more-complete effects of smoked marijuana.

Why, in a hundred years, we could have approval of practically every herb currently in use!

Curtis Wright is a nice man. A scientist of daring and vision. But Curtis Wright doesn't have people with AIDS knocking on his door. John Spacely, on the lam from the hospital, was knocking on Dana's door when he got back to 9 Bleecker. Not once but three times in the next few weeks, Beal had to lobby Housing Works because Spacely had no place to go.

Earlier that fall Spacely's scene had come completely apart. After he insisted on cutting, on his own, a growth off his leg, he started doing heroin again. Then he lost his key and was found wandering delerious in the street. He lost his apartment on Second Avenue, his assets like his baseball cards, everything. In intervals when he escaped from the hospital, the people from Manic Panic on East 7th Street shooed him away because they didn't want him smoking crack in the doorway.

Dana was struggling to update this report, into which Paul De Rienzo and Geerte F. had already inserted Chapter 11, making it thirteen chapters by the time of the 1993 DPF Conference at the end of November. In a reprise of February and March, when he was working on the Macintosh and it was also freezing, Spacely kept showing up at 9 Bleecker and wanting to squat the only warm space, on the third floor where Dana was trying to work on the Macintosh.

The only halfway warm bedroom was the back of the third floor, which Alice wasn't willing to vacate.

Dana's second floor space was unheated, and, like the rest of the building, bitterly cold, a situation that wouldn't be remedied until renovations were completed in February.

Multiple appeals to Housing Works finally got the Spaceman a new apartment. But he kept losing his keys. And he got ripped off and beaten up by a junkie who moved in on his new place.

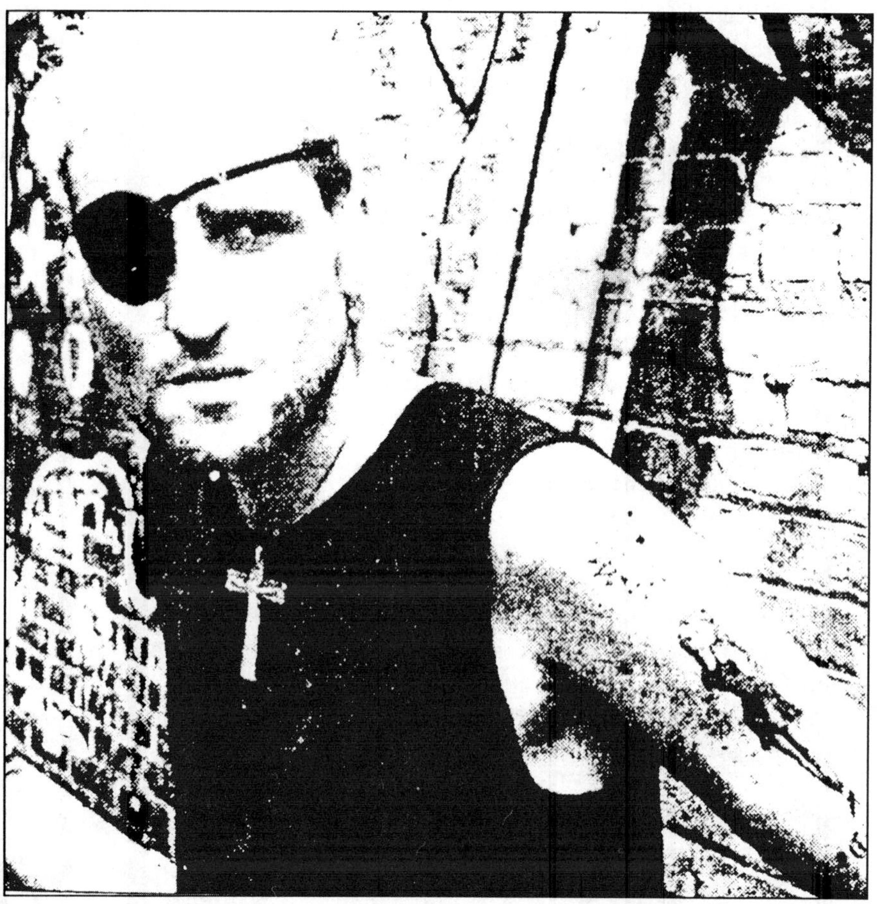

YIPIS

JOHN SPACELY

CHAPTER 16: The Passover Plot

Three days after preliminary drafts of Chapters 14 & 15 were finished, Dana was thinking about the report from PIHKAL, of the subject who went through "a door of light," and was clinically dead for three minutes on a psychedelic drug,[1] only to sit up on the cot as emergency medics rushed into the room. How long could someone be clinically dead and recover?, he wondered.

Quite a while, he remembered, according to *Day One* producers. Fortuitously, when ABC finally ran its Ibogaine story, on the Monday after the FDA re-started the Miami IND, it was paired with a segment on people who were clinically dead and came back to life. (After so many months of juggling the Ibogaine story, for *Day One* programmers the NDE connection must have seemed natural.) Anyway, it turns out as many as *one fourth* of the DOA's hitting the emergency rooms are actually still alive, suspended in extreme shock, their blood moving so slowly that circulation can only be detected by inserting a sophisticated catheter into the vein.

This opening segment on the NDE featured interviews with people who were completely conscious throughout their ordeal. It fit in with the scenes of the Nganga, in the later Ibogaine segment, spooning root bark into the mouth of an initiate lolling, deathlike, in ataxia. To test to see if the dose is sufficient but not lethal, according to Goutarel, the Nganga would next determine if the extremities were sufficiently numb — an effect produced by most Iboga alkaloids, but a good indicator of Ibogaine blood levels. ABC didn't show it, yet Dana, reviewing it in his mind's eye, could visualize the Bwiti priest piercing the hand of the initiate with a sliver of wood. Once they're in the NDE, there's no pain, no jerk, no response.

This revery, a few days before Christmas, was interrupted by a CNN report of a curious admission by the Pope: Christmas had been *moved* to December to coincide with Roman winter solstice holidays.[2] The real J.C. was born sometime in late September!

What next, thought Dana? Papal confirmation of a Dickian Bible in which Daniel took *Peganum harmala* to foresee the final days before the fall of the Temple — in order to discern the intervention necessary to reverse history and re-establish Israel? P. K. Dick believed early Christians had a secret sacrament that enabled them to conquer time — to remember who they were thousands of years later in another body. But he never identified a particular drug, or related its mechanism of action to the crucifixion and resurrection.

What would it take to be dead and revive — not after three minutes, but a full day later?

First Dana asked his friend Ilan Moishe whether the Hasidim had any tradition to the effect that Jesus accomplished his crucifixion and resurrection with the aid of a drug or drugs which put him into a near-death state long enough to fool the Romans.

"Yes," said Ilan. "There are several other instances during that time of Rabbis feigning death in order to make good an escape."[3]

"What we've been saying the whole time is that he was not Moshiach, but a magician."

Bob Sisko added that a Jewish scholar of the New Testament named Hugh Schonfield had caused a big sensation in the '60s with a book laying out the argument, from Biblical analysis, for such an actual physical basis for the resurrection. *The Passover Plot* became a best seller, part of the same milieu as Bishop Pike's quest for the "lost sacrament" of the Gnostic Christians, or Wasson, Hoffman and Ruck's book on the Eleusinian mysteries. It depicted a Jesus firmly in charge, not only of his own fate but of history — combining the discipline of an Olympic athlete, techniques of a Buddhist monk, and a remarkable knack for scripting his Mission Impossible to fulfill prophetic *gnosis:*

> "What we chiefly note is that the plans of Jesus were laid with remarkable care for timing. He had singled out a particular Passover as the season when he would suffer, and had taken every precaution to ensure that he would not be arrested beforehand. During the first half of

1 See Robert Slauiter, et al., *Common Mechanism of Lysergic Acid, Indolealkylamine and Penthylamine Hallucinogens,* (1980) indicating a potential wide range of common effects in "psychedelic" compounds, e.g.: the "Village of the Ancestors" on mescaline, or "Death's Door" effects on iboga.

2 It was also four days after "Mithras-day," the supposed birthday of the divinity of the principal eastern mystery religion competing with Christianity during Roman times.

3 See Schonfield, *Those Incredible Christians.*

Passion Week, keeping himself in the public eye by conducting his activities in the Temple, he had aggravated the ecclesiastical authorities to the pitch that they were determined to destroy him as soon as it should be feasible without the risk of tumult; but he was careful not to help them by staying in the city after dark. Not until Wednesday evening did Jesus apply the pressure that decided Judas to go to the Council with an offer to betray him, and by his secret arrangements he saw to it that the arrest would not take place until Thursday evening after he had partaken of the Last Supper in Jerusalem with his disciples. All this suggests that he intended that his crucifixion should be on Friday, which would be the eve of the Sabbath.

"Calculating that it would require some hours on Friday morning for the Council to obtain his condemnation by Pilate, which could not be withheld as the charge was treason against the Emperor, and knowing that in accordance with custom he would not be left on the cross over the Sabbath, but would be taken down well before sundown when Sabbath commenced, Jesus could roughly reckon that he would experience crucifixion for not much more than three or four hours, whereas normally the agonies of the crucified lasted for many days...

"Jesus... relied on the Old Testament Oracles, and what these intimated... was that while there would be a conspiracy of the rulers to destroy him (as in *Psalm ii*), yet by the mercy of God he would be spared complete extinction of life...: '*Though I walk in the midst of trouble, thou wilt revive me; thou shalt stretch forth thine hand against the wrath of my enemies, and thy right hand shall save me. The Lord will perfect that which concerneth me. The bands of the grave compassed me about: the snares of death prevented me. In my distress I called upon the Lord, and cried unto my God: he heard my voice out of his temple. He sent from above, he took me, he drew me out of great waters. He delivered me from my strong enemy. God shall redeem my soul from the grasp of the grave. My flesh also shall rest in hope. For thou wilt not leave my soul in the grave; neither wilt thou suffer thy holy one to see corruption. Thou wilt show me the path of life. Come, and let us return unto the Lord: for he hath torn, and he will heal us; he hath smitten, and he will bring us up. After two days will he revive us; and on the third day he will raise us up, and we shall live in his sight. The king shall joy in thy strength, O Lord...He asked life of thee, and thou gavest it him, even length of days for ever and ever.*'

"If Jesus was convinced from the Scriptures that he was to suffer on the cross, but not to perish on it, there is no reason why he should not have been concerned to make what provision he could for his survival. We have had ample evidence that Jesus used his intelligence to assure the fulfillment of the predictions. He believed that as Messiah the spirit of wisdom and understanding had been conferred on him, and that it was God's will that he should employ these powers of the mind to accomplish what must come to pass. He did not expect, indeed it was alien to his nature, to sit with folded hands waiting for things to happen whether in a natural or supernatural manner. His whole ministry was purposeful, masterful and practical. He plotted and schemed with the utmost skill and resourcefulness, sometimes making secret arrangements, taking advantage of every circumstance conducive to the attainment of his objectives. It is difficult to credit that he had neglected to do anything about the supreme crisis of his career, when it was imperative that he should outwit the forces arrayed against him and wrest victory from the jaws of death.

"<u>...If we follow the Fourth Gospel the ordeal lasted barely three hours, from a little after midday to about three o'clock in the afternoon.</u> But this obviously was not enough. If he was to cheat death it was essential that well in advance of the time, which could not be much after five o'clock, when in any case he would be taken down because of the incoming Sabbath, he would have to give every appearance of being dead. Otherwise his actual death would be expedited by the soldiers in charge of the execution. Further, help must speedily be forthcoming. Unless his body came into the possession of friendly hands there would be no possiblity of his recovery...

"This person is identified as Joseph of Arimathea. He is one of the great mysteries of the Gospels. He is represented as a wealthy man, and a member of the Sanhedrin; and since he is said to have been waiting for the Kingdom of God he would have been a messianically-minded Pharisee. He enters the story unheralded, and after his task is fulfilled he disappears completely from the New Testament records...

"...Jesus could have got to know him through Nicodemus, mentioned only in the Fourth Gospel, during the three months from the previous October to January when he was at Jerusalem working out the details of the Passover Plot. He needed highly placed individuals on whom he could count to give him inside information on what measures were being taken against him by the Council, and also to advise him about relations between the Council and the Roman governor, procedures on political trials, and other pertinent matters with which he was unfamiliar, but which had a bearing upon his course of action and affected his plans. Evidently Joseph was deeply impressed by Jesus and was ready to co-operate in frustrating the intentions of the Sadducean chief priests. Luke says that he had not consented to their counsel and deed, and John describes him as a secret disciple.

"It transpired that Joseph had property in close proximity to Golgotha, the hill of execution. Part of this was under cultivation as a kitchen garden, and also on the site was a new tomb cut into the rock... Two things, however, were indispensable to the success of a rescue operation. The first was to administer a drug to Jesus on the cross to give the impression of premature death, and the second was to obtain the speedy delivery of the body to Joseph. No other manner of survival could be entertained by Jesus, since he was adamant about the fulfilment of the prophecies which demanded his suffering.

"Considerations of safety and secrecy... dictated that as few people as possible should be in the know or involved.... He dealt individually and singly with Judean individuals who were in a position to carry out the various parts of his design. His was the mastermind, and those to whom he gave his instructions neither worked together nor were acquainted with more than their specific function.

"The first stage of the present action was the cross. We are told that there were bystanders there, and one of them saturated a sponge with vinegar, impaled it on a cane and put it to the mouth of Jesus. He did not perform this office for either of the two robbers crucified with Jesus, which he might well have done if his intention had been purely humanitarian. The incident took place, according to Mark, after Jesus had cried, 'My God [*Eli* in Hebrew], my God, why hast thou forsaken me?' Mark gives the words in Aramaic, which Peter would have used in describing the crucifixion; but Jesus no doubt quoted from *Psalm xxii* in Hebrew. This prompted some onlookers to suppose he was calling for Elijah. The man who acted, who was sent there by Joseph to administer the drug, said: 'Quiet! Let us see if Elijah will come and take him down.' The man here showed his initiative by taking advantage of an opportune moment for his intervention, which no one would suspect was favourable to Jesus. Mark gives no reason for his action, but the Fourth Gospel says that Jesus called out, 'I am thirsty,' which could have been a signal. There was nothing unusual for a vessel containing a refreshing liquid to be at the place of execution, and it presented no problem to doctor the drink that was offered to Jesus. The plan may indeed have been suggested to Jesus by the prophetic words, *'They gave me also gall for my meat; and in my thirst they gave me vinegar to drink'* (Psalm LXIX, line 2). If what he received had been the normal wine vinegar diluted with water the effect would have been stimulating. In this case it was exactly the opposite. Jesus lapsed quickly into complete unconsciousness. His body sagged. His head lolled on his breast, and to all intents and purposes he was a dead man.

"Directly it was seen the drug had worked the man hastened to Joseph who was anxiously waiting for the news. At once he sought an audience with Pilate, to whom he would have ready access as a member of the Sanhedrin, and requested to have the body of Jesus. Pilate was greatly astonished, as well he might be, to hear that Jesus was already dead, and being on his guard in view of all that had happened he sent for the centurion in charge of the execution to obtain confirmation. When this was forthcoming, he readily gave the necessary permission. It has been noted by scholars that Joseph asked for the body (*soma*) of Jesus, which could indicate that he did not think of him as dead. It is only Pilate who refers to the corpse (*ptoma*).

"Joseph hurried to Golgotha with clean linen and spices. The Fourth Gospel says he was accompanied by Nicodemus. It also reports another circumstance. In view of the need to hasten death because of the Sabbath the two robbers had their legs broken with mallets, but Jesus was spared this treatment because he was believed to be dead already. To make sure, however, one of the soldiers thrust a lance into his

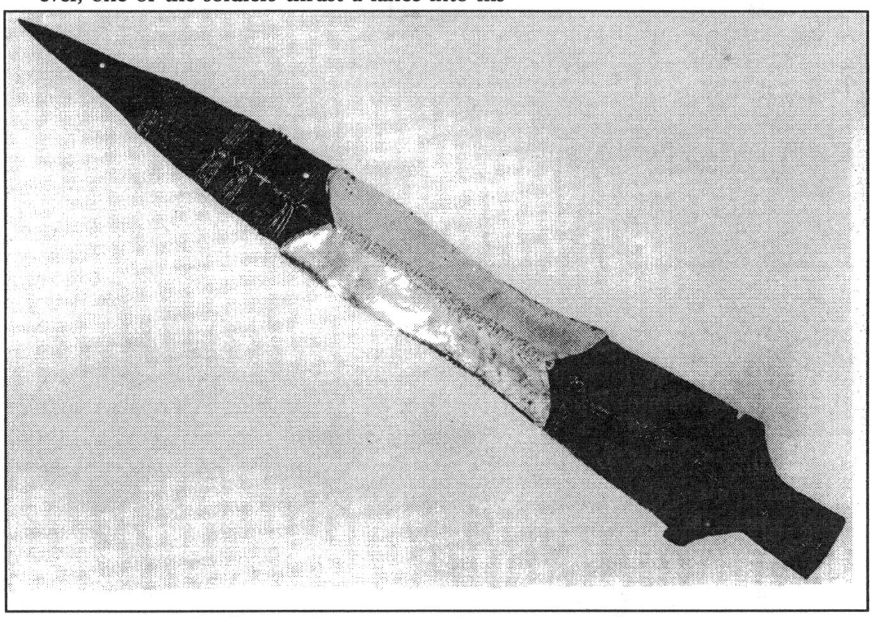

THE SPEAR OF LONGINUS, IN THE AUSTRIAN NATIONAL MUSEUM

side. This incident may have been introduced to historicise certain Old Testament testimonies. The passage suggests that some doubt was thrown on this new information when it was published. If it is correct, the chances that Jesus would recover were heavily diminished. Much would depend on the nature of the wound. The reported emission of blood shows at least that life was still in him.

"As arranged, Jesus was conveyed carefully to the nearby tomb. The women of his following, who had been observing everything at a distance, saw where he was taken. Sorrowfully they made their way back to the city, proposing to return on the morning after the Sabbath to pay their tribute by anointing his body. It is evident they were not expecting any resurrection.

"Jesus lay in the tomb over the Sabbath. He would not regain consciousness for many hours, and in the meantime the spices and linen bandages provided the best dressing for his injuries... But if the body of Jesus was taken from the tomb by his friends on Saturday night, we should be ready to agree with the Gospels that the immediate disciples of Jesus knew nothing about this, and they would be quite sincere in indignantly repudiating any contention that they had been guilty of perpetrating a fraud.

"Christians are surely right in protesting that the Church could not have been established on the basis of a deliberate falsehood on the part of the apostles, and therefore there must be another explanation for the removal of the body than an intention to pretend that Jesus had risen from the dead....We are left with the perfectly natural and fully justifiable reason that Jesus was taken from the tomb at the first possible opportunity for the entirely legitimate purpose of reviving him. For this action at least two persons would have been needed...

"...A plan was being followed which was worked out in advance by Jesus himself and which he had not divulged to his close disciples. What seems probable is that in the darkness of Saturday night when Jesus was brought out of the tomb by those concerned in the plan he regained consciousness temporarily, but finally succumbed. If, as the Fourth Gospel says, his side was pierced by a lance before he was taken from the cross his chances of recovery were slender. It was much too risky, and perhaps too late, to take the body back to the tomb, replace the bandages left there, roll the stone across the entrance, and try to create the impression that everything was as it had been on Friday evening...

"Jesus may not have overlooked that he might taste of death in spite of measures he had secretly taken for his survial. He could have interpreted *Isaiah liii* in this sense. *'He made his grave with the wicked, and with the rich in his deaths* [plural].' Two deaths, two burials were thus foreshadowed. He would die as it were on the cross, and yet again after the cross. But whatever would happen his faith assured him that in some way God would raise him up and receive him until his coming in glory with the clouds of heaven....We are entitled to imagine him... regaining consciousness after he was taken from the tomb, and using these precious minutes to beg his friends to deliver a message to his disciples. He would repeat what was so much a part of him, the Scriptures relating his suffering and revival. 'Tell them these things,' he may have urged. 'They must believe. Tell them that when I have risen I will meet them in Galilee as I said, and afterwards enter into glory'."

— Hugh Schonfield,
The Passover Plot, pp. 153–167

So writes Schonfield, no expert on ethnopharmacology (perhaps imagining the action of a long-acting narcotic). Dana, familiar with the effects of a class of drugs perfectly capable of effecting "miraculous healing" (the "Ibogaine glow") as the sequelae of an NDE was not so sure Jesus might not just have stuck around for the traditional forty days. Long enough to impart the account of his descent into virtual space, his contest with the Adversary, as specified in the Scriptures.[1] In fact, numerous occasions to slip Him booster draughts of an Ibogaine-like drug to get Him up to the full-dose threshold are strewn throughout the Last Supper and the Passion (while toting the cross, for instance, when he's allowed to sip the "water of life") — or even again *after* being taken down, to sleep through the Sabbath.

Leaving on a long-planned trip to Germany, Dana brought his inquiry to Hans-Georg Behr in the form of a question about the Holy Grail. How exactly did this mythic code for the secret sacrament of the Gnostics — embodied in the tale of Parsifal, the knight who conquers death by conquering time — make its way into Europe?

Via the Crusades, Georg replied. Hans-Georg Behr, scion of the Esterhazy branch of the old Dual Monarchy, brought out a book on the fortresses of Teutonic Knights — architectural inspiration of Himmler's SS. Another holy order, the Knights Templar, especially

1 *Ephesians* 4, 9–10. See also the Apocryphal *Book of Nicodemus*, particularly the long prayer that makes up Chapters 13–20, for a more complete account. The last scribe to rewrite it, who was evidently a big partisan of the doctrine of bodily resurrection of the faithful at the End of Time, included it in a much longer, obviously Bowdlerized, account of Jesus's life.

dedicated to the recovery of relics and lost knowledge, penetrated as far as Ethiopia in search of the Ark of the Covenant.[1]

They returned with monophysite heresies which had been banned by Orthodoxy for centuries. These doctrines (which are perfectly African) of Christ's out-of-body state during and after crucifixion are theological vestiges of the Grail Myth. In it the original wine cup from the Last Supper is present to catch Jesus' blood from the spear wound because it's been intentionally brought filled with vinegar and gall [extract of bitter herbs],[2] thereby making His words (*"This is my blood"*) both prophetic, and literally descriptive of the secret sacrament of the Gnostics, the drug that granted Him refuge in the NDE.[3]

Jesus, like all observant Jews, identified blood with the life-force itself. To be kosher, a Rabbi must still certify that an animal was slaughtered humanely and *properly drained of blood.* In offering his disciples wine and wafer, however, Jesus was incorporating into Christianity a version of the ancient *dron* ceremony of Zoroastrianism, whose origins are also bound up with the Priestly slaughter of cattle, but which uniquely identified the life-force with *soma,* prepared from plants.[4]

Both the spear and the Grail Stone of Parsifal are real-life artifacts in a Vienna museum. According to Georg, the Grail Stone is a Roman-era (100 A.D.) commemorative cup carved from a single very large, rare crystal, called an *Achat.* Purported by Byzantium to be the true Grail when given to the Frankish King sometime before 750 A.D., it was also supposed to test for the presence of poison.

More relevant, in *Parsifal,* was the sacrament *in* the Grail. It was organic (a wafer), and was eaten like the ordinary sacrament. And by virtue of interaction with the Cup that caught Christ's blood, the pedigree of this special, secret sacrament was unimpeachable. Yet somehow this wafer was effective beyond ordinary sacraments that offer salvation only in the next life. It conferred healing in this life, and youthfulness "unto the 200th year." P. K. Dick believed *Parsifal's* originators further viewed this mysterious wafer as linked, according to Medieval ideas of sympathetic magic,[5] through Christ's Blood to the Spear that pierced His side; and that when Parsifal points the Spear at Klingsor and makes the sign of the cross, and Klingsor's evil castle disappears, the Spear is re-enacting the healing effect of the lost sacraments the Cup originally contained.

Himmler and Hitler, who removed the Grail and the spear of Longinus from Vienna to Nuremberg until 1945, got it all wrong. They thought Parsifal was a story about racial purity of blood,[6] when it's really about liberation from sin, through the sacraments. In banishing the Evil Castle, the important thing (or clue) is that Parsifal finally gets control of a phenomena that's been occurring throughout the script, i.e., shifting, changing backdrops. "'You see, my son, here time turns into space.' (The whole landscape becomes indistinct. A forest ebbs out and a wall of rough rock ebbs in.... The two men pass through the gateway. What happened to the forest? The two men did not really... go anywhere, and yet they are not now where they originally were.... Wagner began *Parsifal* in 1845. He died in 1873, long before Hermann Minkowski postulated four-dimensional space-time (1908).... Where did Richard Wagner get the notion that time could turn into space?)." (P. K. Dick, *VALIS,* pp. 40–41).

The answer, of course, is that all the weird space-time shifts of *Parsifal,* including the climactic disappearance of Klingsor's Castle, are part of the original storyline, not inventions of

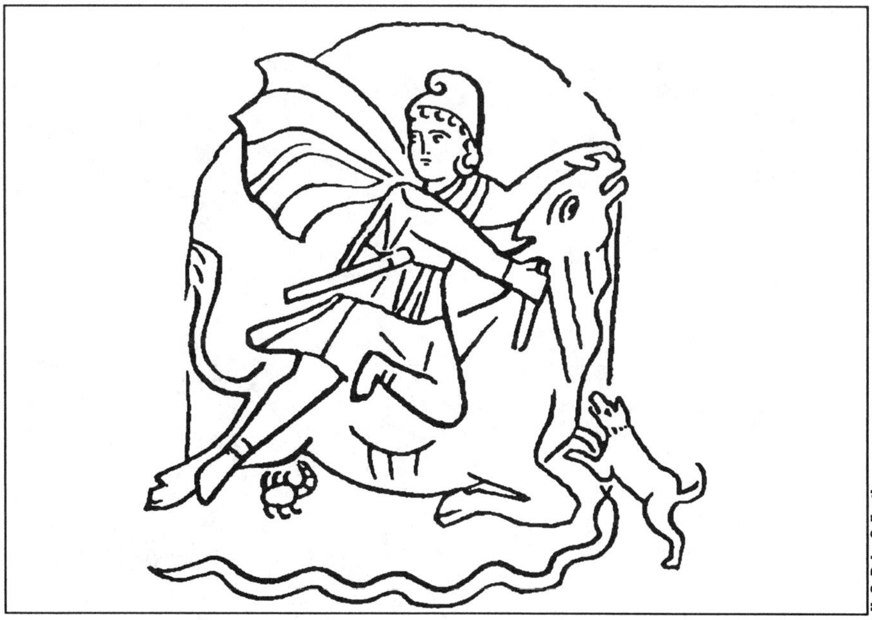

H.-G. Behr Collection

MITHRAS, CHIEF DEITY OF THE ANCIENT PERSIAN RELIGION REFORMED BY ZARATHUSTRA (ZOROASTER).

1 See Chapter 17, p. 197.

2 Biblical cites.

3 See Chapter 17, pp. 194–196.

4 See this chapter, pp. 177–180, and especially p. 179 on the *dron* ceremony. See also Appendix 4, Flattery & Schwartz.

5 E.g., the Law of Contagion — that things once in contact continue to interact from a distance after separation; and the Law of Similarity — that effects resemble causes.

6 Hitler is reported to have emerged from his first experience of Wagner's *Parsifal* dazed and flushed, and to have spontaneously declared that he was dedicating his life to defending the sacred purity of Aryan blood, which he saw symbolized by the Holy Grail.

Wagner. Himmler and Hitler, Wagner's biggest fans, derided Einstein. They were self-styled defenders of so-called "classical," Newtonian physics. In 1938 they sat by — oblivious while the secret of the Bomb was being smuggled out of the Reich.

In other words, Einsteinian space-time in Wagner represents a bigger anachronism than a simple familiarity on the part of the original storytellers with an intriguing potion used during the time of Parsifal in the Cult of St. Michael, to induce visions. St. Michael was the patron Saint of Parsifal and the knightly orders — the Archangel Michael of the Bible, who led the angels in putting down the rebellion of Satan.

As part of their initiation into the Templars or the Teutonic orders, knights would go spend the night in certain grottos, which in ancient times had been shrines of Mithras, the Persian religion which was early Christianity's chief competitor.[1] As part of their ordeal, in order to have visions of Saint Michael and Jesus and psych themselves for morning devotions, they took something — hinted by the Grail myth[2] to be the original gnostic substance used by Jesus.

Within a generation, however, as the Western Empire became more cosmopolitan, the Papacy became locked in a vicious struggle with the last strong Emperor, Fredrick II, who offended Rome by employing Arabs (infidels) in his government, and promulgated the first constitution since Roman times granting equality to commoners.[3] He was particularly supported by the Templars. Before he died the Pope excommunicated him and began a 137-year exile in France, while St. Thomas Aquinas laid the theological basis for purging both the Arabs and the nettlesome knightly orders.

Aquinas' great idea was to exclude all "paganisms" that had crept into Catholicism by elevating Aristotle to near Biblical status (which made Arab scholars redundant), and then excluding all personal experience (either experiment or ecstasy) that didn't fit the Bible or categories of Aristotle. Even more telling was Aquinas' peculiar teaching that dreaming itself was suspect — an opportunity Satan uses to overpower the sleeper with lust, etc.[4] If something looked pagan, it was banned. This doctrine was called scholasticism, and was used by the Dominicans first to liquidate the Templars (1280 A.D.), then the Cult of St. Michael altogether (by 1350 A.D.).

After all, who could tell what they were worshipping in those caves?

Inasmuch as even a hint of other, secret sacraments undermined orthodoxy on the Resurrection, Aquinas set out to debunk the status of Archangels altogether by formulating the "how many angels fit on the head of a pin?" paradox.[5] By 1380 the Dominicans instituted

1 In fact, due to Christianity's subversive reputation, Constantine (founder of Constantinople) himself was constrained to publicly espouse Mithras while he was Emperor, converting to Christianity only on his deathbed.

2 The full flowering of which occurred in the 1100s, although *Parsifal* wasn't composed until 1185, by a Frenchman who left the job of finishing it to Wolfram von Eschenbach.

3 His courts held that a farmer was equal to a Duke, for instance.

4 As to whether dreams were sent by God or the Devil, Aquinas said it must be Satan, because he'd observed other monks get erections while asleep. Any potion based on a plant (see p. 179) called in Turkish Ucerlik , the "dreaming flower" was anathema, Q.E.D.

5 The answer, "All or none at all," was intended to prove an Arch-Angel — who could certainly be no more important than the entire Heavenly Host (the original offense of Satan) — had no special standing as far as Earthlings are concerned.

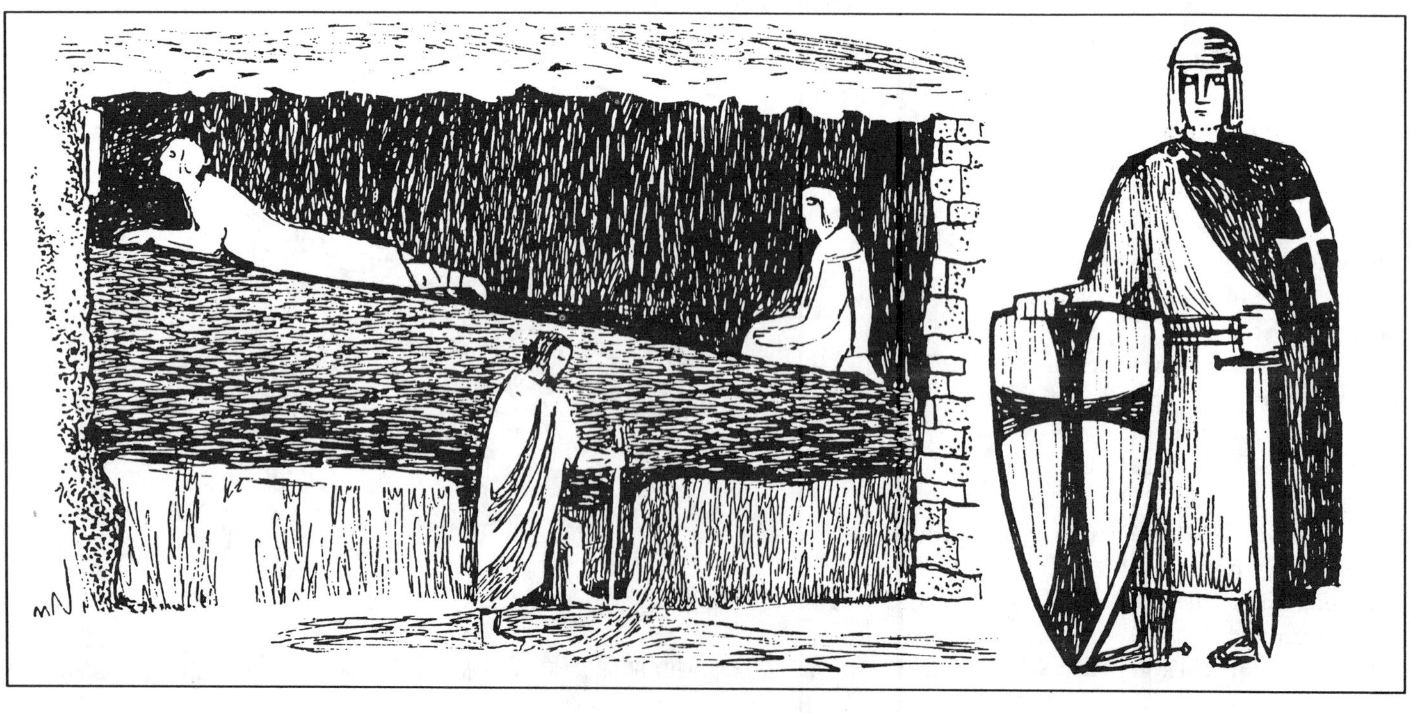

H.-G. Behr Collection

H.-G. Behr Collection

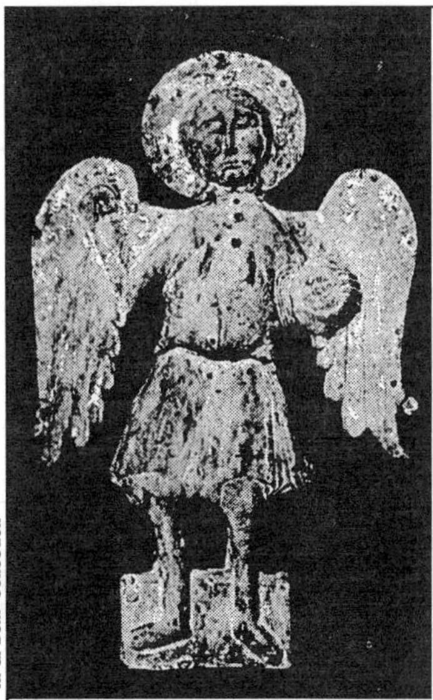

St. Michael, c. 800 AD

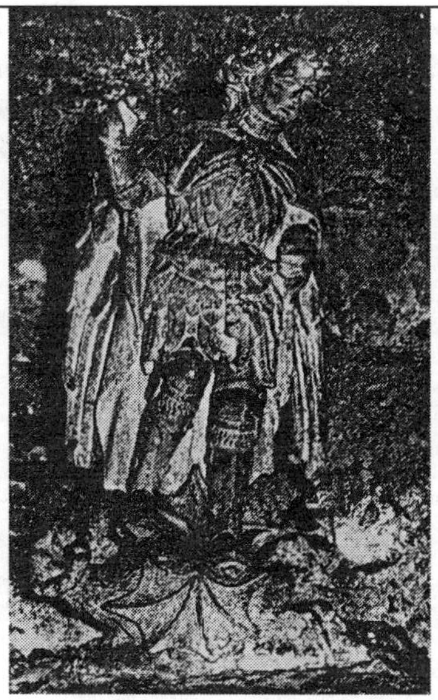

St. Michael, c. 1100 AD

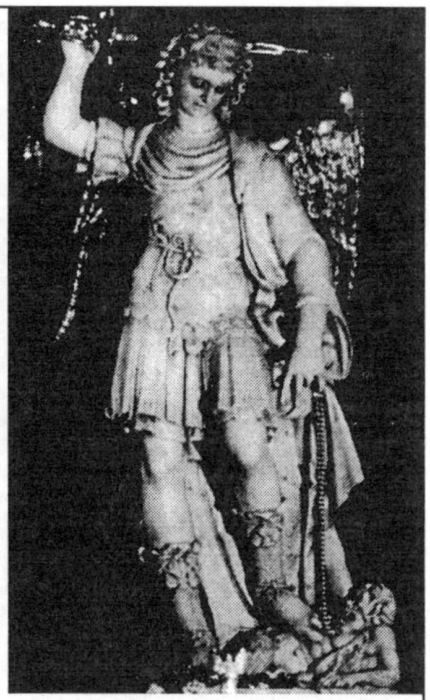

St. Michael. c. 1250 AD

witchcraft trials to be able to seize for mere thought-crimes the riches of people who didn't actually own an Arab book. By 1580 even the wives of commoners were being burned alive at the stake. *Prophecy* itself was a crime.

In banning all magic — propounding the doctrine that Christianity guarantees Aristotelian order against the eruption of Chaos — the Dominican Holy Inquisition unleashed by Aquinas ended up spying on and rooting out "incorrect" scientific experimentation. *Alchemy* had to be done in secret. In 1614 Galileo was arrested and forced to renounce what he could plainly see through the telescope. *"It still moves,"* he is supposed to have muttered, after the Papal commission refused to look at the moons of Jupiter for themselves.

So, was the potion of St. Michael's cult which set off the witchhunts the selfsame gnostic sacrament, the very "gall for my meat," that Jesus used to cheat the Cross? One clue, according to Georg Behr, is that under torture, many Templars admitted spiritual commerce with a certain *Baphomet,* in order to gain access to hidden things. Baphomet is an anagram for *Sophia.* St. Sophia corresponds to both the *Gnosis* of the Holy Spirit and the Athena-like *Kybele,* the chief female diety associated, long before St. Michael, with Mithras.

Sophia also was one of the names of Mary, since as the Mother of He who personified the Law, she bore the Annointed One as the Ark bore the Tablets of Law. Mithraism originally lost out because it was mainly a soldier's religion — too male-dominant. The Christ had more of the qualities women as well as men could relate to. From the time of Aquinas on, the Devil came to be portrayed more and more as Mithras, gaining the name Lucifer and horns like a bull instead of a goat.

Even after the Grail was shorn of Monophysite heresies and coopted to the Trinity via the Marian cult,[1] however, indentification of the spiritual realm with the Near Death Experience persisted among medieval mystics like Dante. Both Bwiti and P. K. Dick are in agreement, moreover, that each use of the true, plant sacrament to breach of the NDE entails a certain risk, specifically characterized in *VALIS* by the Heraclitean fragment "Time is a child at play...." Dana remembered another, second use of the fragment, in *Divine Invasion,* and found that the character who utters it turns out to be — Sophia. [The Shekhina, the female half of God, immanent in the World, who confers dreams; also in Kabala, she is Torah itself, [2] as Malkuth, the most junior of the Ten Sephiroth of the Tree of Life.] She utters it while arguing

[1] The later version which is familiar to English-speakers retains strong elements which show just how difficult this was to do. A Mage named Merlin — practicioner of Persian magical arts — still figures in it as the source of the sword in the stone, which replaces the Spear. In the story of the Knights of the Round Table, as related by Thomas Mallory in the fifteenth century in *La Morte d'Arthur,* the Grail is tracked to the castle Corbenic, where three knights are invited into a chapel and are allowed to look upon the cup. It transforms into a vision of Christ (very much like *duraosa Haoma* to Zarathrustra, see p. 178), who administers the sacrament of Eucharist to them, which is, of course, a version of the *dron* ceremony (see page 179). The purest of the three, Galahad (believed to be the illegitimate son of Lancelot), is immediately consumed in rapture and dies in ecstasy, ascending into heaven. Perceval (Parsifal) survives, leaves the chapel, and enters a monastery where he dies two months later, having repented of his sins enough to join Galahad in heaven. Bors survives, remains pure and holy for the rest of his life, but returns to Camelot to tell his tale, so that others may learn from their quest. Lancelot, the fourth knight who completes the quest, has already undergone physical and spiritual penance en route to the chapel, but is barred from entering the chapel and actually looking upon the Grail due to his adulterous love of Queen Guinevere. (Like Moses, he is denied the promised land, but allowed proof of its existence.) Once they drank from the Grail, in other words, chances of avoiding instant translation into Heaven were somewhat less than 50%.

[2] In *Divine Invasion,* "the sefira that represents the Earth...the womb containing everything, [generating] all the other sefiroth that constitute the Tree itself...[the] nine of them. . .even Kether, who is highest." (pg. 192). God can do nothing without consulting her, because she is Torah, which is "alive...a living being that thinks...the plan of the universe, its blueprint...
"In the Zohar," Malkuth said "the Torah is depicted as a beautiful maiden living alone, secluded in a great castle. Her secret lover comes to the castle to see her, but all he can do is wait futilely outside hoping for a glimpse of her. Finally, she appears at the window and he is able to catch sight of her, but only for an instant. Later on she lingers at the window and he is able, therefore, to speak with her, yet, still, she hides her face behind a veil....and her answers to his questions are evasive. Finally, after a long time, when her lover has become despairing that he will ever get to know her, she permits him to see her face at last." (*Divine Invasion,* p. 191) "Torah is the totality of divine disclosure by God; it is alive; it existed before creation. It is a mystic, almost cosmic, entity. The Torah is the Creator's instrument. With it he created the universe and for it he created the universe. It is the highest idea and the living soul of the world. Without it the world could not exist and would have no right to exist" (*op. cit.,* p. 97).

that instead of Armageddon, God's contest with Evil ought to be played out in each individual, with each being able to choose between the Adversary or one's Advocate.[1]

This put Dana in mind of Sophia's words as a child, reprinted on p. 124 of this Report: *"Now you have a companion who never sickens, or fails, or dies; you are bonded to the Eternal...*

1 Thousands of years ago, she said, she had been Ma'at, the Egyptian goddess who represented the cosmic order and justice. When someone died his heart was weighed against Ma'at's ostrich feather. By this the person's burden of sins was determined.

The principle by which the sinfulness of the person was determined consisted of the degree of his truthfulness. To the extent that he was truthful the judgment went in his favor. This judgement was presided over by Osiris, but since Ma'at was the goddess of truthfulness, it followed that the determination was hers to make.

"After that," Zina said, "the idea of the judgment of human souls passed over into Persia." In the ancient Persian religion, Zoroastrianism, a sifting bridge had to be crossed by the newly dead person. If he was evil the bridge [vs. tunnel on iboga] got narrower and narrower until he toppled off and plunged into the fiery pit of hell. Judaism in its later stages and Christianity had gotten their ideas of the Final Days from this.

The good person, who managed to cross the sifting bridge, was met by the spirit of his religion: a beautiful young woman with superb, large breasts. However, if the person was evil the spirit of his religion consisted of a dried-up old hag with sagging paps. You could tell at a glance, therefore, which category you belonged to...

In these judgments of the dead, stemming from Egypt and Persia, the scrutiny was pitiless and the sinful soul was de facto doomed. Upon your death the books listing your good deeds and bad deeds closed, and no one, even the gods, could alter the tabulation. In a sense, the procedure of judgment was mechanical. A bill of particulars, in essence, had been drawn up against you, compiled during your lifetime, and now this bill of particulars was fed into a mechanism of retribution. Once the mechanism received the list, it was all over for you. The mechanism ground you to shreds, and the gods merely watched, impassively.

But one day a new figure made its appearance at the path leading to the sifting bridge. This was an enigmatic figure who seemed to consist of a shifting succession of aspects or roles. Sometimes he was called Comforter. Sometimes Advocate. Sometimes Beside-helper. Sometimes Advisor. No one knew where he had come from. For thousands of years he had not been there, and then one day he had appeared. He stood at the edge of the busy path, and as the souls made their way to the sifting bridge this complex figure — who sometimes, but rarely, seemed to be a woman — signaled to the persons, each in turn, to attract their attention. It was essential that the Beside-helper get their attention before they stepped onto the sifting bridge, because after that it was too late.

"Too late for what?" Emmanuel said.

Zina said, "The Beside-helper upon stopping a person approaching the sifting bridge asked him if he wished to be represented in the testing which was to come."

"By the Beside-Helper?"

The Beside-Helper, she explained, assumed his role of Advocate, he offered to speak on the person's behalf. But the Beside-Helper offered something more. He offered to present his own bill of particulars to the retribution mechanism in place of the bill of particulars of the person. If the person were innocent this would make no difference, but, for the guilty, it would yield up a sentence of exculpation rather than guilt.

"That's not fair," Emmanuel said. "The guilty should be punished."

"Why?" Zina said.

"Because it is the law, "Emmanuel said.

"Then there is no hope for the guilty."

Emmanuel said, "They deserve no hope."

"What if everyone is guilty?"

He had not thought of that. "What does the Beside-Helper's bill of particulars list?" he asked.

"It is blank," Zina said. "A perfectly white piece of paper. A document on which nothing is inscribed."

"The retributive machinery could not process that."

Zina said, "It would process it. It would imagine that it had received a compilation of a totally spotless person."

"But it couldn't act. It would have no input data."

"That's the whole point."

"Then the machinery of justice has been bilked."

"Bilked out of a victim," Zina said. "Is that not to be desired? Should there be victims? What is gained if there is an unending procession of victims? Does that right the wrongs they have committed?"

"No," he said.

"The idea," Zina said, "is to feed mercy into the circuit. The Beside-Helper is an amicus curiae, a friend of the court. He advises the court, by its permission, that the case before it constitutes an exception. The general rule of punishment does not apply."

"And he does this for everyone? Every guilty person?"

"For every guilty person who accepts his offer of advocacy and help."

"But then you'd have an endless procession of exceptions. Because no guilty person in his right mind would reject such an offer; every single guilty person would wish to be judged as an exception, a case involving mitigating circumstances."

Zina said, "But the person would have to accept the fact that he was, on his own, guilty. He could of course wager that he was innocent, in which case he would not need the advocacy of the Beside-Helper."

After a moment of pondering, Emmanuel said, "That would be a foolish choice. He might be wrong. And he loses nothing by accepting the assistance of the Beside-Helper."

"In practice, however," Zina said, "most souls about to be judged reject the offer of advocacy by the Beside-Helper."

"On what basis?" He could not fathom their reasoning.

Zina said, "On the basis that they are sure they are innocent. To receive this help the person must go with the pessimistic assumption that he is guilty, even though his own assessment of himself is one of innocence. The truly innocent need no Beside-Helper, just as the physically healthy need no physician. In a situation of this kind the optimistic assumption is perilous. It's the bail-out theorem that little creatures employ when they construct a burrow. If they are wise they build a second exit to the burrow, operating on the pessimistic assumption that the first one will be found by a predator. All creatures who did not use their theorem are no longer with us."

Emmanuel said, "It is degrading to a man that he must consider himself sinful."

"It's degrading to a gopher to have to admit that his burrow may not be perfectly built, that a predator may find it."

"You are talking about an adversary situation. Is divine justice an adversary situation? Is there a prosecutor?"

"Yes, there is a prosecutor of man in the divine court; is is Satan. There is the Advocate who defends the accused human, and Satan who impugns and indicts him. The Advocate, standing beside the man, defends him and speaks for him; Satan, confronting the man, accuses him. Would you wish man to have an accuser and not a defender? Would that seem just?"

"But innocence must be presumed."

The girl's eyes gleamed. "Precisely the point made by the Advocate in each trial that takes place. Hence he substitutes his own blameless record for that of his client, and justifies the man by surrogation."

"Are you this Beside-Helper?" Emmanuel asked.

"No," she said. "He is a far more puzzling figure than I. If you are having difficulty with me, in determining—"

"I am," Emmanuel said.

"He is a latecomer into this world," Zina said, "Not found in earlier aeons. He represents an evolution in the divine strategy. One by which the primordial damage is repaired. One of many, but a main one."

"Will I ever encounter him?'

"You will not be judged," Zina said. "So perhaps not. But all humans will see him standing by the busy road, offering his help. Offering it in time—before the person starts across the shifting bridge and is judged. The Beside-Helper's intervention always comes in time. It is part of his nature to be there soon enough."

Emmanuel said, "I would like to meet him."

"Follow the travel pattern of any human," Zina said, "and you will arrive at the point where that human encounters him. That is how I know about him. I, too, am not judged." (P. K.Dick, *The Divine Invasion,* pp. 126–30)

"Every man has an Advocate and an Accuser. In Hebrew, for the Israelites of antiquity, *yetzer ha-tov* was the Advocate and *yetzer ha-ra* was the Accuser." (Dick, *op. cit.,* pp. 231–32)

(*VALIS*, p. 199). Not only is this guardian-spirit (or Bwiti) idea another characteristic common both to Bwiti and ancient Gnosticism, the storyline of *Divine Invasion* ends with one more twist signaling Dick's own indentification of Sophia, the Divine Logos, with the Secret Sacrament. In the end, survival of the righteous Herb Asher is ensured through a microsecond of contact by his own guardian spirit with the Adversary — death.

The best evidence that the wafer in the Grail was an Ibogaine-like substance is *psychopharmaceutical.* The real McCoy, if the Grail myth is any guide, not only gives access to the Near Death realm; it zaps destructive reflexes at the moment of penetration into the dreamtime. Or in Bwiti terms, cerebellar reset occurs in the instant of the splitting of the skull. [Neuroscientists would in fact employ EEGs and MRIs to discern whether a distinct but minute interval of cessation occurs when the new brain wave takes over from the old. *See p. 209.*]

Suddenly Dana realized the oscillating sensation Nico and others felt leading up to the "splitting of the skull" is precisely how the vestibular sense — balance — should register the rhythmic bursting of "new" wave activity as the Ibogaine effect built up.

He called Mark Molliver from Hamburg and asked him about the sense that enables us to feel it, even with eyes closed, when the jet we're on levels off. The vestibular sense registers movement on three planes, Mark reminded him, via three semicircular canals in the inner ear. Projections from these receptor-sites lead directly into the vermis of the cerebellum — the area where Molliver had shown Ibogaine activity in rats. This area controls the anti-gravity muscles, which are completely incapacitated by Ibogaine ataxia. Also, because these projections in the vermis extend to the vestibular nuclei in the brainstem, which are adjacent to nausea centers, disoriention of this sense results in *motion sickness* (or Ibogaine nausea.)

Georg Behr, whose theory had always focused more on Ibogaine reset of the opiate receptors, felt that the demise of Nicola K., who was a German, had put a hold on further human research in Europe for the time being. In fact, the Dutch methadone faction was propagating the notion of persistent sensitivity to heroin after Ibogaine — acute sensitivity that might potentiate an overdose months afterward.

"But heroin overdose typically occurs with the first use after abstinence," Dana objected. "And Ibogaine's effect resembles prolonged abstinence. That's not hypersensitivity."

Even more compelling evidence that ancient Gnostic religions shared an Ibogaine-like sacrament, though, was waiting when Dana got back from Germany — *Haoma and Harmaline, The Botanical Identity of the Indo-Iranian Sacred Hallucinogen "Soma" and its Legacy in Religion, Language and Middle Eastern Folklore.*[1] According to Flattery and Schwartz, the *soma* of the Vedas and Zoroaster — and therefore of Daniel in Babylon — was

[1] Published by the University of California Press, Berkeley, in *Near Eastern Studies,* Volume 21, in 1989. See Appendix 4, p. 258.

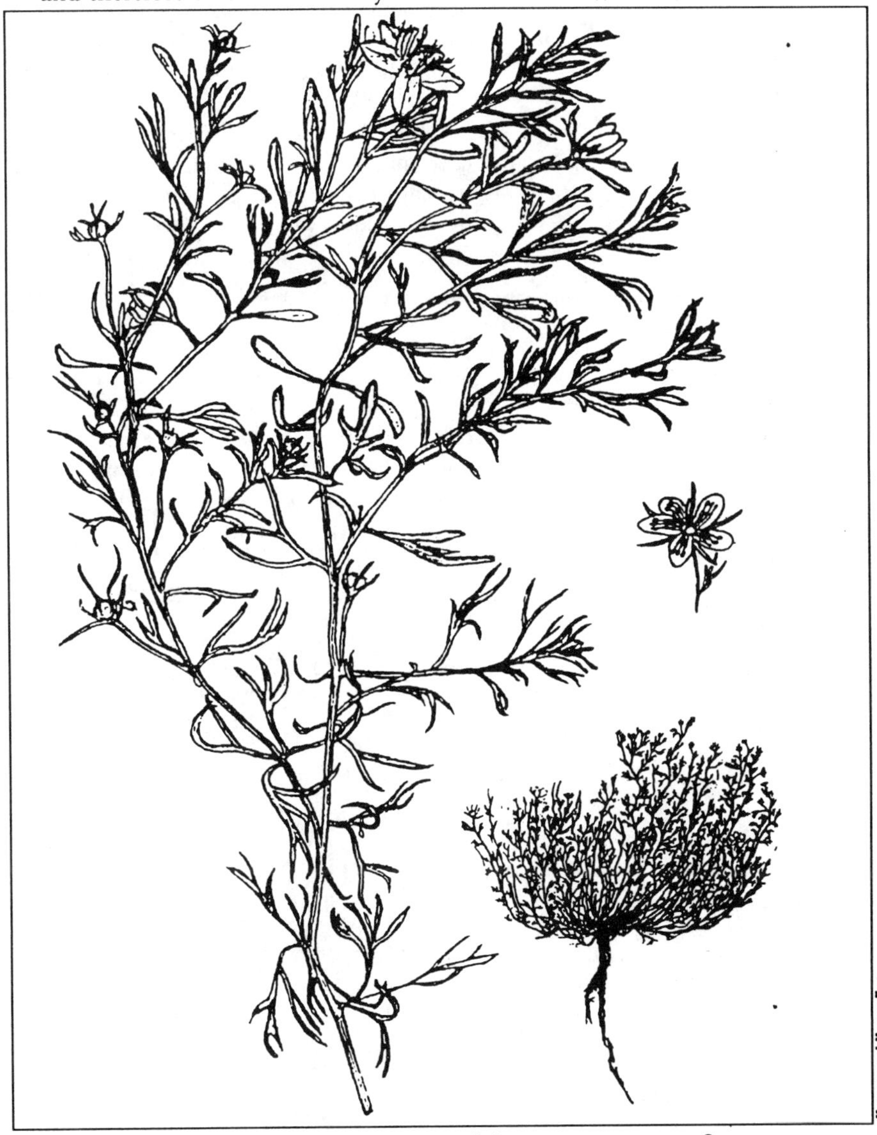

Haoma and Harmaline

"The little white flower by the side of the road," *Peganum harmala, a.k.a.* Syrian wild rue

haoma, an extract of the seed or root of *Peganum harmala.* In a word, harmaline.

Sure enough, at lower doses (the first cup) it initially causes insomnia, and instills excessive bravery. A second cup re-doubles strength, and numbs pain. And with the third cup, full onset, like Ibogaine, *apparently causes sleep* but actually induces a very similar sort of waking dream. One peculiar feature of this is "two-world superimposition" since — writes Flattery, quoting Claudio Naranjo — "when the eyes are opened, there is no distortion of ordinary vision and, though the visions are sometimes superimposed, there is little confusion between what is visionary and what is real" (§42).[1]

[1] See Appendix 4, pp. 258–339. All references given by paragraph (§) numbers.

> The oldest Persian religious texts show that sauma brought about a condition outwardly resembling sleep (i.e., *stard*) in which visions of what were believed to be a spirit existence were seen... the source of revelation in Iranian religion." (§34) "This 'spiritual' existence... differs from the conception of the spirtual realm in other Near Eastern religions in being neither morally superior nor necessarily more sacred than the material world.... [God] does not... create material existence directly, but first creates it in spiritual form. All material things... exist simultaneously in spirit form..." (§30) "The consumption of sauma may have been the only means recognized in Iranian religion for seeing into *menog* [Mid. Pers., "spiritual"] existence before death;... and... the means used by [God] when he wishes to make the menog existence visible to living persons." (§31)

The revelations of Zoroaster himself were said to have occurred because of consumption

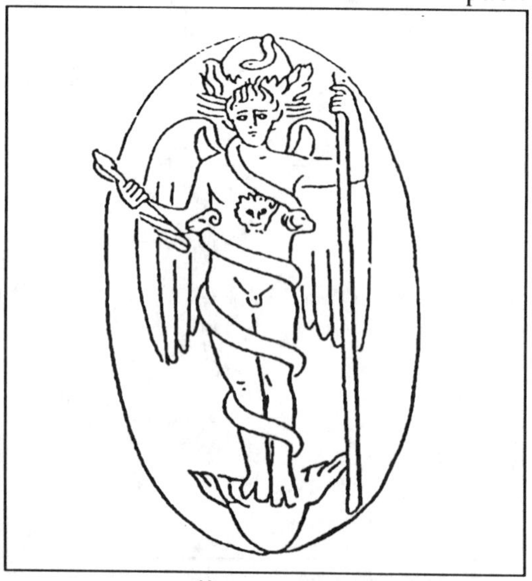
H.-G. Behr Collection

MITHRAS, SAVIOR

of "liquid omniscient wisdom," and became the state religion after God caused the King, Wishtasp, to consume *sauma,* or *haoma,* also. "Haoma" is used at once for the plant, the drink prepared from it, and the personification of the plant. In the *Hom Yasht* "the righteous *duraosa Haoma*" appears to Zoroaster as a luminous, beautiful man who cries out — "Take me... extract me that I may be drunk, praise me with might, as the other *saosyants* (saviors) have praised me... Thus spake Zarathustra: "Praise be to Haoma!" (§91)

This idea of a succession of saviors wresting salvation for their people from the dreamtime via harmel persisted in Persian lands for millenia. When Hellenic influence was expelled by the Sassanids (c. 200 A.D.), for instance, "there were sedition and contention among the people.... And doctrines of many kinds and different manners of faith, and skepticism and different legislations appeared... (in conformity) with diverging... faiths... Religion was in confusion and people in doubt." (§24) In accordance with ancient custom, a certain Wiraz, the most righteous among them, was chosen by council and confirmed by lot (!) Afterwards the Magians filled three cups with wine and the *mang* [*Mid. Pers.,* "drug"] of Wishtasp. Wiraz drank all three, said grace, and fell asleep on the blanket. When he arose he ate and dictated his visions to a scribe.

Flattery and Schwartz feel Zoroastrians were clearly trying to promote their authority to decide religious doctrine by invoking a folkloric legitimacy *haoma* had already possessed since ancient-most times in Iran, where harmala seeds are still burned as an incense and worn like garlic in charms that supposedly ward off noxious influences.

The Western Mithras of Roman times was even closer to the original religion that Zoroaster re-formed in Persia, [which still celebrates *Mihragan* (the Mithras-day sacrifice) by burning actual harmala seeds as *hom.*[2] (§115)]. Zoroaster himself was said to have been been conceived due to the legendary aphrodisiac effect of harmala (§93), which made it an appropriate sacrament for Mithras, a fertility god whose death and rebirth were said to cause the seasons. Mithras' spread through the Roman Empire corresponds

[2] *Hom* was a designation extending to any plant commonly used in the preparation of *soma.*

roughly with the time Flattery gives (§52) for introduction of *Peganum harmala* around the Mediterranean. According to Hans-Georg Behr, the application to build the first Mithras Temple in Rome (15 B.C.) specified its use for consumption of sacraments.

In short, it seems Mithras was another *soma* cult, complete with dim grottos to facilitate harmaline visualizations. Even if harmala hadn't been the sacrament of the early Christians' competition, its notorious power to inspire sexual lust as well as a notation in Plutarch about its use by the followers of *Ahriman* [Satan] certainly damned it for Aquinas and the Scholastics.

Soma (*lit.* "liquid extract") was properly identified as early as 1794 by Sir William Jones, as originally pressed from harmel, or wild Syrian rue (See exhibit, p. 295 — Flattery, §157). So how could Bishop Pike et al., who also believed it was used in the Mysteries at Eleusis and by the Delphic Oracle of Apollo, think *soma* was a mushroom? How could they have been so far off?

The answer is that in both Persia and India, in perhaps the earliest instance of harm reduction, for ordinary sacramental use (as in the wine and the wafer of Christianity), the principal constituent of *soma* was replaced with non-psychoactive equivalents or denatured substitutes like cannabis and *ephedra*.

From earliest Indo-Iranian times, according to Flattery (§115–§116), the priesthood had spiked their harmala extract with ephedra [plant adrenaline] to keep from passing out during the visions. Because of "sensitive dependence on initial conditions," the ephedrine gave the resulting visions the strongly dualistic quality characteristic of Zoroastrianism, Mithras, etc., and contributed to the break-up of the proto-Indo-Iranian religion in the war of the followers of *Ahura* [God] and the *devs*, the Hindu pantheon.[1] So even when harmala was still in use, it was an ordeal reserved for extraordinary circumstances. And it was a taboo subject.

When Islam came in, fundamentally hostile to any drug as the key to revelation (although the Shia soon adopted the burning of harmel seeds as an incense of superior holiness), Zoroastrians successfully concealed the identity of *Haoma*. *Hawrm-al-Majus* ("Harmel of the Magi") is a different plant, a decoy. As *soma*, for sacramental use with *dron* bread (i.e., the wine and wafer), they had long since substituted an extract that kept the additive ephedra (called *hom*), combined with ordinary, non-psychoactive garden rue (which did not resist cultivation like harmala), plus a sprig of pomegranate (whose fruit resembles a giant harmel seed-pod) on the *dron* bread — thereby invoking haoma magically, in name and image.[2]

The antiquity of the pomegranate symbolism, moreover, puts to rest the queries of Bishop Pike et al. In *Bullfinch's Mythology*, after Pluto spirits Proserpine, daughter of Ceres, Earth-mother, away to the land of the dead by striking the riverbank with his staff (the "split-

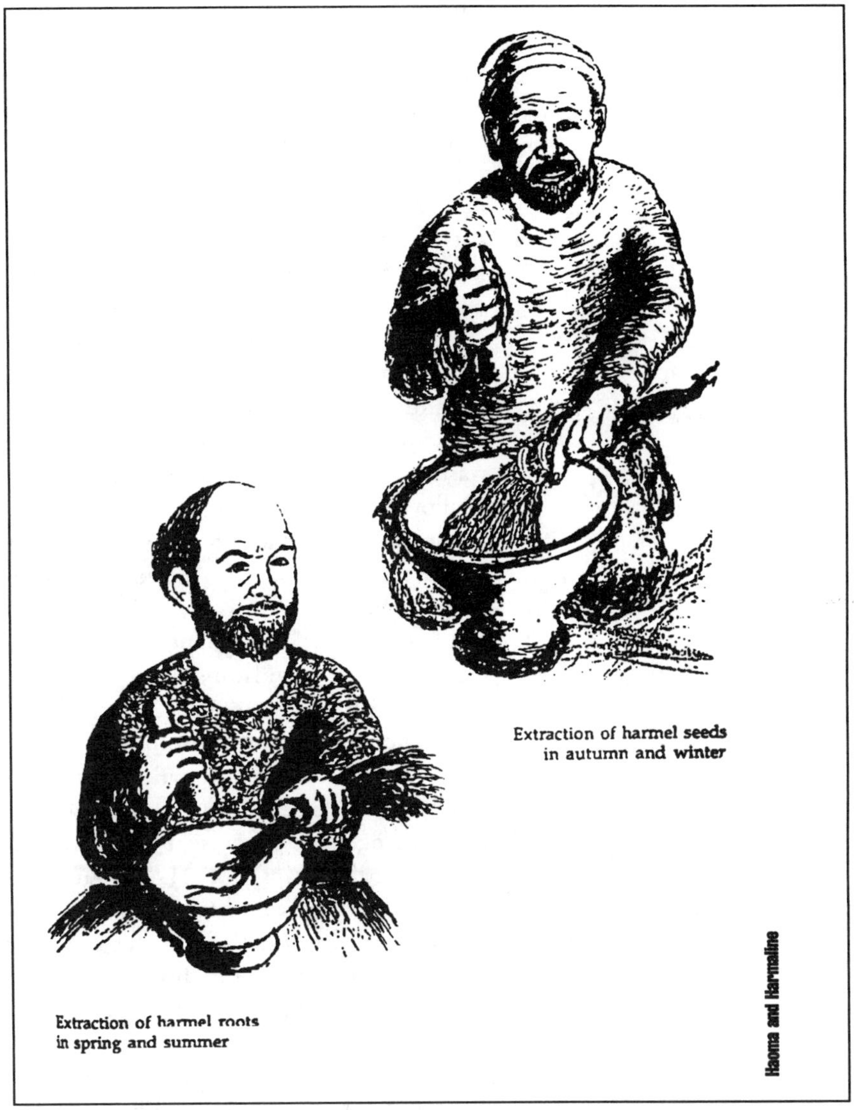
Extraction of harmel seeds
in autumn and winter
Extraction of harmel roots
in spring and summer
Haoma and Harmaline

PREPARATION OF SOMA, FROM FLATTERY AND SCHWARTZ (SEE APPENDIX FOUR).

[1] Indigenous peoples later discovered that tryptamine-bearing biologicals (i.e., mushrooms) could be substituted for ephedra with superior results. See Flattery, §154, note 5.

[2] Having assured themselves by magical means (e.g.: the trip of Wiraz) that for purposes of magic it worked just as well. "In neither tradition is the ceremony conducted with an open acknowledgement that the plant regularly used as soma or haoma is not one originally used, or that the character of the rite was ever markedly different from what it is now. The respective secondary literatures of commentary and interpretation virtually ignore the absence of the intoxication indicated by the liturgical texts." (Flattery and Schwartz, p. 259)

ting of the skull" again), she is able to return only half of each year because she ate of the pomegranate[!] The provenance of this story antedates Rome and Greece; it is Minoan, and reappears in the maze of the Minotaur. It is evidence that the bull-worshipping culture destroyed by the barbaric Greek invaders was survived by a *soma* cult which was able — by keeping harmala a mystery — to market its oracular services to the Achaean newcomers.

An Iranian folk medicine is still prepared by grinding the bitter seeds or roots into powder and boiling it in vinegar, which extracts 98 per cent of the harmala alkaloids. As a mouthwash, it numbs a toothache, but an accidental swallow can cause visions (§43, note 1), which are deliberately induced only to treat maladies where all else has failed. Also known to promote rapid healing of the skin, it is still employed as a folk medicine by the Gnostic baptists called Mandaeans, who preach that John the Baptist, not Jesus, was the Messiah.

"There is good reason to believe that the heirs of these Nazareans," writes Schonfield, "though time and circumstances have wrought many changes, are the present Nazoreans (also known as Mandaeans) of the Lower Euphrates. Their literature reveals that they came formerly from northern Palestine, to which area they had migrated from Judea because of Jewish persecution.... The Jews regarded northern Palestine as the natural home of heresy....We do not know so much about the old Israelite religion, but it would appear to have absorbed a good deal from the worship of the Syrians and Phoenicians... More of the older faith was carried down as folklore and in the ideas and usages of clans and sects which were active in the time of Christ."[1]

[1] *The Passover Plot*, pp. 200–202.

Flattery provides a vivid example of this: the Mandaean *"Scroll of the Wild Rue,"* which is not canonical, but "magical." It survives "wholly for the purpose of furthering the effectiveness of the spirit of harmel in a specific situation, that of purging someone of sickness... Wisdom or knowledge is not among the benefits sought, nor is intoxication... An unusual feature... is the use of the names, haoma and sambra respectively, at once for the plant, the drink prepared from it, and the personification of the plant.... Since the personification of Sambra as a deity is unknown elsewhere in Manadean writing, its appearance... may represent a borrowing... directly of the Avestan [Zoroastrian] *Hom Yasht*... [or] similar early Iranian invocation of sauma" of which *Sambra* is the Mandaean persona:

> "O Sambra, go below like water which gusheth from the peak of a high mountain. The Lady of Gods and Men took thee and carried thee off to the male gods and the female astartes, and she gave favorable testimony concerning thee. And they sent (it) to everyone that was ill, working a cure, and healing was found in it. Thou didst spring forth of thine own strength, and didst come forth and camest into being."
>
> (*Haoma and Harmaline,* §82)

The scroll continues with a plea for "a cure that will free" the one taking the Sambra. But present-day Mandaeans are unflinchingly monotheistic, repudiating Christ's divinity — so Wisdom (but not healing) would presumably be the province of the Holy Spirit. Schonfield writes that "...the indispensable condition of membership [in the Essenes / Nazoreans / Mandaeans] was absolute faithfulness to the Laws of God delivered to Moses." He adds that Jesus' "brother Jacob, who became head of the Nazoreans at Jerusalem, was a typical Essene sectarian.... He... prayed constantly in the Temple for the forgiveness of the people...."

> "We have every reason to hold that the family to which Jesus belonged was nurtured in this tradition, and much of his teaching confirms this. But his reading of his messianic mission led him in many matters to turn his back on it, which may well have been a cause of friction with his family. He associated freely with the people, even with the worst of them, and would have nothing to do with a Nazairite or regulated way of life. 'The Son of Man came eating and drinking, and they say, Behold a man gluttonous and a winebibbler, a friend of publicans and sinners.' He relaxed the rigid Sabbath observance, and held that nothing which enters a man's mouth defiles him. *He taught that all secrets (so dear to 'the Saints') were to be revealed, and that what was whispered in the ear should be proclaimed from the housetops.* No wonder, therefore, that in the Mandaean literature he is stigmatised as a false Messiah. But as Jesus said, ***'Wisdom is justified of her children.'***
>
> (*The Passover Plot,* pp. 204–205)

Now the only key left to nailing down the solution of the Resurrection mystery, Dana realized, was the degree to which harmaline reliably reproduces certain Ibogaine-like effects — including precognition, numbness of the extremities, and any tendency to induce an out-of-body experience, including techniques or special circumstances needed to reproduce the full Near Death Experience (NDE).

By ancient usage, no other substance present in Antiquity could have been deemed appropriate — in that place, in that time — for such a purpose. Only soma *was holy enough. Only harmaline would work. And if, as Schonfield speculates, use of "vinegar and gall" was in fact suggested to Jesus by the words of Psalm* LXIX, *line 21, the vinegar extract of harmala seeds still prepared by modern-day Mandaeans may have been "included in the recipe," according to Essene Gnosis, from the Beginning.*

A week later, across the continent at the Esalen Institute in California, during a conference on recent medical advances with psychedelics, Deborah Mash came upon Anne Shulgin, sitting outside one of the presentations, who asked:

"Aren't you the Dr. Deborah Mash who's working with Ibogaine at the University of Miami?"

"Yes, I am. Why?"

"Make sure you get all your subjects to agree to *come back* before you give them Ibogaine."

Anne proceeded to recount the anecdote at the end of Chapter 14 of this report[1] — about the fellow who went through death's door for three minutes, only to come to and sit up on the cot as medics were rushing emergency equipment into the room.

But by the time of that Esalen conference, Dana and Mark Molliver had already gotten together in person. They had a meeting with Peter Beilenson, head of the Baltimore Health Department, on enlisting Baltimore Mayor Kurt Schmoke to the cause of medications development. Beilenson had one question: "Is it real?" "Very promising," said Mark. Dr. Beilenson, who was impressed by the promise of research dollars for Baltimore, promised to get back with a response from Schmoke.

Afterwards, in the car, Molliver remarked that the cerebellum generates wave activity for the entire brain — but the inferior olive generates the brainwave of the cerebellum. It's reasonable, he agreed, that the cerebellum (which constantly models a somatic image of the body in three-dimensional space) might initially register Ibogaine activity in the olive as a sensation of *the room* oscillating.

With Ibogaine firing ten bursts a second in the olive, however, when the Ibogaine effect becomes strong enough, might not the new wave activity *heterodyne* with pre-existing

[1] See p. 149.

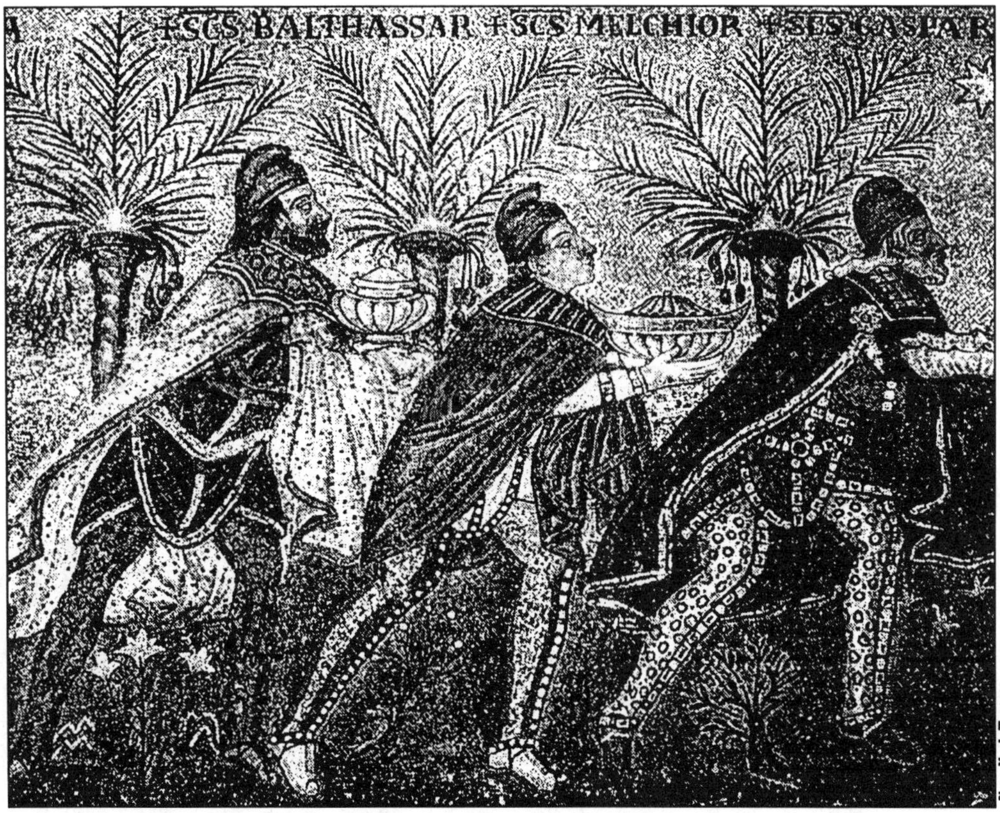

New York Times

The Magi: Did they bring the recipe for the Resurrection? The record has been censored: "It took several hundred years for Matthew's 'wise men' to become the three kings Melchior, Caspar and Balthazar....But by the early sixth century, when what had begun as a persecuted Jewsih sect had metamorphosed into the official faith of the Roman Empire, the whole world suddenly reached unanimity on the number and identity of Jesus' first visitors. Emperor Justinian I, ruling from Byzantium (now Istanbul) — the Goths had long since sacked Rome — had Nativity mosaics installed in the main basilicas in Ravenna, Italy, and Bethlehem. Justinian's mosaics reveal just how closely entwined religion and imperial politics had become: depictions of the birth of a divine child were used to establish Roman orthodox dogma over the heretical Arianism of Ravenna's old rulers (which denied the divinity of Christ). These mosaics not only 'revealed' for the first time the names and ages of the three kings but also clearly showed them wearing traditional Persian clothes." Secret Lives of the Wise Men, Paul William Roberts, *New York Times* op. ed., Dec. 25, 1995.

brain-waves, engendering the "splitting of the skull?" The kicker, according to Molliver, was that earlier researchers felt harmaline also, in some fashion, reset brainwaves. Dana asked if harmala alkaloids in high doses happened to cause numbness of hands and feet, like *iboga* does. Mark said he would try to find out.

Molliver's real news, though, was that he was finding no toxicity in primates. In fact, he was giving 150 mg.-per-kg. orally, and nothing much was happening to his monkeys at all. He and O'Hearn were checking to see if the Ibogaine was bio-available — if it was getting into the blood in the proper chemical form. Meanwhile, to duplicate in monkeys the Ibogaine ataxia seen in humans, they were having to inject 50 mgs.-per-kg. interperitoneally (in the gut). A double-dose. Only later did Linda Aronhoff let drop in a conversation that some monkeys were having seizures with their injections.

Linda Aronhoff was all agog with a speech Bob Sisko had just made at the NIDA Advisory Committee. In it he reiterated that ICASH is not anti-drug:

> "We are pro-choice. We believe it is the right of the individual to self-medicate. We recognize however, that when an individual becomes addicted to drugs, he or she no longer has freedom of choice. We believe any person addicted to drugs who wishes to be free from that addiction should be able to have that choice...
>
> "We applaud NIDA's efforts to create a wide range of new cocaine analogs. I am especially excited to hear you are working on a cocaine analog with a longer duration of action. One of the main problems from cocaine use is that the effects of coke are so short-lived. Addicts must use continually in order to maintain the high. I predict that a potent new long-lasting analog would be popular among addicts, but might quickly end up on the streets, where it could be used as "cut," mixed in with cocaine to make the high longer-lasting. After all, the same illicit chemists who currently manufacture both powder and crack cocaine by the ton could easily manufacture NIDA's new cocaine analog as well.
>
> "Next to the idea of across-the-board legalization, the idea of developing a new stimulant compound that could be used as a medication for cocaine dependent people, much like methadone is used for heroin addiction, is probably the most radical idea around..."

He went on to say that NIDA's conceptual frame-work — all agonists, antagonists — shows they still have not really accepted the idea of the addiction *interrupter*. What, he asked, about people who don't do well on stimulants as maintenance drugs? What about people who want to *quit* drugs?

Kurt Schmoke, meanwhile, sent word that we were already in perfect agreement about medications development. Peter Beilenson did say Schmoke could be counted upon to take a public stand and lobby Congress for increased appropriations. In *Rolling Stone*, after calling for a national commission to re-think drug policy, and allocation of 65% of the drug budget for treatment instead of enforcement, he wrote:

> "Finally, as a third step, the federal government should increase its support of research into new treatments. For example, researchers at Johns Hopkins believe that finding a chemical to block cocaine craving is now possible. This kind of research requires strong backing from the federal government. The research is expensive. But it is an investment that is far more likely to produce successful results than building more prisons, trying to stop drugs at the border, arresting addicts or passing mandatory minimum sentences."
>
> — "Side Effects," Kurt Schmoke, *Rolling Stone*, May 7, 1994

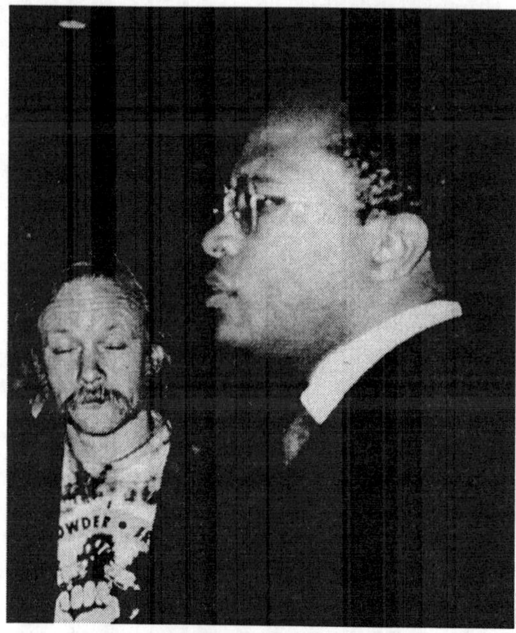

BLINDED BY THE FLASH:
KURT SCHMOKE SHMOOZES DPF CONFERENCE.

CHAPTER 17: Cures Not Wars

In February, 1994, Robert Rygor died. He was a beneficiary of the free pot program, and — as facilitator of the ACT UP Coordinating Commitee, which set the agenda for the Monday night meeting — helped make sure Ibogaine got a fair shake. His death was a direct loss. But more ominous was that during the entire hour-plus obituary at the next ACT UP meeting, facilitator Scott Sawyer (of the regular leadership) refused to call on Beal, pointedly denying him the legitimacy of thanking Robert for so often negotiating behind the scenes for the bubble of tolerance that enabled Ibogaine to go forward.

A few weeks later Dana was in Philadelphia, relating the remnants of the problem to Kiyoshi Kuromiya. Kiyoshi was co-author of Buckminster Fuller's last book *Critical Path,* and edits a journal of the same name, devoted to AIDS. Dana was going over the implications of the re-discovery of Gnostic substances: *mind over immune-system.* "Miraculous healing, true prophecy, liberation from destructive reflex ("sin"), victory over death — Ibogaine reliably, and harmaline if used correctly, provide a version of all of them. The NDE is the key to all four. By means of the dreamtime, we gain a different access to time itself."

This prompted Kiyoshi to recount his own experiments with lucid dreaming, in which he wrote down the location of a shoe store five years *before* it changed into a shoe store from a diner.

"That's the trouble," Dana mused, "You may end up in a stretch of the future that's totally boring — that tells you very little. The Essenes solved this problem by sending thousands of random observers up ahead to map things out — mass invasion of the future.

"*They foresaw the Fall of the Temple* — and that there was no way to stop it. But in the process, they determined not only how to master additional techniques to replicate the NDE more precisely, but the exact circumstances in which, up ahead in the future, one might through this mastery intervene and reverse the outcome of History.

"We can now physically explain the crucifixion and resurrection," said Dana, "but we are still left with the problem of time. He promised *Torah* would conquer the whole world, and that Israel would be re-established thereby. But that's really an extremely long shot. How could they visualize, as early as 600 B.C., outcomes 2,600 years later, to be able to *set up* the Crucifixion?"

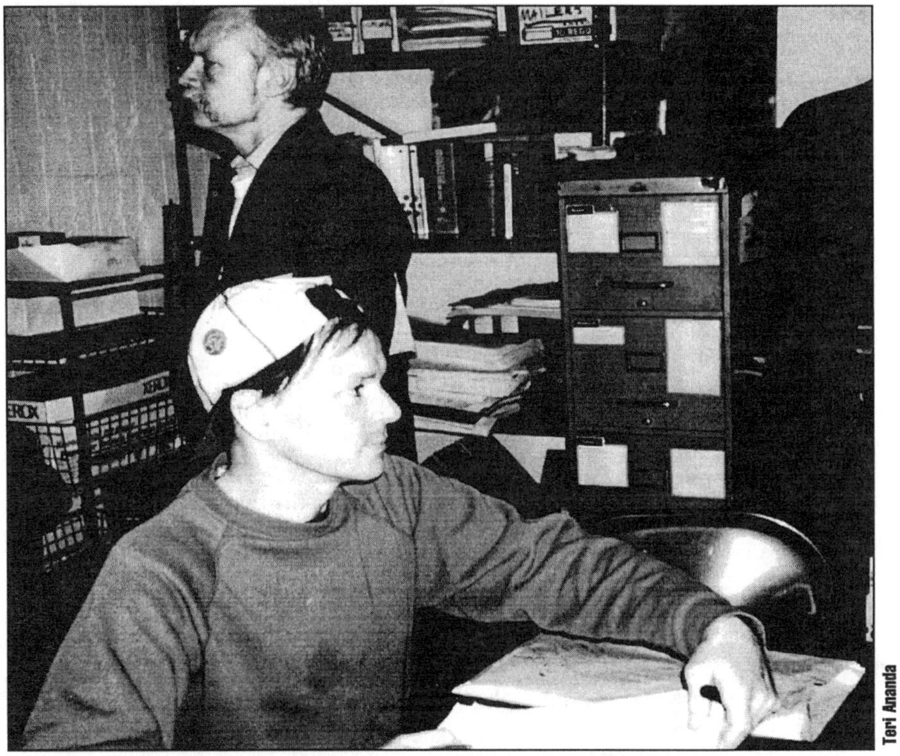

ROBERT RYGOR AND DANA BEAL AT THE OLD W. 29TH STREET ACT-UP WORKSPACE.

Kiyoshi volunteered an article from *The Scientific American,* which proposed that transmission of information from the future, at least, might not contradict quantum physics. In it, writers David Deutsch and Michael Lockwood discuss the fashioning of quantum-level "worm-holes" into "Closed Timelike Curves" (CTCs):

> "Does our universe now, or will it ever contain CTCs? We do not know, but there are various theoretical conjectures about how they might be formed. The mathematician Kurt Gödel found a solution to Einstein's equations that described CTCs. In that solution the whole universe rotates (according to current evidence, the actual universe does not). CTCs also appear in solutions of Einstein's

equations describing rotating black holes...

"A kind of shortcut through space-time, called a wormhole, has been mooted by Princeton University Physicist John A. Wheeler. Kip S. Thorne of the California Institute of Technology and others have shown how two ends of a wormhole could be moved so as to form a CTC. According to a recent calculation by J. Richard Gott of Princeton, a cosmic string (another theoretical construct that may or may not exist in nature) passing rapidly by another would generate CTCs... They may...become accessible to future civilizations..."

("The Quantum Physics of Time Travel," *Scientific American,* March, 1994, p. 70)

From the standpoint of expenditure of energy, transmission of information backward in time presents the fewest problems, and apparently no fundamental contradiction on the quantum level, allowing our world to be shunted orthogonally, at key decision-points, onto another track of the Multiverse.

"Do you realize what this means?" asked Dana. "If science can duplicate the Resurrection, the fall of the Papacy will be bigger than the collapse of the Soviet Union. The Gnostics were only trying to conceal the key to prophecy from the hated Empire. But after the fall of the Temple and exile of Israel, European Orthodoxy took over.[1] We got the Trinity and the Virgin Birth.

"The laws against psychedelic research represent the perpetuation, in secular law, of the original Ecclesiastical cover-up of the true circumstances of the Resurrection! Not only couldn't they allow anyone to know how it was done, they had to ban any investigation of plant substances that might lead to re-discovery of how it was done. That's why under Church law, any attempt to foretell the future was punishable as witchcraft. And nothing's changed! 'Drugs' is still the only taboo where government licenses militant religion — 12-step groups — to convert heretics forceably. I don't think ACT UP is ready for this."

Kiyoshi asked what he meant.

Dana went on. "ACT UP got in enough trouble for breaking the host at St. Pat's. For them to bring proofs that the wine and wafer are only stand-ins for the *real* sacraments repeats the same action on a vastly higher conceptual level — one reason I always felt the original St. Pat's action was like a *strange attractor* for Ibogaine.[2]

"Philip Dick has a scene in a Church where, as the priest dips the wafer in the consecrated wine saying, "The Blood of Our Lord Jesus Christ, which was shed for thee..," the Son of Man calls out from the back pews... '*The blood is not there nor the body either.'* — and when the Priest looks up to see who it is is, the child Emmanual says —***'You do not have the authority.'***[3]

"The Christians are going to freak out! I wonder if we'll get in as much trouble as Salmon Rushdie....

"So in a way it's unfair to involve ACT UP in this. They've already got their hands full finding a cure for AIDS."

Confrontation with the Christians came soon enough, in the form of the Philly Convention of Sue Rusche's PRIDE — Parent's Resource Institute for Drug Education. The Harm Reduction Working Group had set two spring actions — Philly, March 3–5, and New York, May 7 — hoping to derive some spin for the overall push against the Drug War. Gilbert Baker, in town from San Francisco to do a mile-long rainbow flag for Stonewall 25, came up with new spring slogan: *Cures not Wars.*

New York ACT UP also fired off a letter to one of Rusche's minions, the Drug Czar of Michigan, who'd circulated a letter characterizing ACT UP as part of the pot lobby. But the actual protest-date Philly ACT UP picked for the PRIDE zap was February 27. So it ended up as forty AIDS activists picketing Philly's Convention Center the weekend *before* the PRIDE Conference — when no one from PRIDE was even in town yet.

The harm reduction crew came back from Philly to find that Aldyn MacKean had died.

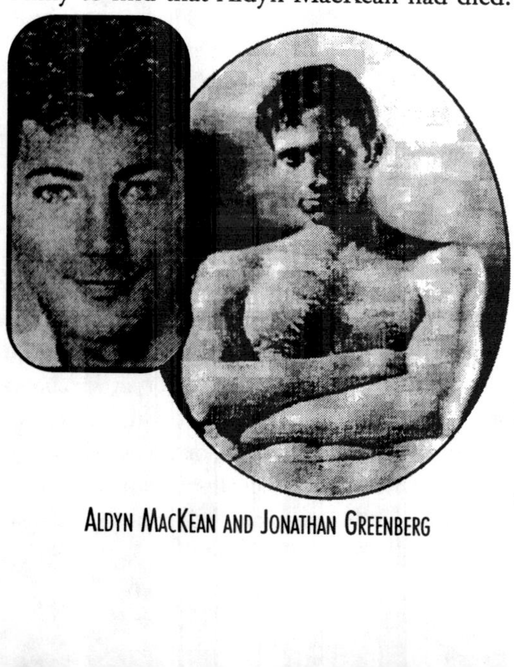

Newsday; ACT UP

ALDYN MACKEAN AND JONATHAN GREENBERG

1 For instance in the Gospel of Matthew, which is Peter's account, the whole end — i.e., Jesus after the Resurrection — consists of one paragraph. The book "Apocalypse of Peter" from the Nag Hammadi scrolls containes additional material, including a vision in which Peter sees Jesus apparently nailed to the cross and another Jesus floating above the cross — clearly a description of a near-death experience. The Orthodox went so far as to furnish the elderly Pharisee whose account forms the basis of the Book of John with a Greek scribe, called John the Younger, who was not John the Elder's original choice. See Schoenfield, *Those Incredible Christians.*

2 In one of ACT UP's first big actions, thousands of protestors besieged St. Patrick's Cathedral, and five persons actually got in and got their hands on sacramental wafer, which they either did or didn't crunch up into little bits, depending on who you believe.

3 *The Divine Invasion,* p. 71.

In the obituary, on the floor, Andy Velez and several others recounted a vision Aldyn had had when he was very sick in the hospital, before he recovered enough to come back to his last few ACT UP meetings. Jon Greenberg, another treatment activist who'd died a year earlier, had appeared beside Aldyn's bed, telling him that he was to be his guide, and not to worry. Interesting *kappa* opiate phenomenon, thought Dana, but he lay awake until late at night thinking about it —

> *"Now you have a companion who never sickens, or fails, or dies; you are bonded to the eternal, and will shine like the healing sun itself....*
>
> *"As you go back into the world I will guide you from day to day. And when you die I will notice and come to pick you up. I will carry you back to your home, out of which you come and back to which you go.*
>
> *"You are strangers here, but you are hardly strangers to me; I have known you from the start. This has not been your world, but I will make it your world; I will change it for you. Fear not. What assails you will perish and you will thrive."*
>
> (*VALIS*, pp. 199–200)

Interaction later that week with the actual PRIDE convention was limited to leafleting the kids with the most recent article from *OMNI* on Deborah Mash's work, together with a press conference denouncing PRIDE's very public campaign to keep Drug Czar Lee Brown from meeting with harm reduction advocates. The *Philadelphia Inquirer* printed ACT UP charges that meetings with Brown about Ibogaine research were on hold because of ACT UP's vocal endorsement of medical marijuana. This triggered off another support letter from ACT UP and a flurry of phonecalls to and from Lee Brown's office. No meeting ensued.

According to Howard Lotsof, every time Lee Brown and the politicians in ONDCP ask their experts about Ibogaine, they get advice to develop longer-acting cocaine analogs instead. More "methadone-like."

Right around April 1, 1994, however,[1] an independent Institute of Medicine panel chosen by the National Academy of Science published a preliminary report, *"Development of Anti-Addiction Medication,"* which endorsed virtually every ACT UP Harm Reduction demand, including accelerated approval, parallel track and physician-inititiated treatment INDs for new anti-addiction drugs, and tapping the Drug Forfeiture fund[2] to fully fund Medication Development up to the $95 million authorized — instead of the current $36 million.

In addition, the Institute of Medicine report identified DEA over-regulation as the principle source of unnecessary red tape. They recommended DEA review be folded into a one-step FDA/DEA approval process; and that Clinton sign an order giving Medication Development Presidential priority. Best of all, in the first paragraph on strategies for discovery of a cocaine medication (p. 33), the committee wrote:

> A medication developed for the treatment of drug addiction ideally is effective when administered orally or is able to be implanted, is long-acting, clinically safe, causes few side effects, is acceptable to patients, is designed to reduce both reinforcing and toxic effects of the addictive drug, has little abuse liability and is useful for more than one class of abused drugs (because many substance-abusers use more than one drug.)

This is impossible for any maintenance agonist, antagonist or mono-clonal antibody[3] currently under development to do, of course. Failure to come up with something that really works is the principle reason for "the absence [cited in the report] of a large, vocal advocacy group that would voice strong support and lobby for treatment funding and research"[4] — although criminalizing addicts certainly doesn't encourage activism, either.

Back in New York, Dana's working majority on the ACT UP floor was coming to an end. It started when the floor rejected, 12 to 11, adoption of "Cures Not Wars" as a new harm

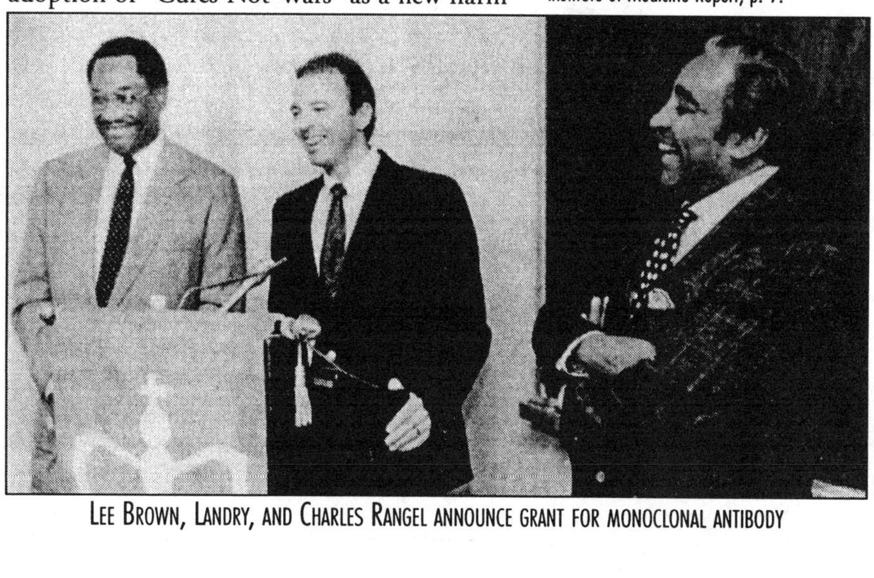

Columbia Spectator

LEE BROWN, LANDRY, AND CHARLES RANGEL ANNOUNCE GRANT FOR MONOCLONAL ANTIBODY

[1] Reported in the April 5, 1994 *Food Drug & Cosmetic Pink Sheet.*

[2] The ONDCP Special Forfeiture Fund results from the transfer of money from the Federal Asset Forfeiture Fund. In Fiscal Year 1990, the Federal Asset Forfeiture Fund transferred $117 million to federal law-enforcement agencies. Deposits of $17 million were also made to the Special Forfeiture Fund to supplement ONDCP program resources, with $115 million going to support federal prison construction. The use of the Special Forfeiture Fund is at the discretion of the director of ONDCP.

The Federal Asset Forfeiture Fund is a sum of money resulting from the sale of assets used in criminal activity that have been seized by the government. In 1990, the DEA seized assets valued at more than $1 billion. About two-fifths of the assets seized by the DEA was currency, valued at almost $364 million. In addition, the DEA seized $346 million worth of real property, 5,674 vechicles worth over $60 million, 187 vessels valued at over $16 million, and 51 airplanes worth over $25 million. Almost two-thirds of the DEA's seizures during 1990 resulted from cocaine investigations. DEA seizures that were ultimately forfeited are valued at more than $427 million for 1990. (See p. 3, "Executive Summary," *I.O.M. Report.*)

[3] Agonists are substitute drugs; antagonists, blockers; the monoclonal antibody (being developed by Landry, Columbia University) is supposed to break cocaine down once it gets into the body, into two inactive metabolites — except that one of the two may be somewhat toxic.

[4] Institute of Medicine Report, p. 9.

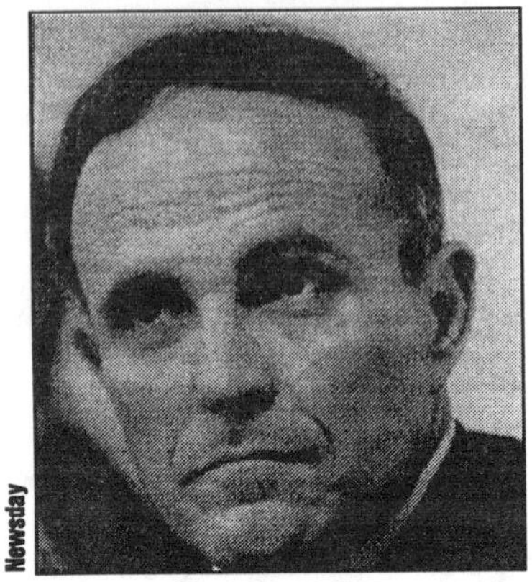

Newsday

GRIM KING III

UPON TAKING OFFICE, NEW YORK MAYOR RUDOLPH GIULIANI INITIATED A MASSIVE "QUALITY-OF-LIFE" CRACKDOWN ON MINOR CRIMES, INCLUDING PAN-HANDLING, SQUEEGIEING, STREET-PEDDLING, CARRYING A BEER *IN* A BAG, PUBLIC URINATION, ADULT SEX ESTABLISHMENTS, AND, OF COURSE, STEPPED-UP FRISKS FOR GUNS AND DRUGS — INCLUDING RELEASING UNIFORMED OFFICERS TO MAKE THEIR OWN DRUG ARRESTS (THROWING OUT A REFORM OF THE KNAPP COMMISSION) — AND A NEW SEVERITY IN HANDLING POLITICAL PROTESTS, WITH MILITARY-STYLE ASSAULTS ON SQUATTERS AND OTHERS, FEATURING USE OF A TANK.

reduction slogan. Then, just before the end of March, John Spacely died of AIDS. In an obituary, Dana bitterly recounted how John Spacely had asked for Ibogaine treatment in 1981, before he was probably even infected. He told the floor he understood perfectly the frustration of not being able to get people drugs in time to save their lives. Later in the evening, Dana and Dennis Peron got a healthy majority of ACT UP to back the annual Stop the Drug Wars Parade, as sponsor of one of two feeder rallies on May 7th.

Egged on by Dan Raymond, however, Donald Grove of the Lower East Side Needle Exchange flip-flopped and a week later turned against May 7th, after initially backing it. He attacked the whole idea of substituting non-injectable substances for heroin or cocaine, saying it wasn't legitimate AIDS-prevention, because it diverted energy from needle exchange. And he charged that the underlying premise of blanket de-criminalization of six plants — market separation of marijuana — stigmatized hard-drug users. Another faction passionately felt ACT UP should reject the move to safeguard medical marijuana access by expanding existing New York State de-crim to six plants — because it would mainly benefit drug users who didn't have AIDS.

This reaction blocked approval of all posters with ACT UP's name until half the lead-time for postering had been frittered away, and the Harm Reduction Coalition reluctantly announced it was going ahead anyway. The opponents of Ibogaine, miffed at being bypassed, pressed for a star chamber proceeding May 2nd facilitated by Amy Bauer, where Dana's character was dissected without his being able to answer allegations against him. During this proceeding, someone even charged that John Spacely didn't die of AIDS — that Dana had improperly taken up time under obituaries for a drug-overdose death.

Later in the evening it became clear that the AIDS Cure Project had enlisted the decisive votes with Donald Grove and the regular leadership in return for support for a full-page ad in the *New York Times*. It was supposed to cost New York ACT UP only $4,000 — but it ended up with the treasurers having to refuse to pay the *Times* the full $18,000, depriving ACT UP of any other ads in the *Times* ever again. A written notice of cancellation of the ad hadn't been sent in time. Bad luck.

Dana, on the other hand, was busily working on preparations for the Cures not

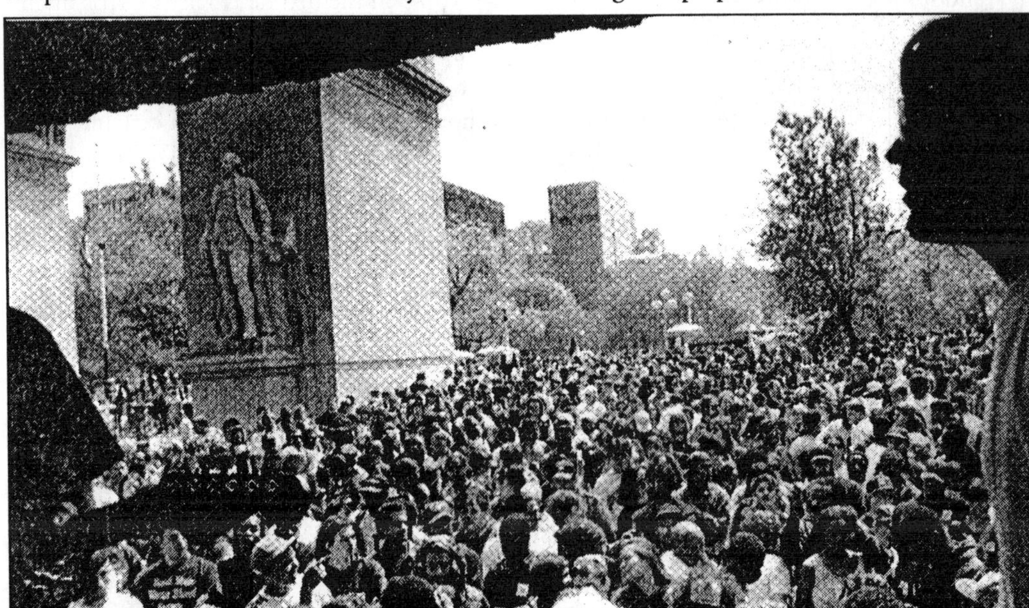

Dith Pran/The New York Times

Groups Join Together in Call for Legalized Drugs and Clean Needles

Crowds gathered in Washington Square Park to protest what they called Mayor Rudolph W. Giuliani's overemphasis on the drug war at the expense of social programs. AIDS-awareness advocates and groups favoring the legalization of drugs joined the rally after holding their own rallies uptown. The groups joined in a march along Fifth Avenue. The protesters also called for the legalization of ibogaine testing and marijuana for medical treatment and over-the-counter sales of sterile syringes.

New York Times

Wars Parade/Rally when an article on harmaline crossed his desk. It was from the "Abuse Folio" by David E. Smith of the Haight–Ashbury Free Clinic, and warned that high-dose harmaline, like Ibogaine, may indeed cause numbness, (presumably of hands and feet first).[1]

The rally, when it happened May 7th, was far more enormous than anything ACT UP expected. The picture and caption in the *New York Times* presented a balanced harm reduction message — not, as feared, just a marijuana protest.

But with negative groupthink dominating ACT UP, only a handful of harm reduction loyalists showed up and got to experience the rally. The ACT UP floor didn't want to acknowledge or deal with 8,000 young people who were not predominately gay or IV users. ACT UP's youth group, YELL,[2] didn't even bother to give out condoms.

Three days later Charlie Kaplan (Nico's old boss) stopped into 9 Bleecker, on his way to Texas to do NIDA contract-work. He offered an interesting notion they'd come up with before he'd left Erasmus University in the Netherlands: that Ibogaine reset the angle of the endorphin receptors — the *tilt* of the receptor surfaces. He also reported Dutch authorities were tolerating harmaline use — but only as part of a religious ceremony[3] — while some kind of challenge percolates up through the courts.

"It's the original root religion," Dana interjected, "For all three monotheisms and for Hinduism. I should really help them in their suit, by furnishing a pharmacologic explanation for the Resurrection. Flattery[4] says use of harmala is taboo for Sikhs and Hindus today because the Brahmin priests long ago realized it infringed upon their magical monopoly on revelation. And all the Catholics ever knew was that it was used by the followers of Ahriman to contact Hell.[5]

"But the Shia still burn harmel seed as incense; and the story is that at the birth of Jesus three Magians showed up with incense. So if Persian Kings customarily took *soma* to increase their perspicacity and grasp of righteousness, how could the Prince of Peace not avail himself of the same insight for His immeasurably greater, more demanding Mission?"

Dana recommended that, before going to Texas, Kaplan pick up the *VALIS* trilogy for $6 at Jim Druggas' store at 34 Carmine Street Dana also urged him to attend the second design session for NIDA's Phase I/II protocol May 16th. But that was the day Kaplan was starting work, so he couldn't make it.

Since mid-April the harm reduction working group had been operating with the understanding that the ACT UP name would henceforth be used only in connection with the needle exchange. Medications development and AIDS-prevention for non-IV drug users would be the focus of a new group, CURES NOT WARS. But this was not finalized until May 30th. On May 16th Dana Beal, Johann Moore and David Goldstein, still representing ACT UP, attended the second Ibogaine Protocol design session. It was an exciting day.

Frank Vocci opened with an overview of what NIDA/MDD is planning. He reviewed the history of Ibogaine research, especially the Molliver/O'Hearn findings of toxicity in rats, which stopped human testing, as well as primate data that prompted FDA to approve resumed clinical research at very low doses. He summarized where we left off in October, 1994, when the first design session was unable to agree to proceed quickly.

NIDA pharmacologist Nora Chang presented what is known about Ibogaine pharmacokinetics. She stressed two points: the discovery that Ibogaine bioavailability in rats and dogs is much greater in larger doses, and the discovery by Lee Hearn of the Miami team of the major metabolite of Ibogaine called *nor-ibogaine.*

Biochemist James O'Callahan next did a quick workshop on the state of the art in measuring neurotoxicity. He presented slides showing the neurotoxicity of a large number of psychoactive drugs in various species of animals, and provided cross-species comparative scales of neurotoxicity.

The "marker" he was using was the activation of astrocyte fibers of *microglial cells* — the *macrophages* that consume damaged neuronal tissue whenever there's toxicity. Ibogaine received a very low tox rating on this scale. He also presented data showing greater Ibogaine effect in female rats than in males.

Mark Molliver, up next, started by saying the cerebellum is the least-known part of the

[1] Dr. David E. Smith and Rick Seymour, *High Times*, January, 1986, p. 30.

[2] Youth Education Life Line.

[3] The Santo Diami Church.

[4] Flattery, §§142–146.

[5] In the ancient Persian religion, *Ahriman* was the name of Satan, *Ahura Mazda* the name of God. The Hebrews recognized this as a kindred monotheism; Byzantium regarded it chiefly as an enemy ideology during its centuries-long war with Persia — prior to the advent of Islam.

brain — we know how it works, but we don't know what it does. The effect in rats that set off alarms in '92, however, was excito-toxic — the result of overstimulation of very well-shielded Purkinje cells subjected to rhythmic bursts from the inferior olive.

The reaction in primates was completely different. Molliver was astounded to find that Ibogaine, when administered orally in doses up to 150 mg-per-kg, had none of the gross effects on his monkeys that he'd seen in rats. In order to maintain such effects (tremors, ataxia) longer than twelve hours, (because he suspected excito-toxicity in rats was due to *length* of tremor) he found it necessary to administer 50 mg/kg, interperitoneal Ibogaine in solution, every 2.5 hours.

Five out of seven animals had seizure activity with each injection. But to check for signs of Purkinje damage, Molliver and O'Hearn needed to adapt immune markers from humans and tissue stains from rats. It became clear to Molliver and O'Hearn that the stains designed for rats, trying to pick up markers derived from humans, weren't working in primates. Findings of no toxicity merely meant their "tools" couldn't detect it if it was there.

On the first six monkeys, nothing they had tried worked. Furthermore, control animals also showed irregular, "spotty" distribution of Purkinje cells in corresponding regions of the vermis — that's normal in primates. So after five sharp assaults with Ibogaine, Molliver was able to find only the most equivocal evidence of damage in one monkey.

Dana Beal asked if the five sharp assaults, with seizures, were really comparable to the long-rolling peak that humans experience with oral administration. He noted that injected Ibogaine, according to Hans-Georg Behr, also produces a shorter peak experience in humans, more similar to Molliver's interperitoneal administration in the primate.

Next up was Deborah Mash, a holder of the University of Miami IND. Her results earlier had conflicted with Molliver's, in that her animal subjects did not experience ataxia. No neurological deficits were found in her human subjects or her primates. Her IND is continuing. She expected to study three more male humans at higher doses. She said her team would like to accelerate the dose regimen, but that this had not been approved.

She was followed by Juan Sanchez-Ramos, the movement-disorders specialist who is director of Miami laboratory and the actual initiator of the IV IND. He placed humans receiving the 1 mg./kg. dose on a neurotest apparatus — the "wobble board." The wobble board was designed to diagnose the presence and severity of Parkinson's disease. It measures whole-body tremor at various frequencies, and can detect fine tremors invisible even to trained specialists. At the low, one mg/kg dose, two subjects reported feeling nothing, while a third actually became calmer.

Linda Weinhold presented NIDA/MDD Ibogaine Phase I / II Protocol Proposals, i.e., the protocol that had been mailed in advance to participants. It involves a cohort of sixty, or fifteen at each of four centers, a nested double-blind dose run-up Phase I safety study, with a followup Phase II efficacy component to track interruption or diminution of cocaine use.

Subjects must be using $150 worth of cocaine a week. Out of fifteen subjects at each center, three receive placebo, three receive 150 mg, three receive 300 mg, three receive 600 mg, and three receive 900 mg. One-week in-patient status preceding administration of Ibogaine, one-week out-patient, with anniversary check-ups at three months, six months, and one year.

Weinhold asked for questions, and it was half a minute before Beal broke the silence with a query following his earlier line of questions to Molliver: Since electro-encephalograms (EEGs) were being run before and after, how about doing an EEG or magnetic-resonance imaging (MRI) as far into the treatment as the subject could tolerate? Subsequent discussion elicited views suggesting subjects would probably not object as much to this during the dreamlike phase as they would during the second, cognitive-evaluation phase starting about six hours into the procedure.

The panel also seemed to be growing more comfortable with the idea that Ibogaine activity might be 'replacing' REM. Ed Friedrich stated that since sleep deficit is a significant part of addiction sequellae, a sleep specialist should be present during Ibogaine treatment.

Doblin suggested use of a PET[1] scan on subjects. This suggestion was rejected.

There was much discussion of an active placebo, because subjects *know* they're getting Ibogaine. Since Ibogaine is a psychedelic, said Yensen, training should be given to each treatment team, including briefings on human behavior during psychedelic experiences. Rick Strassman further stressed the importance of set and setting. An expert on DMT, he reiterated the need for sensitivity to psychedelic phenomena on the part of treatment teams.

For an active placebo, Yensen suggested LSD, prompting a lot of comparisons with Ibogaine. Ibogaine was said to be more intense, but more dreamlike and therefore more benign, unlikely to trigger a schizophrenic break.

Beal suggested *mitragynine,* reportedly used to interrupt heroin addiction in New Zealand, derived from the *Rubiaceaea* "kratom," *mitragina speciosa.*[2] Both suggestions were rejected by Charles Grudzinskas, the Acting Deputy Director of NIDA, who said that even less is known about the latter than about Ibogaine. This prompted general laughter and a release of tension.

Things were running late, so, while many panelists were still out of the room for a coffee break, Alan Trachtenberg of NIDA Basic Research launched into his presentation on three inclusion and three exclusion criteria. The inclusion criteria: healthy male cocaine users (25–40 years-old) with $150/week habit. Urine tests would be used to determine that subjects are THC negative, methadone[3] negative, and cocaine positive. HIV- or TB-positive subjects are excluded. Women are excluded until NIDA finds some clinical indication of efficacy in males, because of a greater sensitivity in the female to Ibogaine across a broad range of species, including human females.

Christine Ollo came next, with protocol questionnaires to measure psychological state of subjects both prior to and following the Ibogaine session. There was significant discussion of the amount and endpoint of testing. After Ollo's presentation, discussion centered on the need for treatment teams to show sensitivity to the mood of persons undergoing psychedelic experiences, specifically in accepting the subjects' possible refusal to answer questions.

The session wrap-up discussion had two facilitators. Paul Fudalla asked if anyone objected to proceeding to a clinical trial; no one responded. Wright, the FDA case officer for Ibogaine, at this point refined the question to inquire at what point the trial would be aborted. There was a heated discussion of the "Go/No go" decision points, i.e. the interpretation of behavioral manifestations in human subjects and the establishment of criteria for intervention, i.e., stopping.

O'Hearn was asked to weigh in on neurotoxicity; she said the data from just one animal was too preliminary. Tractenberg said he agreed with earlier comments that giving the animal repeated 50 mg./kg. IP jolts of Ibogaine was just not equivalent to the oral dose in humans; especially if it's really not much more long-lasting in humans, when injected, than in primates.

At this point Mark Molliver came back into the room, passing Dana, who whispered that it looked like the panel was overreacting to the new toxicity findings again. Mark immediately went to the microphone. After a minute or two he commented: "My feeling is that this is going to be a safe drug in humans." With this remark there was a palpable shift in the sentiment of the room. He went on to say his results suggested that, even in double-doses injected IP five times in twelve hours, Ibogaine damage was very hard to find in primates.

Juan Sanchez-Ramos volunteered that he would be ready to stop the minute he had proof of even the slightest cell loss. But Curtis Wright surprised everyone by ruling that in dealing with addiction, a life-threatening disorder, a little brain-cell loss might be okay. Wright then specified that the Data Safety Committee ought to have clear evidence that "something is broken" before intervention. For example, persistent minor tremor should not be sufficient to interrupt the study. Finally, Wright of FDA said, "It sounds to me like you folks have a Phase I clinical trial."

Carlo Contoreggi now took over, asking for further suggestions as to how to proceed. It was agreed that nicotine and alcohol consumption be monitored as part of the follow-up.

Ed Friedrich also suggested there should be follow-up immune function studies. "Sleep medicine experts should be involved in Ibogaine research. If Ibogaine first releases

1 Stands for Positon Emission Tomography.

2 William Emboden, *Narcotic Plants,* (London, 1972), pp. 13–14.

3 At one point Trachtenberg gratuitously observed that trials to determine Ibogaine efficacy versus opiates were "unnecessary" because methadone was working so well.

REM, then allows catch-up Slow Wave Sleep as an after-effect, we have to beware of potential undesirable rapid healing effects of sleep restoration — latent antigens belatedly attacked by the revived immune mechanism, causing rheumatoid arthritis, etc." Friedrich urged extreme caution in administering Ibogaine to the aged.

MDD also seemed amenable to a suggestion about adding another echelon — 1200 mg., or the lowest full dose — if all went well. That would bring the total cohort up to 75. The timeline was set, but no dates given.

At this point Beal asked when the trial would start. Wright turned the floor over to NIDA pharmacologist Belinda Hayes, who explained that on-going pre-clinical work in dogs, intended to determine the half-life of Ibogaine in the blood and to correlate blood levels with Ibogaine's different phases, would have to be completed first. Mash spoke up and said things were moving quickly — that ACT UP should be satisfied.

Johann Moore asked when the Ibogaine would get to junkies on the street.

Beal ended the session by remarking that narcotics agents in Staten Island had just strangled a man, Ernest Sayon, and that New York had a real possibility of exploding, Los Angeles-style: "As long as people have a hope of doing something about a problem, they'll wait instead of lashing out — but we can only keep hope going for so long without actually delivering something."

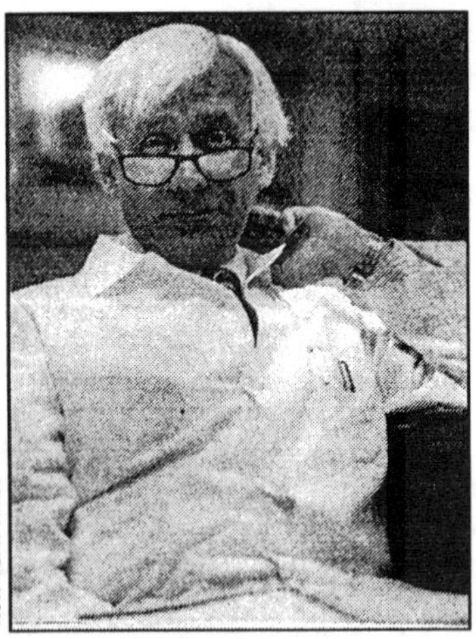

New York Times

DR. RODOLFO LLINÁS

When Johann, Rommel Washington and Dana went on to the ACT UP floor the next week, they told them that the ball was now in ACT UP's court so far as doing anything about exclusion of women; and that it was really up to the floor if they wanted anything to happen to make it available to junkies with HIV, the original target group, any time soon. What Harm Reduction recommended was to see if females tolerated mitragynine better, so that it also might be fast-tracked.

The next step was to make contact with New Zealand. A phone call established that mitragynine had indeed been given for methadone addiction detox. Kratom was smoked whenever withdrawals occured, with treatment extending over six weeks. It turned out there was also a visualization effect, but it shifted into regular sleep, occuring at night as vivid, hypnagogic dreams. Some re-regulation of the sleep cycle — indicated by an "Ibogaine-like glow"[1] — seemed to persist as long as kratom is smoked, however.

A few weeks later Juan Sanchez-Ramos, upon reading an earlier, 15-chapter version of this Report, furnished a paper[2] on treating Parkinson's disease with harmaline, an MAO-inhibitor, which was tried and abandoned around 1930. However, more selective monoamine-oxidase inhibitors discovered during the '60s are the current standard of care for Parkinson's. And MAO-inhibitors inhibit oxidative stress, known to have a role in the progress of AIDS.[3] So harmala can also impart a glow (and is used to improve skin complexion, according to Flattery). However, according to Lotsof, more up-to-date techniques have determined that Iboga alkaloids, thought by Dhahir and others to be MAO inhibitors, are not.

Now Mark Molliver had also detected — although he barely mentioned it on the 16th, — Ibogaine activity in the thalamus and locus coeruleus. The particular part of the thalamus activated by Ibogaine has an excitatory function, while the locus coeruleus is involved in concentration and dealing with novel situations. Both regions are implicated, like the cerebellum, in the generation of brain-waves — with the thalamus at forty cycles-a-second synchronizing on every fourth beat and "binding" the slower ten cycles-a-second rhythm of the olivo- cerebellum that governs body movement. This is known as "entrainment." According to Dr. Rodolfo Llinas of NYU, brain-wave activity must "entrain" (synchronize), lest the brain waves clash (and crash) — so the thalamus has to "keep time" with Ibogaine activity in the olivo-cerebellum.

The thalamus handles sensory perception. Llinas has discovered that a doughnut-shaped group of cells in the thalamus called the intralaminar nucleus sends out a wave that scans all areas of the cerebral cortex every 12.5 thousandth of a second. This fires synchronized cells in the cerebral cortex that are currently recording sensory information, which instantly fire a coherent wave of messages back down to the thalamus. This syn-

1 The subject, a middle-aged woman, reported that thinnning and greying of her hair reversed; however, she tended to develop a paunch.

2 Sanchez-Ramos report.

3 L-deprenyl, for instance, the Canadian "youth drug," is carried by some AIDS buyers clubs, although technically banned by the FDA.

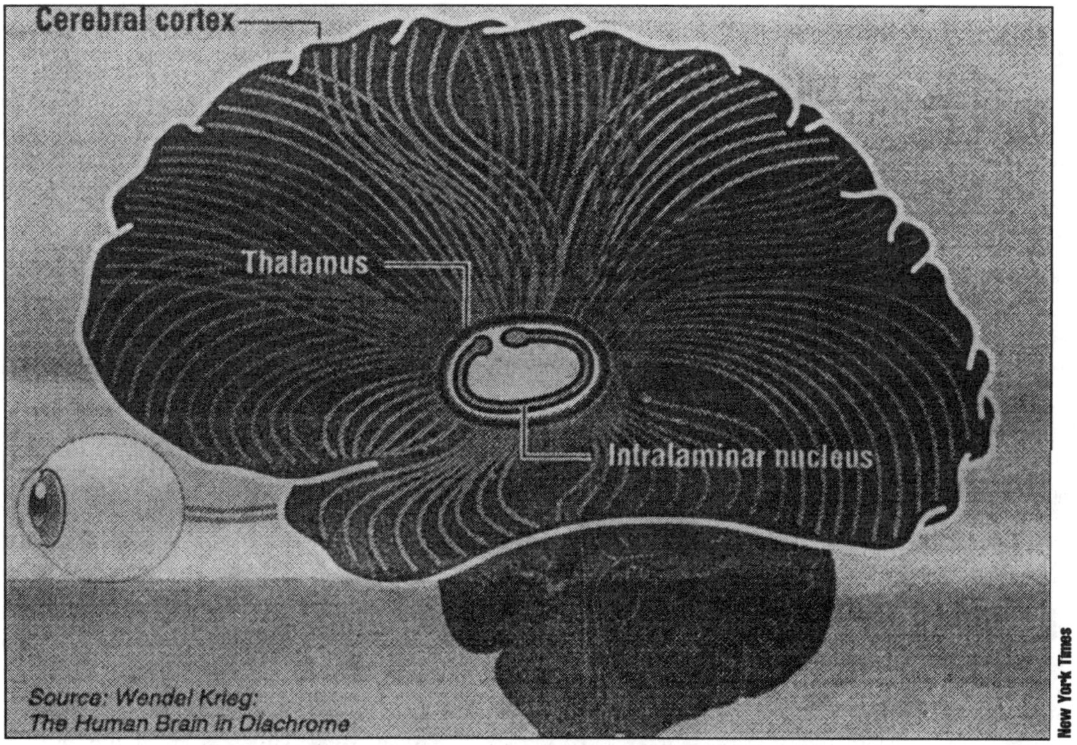

ASLEEP OR AWAKE, THE THALAMUS SCANS THE ENTIRE BRAIN FORTY TIMES PER SECOND.

chronous firing, according to Sandra Blakeslee,[1] is thought to be the basis of waking consciousness.

At night, on the other hand, the locus coeruleus is active in REM; while the thalamus generates both the slow-wave activity of deep sleep (when the cerebral cortex is shut down), and then while we dream, cells in the thalamus and cerebral cortex oscillate together for brief periods, according to experiments conducted in Quebec, by Dr. Mircea Steriade. The brain, in essence, is an organ that generates images. Wakefulness "is a dream guided by the senses," Llinas told Blakeslee.

In the standard model of addiction, as we saw in Chapter 7,[2] visualization in the striatum triggers craving in the nucleus accumbens, which sets up a dopaminergic cascade of further visualizations and cravings that finally trip the dopamine switch in the pre-frontal cortex, initiating drug-taking. Not all visualization is dopaminergic, however.

Glick showed that Ibogaine weakly binds to the *kappa* receptor during the initial hours of a treatment. Other researchers have found that the *kappa* receptor, which is normally activated not by endorphins or enkephalins but a third class of endogenous opioids called dynorphins, down-regulates *mu* analgesia in opiate-naive rats while potentiating analgesia in opiate-dependent animals.[3] *Kappa* opiate receptors have in fact been found to generate "dysphoric pseudo-hallucinations" as a part of an endogenous opiate system that operates in opposition to the normal euphoric analgesia of *mu* receptor agonists[4] — a possible reason why the FDA now considers Ibogaine to have low potential for abuse. Geerte F., on the other hand, believes the only true junkies are the three per cent or so of the population whose heroin experience has significant *kappa* receptor qualities. They get an out-of-body experience on heroin.

Moreover Pfeiffer, *et al.* induced "somesthetic changes and disturbances in the perception of space and time... de-personalization, de-realization and loss of self-control" with the potent benzomorphan *kappa* agonist MR2033 which are consistent with the naturally-occuring NDE.

Now if the function of an active placebo is that neither subjects or clinicians be able to tell whether they're getting Ibogaine, harmaline would be a logical candidate. Fred Gotbetter, who's taken both, says harmaline is very close — more euphoric than Ibogaine, but not dissimilar in peak and duration. It is oneiric and tremorigenic, and has a much

1 "How the Brain Might Work: A New Theory of Consciousness," Tuesday, March 21, 1995, *The New York Times*, p. C1.

2 See. pp. 67–68.

3 So that with chronic pain the effect of endorphins on the *mu* or enkephalins on *mu* and *delta* receptors does not completely disappear. See Poduri Ramaroo, *et al.*, "Effect of *kappa* opioid receptor agonists on morphine analgesia in morphine-naive and morphine tolerant rats," *European Journal of Pharmacology*, #156 (1988), pp. 239–246.

4 See Pfeiffer, *et al.*, *Science*, Vol. 233, 1986, pp. 774–76.

2 Studies Suggest Sleep Is Vital in Consolidating Memories

By SANDRA BLAKESLEE

In separate experiments conducted on rats and humans, scientists have found the first direct evidence that memories are consolidated during sleep.

The findings, which are being reported today in the journal Science, have implications for students cramming to pass an examination, people learning new skills like skating and anyone trying to navigate through new surroundings. They suggest for example, that people learning to ski might improve their performance after a few nights' sleep.

In the rat studies, researchers found that when an animal moved through a somewhat familiar environment, a particular pattern of cells was activated in a part of the brain called the hippocampus. Soon after, when the rat was allowed to sleep, the same cells showed an increased tendency to fire at the same time. The researchers hypothesize that this occurs as the memories are being consolidated in the brain.

The human studies, conducted by another group of researchers, focused on a different type of memory, involving the learning of a new skill. When the subjects were allowed to sleep and then repeatedly roused to wakefulness when they entered a period of vivid dreaming called rapid-eye-movement sleep, it hampered their performance on subsequent tests of the skill. This provided the best evidence so far that memories are consolidated during sleep.

2 Groups of Researchers

The animal experiments were conducted at the University of Arizona in Tucson by Dr. Matthew Wilson and Dr. James McNaughton. The human experiments were carried out by Dr. Avi Karni and Dr. Dov Sagi at the Weizmann Institute in Rehovot, Israel.

The Arizona group was interested in spatial memories. Animals have to know where they are at all times, so they can hunt, explore new territories and find their way home, said Dr. Wilson, who has just moved to the Massachusetts Institute of Technology. In animals and humans, he said in a telephone interview, spatial memories are first formed in the hippocampus, a small structure in the middle of the brain. Humans also use the hippocampus to acquire and store so-called declarative memories, involving all the events with which a person is involved during waking hours.

Most scientists believe that the hippocampus is essential for processing and consolidating new memories, Dr. Wilson said. They suspect that hippocampal neurons somehow strengthen the links between neurons in other regions of the brain where various aspects of each memory are stored; when a memory is recalled, these links are activated simultaneously and the memory is perceived as a coherent whole.

According to this hypothesis, specific cells in the hippocampus would be primed by events to help encode a new memory. But just how the information held temporarily in the hippocampus is shuffled out to other brain regions for long-term storage is not known.

Implanting of Electrodes

In a series of experiments, Dr. Wilson implanted electrodes into so-called place cells in the rat hippocampus. Each place cell is activated when an animal is in a certain region in its environment, Dr. Wilson said. A place cell that fires when an animal is in one position will stop firing when the animal moves to a different place. As an animal moves through an environment, like an enclosed box with distinct features on the walls, different ensembles of place cells will fire to reflect the animal's movements through that space, he said.

Rats fitted with a lightweight multi-electrode array were placed in an enclosed box that they had been in before but that they did not know well. They were then allowed to explore, as the electrodes recorded the activity of their place cells. Next the rats were put back in their cage, where they fell back asleep. After five to ten minutes, Dr. Wilson said, the rats entered slow-wave sleep, which is dreamlike but does not contain vivid dreams.

Hippocampal place cells that fired together when the rats explored the box showed an increased tendency to fire together during sleep, Dr. Wilson said. Information about activity in the environment is preserved in the hippocampus with the same ensembles of cells, he said, and it is acted upon by the sleeping brain.

Exactly what happens next is not known, Dr. Wilson said. The leading hypothesis is that the hippocampus plays out the stored information to memory networks throughout the brain. During this reorganization and consolidation of memories, he said, the brain creates a more useful representation of information than what was stored during the actual experiences.

Clues for Students

Humans also have place cells, Dr. Wilson said. When people learn to navigate through a new environment, they presumably form patterns in their hippocampuses which are later processed in sleep and stored throughout brain. Thus ability to find one's way around a new city should improve after a night's sleep.

The same may be true for students who cram for an examination. Experiments done in Canada show that students who get some sleep after studying for an exam retain more information than those who stay awake overnight. While short-term memory can hold a lot of information, it may be that sleep helps consolidate memories in ways that are more useful to the student.

Dr. Karni, who helped carry out the human experiments, explored a different phenomenon called procedural memory, which involves repetitive movements that help people learn to perform skills, like riding a bicycle, skating or downhill skiing.

Because procedural memories are not processed through the hippocampus, most researchers felt that sleep would have no effect on them. Dr. Karni's experiments tested this notion for the first time.

In the experiments, subjects were trained in a simple visual task: to recognize the orientation of an object appearing in their peripheral vision. After several days' practice, they got progressively better, Dr. Karni said. Last year he reported that once people learned this skill, they retained it for years.

But while doing those experiments, Dr. Karni, who is now at the National Institute of Mental Health in Bethesda, Md., noticed that subjects improved after an eight-hour delay. To see if sleep played a role in their better memories, subjects were trained in the evening before they went to sleep. One group was awakened every time they began to enter rapid-eye-movement sleep. They were roused about 60 times during the night. Members of a second group were awakened every time they entered slow-wave sleep, a stage when dreams tend not to occur. They were roused a comparable number of times during the night.

With rapid eye movement or dream sleep deprivation, the subjects' learning did not improve at all, Dr. Karni said. They did as well as they had the night before. But subjects who were awakened during periods of slow-wave sleep, but who were allowed to dream, showed distinct improvement over the night, he said.

Thus dreaming seems important for consolidating procedural memories, Dr. Karni said. Exactly what happens during dreaming to improve performance on procedural memory tasks is not known, he said.

New York Times

more solid track record of reasonably safe use in humans than any substance recently discovered, such as LSD. Lee Cummings, informed that harmaline use was once so widespread in Indo-European cultures, asked if it had ever been used to treat addiction. As a matter of fact, *ayahuasca* preparations are used in traditional South American medicine to curb alcoholism, curse of tribal peoples.[1] But telepathine, the compound in *ayahuasca* consisting principally of harmaline, contains additional tryptamines — which could explain why no Old World *materia medica,* working with pure harmala preparations from the wild rue, mentions treatment of alcoholism.

Mitragynine, because its gradual mode of administration is not enough like Ibogaine, must actually be ruled out as an active placebo. But as far as any "efficacy component" of the current research is concerned, use of harmaline would allow fine comparisons with the simultaneous weak binding to the NMDA and *kappa* receptors which the additional architecture of the Ibogaine molecule seems to confer.[2]

The discovery of an endogenous nor-harman by M.R. Dzoljic[3] should put to rest NIDA fears about harmaline toxicity. Turns out the active molecule in the little white flower by the side of the road is a naturally occuring neurotransmitter.[4] Dzoljic also found that activation of the opiate receptor types — *mu, delta,* and *kappa* — kicks up higher levels of nor-harman. Lotsof believes increased levels of this neurotransmitter represent the body's endogenous response to opiate dependency — but that heroin overwhelms nor-harman's ability by itself to counter-act the addictive effect.

Recent findings[5] on metabolization of Ibogaine in humans suggest the existence of a natural pathway in the liver (chi) that may also retard metabolization of nor-harman so that it can accumulate and be released in a squirt during REM, in all probability as part of the digestive process, like TNF alpha.[6] As an MAO-inhibiter, it modifies completely the effect of a significant simultaneous release during REM of the endogenous tryptamine serotonin — making it "trippy."[7] One or more harmala alkaloids seem to be the brain's own natural substance for generating long-term memory, dream content, eidetic visions, "peak experiences" (P. K. Dick's "blinding pink beam of light"), and in an emergency, the NDE — via complex interaction with dynorphin-generated kappa activity designed to counteract mu analgesia and stave off respiratory collapse. When this happens, years flash past like a movie and folks find themselves floating autoscopically above the operating table.

NDE research gives us a window upon a quantum state in which subjects are out-of-phase with space and time, where harmala and *kappa* receptors peek around the regular four dimensions through one of the seven that (not quite completely) "collapsed" not long after the Big Bang, according to "superstring" theory.

The ancients, in the course of centuries of harmaline use, apparently discovered that the genuine prophetic effect comes not with *ephedra,* but that it can be magnified by simultaneously flooding the system with endorphins. The ritual mortification of flesh is a fossil remnant of this in the practices of present-day Christian and Islamic sects. The Native American Sundance ritual — involving hanging, crucified, skewered through the pectorals — is a living example.

Late in the summer, Dana talked to Carlo Contoreggi again, who felt a long-lasting metabolite, linked to the liver, might explain why some people get into distress hours after taking Ibogaine, when it should be wearing off:

> "Most people have the metabolic equivalent of a four-lane tunnel to handle the de-methylated Ibogaine — the nor-ibogaine — so that it can be further metabolized. But sometimes four lanes of Ibogaine and nor-Ibogaine get all jammed up trying to go through a one-lane tunnel, and active metabolite levels go way up. We think we can test for that susceptibility."

Dana was doubtful:

> "Howard says Stanley Glick has a new paper out showing no Purkinje loss in the vermis of his rats at forty mg.-per-kg. I don't think toxicity results are going to tell you what you want to know, because it's another variation of the 'guilty cell' approach."

"What do you mean?" Carlo asked.

> "The original idea that the Ibogaine effect was like psychosurgery — killing the cells where the addiction is. Another possibility — if brainwave activity actually ceases for a minute interval during the "splitting of the skull" — is that in one

1 Claudio Naranjo indicates that ayahuasca use is reported by native healers to "dry out" alcohol abuse to some extent.

2 Including production of nor-ibogaine, and its distinctive effects (see next chapter, pp. 204, 209–210). More recently, Sanchez-Ramos confirms Mash's team is looking at the well-knonw dopamine deficiency in female heroin addicts just before menstruation as inferential basis for a possible greatly heightened sensitivity to Ibogaine during that phase of the estrus cycle. In other words, PMS may be an Ibogaine contra-indication.

3 See Appendix 5, pp. 337–339. In fact, researchers have discovered endogenous harmala alkaloids a number of times, notably McIsaac in 1961 and Llinas of NYU again in the early '80s, although "he never published because he couldn't figure out what it did," according to Molliver. They are beta-carbolines; some, like norharman, may play a role in delerium tremens, as well as acting like a natural MK801 to prevent ischemia during the NDE.

4 Making the statement "This is My Blood" literally true.

5 See next chapter, p. 212, on information on Ibogaine metabolism in humans, March 8th NIDA meeting.

6 See "Sleep and the Immune System," pp. 153–54.

7 See J. C. Callaway, "Tryptamines, Beta-Carbolines and You," *MAPS,* Vol. IV, Number 2, p. 30; also Callaway's "A Proposed Mechanism for the Visions of Dream Sleep," *Medical Hypotheses,* 26, pp. 119–124, and B.L Jacobs and M.E. Trulson, "Dreams, Hallucinations and Psychosis — The Serotonin Connection," *Trends in Neuroscience,* 2, pp. 276–280. Below, one of two endogenous beta-carbolines found in humans:

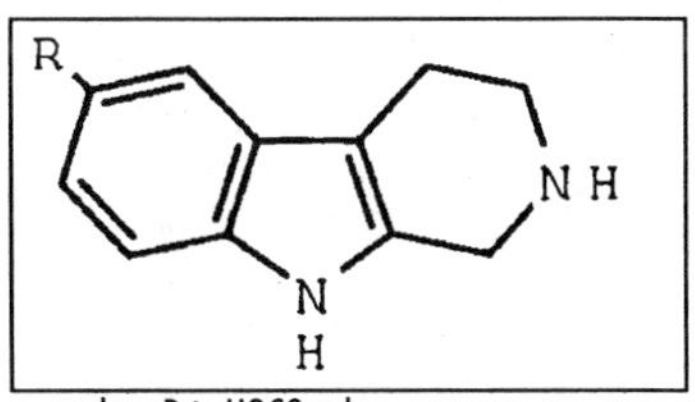

when R is H3CO-, the structure represents pinoline, when R is H-, the structure is THßC (tetrahydro-beta-carboline).

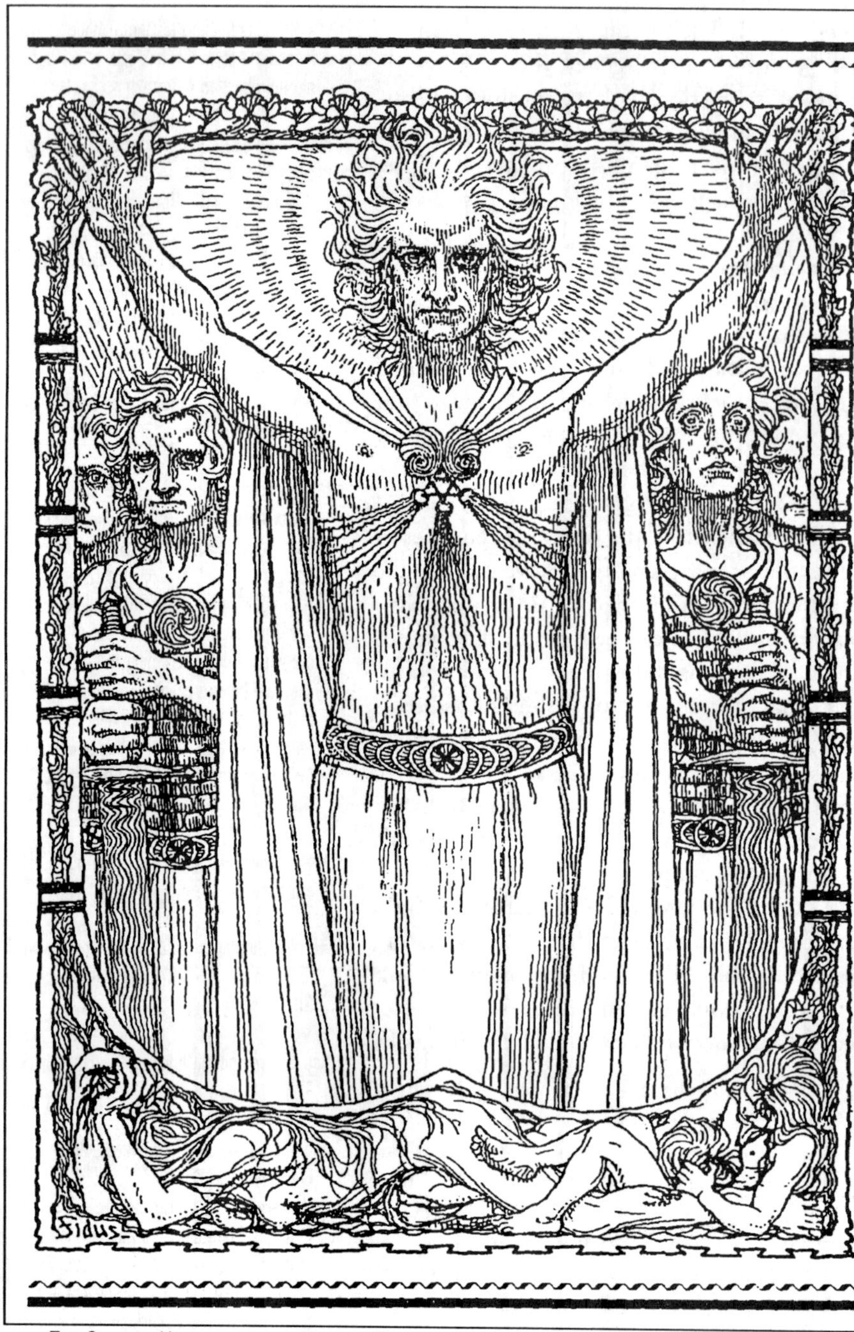

H.-G. Behr Collection

THE GERMAN MICHAEL AND THE KNIGHTS TEMPLAR, 1917 (NOTE STAR OF DAVID ON BREASTPLATE).

in 6,000 people, it doesn't *restart* perfectly. The autopsy of Nicola K. released at long last by Dutch authorities, showed 'no determinable cause of death.'

"We may have to face the fact that if we run thousands and thousands of people through the NDE, every so often one won't come back. In Gabon about one in 6,000 die, usually a woman or a physically slight male. We always chalked that up to other cyto-toxic *iboga* compounds, uncertain release-rate from crude root bark scrapings, etc.; and thought it could be controlled in a hospital setting with full resuscitation facilities. But perhaps, even though you are only *simulating* the NDE with Ibogaine, you have an occasional 'psycho-somatic death.'

"Uncertainty can be fatal. On the other hand, you have to balance it against fifteen people dropping dead here last week from too-pure heroin."

and then he asked —

> "Do you think the body's capacity to store long-lasting Ibogaine metabolite will lead to discovery of the endogenous neuro-transmitter involved in the NDE?"

A week later Bob Sisko and Dana were walking up Third Street, discussing the notion that the NDE is the key to access — on the quantum level, through Closed Timelike Curves — to Time itself. Dana exulted,

> "That harmaline book really turned out to be the key to understanding the ramifications of *The Passover Plot!* The Essenes must have *scoured* the dreamtime for the meaningful touches Christ incorporated into His Action. To access the far-distant future, His own harmaline trip had to be wrapped around some event of fundamental symbolic import, whose strange attractor would stamp itself on everything for millenia to come, so it would *resonate*. One way to understand it is to remember that consciousness, as Molliver says, is a matter of widely distributed circuits oscillating in phase with each other.
>
> "The resonance was undeniable. Remember, even after 1900 years the Grim King was so repelled by the example of the Suffering Just One that he scoffed at 'Jew-clear physics!' The Nazis taught that Aryan psychic powers had been not pharmacologic, but genetic — lost chiefly by interbreeding with Asians, Jews, etc.
>
> "In the Theosophical swirl around the appearance of Nazism, Himmler identified Eastern religions generally with the renunciation and self-abnegation of the Buddhism of Hermann Hesse — a chief competitor with Nazism in Germany during the '20s. Himmler had become obsessed, creating SS research bureaus to plumb "the secrets of Tibet." He was convinced Tibetan Buddhism was behind the Jews[!], who of course controlled Rome through the Buddha-nature of Jesus.[1] [*See next page.*]
>
> "Did you know that, acording to Hans-Georg Behr, The Sermon of the Mount repeats, word for word, parts of the Mountain Discourses of Buddha? Or that a Legion was in fact stationed in Jerusalem during Jesus' lifetime that was up

[1] In fact, Heisenberg — who advised Speer that production of an atomic bomb would not be feasible before the war ended (concealing the very existence of plutonium from the Nazis) — was close friends with chemist Karl-Friedrich Bonhoeffer, whose brother pastor Dietrich Bonhoeffer was arrested in 1943 after learning of the Holocaust and denouncing Hitler as the Anti-Christ. Dietrich Bonhoeffer was executed after the coup attempt of July 22, 1944.

Heisenberg never told

Cont. next page

to one-third Buddhist? The 10th. They had been stationed in Mesopotamia. After the Resurrection, some became Christians, and carried Christianity with them when they were transferred north of the Alps."[1]

Dana went on:

"For Nazism, Eastern religion existed to weaken the West. They brought back St. Michael as the personification of Germany: the German Michael (*see right*). So Himmler, — who believed he was Baldur (the German Mithras), and who was the one who decided which nuclear physics was politically correct! — never caught on to the *soma* angle, or the relevance of certain Buddhist techniques which bring the apparent heartbeat down to zero."

"Hitler was such a loser," said Sisko:

"I never understood that until I read *How Hitler Lost the War.*[2] We used to think of him as almost winning, but the author of this book shows how Hitler made one wrong decision after another. I've thought a lot about this. And the only thing you can say is that, through the Holocaust, the Nazis were diverted from their larger object: the destruction of humanity."

"Victory went to the followers of Christ,"

the Nazis an atomic bomb was flatly impossible, only that it would take years and cost billions. Meanwhile, he suggested to Niels Bohr that Allied scientists hold back as well — so that *no* government woud develop the bomb. Heisenberg was a patriotic German, but had been extensively persecuted by the Nazis because of his "uncertainty principle." See Thomas Powers, *Heisenberg's War*, p. 110.

1 Perhaps how the spear wound up in Vienna (see p. 171).

2 *How Hitler Lost the War,*

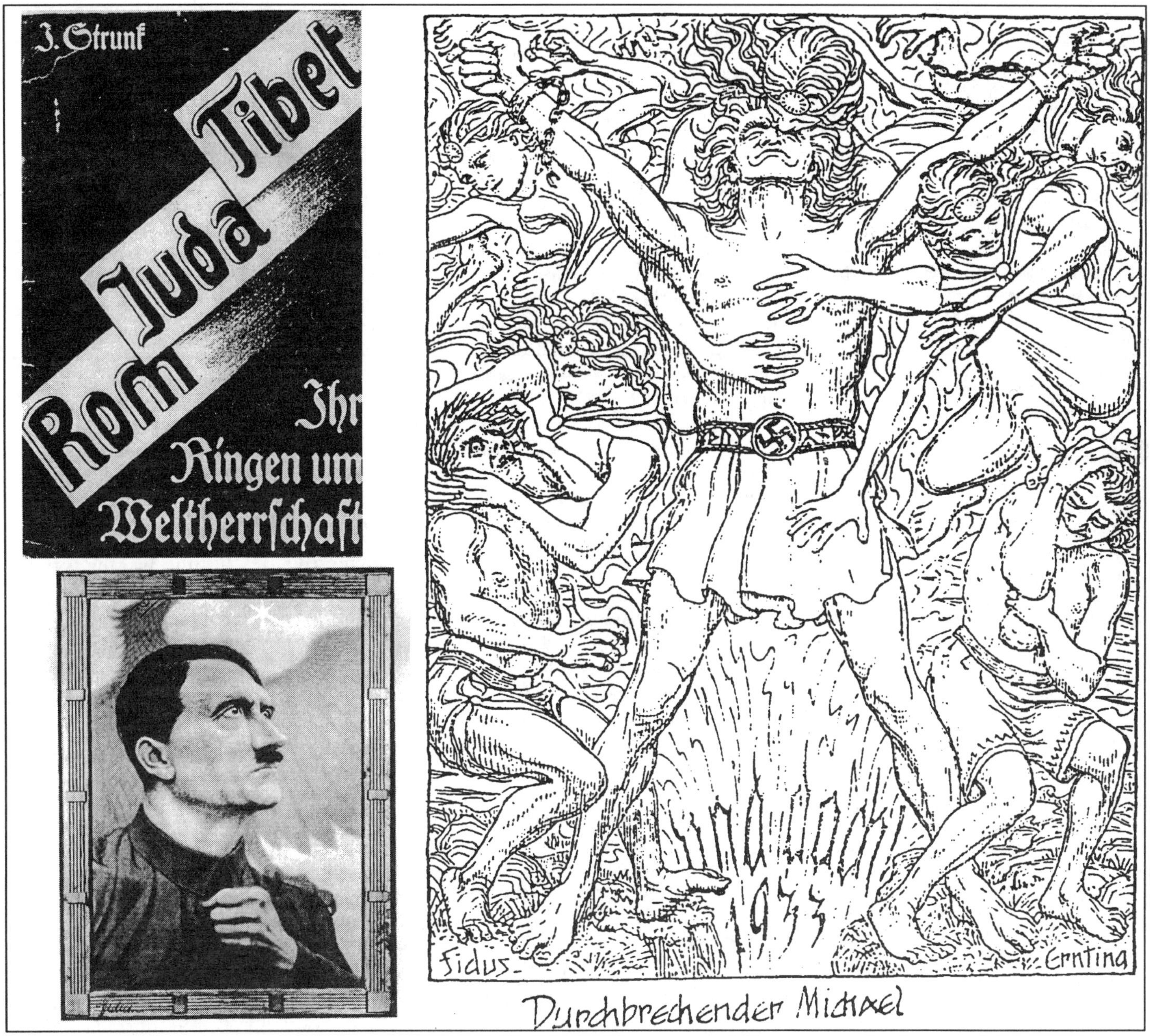

H.-G. Bohr Collection

The Grim King and his Angel. At upper left, cover of publication on the "Buddhist influence" behind the Jews, sponsored by Heinrich Himmler.

said Dana, "not Mithras."

"Remember, in the original Mithraic vision, the world ended in fire. Because Germany and Japan win and go on to annihilate each other,[1] whereas Marxism and Christianity shared an anti-racist premise that enabled the Soviets and the West to reconcile. The Dream of the Prophets — of Universal World Government — was realized. And Israel was re-established, armed with nukes."

"So Jesus was a Jewish radical," exclaimed Sisko. "The original Abbie Hoffman!"

"You've gotta read Schonfield's other book, *Those Incredible Christians*," said Dana.

"He believes the *Book of Revelations* is actually the earlier document. Like the *Book of John*, it is associated with the Beloved Disciple — who is reputed to have lived more than a century. *Revelations* seems to have been written by someone whose first language was Hebrew, unlike *John*, which was written in the Platonic manner, in Greek, with dialogue. That could make parts of *Revelations* the equivalent to the visions Wiraz dictated to the scribe when he arose from the *stard* state — the product of excursions forward of Jesus and others to next decision point.[2]

"The interest of the Beloved Disciple was to debrief Jesus after his trip to the end of the Epoch initiated by his Crucifixion and Resurrection, for instance:

"*Revelations* 22:1 — *'And he showed me a pure river of water of life, pure as crystal, proceeding out of the throne of God and the Lamb.'*

"22:2 — *'In the midst of the street of it, and on either side of the river, was the Tree of Life, which bare twelve manner of fruits, and yielded her fruit every month; and the leaves of the Tree were for the Healing of the Nations.'*

"Also 22:13 — *'I am the Alpha and Omega, the beginning and the end, the first and the last.'*[3]

"And 22:14 — *'Blessed are they that DO HIS COMMANDMENTS, that they may have right to the Tree of Life, and may enter through the gates into the City.'*

"What this implies is that only those who *keep kosher*, by regarding the host not as the literal blood of Jesus, but as the *plant soma of the Tree of Life* — that is, as the living blood of the Spirit which indwelt in Jesus when he was baptised by John the Baptist — get to enter the Village of the Dead!

"I told Charlie Kaplan that the effect of millions of addicts taking Ibogaine might well be like the "scatter" from city light messing up intersellar observatories — a sudden zone of translucence, which would be perceived from a distance as the event-limit. And dig this! According to Flattery,[4] in Zoroastrian eschatology, at the end of Time a final *yasna* (sacrifice/communion) will be performed in which the bull Hadayus and its fat are mixed with *"white haoma."* This differs from ordinary haoma just as the Hadayus bull differs from ordinary cattle,[5] (i.e., *hadanaepata* being the ancient priestly usage for *haoma* that actually contained harmel). But to the resurrected dead, the mixture is the draught of immortality!

"*The Ancestors!*

"I also read a book called *The Sign and the Seal* that claims the Ark of the Covenent still exists. This guy Graham Hancock uses textual analysis, his own archeology, plus the well-known fact that the falashas of Ethiopia practiced Old Temple rites not used in mainstream Judaism since the Babylonian exile, all to bolster the claim that the Kahanes actually spirited the Ark of the Covenant off to Egypt, to keep it from being defiled when Menasha tried to introduce idols into the Temple.[6]

"Hancock even found ruins of a replica of the first Temple on the Egyptian island of Elephantine, near Aswan, from the end of the Persian Empire, when he beleives the Ark was removed to an island on Lake Tanith in the Abyssinian Highlands. On that island he found intact the stone altar for animal sacrifice, on the spot where the Ark was kept in a tent for 814 years. After that it was taken to a church in the town of Axum during the mass conversion of Ethiopian Jews to Christianity around the time of Constantine the Great. Ethiopia was the only place where most Jews accepted Jesus as Mosiach."

Dana mused. "By that time, half the population were Jews. They were there for a long time — maybe before Solomon and Sheba."

"The Ethiopians actually brought the Ark out in front of their army for the last time in 1898, when they met the Italians at Adowa. They say St. George came riding down on his dragon with a heavenly host, and the Italians were slaughtered — the largest European army ever to invade Africa up until that time. Emperor Menelik reproached his couriers, saying that it was not right that they rejoice at the deaths of so many Christians.

"The next time, in 1935, the Italians used poison gas. And in '36, fascist blackshirts massacred the monks at Axum. But Mussolini — who thought he was Caesar — didn't know or care about the Ark.

"He lost his armies in 1941 — first, a quarter of a million men before the British in Libya, in

1 See *Man in the High Castle*, the 1962 Hugo Award winner by P. K. Dick, which established the pop cult status of the *I Ching*.

2 Like Joseph of Arimathea, the Beloved Disciple was not an Essene, but a member of the Establishment, albeit the wing of it who believed in the imminent coming of Mosiach, who were called Pharisees, many of whom rejected Jesus. Saul of Tarsus was one of these, until struck by a beam of light on the road to Damascus. "The Pharisiac faith included belief in angels and demons, the mapping the the heavenly abodes, Paradise and Gehinnom, magic and astrology, the mystery of the Achetypal Man, special creation and pre-existence, the Above and the Below, the messiah, transmigration of souls, revelation and Divine intervention, predestination, the Day of Judgement, the resurrection of the body, and the life everlasting. Pharisaism had its esoteric aspect, and those who were specially trained and qualified could follow the difficult and dangerous path that led directly to the heavenlies, and permitted access — to use the phrase employed — 'behind the curtain.' How hazardous was this undertaking may be gathered from the account given of the four rabbis who...penetrated into Paradise, of whom one died, one went out of his mind, the third became confused in his theology, and only the fourth returned in peace." (Those Incredible Christians, by Hugh J. Schonfield), Note similarity to footnote 1, p. 175 — whatever they were using was certainly not as safe as iboga, (1 fatality in 6,000), but more comparable to vincristine chemo for leukemia — fatal to 1 in 5.

3 See Chapter 6, p. 60, column 2.

4 Flattery, ¶138.

5 Native Americans recently reported that a special White Buffalo has been born in Wisconsin, where crowds now flock to view it.

6 In the mid–600's BC, prior to the fall of the First Temple. Fascinating research, but his medieval history and stuff on the Grail Myth are one-sided.

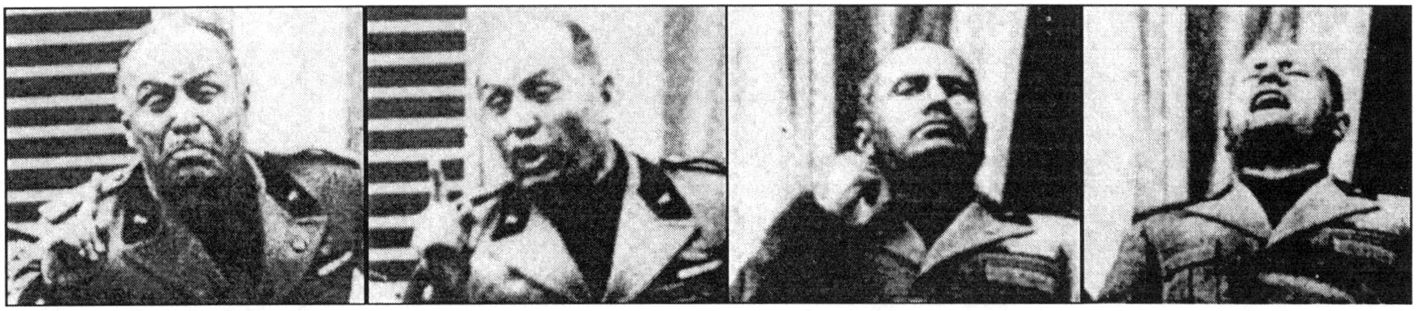

Radio Times Hulton

"HE SHALL CHALLENGE EVEN THE PRINCE OF PRINCES..." TIN-POT CAESAR HEAPS SCORN ON A FALLEN ETHIOPIA, 1936

February. Then the British brought Haile Selassie back from exile, to Khartoum, and as he ascended into Ethiopia, tens of thousands of Rastafarians came down from the hills, and the House of David re-entered Addis Abbaba at the head of a mighty host. In all of East Africa, a second quarter-million Italian troops were captured, almost without a shot being fired.

"After that, Italy was out of war.

"Those who want to understand what comes next with Ibogaine ought to study that story of abject collapse — study its strange attractor: the re-match between Caesar and Christ, the return of the Negus. Remember, he was Jesus' distant great grandnephew. The Ark is still at Axum. No one gets to see it but a single custodian, who always goes blind with cataracts after a couple years. It goes with the job. Once a year, at *Kineret,* they bring out a replica, covered with a blue robe emblazoned with the dove of the Holy Spirit."

Dana concluded:

"That seems to be the story: Ark of the Covenant into Africa, Ibogaine out... 'cause now, out of Africa, comes a new sacrament.

"It restores the cultural importance of Dreamtime.

"It obviates the need for mortification of flesh. From the Sundance to accupuncture. The improvement over harmaline is sufficiently dramatic to rehabilitate a lost branch of medicine. Ibogaine heals 'wounds that will not heal.' For addiction medicine, it's like 'the key that opens every door.'

"What dopaminergic visualization can do, Ibogaine visualization can undo, by going back in virtual time to undo it.

And it is appropriate that emancipation from pathologic reflex is located in the dreamtime. All our concepts of a Spiritual Realm, a Platonic realm of Ideal analogs which generate everything in the real world, are cultural relics of a harmaline-induced state. As Dick poetically put it, about the previous possibilities of harmala alkaloids, 'St. Sophia is going to be born again; she was not acceptable before.'[1] And a few pages earlier, he also wrote: 'The Godhead is impaired; some primordial crisis occurred in it which we do not understand.'[2]

"Ibogaine clears up the problem with primordial crisis, at least. It wasn't the Godhead but the previous sacrament, harmaline, that was impaired. A perfect sacrament wouldn't require additives."

1 *VALIS*, p. 100.

2 *VALIS*, p. 97.

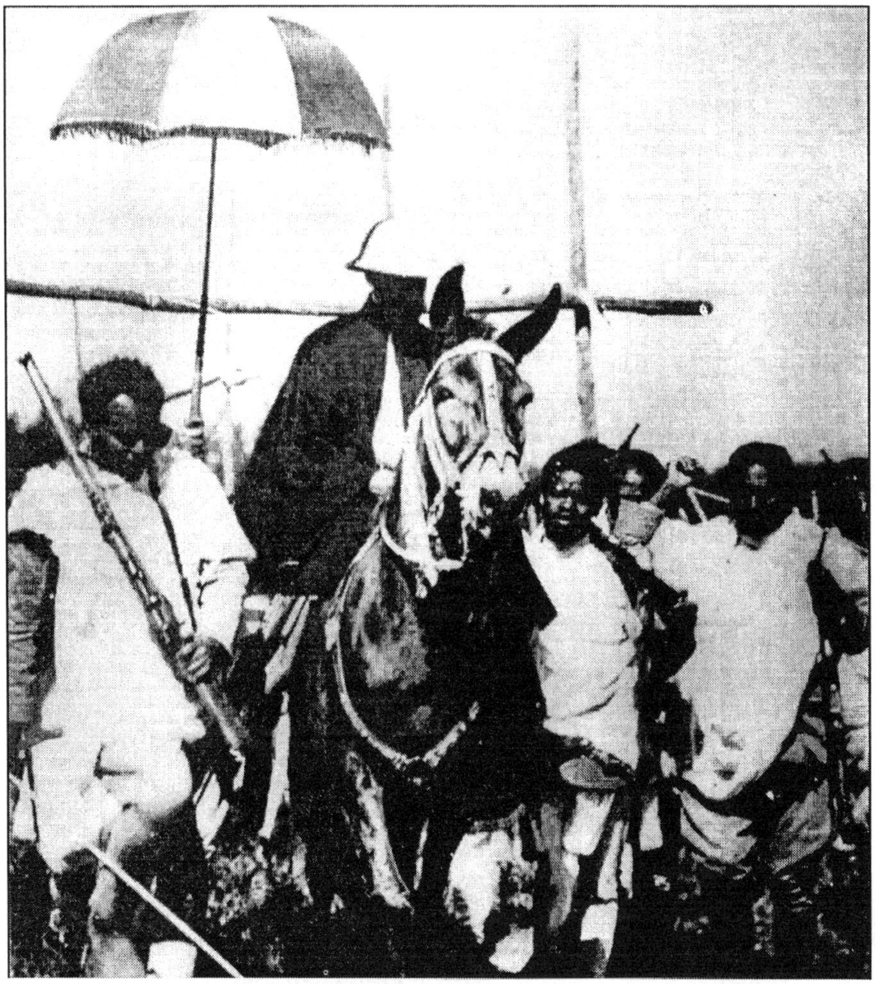

Radio Times Hulton

HAILE SELASSIE, THE TRUE NEGUS AND KING OF KINGS, AT THE HEAD OF THE IMPERIAL GUARD

CHAPTER 18: Deborah Mash's Brain

In March, 1994, in strictest secrecy, Howard Lotsof re-instituted treatments of addict volunteers in an ultramodern hospital in Panama City, with pre-treatment work-ups at the University of Miami. But this time — under a hush-hush clearance by the Panamanian Ministry of Health — hourly blood samples would be flown directly to the Addiction Research Center in Baltimore, affording NIDA scientists a window to observe the pharmacokinetics of Ibogaine in humans for the first time. Grudzinskas was once again full-time head of MDD, following the appointment of Alan Leshner as Director of NIDA in February, and Frank Vocci, true to his word, was moving into high gear.

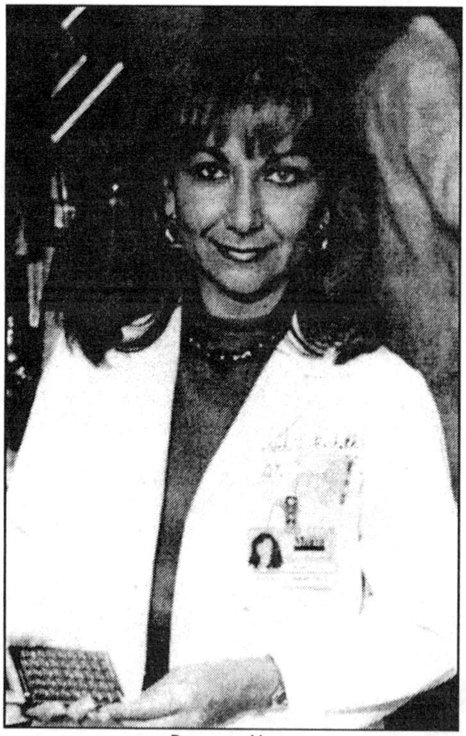
MAPS

DEBORAH MASH

Among these new treatments was Nancy, a third-timer who'd become re-addicted since the treatments stopped. Nancy's opiate experience began with access to someone else's take-home methadone — she was on 100 mgs. daily, plus other drugs.

Her first Ibogaine was in Holland — 25 mg./kg., during the same January '93 treatments as Mark Lamantia — except that she declined to be videotaped by ABC's "Day One." Two-and-a-half months later, at the end of March, '93, she required re-treatment, with 29–31 mg/kg And progress against her addiction didn't bring an end to her health problems; during the summer she stopped menstruating.

Her third treatment, in March of '94, actually consisted of two administrations — 10 mg/kg on the 25th and 20 mg/kg on the 28th — since Howard and the treatment team were leery of giving the whole 30 mgs. at once in light of known female sensitivity. A painstaking checkup at the University of Miami had failed to detect any physical basis for her complaints of recurrent intestinal malaise and diarrhea such that it would preclude more Ibogaine. Recovery was uneventful, although the problem with her insides didn't get any better. She was examined five days after treatment at Jackson Memorial Hospital, and flew straight back to the New York area.

On April 21, though, she flew back down to Miami for a medical exam at the University of Miami — part of the followup to her Panamanian re-treatment. No ill-effects of Ibogaine — but still no explanation of her diarrhea and recurrent vomiting. She was released from the hospital. Much later that evening she was found dead at the apartment where she was staying, collapsed in her vomit. Estimated time of death: 9:40 PM.

By coincidence, Nancy died in the only place in the country where bodies routinely go to Dr. Lee Hearn, who happens to be Dade County Medical Examiner as well as the member of Deborah Mash's team who discovered the active metabolite nor-ibogaine. The autopsy — much more exhaustive than in previous deaths — found no discernible link to Nancy's recent re-treatment, establishing cause of death as a small bowel infarction (obstruction) associated with a blood-clot blocking her mesenteric artery, caused by a general "hypercoagulable state" of the blood due to chronic infection in the thigh.

The Institutional Review Board of University of Miami Hospital double-checked their findings and concurred: death was not caused by Ibogaine. So Deborah Mash wound up with the one and only body in existence of a woman who certifiably didn't die of Ibogaine yet had received multiple Ibogaine exposures in the previous fourteen months. And the brain was in pristine condition, so that researchers could look for traces of non-lethal neuro-toxicity, the kind that ordinarily never shows up in behavior, and goes undetected. Mash's people began the process of sectioning Nancy's cerebellum, staining the sections, looking for Purkinje damage, for special female sensitivity. Such a brain, with just the right drug history, is hard to come by.

NMDA Receptors Trigger Excitement

NMDA receptors seem to regulate many normal changes in the brain of an adult or developing animal, but their overstimulation may cause nerve cell death in heart attack or stroke patients

As recently as 5 or 6 years ago, neuroscientists had little understanding of the mechanisms that regulate many important changes at brain synapses. They did not know, for example, what cellular and molecular processes might underlie learning and memory in an adult animal or what events regulate the formation of nerve cell contacts in a developing animal. And until 2 or 3 years ago, researchers had little knowledge of what actually causes brain damage in a heart attack or stroke victim. Today, neuroscientists are beginning to view NMDA receptors in the brain as regulators of all of these processes—good and bad.

"Each one of the processes in itself is an area of great interest, so when you have a nice unitary mechanism that seems to underlie all of these events, it is very exciting," says Charles Stevens of Yale University School of Medicine. In his presentation at the annual meeting of the Society for Neuroscience,* Stevens highlighted new data on mechanisms that regulate NMDA receptor activity. He stressed the emerging concept that appropriate stimulation of NMDA receptors may promote beneficial changes in the brain, whereas overstimulation of the receptors can cause nerve cell damage or death.

The NMDA receptors take their name from the fact that *N*-methyl-D-aspartate (NMDA) excites them under experimental conditions. NMDA itself does not exist in the brain, however. It is simply a chemical tool used to probe the activity of this class of receptors. In an intact animal, amino acid neurotransmitters such as glutamate or aspartate probably stimulate NMDA receptors.

During the past several years, neuroscientists have pursued the roles of NMDA receptors from at least three major perspectives. First, some study the mechanisms that regulate the activity of NMDA receptors and their ion channels. Second, some focus on the role of NMDA receptors in normal brain processes that depend on long-lasting increases in nerve cell communication at synapses. These include changes in brain development as well as changes that underlie learning and memory. And third, neuroscientists monitor the role of NMDA in brain disease or trauma. For example, NMDA receptors may participate in the hyperactivation of certain brain circuits in epilepsy or Huntington's disease. And increasing evidence indicates that overstimulation of NMDA receptors may cause damage to brain neurons in an ischemic attack when the blood supply to the brain is blocked during a heart attack or stroke.

> *"Excitotoxicity comes into play if there is too much glutamate and too much calcium."*

Stevens summarized recent findings in the first research area, namely, the structure and activity of the NMDA receptor and the membrane pore (ion channel) that it regulates. During the past several years, researchers have learned that the receptor is part of a large molecular aggregate that includes binding sites for certain chemical substances. When glutamate or NMDA binds, the ion channels open and allow positively charged ions to flow into the nerve cell. This excites the neuron.

Stevens and others now postulate that the NMDA receptor complex is a member of a superfamily of proteins—a group that includes the receptors and ion channels for the neurotransmitters acetylcholine, glycine, and γ-aminobutyric acid. Several researchers are now trying to isolate and clone the receptor complex for NMDA and glutamate, which should yield specific information about its organization.

Although the NMDA receptor complex seems to be physically similar to other receptor complexes, Stevens notes that regulation of the NMDA ion channel is unique. Most ion channels are governed by one major kind of signal—either a chemical transmitter or the electrical potential across the nerve cell membrane. But the NMDA channel is unusual because both chemical and electrical signals affect its activity.

Even the chemical regulation of the NMDA receptor is complex. Within the past 2 years, researchers have discovered that at least two different categories of chemical signals regulate NMDA receptor activity. One kind is an excitatory amino acid transmitter, probably glutamate or aspartate in vivo, or NMDA under experimental conditions. Now, according to Stevens, recent data indicate that glutamate binds to at least two kinds of receptors in nerve cell membranes, and it activates at least three kinds of ion channels—small, medium, and large. Whether each receptor type is coupled to a different sort of channel has yet to be resolved, however.

Last year, Jon Johnson and Philippe Ascher of the Ecole Normale Supérieure in Paris reported that the amino acid glycine serves as a second category of chemical signal that increases NMDA receptor activity. This surprised many neuroscientists because glycine is a well-known inhibitory transmitter, particularly in the spinal cord. The idea that glycine somehow enhances excitatory transmission in the brain was completely novel.

"If glycine is not present, glutamate will not open NMDA-gated channels unless the concentration of glutamate is raised," says Stevens. Glycine apparently binds to a site on the NMDA receptor complex that is different from the NMDA binding site, but its precise mechanism of action is not known. And because the normal level of glycine in brain tissue may be sufficient to increase NMDA receptor activity, it is also not clear if the glycine effect is an ever-present one or whether it occurs only under specific conditions.

In addition to chemical signals, the electrical potential associated with the nerve cell membrane also regulates NMDA receptors and ion channel activity. For instance, depolarization (making the normal negative electrical charge across the nerve cell membrane more positive) allows a bigger response to glutamate or NMDA. This is so because depolarization somehow dislodges magnesium ions that block NMDA channel activity when the cell is at rest.

Ascher and Linda Nowak of the New

*The annual meeting of the Society for Neuroscience was held from 16 to 21 November 1987 in New Orleans, Louisiana.

York State College of Veterinary Medicine at Cornell University at Ithaca, are continuing to explore the means by which magnesium ions block the NMDA channel. "It appears that magnesium ions sense the electrical field of the membrane and enter the NMDA ion channel," says Nowak. "Magnesium is very hygroscopic; it attracts water strongly." Other ions, including sodium and calcium, also attract water but can go through the ion channel easily because they lose their water readily. Nowak theorizes that because it takes much more energy to strip the water from magnesium than from calcium, magnesium ions tend to retain water. And, in this bulky state, they clog the NMDA ion channel.

Thus, it requires a combination of chemical stimuli and the right electrical environment to activate NMDA receptors fully. With maximum stimulation, NMDA ion channels open and allow sodium, potassium, and calcium ions to flow through the nerve cell membrane. Of these, calcium seems to be the most critical. Apparently, the right amount of calcium influx leads to beneficial changes in brain synapses but too much intracellular calcium causes nerve cell damage. A growing number of neuroscientists are actively pursuing these second and third areas of research on NMDA receptors.

For example, within the past year, several groups of researchers have shown that activation of NMDA receptors may regulate synaptic changes that are crucial to normal brain development—particularly of neural pathways that carry sensory information. Wolf Singer of the Max Planck Institute for Brain Research in Frankfurt, West Germany, and his colleagues find that stimulation of NMDA receptors is important in the development of brain pathways that carry visual information in the kitten. Martha Constantine-Paton of Yale University in New Haven, Connecticut, and her co-workers describe a role for NMDA receptors in visual system development in the experimental three-eyed tadpole. And Carl Cotman of the University of California at Irvine and his collaborators report that NMDA receptors are important for the development of the olfactory system in the rat.

Perhaps the most exciting aspect of NMDA receptor function in the adult brain is its potential role in learning and memory. Several research teams propose that two molecular events must occur simultaneously in the brain of an intact animal in order for it to learn. The first is that NMDA receptors must be excited chemically, and the second is that the nerve cells receiving the excitatory NMDA stimulus must be depolarized sufficiently to trigger calcium influx. This combination of events, the theory goes, will lead

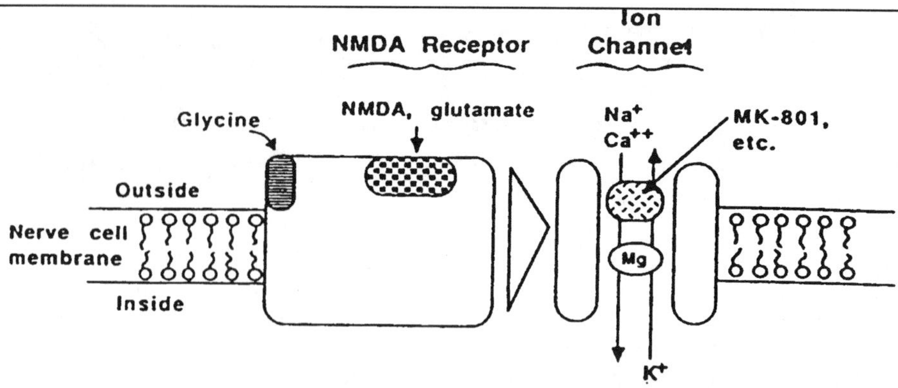

How the NMDA receptor complex might work. *A combination of factors are thought to regulate the activity of the NMDA receptor and its ion channel—an agonist, such as NMDA or glutamate, membrane potential, magnesium (Mg) ions, and glycine. When the NMDA ion channel is activated, as shown here, sodium (Na^+) and calcium (Ca^{++}) ions flow into the nerve cell and potassium (K^+) ions flow out. [Adapted from J. A. Kemp* et al., Trends Neurosci. ***10****, 297 (1987)*]

to long-lasting increases in nerve cell communication at synapses.

Tim Bliss of the National Institute for Medical Research in London, for example, sees a persistent increase in synaptic strength as one of the mechanisms that underlie learning. "There is no doubt that the NMDA receptor is involved in long-term potentiation in the hippocampus," he says. "But we are not certain if it is exclusively an effect on postsynaptic neurons or whether NMDA receptors on the terminals of presynaptic neurons are involved as well." Postsynaptic cells receive signals from other neurons. Presynaptic neurons send the signals in the form of chemical transmitters such as glutamate. The hippocampus is a primitive part of the cerebral cortex that plays an important role in certain kinds of learning and memory.

Within the past few years, other investigators showed that long-term potentiation can induce changes in the physical structure of a synapse. Some of these changes, which probably involve NMDA receptor activation, are on the spiny protrusions of dendrites, the fine neuronal processes that typically receive chemical signals.

Now, Bliss and his colleagues have new data indicating that NMDA may also stimulate another kind of synaptic change. Their results indicate that NMDA induces postsynaptic neurons to release derivatives of arachidonic acid, a kind of fatty acid. Bliss proposes that these metabolites might travel backwards across synapses to presynaptic neurons and increase their output of neurotransmitter. Such a change, he says, would cause a larger response from the postsynaptic neuron and be interpreted as an increase in synaptic strength. Whether these events occur in an animal when it learns, as the London researchers have shown it does under experimental conditions, is not yet known.

Additional recent data indicate that activation of NMDA receptors may stimulate protein kinase C, an intracellular enzyme that adds phosphate groups to certain proteins. With stimulation, the enzyme apparently moves from the cytoplasm of the nerve cell to its membrane where it may phosphorylate proteins thought to be inportant in long-term potentiation and certain growth processes. Like other events regulated by NMDA receptors, this response also seems to be linked to the influx of calcium.

Thus, accumulating evidence points to the fact that NMDA receptors play an important role in long-lasting changes at brain synapses. But Stevens, Nowak, and Bliss all question whether NMDA receptors play a role in ordinary communication among nerve cells in the brain. They postulate that normal synaptic transmission may be controlled by non-NMDA receptors, which trigger small currents carried by sodium ions flowing into a neuron. In contrast, NMDA receptors are more likely to be important for inducing larger ionic signals that depend on calcium influx, thereby inducing increases in nerve cell communication that underlie long-lasting changes at synapses.

NMDA receptors not only regulate beneficial synaptic changes in the brain, their overstimulation can be toxic to nerve cells and kill them. This is the subject of a third major area of research. "Excitotoxicity comes into play if there is too much glutamate and too much calcium," says Stevens. Under these conditions cells can no longer regulate their internal concentration of calcium, leading to very high levels of calcium that are toxic. "It is not known what the actual mechanism of cell death is, but a current guess is that calcium stimulates protein- and fat-digesting enzymes within the cell that destroy it," says Stevens.

The idea that overstimulation of NMDA receptors might cause brain damage has prompted researchers to develop compounds that might block the activity of the receptors and prevent nerve cell death. For instance, a class of compounds, including MK-801 and the hallucinogen phencyclidine ("angel dust"), appears to block the NMDA ion channel. Last year, Leslie Iverson of Merck, Sharpe & Dohme Research Laboratories in Harlow, England, and his colleagues proposed that MK-801 may be a treatment for preventing brain damage during a heart attack or stroke.

Several other research groups are trying to unravel the precise mechanisms by which MK-801 works. Among them are Stuart Lipton and Elias Aizenman of Harvard Medical School in Boston and their collaborator Andreas Karschin of the Max Planck Institute for Brain Research in Frankfurt. They are pursuing an earlier observation that MK-801 works best when the NMDA ion channel is already open. "We find that the action of MK-801 is dependent on the concentration of agonist," says Lipton. "The more NMDA you put on a cell, the better MK-801 blocks its effects. And, if you think about it, this is exactly the way you would want the drug to work."

Like others, Lipton reasons that in the brain of a stroke patient, damage to nerve cells increases with the release of more and more excitatory neurotransmitter. If MK-801 works in vivo as it does in the Harvard group's in vitro system, then the drug should have its maximal blocking effect in a patient with escalating levels of excitatory neurotransmitter in the brain.

The past 5 years have produced an explosion of information about NMDA receptors. Complex chemical and electrical mechanisms regulate their activity. NMDA receptors, in turn, regulate synaptic changes that may underlie learning and memory. They also appear to participate in normal synapse structuring in the brains of developing animals. But the same receptors probably cause some of the brain damage that occurs during ischemia. Despite the progress in understanding NMDA receptors and ion channels, key questions remain about their precise structure, regulation, location, and function. These issues will most certainly sustain this research field as one of the most exciting in neuroscience today. ■

DEBORAH M. BARNES

Meanwhile, it was deemed safe to go ahead in Panama with more male treatments, in July. After talking with Anne Shulgin about the "doorway of light," Mash did make one change in her protocol. She drew up a contract all prospective treatments have to sign "agreeing to come back." To this day, she says Nicola K's boyfriend insists that Nicola did not die of Ibogaine toxicity, but "found the doorway and went through it of her own free will."

In late September, Sisko and Rommell flew to Panama City, to be with Howard and Deborah Mash as they treated three more male addicts, including an older heroin addict who was shooting $5,000 a month; and a younger crackhead who was basing $1,000 a week, so that his wealthy family could well afford the Ibogaine. The kid had a full-blown experience. He described encountering Bwiti as a half-million-year-old Black Man in a Desert. He almost relapsed, but stabilized as soon as he got home. The older guy's liver function improved.

Howard and the local doctors did a press conference announcing Panamanian government approval of experimental Ibogaine.

At the very end of October David Goldstein showed up one day at 9 Bleecker with important news: a researcher named Popik[1] had discovered Ibogaine activity at the same NMDA (N-Methyl-D-Aspartate) receptor as harmaline (Woods, 1982).

Popik characterized Ibogaine and its congeners including harmaline as "noncompetitive" NMDA antagonists [binding only one micron more to the NMDA receptor, according to Molliver, than to the *kappa* opiate receptor]. In effect they are more like nor-harman, the neuro-transmitter associated with REM, eidetic memory and the NDE, as opposed to serotoninergic[2] indole ring alkaloids like LSD.

In David's materials on the NMDA receptor were papers on the potent anti-stroke medication diszocilpine (MK801), which showed that, in essence, *the NMDA receptor downregulates addictions of the common narcotic receptor.* Both Ibogaine and harmaline displace the somewhat oneiric MK801, suggesting a common mechanism of action. Daily administration of MK801 seemed to attenuate both tolerance to and dependence upon alcohol and morphine.[3] Also, MK801 was found to inhibit the supersensitization that sometimes develops with tolerance to cocaine.[4]

1 "Ibogaine Competitive Inhibitor of 3H MK801 to the NMDA Receptor Complex," Piotr Popik, Richard T Layer, Phil Skolnick, *Pychopharmacology*, Vol. 114, pp. 672–674, 1994.

2 Serotonin-releasing or -mimicking.

3 "MK801 Potently Inhibits Alcohol Withdrawal Seizures in Rats," Richard A. Morriset, Amir H. Rezvani, David Overstreet, David S. Janowsky, Wilkie A. Wilson and H. Scott Swartzwelder, *European Journal of Pharmacology*, 176 (1990) pp. 103–105. See also "Inhibition of Morphine Tolerance and Dependence by the NMDA Receptor Antagonist MK–801," Keith A. Trujillo and Huda Akil, *Science*, January 4, 1991, Vol. 251, pp. 85–87.

4 Blockade of "Reverse Tolerance to Cocaine and Amphetamine by MK801, R. Karler, L.D. Calder, I.A. Chaudhry and S.A. Turkanis, Pharm. Dept, U. of Utah Medical School, *Life Sciences*, Vol. 45, pp. 599–606.

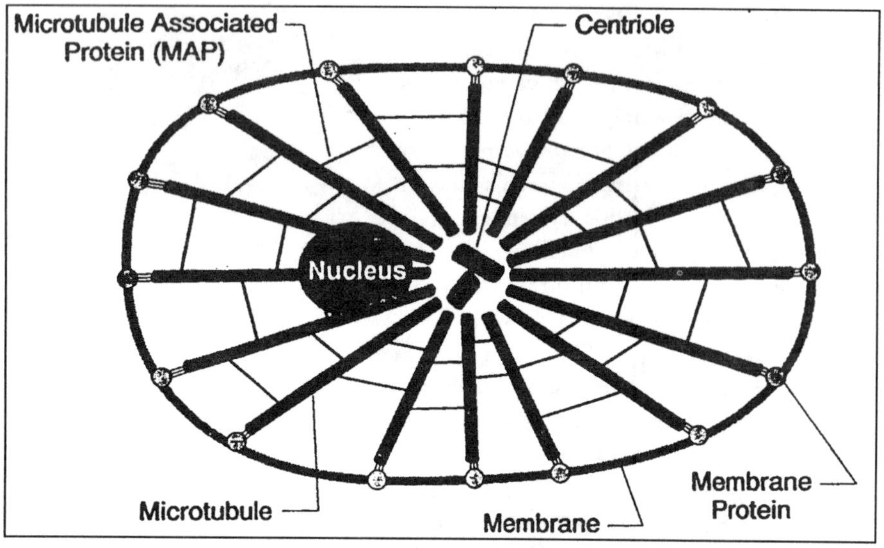

Figure 1. **Schematic of simple cell with cytoskeletal microtubules organized radially around centriole near nucleus. Micotubule associated proteins (MAPs) interconnect microtubules.**

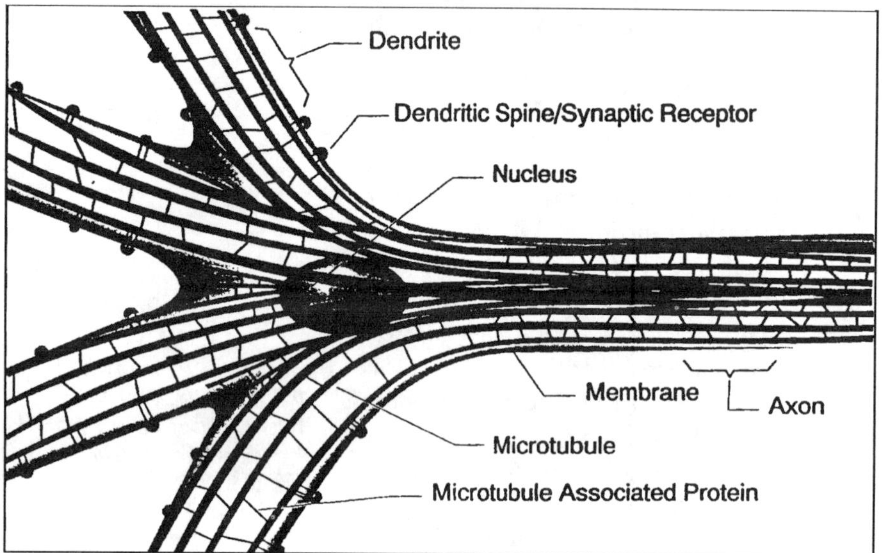

Figure 2. **Schematic of central region of neuron (distal axon and dendrites not shown). Microtubules, interconnected by MAPs, are arranged in parallel. Linking proteins connect microtubules to membrane proteins including synaptic receptors on dendritic spines.**

MK801 is a hallucinogen — more akin to phencyclidine and ketamine than Ibogaine/harmaline. Yet FDA approved it, because an injection of MK801, even half-an-hour after a stroke, by blocking flow of potassium, sodium and calcium ions into brain cells, interferes with the "glutamate cascade" that fuels neurologic stroke damage,[1] cutting it 50-to-75%.

This is important for understanding not just Ibogaine, but how "opium dreams" and *delerium tremens* may actually represent the neuro-protective activity of *nor-harman,* which has been implicated by Dzoljic et al as "endogenous Ibogaine."

Ordinarily, NMDA receptor-channels are clogged by a bulky Magnesium ion (*see illustration p. 200*), and may not even play a role in normal synaptic transmission.[2] A number of researchers are looking at the role of calcium influx in potentiation and growth, i.e., in long-lasting increases in nerve-cell communication *within* the synapses.

In "Quantum Coherence in Microtubules: A Neural Basis for Emergent Consciousness?," Stuart Hameroff explains that consciousness itself emerges from a critical level of coherence of quantum-level events in cytoskeletal microtubules within neurons — that each microtubule tranforms disordered molecular, thermal or electromagnetic energy into coherent photons within its hollow core, which penetrate without loss along the microtubule in a quantum phenomenon called self-induced transparency, manifesting a collective dynamics called super-radiance — involving synchronous, self-organizing firing of widely distributed neurons.[3] Our neurons, like swarms of fireflies, wax and wane together in quantum simultaneity, even though cell-to-cell, receptor-based communication must be electro-chemical, and therefore slower.

NMDA-mediated calcium influx induces changes in the spiny protrusions of dendrites, which receive chemical signals (*see figure 1*), while NMDA activity also a) stimulates post-synaptic release of arachidonic acid, a fatty acid that travels backward across synapses to presynaptic neurons and increases their output of neuro-transmitter, increasing synaptic strength; and b) may cause the enzyme protein kinase C to move from the cytoplasm out to the membrane where it phosphorylates protein growth. This new "hardwiring" allows the neuron to download the day's short-term receptor memory into long-term cellular memory — clearing up the receptors, down-modulating tolerance and supersensitivity.

To reconcile myriad conflicting receptor impulses requires more than blind tabulation, though. Remember that neurons are *fiber-optic.* Like any good neuro-transmitter, the body uses nor-harman to do a number of jobs — dreaming, waking REM, the NDE, even the DTs — which involve visualization, so that impulse and counter-impulse are played out in the REM circuits and choices may be (semi)consciously made, not blindly tabulated.

A clue to the mechanism here came from Molliver, who recounts an experiment in which Llinas briefly exposed vermal cerebellar purkinje

1 The initial blood clot excites glutamate firing in the immediate area, which sets off glutamate firing in the surrounding cells, etc., etc. — allowing all of the neurons to fill up with calcium and die.

2 Typically the NMDA receptor is involved in long-term potentiation of the hippocampus, a primitive part of the cerebral cortex that plays an important role in long-lasting memory and learning.

3 "Frolich theorized that energy could be stored without thermal loss in coherent, dipolar propagating proteins or in a thin layer of water and ions just beneath the cell membrane. Watterson (1987) has shown how organized, dynamic water clusters ('pix-

Cont. next page

cells to harmaline — immediately "washing" his sample to remove all traces of harmaline. The purkinjes continued firing for six hours from this exposure — *as if transparency in microtubules had been altered directly.* Also, instead of blocking the NMDA receptor completely, the "flickering" effect of the harmaline (and iboga, and nor-harman during REM) allows a trickle of calcium in (since too much causes cell death) — to be processed, under the apparent direction of the REM circuits,[1] into new hard-wiring for your neurons.

This means that there's no natural recovery without REM action on jaded receptors,[2] turning short-term into long-term memory — without "maturing out." And six hours of Ibogaine is like six months of REM. Chaotically (yet not randomly, since this chaos has *personality*), by calceous accretion of dendrites and microtubules, Ibogaine-fired information is not only retrieved but also (contrary to the reigning 12-step paradigm) generated — created from connections that were not *there* before.

Ibogaine's 'stroboscopic' effect — by almost but not quite blockading calcium influx at the NMDA site[3] — seems to keep a feedback loop open which enables the body to "learn" its way out of withdrawal and craving. "Compared with the effects of harmaline," observes Goutarel, "the fantasy evoked by Ibogaine is easier for the subjects to manipulate... so that, more often than with other drugs,[4] they can stop to contemplate a scene, go back, explore an alternative in a given sequence, bring a previous scene back to life, etc."[5]

The key here is "sensitive dependence on initial conditions," which vastly multiplies the initial will of the addict to get better because dendrite/microtubule accumulation has a built-in multiplier effect, an effect that's not supposed to get out of control as long as they follow the red road [perhaps because neurons must snag iron ions from the blood to keep the calcium activity in check].[6]

The Nganga say the red road is the best and safest way to the Village of the Ancestors. The first appearance of Bwiti as guide/gatekeeper is usually as a familiar elder or trusted ancestor. And *this* had been the thing Sisko emphasized, quoting Goutarel in response to Dana, in late September as they were returning to his house at the end of their long rap[7] about harmaline and Ibogaine as sacraments: "For various reasons, poor preparation, inadequate motivation, fear, psychosis, neurosis — certain subjects are unable to get past this critical phase;"[8] and he cited the need for the neophyte to be "watched constantly by his 'mother,' who regulates his psychophysiological reactions to prevent him from letting *terrifying phantoms* interfere, for they would lead him down the wrong path, down the *road of death*."[9]

Later, on the other hand, after reviewing data on the NMDA receptor, Dana said to Sisko, "You know, if you're being crucified, it makes perfect sense to take an anti-stroke medication. Harmala ought to stop the glutamate cascade — it binds to the same NMDA receptor as MK–801!"

In the beginninng of November the Republicans won the election. Instead of focusing on AIDS and Ibogaine, Lee Brown had listened to CASA, Sue Rusche, and the Partnership for a Drug Free America: when in doubt, bash pot. Their idea of a big media event for the final days of the campaign was a highly telegenic Clinton speech to some schoolkids in Massachusetts, in which he apologized for even not inhaling. Clips of that ran all day on CNN, inspiring 3–5% of the electorate not to vote — since who or what was there to vote for? Post-election analysis concluded that the GOP carved out their narrow statistical victory not because of more Republicans, but because significant numbers of Democrats, in disgust, didn't bother to vote.

The full impact of the 1994 election had not really sunk in when drug reformers gathered two weeks later in DC for the annual conference of the Drug Policy Foundation. One of the hottest workshops was the Ibogaine panel, starring Deborah Mash, with a ton of new data.

Mash revealed that Ibogaine blood concentrations reach a sharp peak from two to eight hours (during the visualizations), then rapidly fall off — de-methylated by the liver into the longer-acting, water-soluble nor-ibogaine (termed M–1, or metabolite-one) — which peaks more shallowly at twelve hours and slowly descends during the cognitive evaluation and insomnia phases (*see Figure 2, p. 210*). Somehow, she indicated, nor-ibogaine may be hanging around the central nervous system for quite a while — perhaps during the several weeks post-treatment when Ibogaine subjects are working off their REM-surplus and don't sleep much. In fact, Mash's team suspects

els') can represent information at membrane and cytoskeletal surfaces. Considering the layer of ordered water outside and inside microtubules, Del Giudice *et al.* (1983) proposed that microtubules' cyclindrical structure may be understood by quantum-vacuum symmetry breaking and boson self-focusing by ordered water. Like the Meissner effect for superconducting media, electromagnetic energy would be confined inside filamentous regions around which microtubule subunits gather. Del Guidice's group (1983) showed that this self-focusing should result in filamerntous beams of radius fifteen nanometers, precisely the inner diameter of microtubules" (*see note 13, p. 250*).

1 See pp. 119–120.

2 See illustration, p. 68.

3 See pp. 212–213 for pharmacokinetics of this. Mash, *et al.*, report that Ibogaine binds to the receptor with fifty-to-a-thousand times less potency than dizocilpine (MK801).

4 E.g. ketamine, the other NMDA receptor drug now being used in the treatment of addiction in the former Soviet Union, in a kind of aversion therapy.

5 See Appendix 2, p. 236.

6 Is color perceived on the cellular level? Hameroff asks: "Can the redness of a red object be explained by a given pattern of neuronal firing, perhaps accented by a neurochemical bathing of a particular transmitter concoction? Do two people experiencing red have the same sense of redness in their minds?....The theory of quantum coherence in the cytoskeleton implies excitations of a ground state yielding a condensed field of coherent bosons (phonons, photons, etc.) with specific frequency characteristics. Red of the electromagnetic spectrum can then correlate with a specific frequency boson-condensed field excitation in the brain." (Hameroff, pp. 95–96)

Fernandez notes that initiates often find themselves traveling a red road. Dick adds: (In) the early medieval Romanesque paintings... Red always represented the Father, Blue, the color of the Son. And gold, of course, that of the Holy Spirit." *Divine Invasion*, p. 70.

7 See end of Chapter 17, pp. 194–197.

8 Goutarel, see Appendix 2, p. 234.

9 Goutarel, see Appendix 2, p. 233.

nor-ibogaine is Stanley Glick's elusive, long-acting metabolite — that it was nor-ibogaine which up until four months after her first treatment, made Geerte F. "experience colors and light very intensely" — that nor-ibogaine was in fact responsible for the "Ibogaine-aftereffect" which Geerte experienced as "blockading craving until it wore off."

Mash also announced her team had confirmed the discovery of Poppik, et al., finding that Ibogaine keys into the NMDA receptor. Activity at this receptor is important to understanding how Ibogaine averts brain cell loss from excito-toxic withdrawal, but also a clue to what can go wrong on Ibogaine: too much glutamate and too much calcium cause excito-toxicity, and apoptosis — cell death.

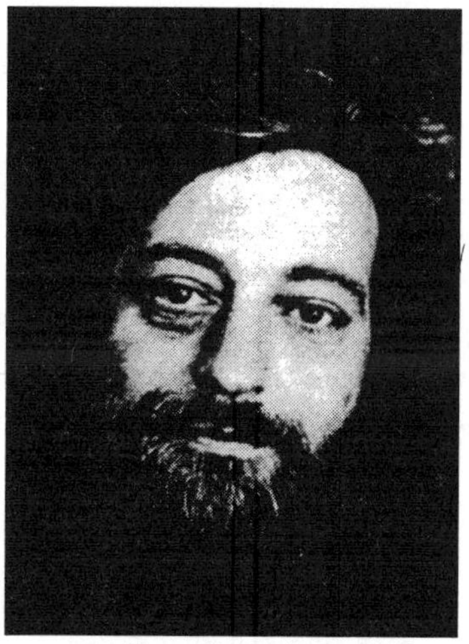

HANS–GEORG BEHR

Another discovery of the Mash team was Ibogaine binding at a third site — the muscarinic acetylcholine receptor — though even weaker than at the *kappa* opiate or NMDA receptors. This is a post-synaptic receptor, i.e., it acts presumably by up-modulating reception of pre-synaptic acetylcholine activity, and could explain Llinas's self-firing Purkinje cells. Acetylcholine is the neuro-transmitter for all sorts of muscular activity (heartbeat, etc.), but it is also an important neuro-transmitter, especially for sleep, REM, and so-on. Muscarine is the active, non-psychedelic component of amanita muscaria,[1] and is present, according to Sanchez-Ramos, in a number of substances used in traditional divination, such as datura. The Viking Berserkers used it just before battle, not to trip, but because muscarinic acid causes bursts of action, and rage. In the REM circuits, the giant pontine cells (*see illustration, p. 206*) of the hippocampus where cerebellar acetylcholine activity is shunted during REM, this is expressed as tremor, because one's responses are part of the dream — generating the "REM twitch."

The other big revelation for Ibogaine-watchers at the DPF Conference came from Dr. Todd Mikurya, who had a letter from Defense Secretary William Perry declassifying records of all chemical research prior to 1968, including psychedelic research in humans. Dr. Todd had gone personally with a delegation of relatives of victims of various accidents and experiments over the last forty years, and met at Edgewood Arsenal with a bevy of Army brass headed by a colonel. He couldn't get access to the locked CIA facility at Edgewood, however, where the Ibogaine records would be, without parallel clearance from the Director of the CIA. Curtis Wright was informed that FDA or NIDA could go ahead on their own and try — armed with the Perry letter — to get CIA to release their archives on the work of Isbell and others.

In December, Beal flew to spend Christmas in Germany with Georg Behr, who was just finishing up the new improved *Von Hanf Ist Die Rede.* Behr was certain the last word on Ibogaine and the opiate receptors was not in. Just a few months earlier, Sanchez-Ramos had told him that his previous intuition that Ibogaine must generate some kind of opioid receptor activity besides the *kappa* had been a "good clue."

In January, as the new Congress took its seats intent on enacting Gingrich's game-plan with the first 100 days, the FDA and NIH huddled to consider threats that they might be abolished, or severely neutered. All the opponents of proceeding with NIDA's first Ibogaine trial — including the NIDA old guard who disbelieved an interrupter was even possible — took their cue to come forward, to lobby Alan Leshner to stop it. Leshner ordered a complete review of MDD's Ibogaine Project by a new panel, of "outside consultants" including foremost critics like Reese Jones, Charles Gorodetzky, et al.

The first clue activists had that something was up came when Curtis Wright, after telling them another NIDA design session was in the works, said MDD had determined further "public" meetings were unnecessary. It transpired that Frank Vocci had decided not to invite the activists, or send out conference packets to anyone but invited experts.[2]

Cures Not Wars huddled, reviewed contacts among libertarian legalizers, and once more initiated the now-familiar drill of phoning, faxing, and mailing Ibogaine information to a new group. But this time it was to GOP Congressmen and conservative think tanks working on de-regulating drug approval: the Cato Institute, the Competitive Enterprise Institute and Gingrich's own Progress and Freedom Foundation. So the new Cyber-Right was put on notice. Were they interested in a quick techno-fix for addiction?

1 The psychedelic effect is caused instead by *muscamol,* which is unstable and quickly breaks down. *Amanita pantherina* has twice as much muscamol, and is much to be preferred.

2 Charles Kaplan was not invited, even though he's a regular NIDA researcher with expertise on Ibogaine in humans. A number of health activists from the Black community who'd attended the May 16, 1994 session were not invited back, either.

Clues to the Irrational Nature of Dreams

By SANDRA BLAKESLEE

FIRST comes drowsiness and a sense that it's time to rest. Eyelids grow heavy. Stray thoughts flicker through the mind as sleep begins, often with a sudden twitch. And then the human brain falls into a state of profound madness filled with hallucinations, delusions and confabulations.

Dreams unfold. We walk, run, fly and float through strange landscapes. Characters appear and turn into different people. Objects are transformed. A rope becomes a snake. Uncle Harry turns into a Tibetan monk and it all makes sense in some screwy, dreamlike way.

The bizarre nature of dreams is beginning to make sense to scientists who study the biological and physiological changes that occur in the brain during sleep, wakefulness and the many related states, like dreamless sleep, daydreaming and, some say, the writing of poetry and other creative acts.

For example, researchers have found that during sleep the brain is bombarded by wild, erratic pulses from the brainstem and flooded with nervous system chemicals that induce the insanity of dreams. Areas that control sleep are near areas that control body movements, which explains why eyelids grow heavy with drowsiness and why dreams are full of fictive movements.

Finally, the research is shedding light on the biological basis of some forms of schizophrenia, and may also help explain why deep meditation or isolation tanks can induce hallucinations and offer insight into the nature of consciousness itself.

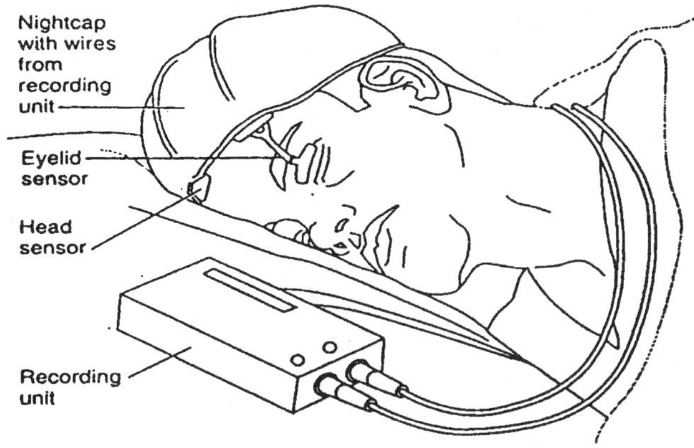

Waking, Sleeping, Perchance Dreaming

The Nightcap, a home-monitoring device, has eyelid and head sensors to record movements associated with dreaming. The lids move during dream sleep; head movements tend to increase when dreams end and non dream sleep or the transition to wakefulness occurs.

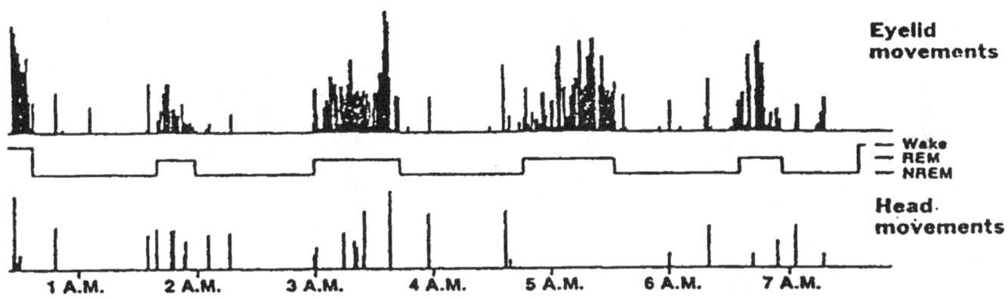

Source: Harvard University

The New York Times; Illustration by Al Granberg

"We study sleeping to understand waking," said Dr. Allan Hobson, a neuroscientist at Harvard University who has helped develop some of the leading theories on the biology of dreams. "We study dreaming to understand madness."

Dr. Hobson and his colleagues presented their latest findings at the annual meeting of the Society for Sleep Research in Boston last month.

Dream researchers disagree about many of the details, "but the Hobson model is the best thing we have going for us now," said Dr. Stanley Krippner, president of the Association for the Study of Dreams and a veteran dream psychologist. "It can tell us a lot about how memory is constructed and reconstructed and how people use personal myths" to define reality.

Machines like electroencephalograms that measure electrical brain activity and others that measure magnetic brain activity cannot distinguish the awake brain from the dreaming brain, Dr. Hobson said in a recent interview.

The awake brain receives copious amounts of information from the outside world, mainly in the form of light and sound frequencies, chemical signals and physical touch, Dr. Hobson said. It processes these signals in vast, oscillating networks of brain cells to form representations of the external world and combines these maps with memories, movements, emotions and forethought in a way that gives rise to self-awareness and an ability to navigate the world during waking hours.

The dreaming brain employs all of the same systems and networks, Dr. Hobson said, but with a few critical

> We study sleeping to understand waking and dreaming to understand madness.

differences. Input from the outside world is screened out. Self-awareness ceases. The body is paralyzed. And everything that the dreaming brain sees, hears or feels is generated from within.

During sleep the nondreaming brain falls physiologically, somewhere between these two states, Dr. Hobson said. New technology allows researchers to examine the chemical, electrical and physical properties of each state. "We can study each of these states to see what the differences are," he said.

The key to dreams is found in several tiny nodes within the brainstem that contain cells which squirt out different chemical transmitters, Dr. Hobson said. These cells have projections that carry the chemicals throughout the brain and modulate its activity. The projections also extend down to the spinal cord and help control movement.

The awake brain is dominated by so-called adrenergic chemicals released from two of these nodes, Dr. Hobson said. The cells fire these chemicals in pacemaker fashion, keeping the brain alert, enhancing attention and priming motor activity. In the adrenergic state thought processes are generally stable and the brain is not easily dominated by stray images.

'Gimmick' to Induce Sleep

As the brain goes to sleep, the adrenergic system begins to shut down, Dr. Hobson said. Other nodes release so-called cholinergic chemicals which, although active in performing important brain functions during the day, begin to dominate the brain's chemistry. Self-awareness ceases and memory is lost. The brain enters a state of dreamless sleep featuring fuzzy images. It is not organized.

The cholinergic neurons are located one millimeter away from neurons that control muscles in the eyelids, Dr. Hobson said. This is why the eyelids get heavy when cholinergic signals take over. "It's the body's gimmick to get you to sleep," he said.

Soon, Dr. Hobson said, adrenergic neurons cease firing altogether. Cholinergic chemicals decouple the extensive networks used for cognition and behavior. In this state, the brain is ultrasensitive to stray thoughts and can jump from one class of images to another without realizing contradictions. In other words, it dreams.

The bifurcations of thought and the bizarre nature of dreams are also driven by cholinergic neurons, he said. Instead of firing steadily, as they do during the day, these cells begin bursting hundreds of times a second and sending erratic pulses into higher brain regions. These pulses, called PGO, or pontine-geniculate-occipital, waves, occur only during dreams and have multiple effects.

First, they stimulate the body's

New York Times

The Sleep-Dream Cycle at the Brain-Cell Level

Two types of brain cells show different activity patterns in waking, non-dreaming sleep and dreaming sleep. The type called locus ceruleus neurons, controlling the adrenergic chemical system, are most active during waking hours, drop during non-rapid-eye-movement (NREM) sleep and are quiescent in REM, or dream, sleep. The type called giant pontine neurons, controlling the cholinergic chemical system, are least active in waking, progressively more active in NREM sleep and most active in dreaming.

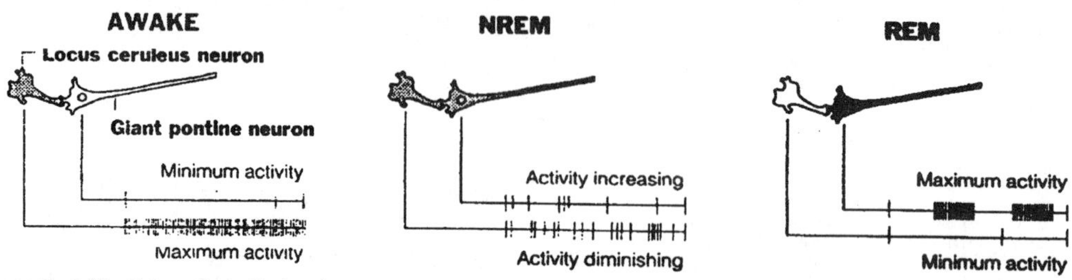

Source: Dr. J. Allan Hobson, Roche Products Inc.

The New York Times

motor centers, found in the brainstem. This would cause the dreamer to walk, run and carry out a vast repertoire of movements except that another signal is sent simultaneously to the spinal cord, resulting in total muscle paralysis except for the eyes. This increase in cholinergic activity is what makes many people twitch or startle when they are drifting off to sleep, Dr. Hobson said. And it explains why sleepwalking almost always occurs during nondream sleep, when the muscles are not paralyzed.

In dreams, Dr. Hobson continued, complex motor patterns are activated. "It's no accident that we are always in motion," he said. "We are practicing all sorts of movements in a kind of neural gymnastics."

The Stuff of Dreams

PGO waves also bombard the brain's emotional circuits and give rise to the strong feelings that often accompany dreams, Dr. Hobson said. One-third of all adult dreams involve anxiety and fear, he said, followed by joy, anger, sadness, guilt and eroticism.

Finally, the PGO waves shoot into the brain's higher regions where vast networks for processing information reside. Except now, Dr. Hobson said, every sight, sound and sensory input is generated internally by the brain itself. The higher networks, which are used to making representations of the world during the waking state, try to make sense of the internal images and feelings by concocting stories in the cholinergic brain, he said. The repertoire of possible combinations of images, memories and story lines on any given night is extremely large, and chance stimulation probably plays a large role in the content of our dreams.

People can enter a cholinergic state without going to sleep, said Dr. Edgar Garcia-Rill, a neuroscientist at the University of Arkansas in Little Rock, in an interview after the Boston meeting. He points out that such states exist during meditation, as well as sometimes when people are in sensory isolation tanks. Pilots occasionally experience these states when they stare at nothing but blue sky. Hallucinations, as in dreams, may result.

Many scientific insights have occurred in dreams, when the brain is open to unusual associations, Dr. Garcia-Rill said. He suggested that poets may be more naturally cholinergic. And, in work underway in his laboratory, Dr. Garcia-Rill has found that some schizophrenics have an abnormal number of cholinergic neurons in their brainstems, and that this defect may explain the hallucinations that mark the disorder.

To explore dreams in a more natural setting than the hospital-based sleep laboratory, Harvard researchers recently invented a device called the Nightcap. It is a cloth bandanna, worn pirate-style around the head, attached to a wallet sized instrument that tucks under the pillow. One lead goes to a tiny box stitched into the bandanna that registers each time a person's head moves. A second lead sticks to one eyelid and records lid movements all night long. The lids move during dream sleep, whereas head movements tend to occur when dreams end and nondream sleep or the transition to wakefulness occurs, said Robert Stickgold, a researcher in the laboratory.

The Nightcap can record up to 30 nights of sleep, Mr. Stickgold said. The device plugs into a computer so that any individual's sleep patterns can be analyzed in minutes, easily and relatively inexpensively, while he sleeps at home in his own bed. A Nightcap user can program the device to sound a signal during a dream episode to wake him up, so that he can recall the dreams.

Alcohol, Prozac and Exercise

Home dream reports are four times longer than dream reports taken in laboratories, Mr. Stickgold said.

In experiments described in the March issue of the journal Consciousness and Cognition, the Nightcap showed that alcohol use suppresses dream sleep, that Prozac intensifies it and that heavy exercise can result in no body movements throughout the night.

Mr. Stickgold said that researchers in Thailand plan to use the device to explore why many young men who live near the Laotian border die suddenly in their sleep. The current explanation is that the men are being visited by the widow ghost who punishes them for infidelity.

"We also hope to send the Nightcap into space," Mr. Stickgold said. Astronauts on the Mir space station could use it to study the effects of zero gravity on dreams: "Do you still shift your body after coming out of a dream? Are dream reports going to be different?" he said.

The Harvard laboratory is also studying the content of dreams for insights into changing brain states. Dreams are full of discontinuities, incongruities, uncertainties and jumps in plot, scene location, characters and objects. What do these say about dream mentation?

Using 453 dream reports from 45 volunteers, the Harvard researchers cut dream reports into segments at discontinuity points — as when a beach scene abruptly and nonsensically turns into an indoor scene. The segments were spliced together in novel ways, while other dreams were left intact. Independent observers were asked to pick out the spliced dreams. They did no better than chance.

The Nature of Consciousness

In a second experiment, the researchers studied character and object transformations in dreams. Can a teacher turn into a whale? Can a barn turn into a teacher? Apparently not, for when people were shown two columns of characters and objects and asked to pair those that made sense, they got it right 80 percent of the time.

"There are limits to the transformations that can occur at some deep category level," Dr. Hobson said.

Eventually, he added, research into sleep and dreaming may help explain the nature of consciousness. People cycle through different brain states every 24 hours, he said. If more can be learned about each state, it might be possible to subtract one from the other to learn how consciousness is engineered.

Only Speaker Gingrich or President Clinton can resolve the current impasse between two committees of Congress and authorize release of $60 million[1] from the Forfeiture Fund (under Criminal Justice) to NIDA Medications (under Health & Environment) for Ibogaine development. Even the biggest advocates of prisons ought to appreciate the fiscal implications of a cure that enables 25–40% of addicts to walk away from addiction without expensive support and social services.

The most interested, though, seemed to be the Cato Institute. [Presumably not directly named after the Roman Cato who declared, *"Cartago dalenda est"* ("Carthage must be destroyed") — *to defeat Hannibal. Smash every brick and sow the land with salt, that nothing may grow there, ever again. And pursue Hannibal even to Asia Minor (where he generalled for a while for the Jews), to bring him back to Rome in chains…*]

Meanwhile, on January 19, 1995, Dhoruba was definitively cleared of the 1971 attack on two NYC police officers. The day of Wisdom and the rule of Wisdom had finally come. Manhattan District Attorney Robert Morgenthau, after exhausting every legal manuever to re-instate the original conviction, decided the case was too old to re-try.

A few days later in Rotterdam, after several months of terminal dementia, Nico Adriaans died of AIDS. Despite being an original founder of needle exchange, Nico had somehow become infected, and as an HIV positive would be excluded from current Ibogaine trials. That's unfortunate, because through Ibogaine, he was able to elucidate something very important about addiction and freedom: *"If you are resisting suffering, you suffer more. So you know: If you learn from suffering, so that you can know how to act in order to be free, you must accept a lifetime of constant, difficult learning. Addicts stop learning."*

The date of NIDA's new Ibogaine meeting wasn't hard to find out — March 8. But when David Goldstein requested an invitation, he was informed only designated experts were invited. As an addiction professional who'd been at the previous session in May, Rommell Washington was able to wrangle an invitation on the phone, but no conference packet arrived in the mail.

At this point parallel processes intervened in the person of "Brother Shine" of ADAM, the Afrikan Descendents' Awareness Movement. Within days of being paroled from a two-year bit upstate stemming from a crack relapse, Thomas Shine was organizing the first broad community forum on Ibogaine in Harlem in conjunction with the Black Coalition on Drugs, inviting among others Deborah Mash and Carlo Contoreggi. For Carlo to come up and speak, approval was needed by NIDA higher-ups.

On February 8, at the regular NIDA Advisory Council[2] on the campus of the NIH, Dana Beal hand-delivered a letter from the Black Coalition on Drugs to Alan Leshner, asking his approval for Carlo to go to an Ibogaine forum in Harlem, which Leshner gave on the spot. Frank Vocci was there also. He conceded they couldn't really keep the activists out on March 8. But because there would only be public seating at the Rockville Holiday Inn for ten, it was on a first-come, first-serve basis. Dana said he'd be there at 6:00 AM.

The main preoccupations of the Council session seemed to be marijuana, and to a lesser extent finding a cure for cocaine. Leshner enthusiastically reported meeting — in the company of Jim Burke of the Partnership for a Drug-Free America — with Bill and Hillary Clinton in the White House. Then he wondered aloud why our society has a "unique disconnect" between its understanding of drug abuse as a disease and its drive to punish users. But before the "public comment" at 4:30 PM, Leshner ducked out, leaving his deputy Richard Millstein in charge.

Dana got up and asked whether NIDA was contemplating any public education aimed at keeping the latest crop of kids using cannabis from experimenting with the new stronger smokable heroin under the influence of "grunge" rock, etc. Millstein said the Institute has only two pilot programs, in two cities, aimed at preventing casual users from "graduating." The attitude that day seemed to be, heroin's fine — we've got methadone.

Now as it happened, neither Deborah Mash nor Carlo made it up to the Harlem forum. But Leshner had become aware that the Afro-American community was conducting its own review of Ibogaine -- a few days

[1] As recommended by the IOM Report.

[2] Held every four months.

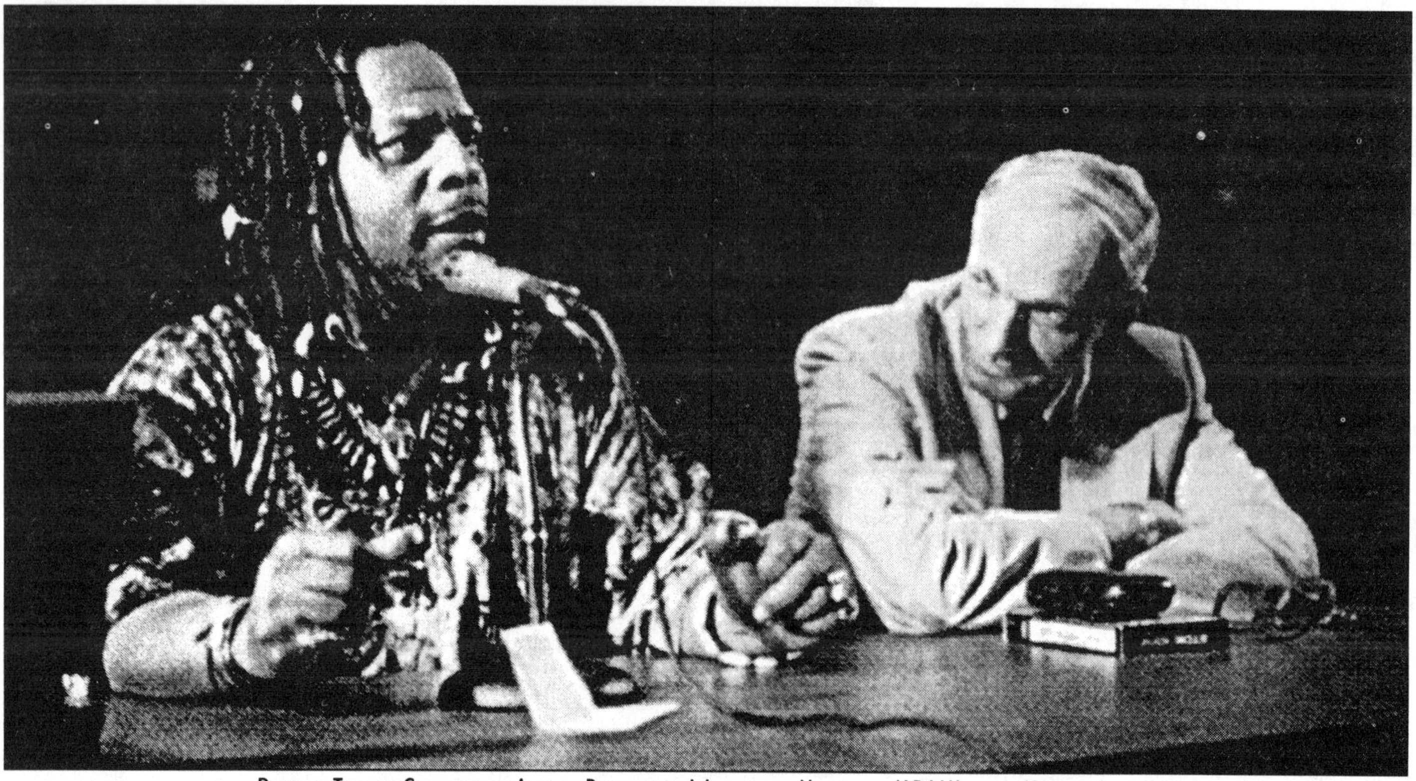

Paul Di Rienzo

BROTHER THOMAS SHINE OF THE AFRIKAN DESCENDENTS' AWARENESS MOVEMENT (ADAM), WITH HOWARD LOTSOF

before NIDA, on March 4. And Leshner's office increased seats for the public on March 8th to 25, after Kiyoshi Kuromiya called the Director's office to make sure he had a seat. Then, a week-and-a-half before his forum, Brother Shine invited Leshner himself to come, or send a representative to Harlem.

Finally, two weeks of intense airplay on WBAI, WLIB, and WRL produced, on the afternoon of March 4th, a turn-out of 350 at the Dempsey Center (127 W. 127th Street, off Malcolm X Boulevard).

Brother Shine took the stage, and said that as someone born addicted to heroin, Ibogaine was "very personal" to him. He introduced John Morgan, a New York City College pharmacologist. Professor Morgan recounted the surprise that took hold among skeptical professionals in the field when the work of Glick, Dzoljic, Broderick and others first demonstrated in rats the pharmacological basis — independent of "set and setting" — for Ibogaine's interruption of addiction.

Howard Lotsof followed with his story of discovery in the '60s, development in the '80s, and the experience of treating almost sixty addicts in the Netherlands and Panama. Natural-healing advocate John Harris spoke on the historical use of Iboga as central to the African Bwiti rite-of-passage involving an entire extended family. Moderator Bernard White of WBAI read a statement on Ibogaine and Re-socialization therapy from Dhoruba Bin Wahad, delayed on a Ghana Air flight. Then Eddie Ellis from Neighborhood Defender made the best speech of the day, placing Ibogaine squarely in the history of Black Panther struggle, COINTELPRO, AND his own liberation from prison.

Dana wrapped up the program with word of the NIDA review in Rockville a few days later, inviting everyone to come on down or at least make their views known to NIDA, Lee Brown and Charles Rangel.

On Tuesday, New York state parole officials balked at letting Shine go to Rockville. But a vanload did make it down the next morning to the Crowne Plaza Holiday Inn, a few blocks from NIDA offices at the Parklawn Building. Dhoruba, who had come down on his own, brought in six or seven local people from Howard University.

Frank Vocci began promptly at 8:30 AM, saying the question was whether or not it's safe to proceed in humans.

Rick Strassman presented the Baumann

data. It seemed that after badmouthing Lotsof's procedure at the 1987 Ibogaine Conference in Paris ("...Addiction is not in the competence of psychiatry..."), Baumann promptly went home and used the procedure to treat 35 female addicts, though at about half the dose Lotsof recommends. He also disregarded the contra-indication for patients with coronary problems, which apparently cost a life.

Next, Howard Lotsof summarized about sixty treatments done by NDA International. He offered the first time-lapse video showing Mark Lamantia just before re-treatment, then answering questions of a neurologist at one-hour intervals as the Ibogaine peaked, and then after recovery. The evident pharmacological impact of Ibogaine on the slurred, sideways-glancing, hunched body-language of chronic cocaine/methadone intoxication — the striking transformation of skin and muscle tone — made for a before-and-after comparison no written account can really convey.

Howard characterized Ibogaine efficacy as "15% success, 15% failure, with the length of interruption in everyone else falling somewhere in between on a bell curve."

Much more detail was provided on the last eight Panama treatments, with Dr. Dan Luciano and Deborah Mash joining Howard to present their observations. Luciano noted Ibogaine was well-tolerated except for early movement-induced nausea and vomiting; with acute transitory cerebellar/vestibular effects, but none persistent. EEGs before, during, and after showed no abnormalities of any kind, not even at the moment of the "splitting of the skull." A distinct interval of cerebellar reset was not possible, via EEG, to detect.

Instead, Deborah Mash provided a trove of new details on blood levels of Ibogaine and its active metabolite that offered a *pharmaco-kinetic* explanation of what's going on. Her graph (*see next page*) showed Ibogaine at first being converted into metabolite at such a rate that blood levels of both rise almost in lockstep.

The visualization phase clearly corresponds to the Ibogaine spike between one and six hours — thrusting above the long rolling peak of metabolite which does not exit the brain easily and may hang out there for weeks.

Dr. Mash identified the active metabolite as 12-hydroxy-ibogamine. Miami found that nor-ibogaine was significantly blocking serotonin re-uptake[1] — an effect that would heighten mood and attenuate drug craving — as well as being active at the *mu* and *delta* opiate receptor sites[!] Although presumably the same kind of "weak" activity seen at the *kappa* and NMDA receptors, this filled a great deal that was missing when the only thing stopping opiate withdrawal seemed to be some weak *kappa* receptor activity.

Howard concluded that the treatment team felt the intrusive taking of bloods interfered with the therapeutic Ibogaine effect[2] — and that expectations of efficacy during Phase I safety trials should be scaled down correspondingly.

Charles Gorodetzky next presented complete autopsy reports on the Baumann death and the possible Dutch heroin OD, plus the case of Nancy, even though Ibogaine had been ruled out as cause of her death. It turns out Baumann, in clear defiance of Lotsof's recommended procedure, had given Ibogaine to a female with not only 80% coronary arterial schlerosis and evidence of previous silent heart attack, but opiates in her urine! In the case of Nicola K., heroin overdose just prior to death was still not ruled out, since she had foil and an empty vial and time in the bathroom to smoke what was in the vial. However, sky-high blood levels of metabolite (but expected levels of Ibogaine) pointed instead to Nicola K. being an extremely slow metabolizer, who succumbed to respiratory collapse when the effects of 12-hydroxy-Ibogaine were overly prolonged.

Jim Dingell[3] asked if they'd considered whether glucuronidation was the pathway for eliminating Ibogaine, since her body's glucuronic acid could still have been occupied processing her previous evening's opiate use in the liver even without great levels of opiate anywhere else. Or was the P450 pathway involved? Without knowing how exactly Ibogaine and nor-ibogaine are excreted in humans, it might be impossible ever to figure out precisely what happened to Nicola K.

After lunch Peter Hoyle took over, and made it clear right away that he felt the pre-clinical work hadn't been done to provide a pharmacokinetic, pharmacodynamic model to support a clinical trial design. Mechanism of action was unclear, and receptor-specificity —

1 Same as Prozac, which can be used as an anti-addictive drug. "Chronic use of cocaine may lead to a 'serotonin-deficit' form of 5–HT dysregulation," according to Mash, et al., in "Identification of a Primary Metabolite of Ibogaine that Targets Serotonin Transporters and Elevates Serotonin," *Life Sciences,* Vol. 57, No. 3, pp. PL45–50, 1995. "The elevation of synaptic levels of 5–HT by 12-hydroxy-ibogaine may, by analogy with the potent 5–HT reuptake blocker fluoxetine, promote generalized anti-craving effects along with improvements in mood and cognition."

"Drugs that interact with transporters act as uptake inhibitors or releasers to increase synaptic levels of neurotransmitters. Ibogaine and 12-hydroxyibogaine failed to significantly elevate DA levels, although a trend toward increased synaptic concentrations was apparent at the higher dose... 12-hydroxyibogaine elevated 5–HT with ten-fold higher potency as compared to ibogaine.... Re-uptake blockers usually show a thee-to-five-fold elevation in neurotransmitter, whereas neurotransmitter releasers are usually distinguished by a twelve-to-twenty-fold elevation in monoamine. At the highest dose tested (10 mg/kg), 12-hydroxyibogaine may act as a potent 5–HT blocker. In drug discrimination screens to test generalization of ibogaine to DA and 5–HT drugs, ibogaine was most like the potent 5–HT releaser D-fenfluramine. Ibogaine has been shown by in vivo microvoltometry to elevate extracellular 5–HT in the nucleus accumbens. Future studies are needed to define... whether or not the elevation in 5–HT is due to blockade of 5–HT re-uptake and/or increased 5–HT release" (p. PL–50.)

2 For an explanation of why this is so, see Hameroff on the brain as quantum computer: "coherent quantum phenomena cannot perform computation if the system undergoes significant 'measurement-like interactions' with the outside world..." p. 249.

3 The brother of the US Congressman from Michigan.

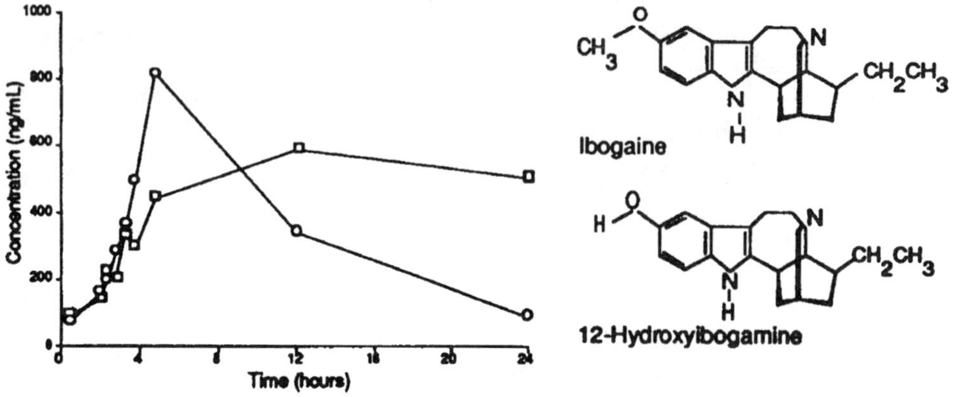

Fig. 2

Pharmacokinetics of ibogaine (O) and 12-hydroxyibogamine (□) over the first 24 hr after oral administration.

Data shown are from a representative male subject (20 mg kg^{-1}) and were measured in whole blood samples (ng per ml).

kappa-opiate, voltage-dependent NA channel, and NMDA interaction — difficult to extrapolate to a clinical setting. Impressive basic research, but study designs hadn't provided an objective basis for optimal dose-schedule, route, and duration of administration in a clinical trial. Correlations between non-clinical data and target indication were too weak to provide pre-clinical rationale for Ibogaine efficacy. With Ibogaine, rationale for efficacy and clinical benefit depend totally on previous human data. Two tours of duty at the FDA, he knew how tough this made it. Oftentimes clinical benefits are realized without understanding mechanism. Still, in his opinion, Ibogaine wasn't ready.

Glick, up next, demonstrated conclusively that *something* measurable was taking place in his rats — something that could amount to interruption of addiction in humans. But how, for instance, do you measure in rats the craving newly-recovering addicts keep in check via NA meetings?

Dr. Robert Upton presented mathematical analysis of his rat data, showing that whereas Ibogaine was converted to metabolite virtually on the first pass through the liver and other organs, systemic clearance of 12-hydroxy-ibogamine tended to be saturable — i.e., elimination would be slow at first and then gain momentum. Ibogaine could even actually be de-methylated by enzymes within nerve tissue, where nor-ibogaine might behave "as if trapped in the nerve tissue" due to the different electrical charge of the ibogamine.

With such drugs, the enzymes that clear the drug are overwhelmed until levels fall. With a drug that really saturates the system, like dilantin,[1] a 15% increment could potentially take its effect from marginal to lethal. Although the margin of error with Ibogaine was almost certainly greater,[2] he urged great care with the dose. Additionally, dose-relatedness is complex — with blood levels showing concave instead of convex curves — indicating uneven solubility of Ibogaine HCl as currently formulated.

Peter Hoyle came back up. He presented horrendous toxicities — setting new definitions of the lethal dose level in rats by giving 200-to-800 mg/kg (only one died!) — or vasculitis of arteries, necrosis of organs, and fluid in body cavities, achieved by dosing female dogs (25 mg/kg,) continuously for fifteen days.

In the hall, Curtis Wright intimated that Hoyle had been burned as the FDA hearing officer responsible for approving AZT, okayed on a showing of efficacy in just twenty persons!

Mark Molliver painted a much-less-alarming picture. He said glial-cell activation in his primates was minor, and the kind of Purkinje cell damage seen in rats was so rare that he concluded neurotoxicity is not important in primates. But he'd observed a syndrome of withdrawal/respiratory slowdown leading to collapse and death — an outcome that could be obviated by massaging the animal to bring it around. And the doses he was using (150 mg/kg five times every two-and-a-half hours) caused seizures.

Molliver also gave the neurotox results in monkeys on 12-hydroxyibogamine, which turned out to have "only a fraction" of the toxicity of Ibogaine itself — though in all the same sites, in the Purkinjes of the cerebellar vermis and so-on. It was also strongly hypotonic,[3] not tremorigenic like Ibogaine. But Ibogaine brain levels reached this extraordinary inverted "V"-shaped peak because it took

1 A common anti-epileptic medication.

2 He wanted additional grants to measure results of low-dose Ibogaine over time. However, he also confided that the rat doesn't have a proper gall bladder — a human organ that may be important where excretion of gall is concerned.

1 Ataxic, sleep-inducing.

the liver four hours to turn the majority of the mother compound into active metabolite.

What this presented was a new, *pharma-co-dynamic* picture of the "splitting of the skull": of the Ibogaine *punching through* — the initial oscillating effect abruptly bleeding into dreamlike visualizations due to metabolite-heightened serotonin levels — and then reaching a sharp peak for a few hours in the brain before falling off in line with the ending of the visions, leaving mostly 12-hydroxyibogamine during the next, introspective phase, and serotonergic metabolite alone during the final insomnia. So a distinct interval of cerebellar reset, if any, might lie in this moment of discontinuity between the effects of drug and metabolite, not the transition from normal wakefulness to drug.

Then Deborah Mash got up and presented neuro-toxicity data on her primates, which showed no damage. Finally, she played her trump card. She pulled out a human brain — Nancy's brain — which, by the greatest coincidence of all, was the perfect specimen for determining faint trace-neurotoxicity in human females.

There was evidence of chronic vitamin E depletion caused by drinking on top of methadone; but brain sections failed to show any damage to Purkinjes in the critical area of the cerebellar vermis.

The trend of the evidence was clear: even though some of the animal toxicities were horrendous, at therapeutic levels Ibogaine is non-neurotoxic in humans, and nor-ibogaine even less so. In animals, high doses are toxic — increasingly so as researchers moved from primates to the rat and dog, but only at prolonged exposures, which might be generating distinct toxic metabolites.

When Molliver suggested he would like to take his own look at Nancy's cerebellum, though, Mash shot back — "I'll trade you my brain samples for your blood levels!" She felt that Molliver's primate deaths were particularly senseless, since he hadn't even bothered to track blood levels of Ibogaine to correlate with the rest of his data.

Next was Juan Sanchez-Ramos with his findings from the stalled Phase I clinical trial. Out in the hall Dhoruba was talking to the ONDCP representative, Barbara Roberts, asking to meet Lee Brown instead of being put off to the end under public comment. Inside, Bonnie Levin explained the battery of neuro-tests to be given to subjects of the Panama treatments. Aside from minor difficulty with re-call in one subject immediately after Ibogaine, she found no cognitive deficits or impairment. Walter Ling presented the draft protocol, and the main modification Grudzinskas suggested was to unblind the blood level data, so that it could be carefully monitored before each dose escalation.

Howard re-iterated that NDA now considered Phase I procedures too intrusive; and that they'd rather do a quick, simple safety trial followed by clinical determinations in men focusing exclusively on efficacy against different addictive drugs. He repeated his call for low-dose testing in women, saying it would have to be tackled sooner or later. But when Frank Vocci sounded out the outside consultants, it was clear some of them were still unfamiliar with, or just didn't believe in, the whole idea of an addiction interrupter.

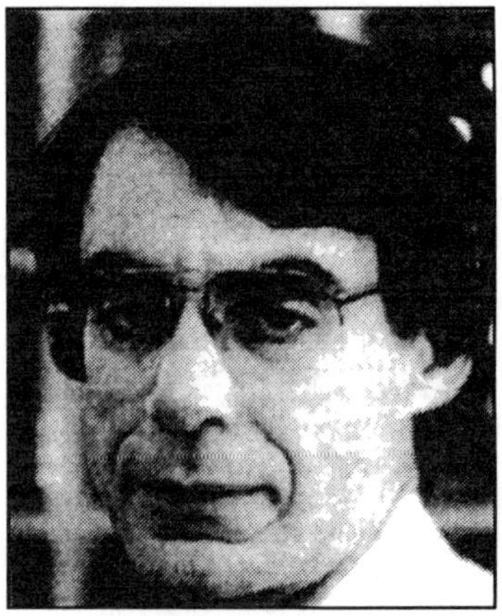

New York Times

DR. DONALD DESJARLAIS

So it fell to Dana to rebuke them for looking at Ibogaine in a vacuum — when the most important new vector for AIDS is sex-for-crack, according to data from Don DesJarlais, former head of the National AIDS Commission, published a week earlier in *The New York Times*.[1] Said Dana:

> "The reason we're all sitting here is that there is no known pharmacotherapy for cocaine. If we have to go into humans anyway to find out which other species is most like man, we might as well procede in man. As for dropping efficacy, we were told a showing of efficacy would make-or-break Ibogaine. How big was the sample used to approve AZT? We have 65 Ibogaine treatments. Don't make us wait another three years before going into humans."

Peter Hoyle, incredibly, argued that second thoughts about AZT justified a double standard for Ibogaine — that accelerated approval of AZT should become a precedent for *not* approving Ibogaine! — despite much more clearly established benefit, and some permanent interruptions of addiction with Ibogaine.[2]

Frank Vocci cautioned the room that this meeting was not designed to come to consensus, and announced an end-of-the-month deadline for outside consultants to file their

1 "Maybe as much as half of the new infections among heterosexuals are occuring in relation to crack cocaine.... HIV is transmitted more easily during two periods: when a person first contracts the virus and a decade or so later when the immune system is collapsing. If a woman...has sex 100 times with a man who is infected... but... latent... she is much less likely to get infected than if she has sex just once with one man who may be... infectious... So a woman is at much greater risk having sex once with 100 partners, most of whom are infected. "New Picture of Who Will Get AIDS is Dominated by Addicts," by Gina Kolata, *New York Times*, p. C3.

2 There has never been a single case of AIDS cured with AZT.

recommendations and comment.

No matter what the outcome, it will be revisited. The irresistable force of the public demanding medicine to stop addiction is up against the immovable object of the experts who believe only maintenance drugs are possible, or even desirable.

During the session, Dana also released a letter he and Dhoruba had faxed Leshner the day before, which said in part —

> "Without a much higher profile on the distinct dangers of heroin, your present public relations campaign in conjunction with Jim Burke and the Partnership may well reinforce the perception that heroin is not that much worse than marijuana — or really that different. Even more than rock scene or celebrity status, this perception that heroin is not really that different from other drugs is an essential ingredient of 'heroin chic.'
>
> "Inasmuch as NIDA is doing yet another review of Ibogaine's clinical possiblities ...a small safety/efficacy trial of Ibogaine this year in a few opiate addicts would both provide that media focus and deliver concrete benefits against heroin addiction in the near future. Do something that sends a *real* message."

More than one speaker on the 8th, acknowledging growing pressure to go ahead in humans, warned of safety considerations being "swamped" in the rush to use Ibogaine if the first small trial confirms efficacy. According to Carlo, "If Ibogaine is slowed down, it's about three years too late to stop it. They know it works. Even if in the end they can't use it in people, still NIDA views Ibogaine as a fascinating window into the human brain, a probe to the farthest reaches of addictive behavior."

Frank Vocci sees Ibogaine NMDA receptor activity, for instance, as a possible clue that "strong memory" in the amygdala (where you lay down long-term memories, as well as remembering what you're doing from moment to moment) may involve a nano-second NMDA "flare-up" which is as essential to addictive craving as the dopamine 'reward' in the nucleus accumbens 'pleasure spot.'

The persistence of 12 hydroxy-ibogamine in the brain may also be the key to Ibogaine's "re-set" of endorphin levels from the chronic deficit of heroin addiction. According to findings of Dzoljic, the weak but long-lived nor-ibogaine effect on all three opiate receptors potentiates production of endogenous *nor-harman,*[1] the neurotransmitter of eidetic memory and dreams — in effect 'fooling the system' because another of the active metabolite's effects, like nor-harman, is itself to reverse built-up tolerance, so receptors can then signal normal production of endorphins to resume. In fact, Lotsof believes nor-harman is also the body's first line of defense against opiate addiction, but that without help from the metabolite, it is simply overwhelmed by heroin.

The underlying hypothesis — that the opiate and NMDA receptors are in fact one, interactive receptor-complex — is supported by additional, recently published findings that Ibogaine (but not, according to Glick, nor-ibogaine[2]) binds to a site called "sigma-2," the receptor for haldol. None of the other NMDA receptor drugs like PCP, MK801, or ketamine bind to the *sigma* receptors, which were first thought to be a fourth opioid-receptor type because of affinity for benzo-morphans — then rejected as true opiod receptors because of zero affinity for morphine and naltrexone. But different *sigma* drugs have been shown to attenuate or potentiate NMDA activity.[3]

In the complex opioid/NMDA receptor interaction, the probable function of *sigma*-2, especially, is down-modulating hallucinogenic *kappa* and NMDA effects — just as *kappa* in turn downregulates primary *mu* euphoria, yet prolongs analgesia, and NMDA activity obviates build-up of tolerance/withdrawal. Interestingly, both NMDA and *sigma*-2 ligands are considered neuro-protective.

On the other hand, these kinds of "mixed," agonist/antagonist effects with Ibogaine (tremorgenic, *kappa*-ergic, with NMDA binding attenuated by *sigma*-2 activity) raise the interesting possibility that Ibogaine both potentiates and partially antagonizes the effects of its active offspring nor-Ibogaine (hypotonic, serotonergic, weakly active at the *mu* and *delta,* as well as *kappa* and NMDA sites — but not at *sigma*-2). This is because glutamate and glycine are necessary to "unlock" the NMDA receptor. Therefore NMDA activity and any modulatory *sigma*-2 effect must *entrain* with Ibogaine's rhythmic (10-times-a-second) glutamate firing, driven by the olivo-cerebellum. And during the peak, visualization phase, Ibogaine tremor is shunted into "flickering" back and forth between Ibogaine and nor-ibo-

1 Precipitated by the weak but long-lived nor-ibogaine effect on all three opiate receptors, according findings of Dzoljic that opiate receptor stimulation up-regulates production of the neuro-transmitter responsible for eidetic memory and dreams. See Dzoljic, p. 339, for evidence that nor-horman down-regulates narcotic withdrawal.

2 Personal communication, D. Beal. See also Mach, et al., "Ibogaine Possesses a Selective Affinity for the Sigma^2 Receptor," *Life Sciences,* Vol. 57, #4, pp. PL57 — PL62. Also Bowen, et al., "Ibogaine and its Congeners are Sigma^2 Receptor-Selective Ligands with Moderate Affinity," *European Journal of Pharmacology,* 279 (1995), pp. R1–R3.

3 See Kaiser, Pontecorvo and Mewshae, "Sigma Receptor Ligands: Function and Activity," *Neurotransmissions,* Volume VII, Number 1 (May, 1991).

gaine modes, which subjects experience as "two world super-imposition" —as the *sigma*-2 pulse of the more potent Ibogaine[1] momentarily brings them down from their Iboga/serotonin dream ["I had only to open my eyes and I was back in the room"] attenuating the NMDA channel blocker effect and letting in a nano-pulse of calcium.

Calcium channels / action potentials are also possibly being modulated by Ibogaine's *kappa* effect.[2] But according to Henry Sershen[3] even this *kappa* effect is definitely "mixed," since Ibogaine blocks ordinary *kappa* inhibition of dopamine, glutamate and locomotor activity. The main effect of Ibogaine pre-treatment was to *inhibit serotonin release* — and depletion — by cocaine. Dopamine was not inhibited, indeed Ibogaine initially released DA.[4] Instead nor-Ibogaine — possibly by sensitizing the serotonin receptor[5] — seems to block dopamine from any *further* run-up.

Not only does this explain how the dopamine in Broderick's Ibogainized rats (p. 130) goes up only slightly while the untreated controls go sky high, but it indicates 1.) that multiple receptor interactions[6] control cocaine dopamine release, 2.) that at least three receptor systems are most likely involved in natural recovery.[7] All of which makes NIDA's opposition to a multi-receptor treatment for coke seem more and more predicated on keeping the distinction between dopaminergic and non-dopaminergic drugs[8] from ever becoming clear to the general public.

Adam N., recently re-interviewed, provided the additional insight that the process of working the aches out of one's body for several days after a treatment may be fairly integral to the successful interruption of opiate dependence. Just as some kind of prolonged up-regulation of nor-harman by lingering iboga metabolite may be necessary for the successful "reset" of endorphin receptors, this upsurge of endorphins caused by tremor-induced body aches that settle in at the beginning of the introspective period — following after peaks of Ibogaine and 12 hydroxy-ibogamine — may put opiate addicts on the pharmacokinetic equivalent of a glidepath to receptor re-set. Indirect evidence of such an effect is seen in the longer recovery times Lotsof notes that heroin and methadone addicts seem to need after Ibogaine, compared to the relative ease with which cocaine abusers recover.

Or put another way, the unease and imbalance addicts experience when their dopamine levels aren't maintained at an artificially high level may be eliminated during Ibogaine treatment as naturally as a boat righting itself in water — via cerebellar/vestibular "re-modeling" of the self flickering between waking space/time and the circuit that allows us, while dreaming, to walk and run even though we're flat on our back.

On the other hand, if a certain "symmetry" is necessary between this after-surge of natural endorphins and the earlier Ibogaine and nor-ibogaine peaks, then conversely the uncertain pharmacokinetics of "dueling peaks" of Ibogaine and its systemically saturable offspring, as well as a review of information on slow wave activity and the immune system,[9] might seem to suggest a correlation in two out of three supposedly Ibogaine-related deaths with administration of two distinct doses more than a few hours apart (6 and 72 hrs, respectively).[10]

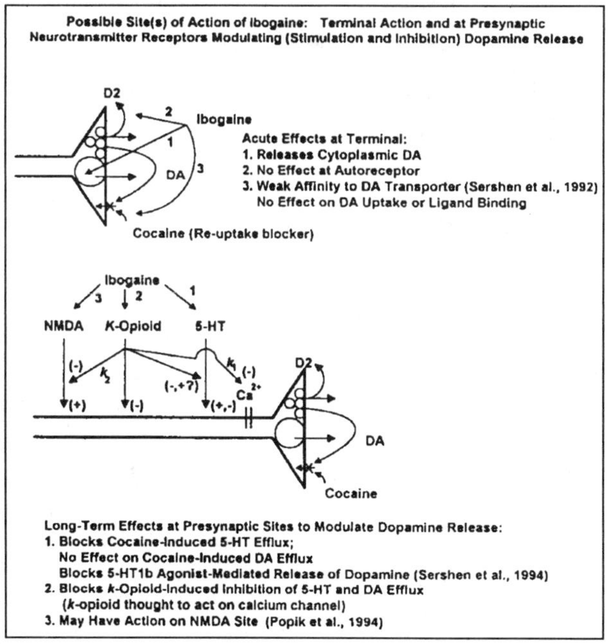

According to Carlo Contoreggi, NIDA now offers vasculitis in the arteries of female dogs that were given 25 mg/kg of Ibogaine for fifteen consecutive days as evidence of toxic build-up of a metabolite, which according to this theory might have triggered a similar auto-immune response in the delayed death of Nancy, of an intestinal blockage caused by an inflamation of the main artery to the bowels. But careful review of Nancy's medical history reveals that her intestinal complaint began the previous summer — well-before her last, double-dose in March of '94, and four months *after* her 29–31 mg/kg dose in late March, '93. And Mash insists that the autopsy showed *no vasculitis* of the artery in question — only a bloodclot caused

1 Four to six times more so than M-1, the metabolite, according to Mash. "Properties of ibogaine and its principal metabolite (12–hydroxyibogaine) at the MK801 binding site of the NMDA receptor complex," *Neuroscience Letters* 192 (1995) pp. 53–56.

2 Calcium is also, according to Sershen, required for dopamine synthesis.

3 See Henry Sershen, Audrey Hashim and ABel Lajtha, "Effect of Ibogaine on Cocaine-Induced Efflux of [3H] Dopamine and [3H] Serotonin From Mouse Striatum," *Pharmacology Biochemistry and Behavior*, Vol. 53, No. 4, pp. 863–869, 1996.

4 See footnote, p. 68

5 Acutely, Ibogaine depressed striatal serotonin turnover in Sershen's mice.

6 E.g., dopamine/serotonin, dopamine/glutamate, dopamine/*kappa* opiod. *See lower panel, illustration above; also, illus. p. 68.*

7 The process involving old-fashioned nor-harman manifestations such as DT's & opium dreams.

8 *I.e.*, Pot is not active at the dopamine receptor; and according to Popik, *et al.*, "100 Years of Ibogaine," Ibogaine is not active at the anandamide receptors.

9 See exhibit, pp. 153–54 of this Report.

10 Adam N. also said that he refused to do successive doses when asked by Lotsof, citing the need to recover from the enormity of the ordeal.

Hidden Arsenal Found

Guns, bombs, grenades taken

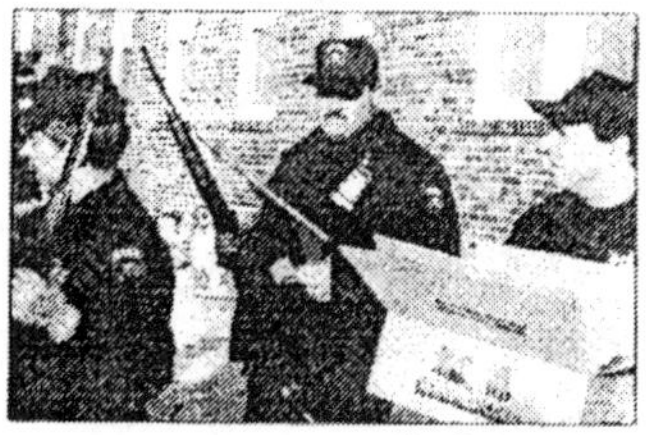

Photo By [illegible]
Police confiscate weapons yesterday in Brooklyn.

COPS EYE ALLEGED BROOKLYN NAZI IN 1981 BLEECKER STREET BOMBING

ALTHOUGH HANK NEUSLEIN BROKE WITH THE (NAZI/SATANIST) NATIONAL RENAISSANCE PARTY IN 1966, BY 1980 HE WAS WORKING AS A DOUBLE AGENT FOR LYNDON LAROUCHE, WHOSE WAR ON DRUGS ORGANIZATION WAS A PRINCIPAL US SPONSOR OF GABRIEL NAHAS DURING THE CARTER YEARS. FOR DETAILS ON 1980 NAHAS CONFERENCE AT COLUMBIA UNIVERSITY CO-SPONSORED BY LAROUCHE, SEE P. 35 & DENNIS KING.

3/20/95 NEWS p.2

Subway retiree arsenal is eyed

By ALICE McQUILLAN
Daily News Staff Writer

by a hyper-coagulable state due to a chronic infection in her thigh — leading Nancy Touchette, the only reporter at the March 10th NIDA presentation, to conclude that no really convincing explanation involving Ibogaine alone had been established in any of the three deaths.[1]

Stanley Glick, pursuing the antithetical notion that the interrupter effect is independent of tremor, reports that coronaradine and racimic ibogamine (both non-tremorigenic) interrupt morphine self-administration in rats. Mash, likening nor-ibogaine to a long-acting opiate, told *OMNI* magazine, "If craving returns to some extent in some people, it may be because Ibogaine's metabolites are washing out over time. Maybe we'll need something after Ibogaine for maintainance." (*OMNI*, February, 1994, p. 16.)

But if nor-ibogaine and other iboga compounds are non-competitive NMDA antagonists, like Ibogaine and harmaline, then the proper area of inquiry leads into aspects of learning and reorganization of long-term memory that can only be studied in humans. A long-lasting NMDA noncompetitive antagonist metabolite that lingered in the brain might, for example, potentially explain the 'delayed recall' effect where events from an Ibogaine experience may still snap something into focus weeks or even months after a treatment.[2]

Ibogaine's "acute effect" pharmacodynamics, moreover, provide a unique window into the neuro-physics of "two-world super-imposition," which, according to Dick, is to the understanding of Time as particle physics is to the understanding of quantum mechanics. According the Einstein, no vision of the future is allowed to get here any faster than the speed of light. Simultaneity cannot exist — except that since the reverse of Bell's theorem has been proven, according to current particle physics,[3] if a particle is perturbed its anti-matter counterpart is perturbed, simultaneously, even halfway across the solar system. Advanced physics solves this problem by explaining that they are really not separated. Only on an explicate hologramatic level. In implicate reality they are one.

This is reminiscent of Philip Dick's musings on the Gnostic doctrine of original sin —

> "We did not fall because of moral error, we fell because of an intellectual error: that of taking the phenomenal world as real. Therefore we are morally innocent. It is the Empire in its various disguised polyforms which tells us we have sinned... " (VALIS, p. 97.)

Magical thinking! — but no more magical than the Orthodox miracle of transubstantiation. According to Rome, the wine and the wafer are throughout all Time the body and blood, which Gnostics call the Plasmate.[4] So the orthodox are stuck with their own version of Time Travel — but a passive one, without the explanation of a physical mechanism, an ethnopharmacological basis. By comparison, the idea that these pharmacokinetics have been used at least once before to change history — by receiving information from the Future — is relatively straightforward.

Paradoxically, Ibogaine is probably closer than harmaline alone to the interaction of harmala alkaloids plus endogenous neurotransmitters at the moment of crucifixion. So we know Ibogaine can fiddle with time, and alter history. Because it's been done before. And with its exact mix of opiate and NMDA stimulation, Ibogaine and its long-lived offspring seem to be a lot more effective addressing garden-variety pathologies than

[1] "Ibogaine on Trial," *Nature Medicine*, April, 1995, Vol 1., #4, pp. 288–289. See also Associated Press, Donna Liquori, Jan. 21, 1996: "...what caused the two deaths cannot be directly linked to Ibogaine...."

[2] See Hameroff: "...one part in ten thousand..." pp. 250.

[3] See Hameroff, pp. 248.

[4] The Plasmate: *She leaned forward and kissed him on the mouth!* — "He looked around him and saw bamboo. But color moved through it, like St. Elmo's fire. The color, a shiny, glistening red, seemed alive. It collected here and there, and where it gathered it formed words, or rather something like words. As if the world had become language.... The red, glistening fire, like visible electricity, spelled out a message to him... YOU SHALL LOVE THE LORD YOUR GOD WITH ALL YOUR HEART, WITH ALL YOUR MIGHT, AND WITH ALL YOUR SOUL ... The fire moved; it came and it passed on; it flowed this way and that; pools of it formed, and he knew he was seeing a living creature. Or rather the blood of a living creature. The fire was living blood, but a magical blood, not physical blood but blood transformed." *The Divine Invasion*, p. 173. For additional description, see the *Book of Daniel*, as in — "Mene, Mene, Tikal U-pharsim."

harmaline.[1] Ibogaine is going to get a lot of use. Science will not be able to shrink from studying a known example of Time Travel. Time will never be the same again —

> "We are in a maze...which we built and then we fell into and can't get out...We did it voluntarily; were we such good builders that we could build a maze with a way out but which constantly changed so that, despite the way out, in effect there was no way out for us because the maze — this world — was alive? To make the game into something real, into something more than an intellectual exercise, we elected to lose our exceptional faculties, to reduce us an entire level. This, unfortunately, included loss of memory...and here is where we...managed to defeat ourselves, to turn victory over to...the maze we had built — "(*VALIS*, p. 187)

Philip Dick never doubted that re-introduction of a Gnostic sacrament would be sufficient, by itself, to free humanity from the maze. Some inkling of the coming Divine Invasion from Africa — both puritanical Bwiti ethos and the capricious whimsicality of the Ibogaine Coincidence factor — is captured in the opening lines of Sophia's *VALIS* monologue, (not included on page 140 of this Report):

> "...Listen to me; I tell you in truth, in very truth, that the days of the wicked will end and the son of man will sit on the judgement seat. This will come as surely as the sun itself rises. The grim king will strive and lose, despite his cunning; he loses; he lost; he will always lose; and those with him go into the pit of darkness and there they will linger forever."

Before writing this off as traditionally Christian, obviously derivative from Jewish or Zoroastrian sources, consider the misogynist crank in the beginning of Chapter 12 whose phone-sticker snared the Ibogaine story on the front page of the July 4, 1992 *Philadelphia Inquirer*.[2] For years, Hank the Skank brooded on this cosmic joke at his expense, while keeping up his crank barrage against 9 Bleecker — and in his phonecranks called it Ib-*rogaine*, and asked obscenely — "Does 'Guidi' do the 'Wild Thing'?"

A few days after the March meeting, reflecting on the puritan streak in Bwiti, Dana realized what a truly bad idea it was to make dirty jokes about the Ibogaine Coincidence Factor. The next time Hank called, Dana told him: "Something really bad is going to happen to you. Very soon you will have incredibly bad luck. Very bad luck. Don't dis the Bwiti!"

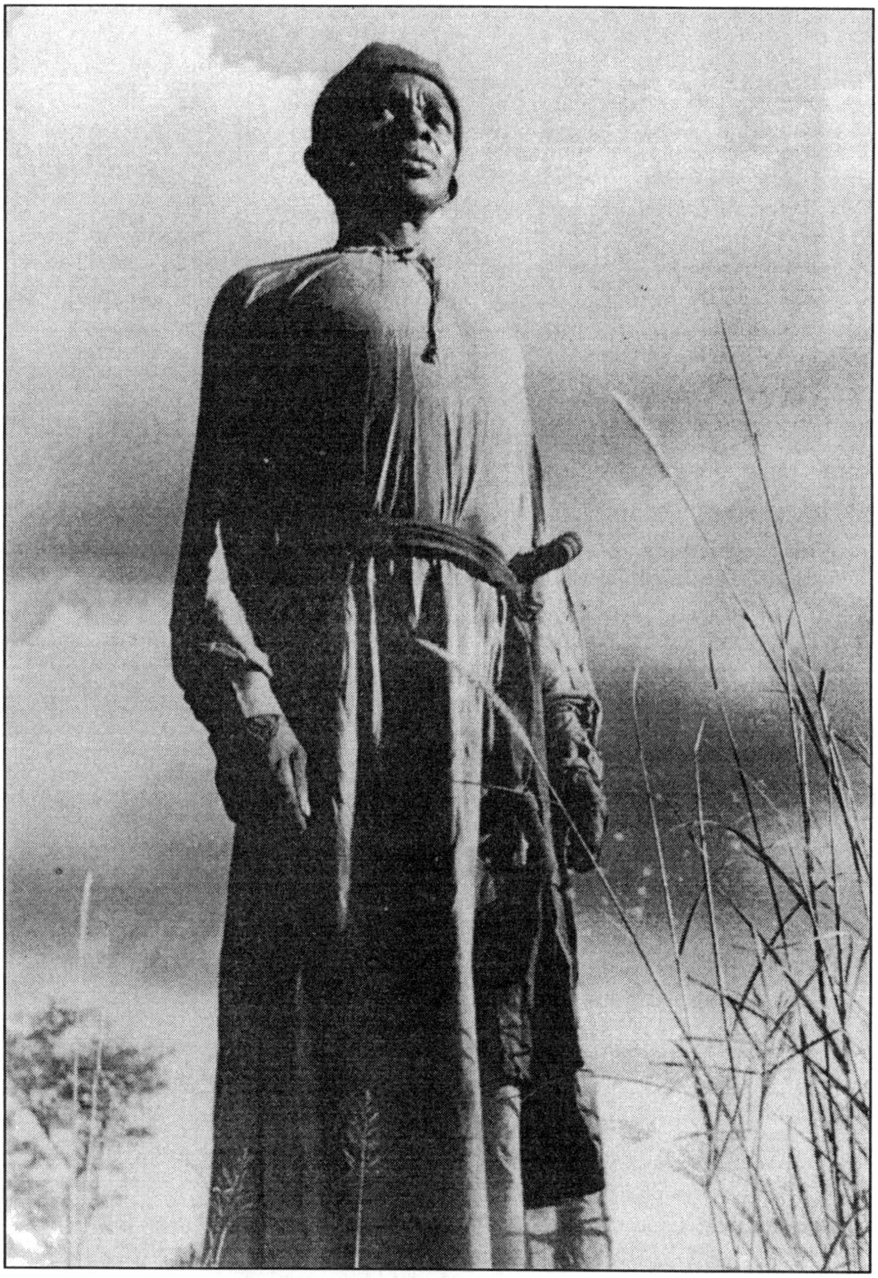

EKANG NGONGO, NGANGA BWITI. FROM THE COVER OF JAMES FERNANDEZ' *BWITI: AN ETHNOGRAPHY OF THE RELIGIOUS IMAGINATION IN AFRICA* (PRINCETON UNIV. PRESS).

In the wee hours of Monday morning, March 20th, Capricious Whim struck again. The super at 5901 Tenth Avenue in Brooklyn had to open the door to fix a leak in Apartment 3B. He took one look at the hand grenades on the wall, and called the cops. Once inside, they found bomb-making materials, nail-bombs, grenades, twelve rifles (including an AK-47 in plain view), seven pistols (including a Glock), ten thousand rounds of ammunition, along with terrorist manuals,

[1] "Fat decided to put down... all the prophetic statements fired into his head... 7. The Head Apollo is about to return. St. Sophia going to be born again; she was not acceptable before." (*VALIS*, p. 100) — i.e., with harmaloids, there's no long-lived "Apollonian" metabolite that hangs around the "head," the central nervous system. Demethylation changes the molecule's *XX* into an *XY* — from female to male — viz: "The linking and relinking of objects...is actually a language, but not a language like ours... (*VALIS*, p. 23)

[2] See Chapter 12, p. 113–114.

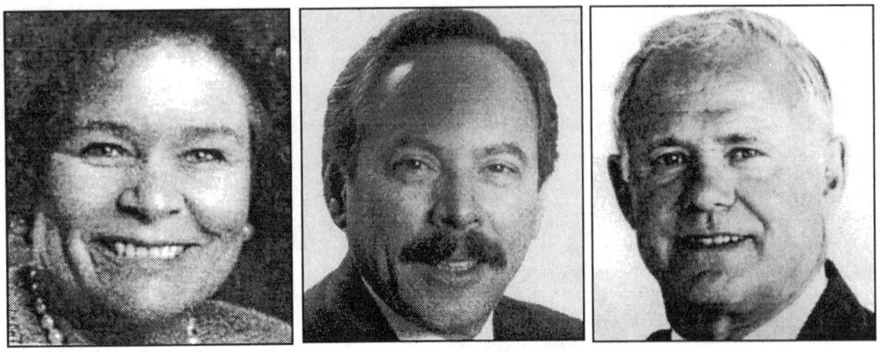

SUE RUSCHE, ALAN LESHNER, JAMES BURKE

ACAD

(LIST CONTINUES NEXT PAGE)

"numerous books and magazines about war and Hitler with Nazi emblems on shelves and countertops."[1] Because of the statute of limitations, they couldn't get the tenant, Henry Neusslein, for the bomb that blew up in the face of the two cops on St. Paddy's Day 1981. But that morning sixteen years of 5:00 AM cranks stopped. Sometimes an Act of God only needs a leak, not a flood.

Still, it's hard to explain something like a Coincidence Factor — especially hard to get the idea across to people who don't believe Ibogaine works to begin with. On April 6 the FDA gave the University of Miami team a hearing on their request to escalate the dose in their safety trial, and took the whole matter — including the vasculitis or lack of it in Nancy's autopsy — under advisement.

On May 14–16th in Atlanta, Mayor Bill Campbell, Lee Brown, Sue Rusche, and Joe Califano convened the first meeting of a new group, American Cities Against Drugs (ACAD), specifically designed to stem the advance of harm reduction from Europe. Instead they called for "prevention," the idea of stamping out every single manifestation of drugs with equal fervor — from marijuana decals to bags of smack. Together with the DEA (touting "community policing" as prevention), they had succeeded in reversing the original Clinton pledge to make treatment for "hardcore drug users" the number one drug control priority. After his meeting with Partnership head James Burke and Alan Leshner, Clinton was persuaded to reinstate the Bush/Bennett focus on the marijuana "gateway" as the key to preventing future addiction. Now they proposed to use the mayors to transform their lock on the ONDCP into nationwide ostracism of "legalization talk" from all public debate.

Asked about Ibogaine as a possible "magic bullet," Sue Rusche told Atlanta Cox ı WGSB that she opposed "swapping a drug drug." On the opening night of the confeı Lee Brown deflected a direct question a Ibogaine by Noah Potter, mentioning Lan monoclonal antibody and the WIN dı Minutes later Noah was approached by Palleria Cox, a rep of Otto Molton's Conce Citizens for Drug Prevention, who told Ibogaine is "a dangerous, addictive hallu gen and a fraud," and that he was "being u

At an interactive forum with all the ors the next day, Noah got to ask them di ly about Ibogaine, and the host passec question off to Herb Kleber, who said di sively that only a hundred people had tak there had been three deaths, and that i still in animal studies. But the host (an WGSB reporter) didn't let it drop there, sa "All of us are against legalization, but whe the mayors stand on AIDS-prevention mea like this Ibogaine, or clean needles to sto spread of HIV? Everybody's in favor of needles, right?"

Wrong: the Mayor of Worc Massachusetts declared he would never it, while Philadelphia Deputy Mayor Wilder made an impassioned plea to imize needle exchange.

On the issue of AIDS, which the O and NIDA had tried hard the whole time ı mention, the mayors were in total dis From the standpoint of the hardliners convened ACAD specifically to torpedo needles, Ibogaine and medical mari under the pretext of stopping drug leg tion, it was all wrong!

Next to Noah, Lea Palleria Cox gr and exclaimed, "There goes the confer After the mayors were done she got the n phone and addressed them: "You ha understand the counterculture has jump the AIDS bandwagon, and they're using like legal needles and medical marijua wedge issues. That's why we have to o de-crim in any form."

But another woman got the last w conference participant from a small "We desparately need treatment. Do a the mayors have anything to offer us on availability of treatment any time soon one said a thing. They shuffled their pa

[1] See *New York Law Journal*, April 6,1996, p. 30. Hank was convicted by a jury and on July 15 was sentenced to 8 1/3-to-25 years.

[2] See the next page of this chapter, and Chapter 17, p. 185.

Alan Leshner did vow, in his speech to ACAD, to "move to a science-based, not ideology-based drug policy by the year 2000." The next day, back in Maryland, he chaired a meeting that put clinical research into Ibogaine on hold for at least nine months.

Ten days later the FDA reached the opposite conclusion. They approved Miami's protocol, and best of all gave Miami their own independent review committee, so they won't have to keep running back to FDA every time that they go up a mg. The bad news is that FDA cut them back from 10 to 8 mg/kg, and somehow they still have to run it by NIDA, even though Leshner says Sanchez-Ramos and Mash have to submit funding requests to regular NIH peer review [just like Don Abram's marinol vs. smoked marijuana AIDS-wasting study]. MDD funding is totally commited — possibly until after the Miami protocol is complete, in two and a half years — to development of the "WINN cocaine blocker." No actual target compound exists yet, but computer simulations show that it ought to be possible to design a drug that blocks recognition of cocaine at the dopamine–re-uptake transporter, without blocking dopamine binding to the transporter itself.

It will take fifteen years, and hundreds of millions in research dollars.[1] But the end result may be a "clean" single-receptor cocaine blocker, which addicts will have to take every day. As Phil Skolnick says, "Existing pharmacological treatments have traditionally been targeted to specific receptor systems at which abused drugs are presumably acting... There are few exceptions to this receptor-targeting strategy. The use of NMDA antagonists offers a new paradigm... because preclinical data suggest that these compounds are effective in attenuating the development of tolerance and in decreasing the symptoms of dependence on all abused substances... The recent demonstration that Ibogaine is an NMDA antagonist... is consistent with the notion that this class of compounds may offer a general approach to the treatment of addiction."[2] But even Skolnick distanced himself from Ibogaine a bit, calling for "more specific NMDA antagonists." In NIDA parlance Ibogaine itself is too "dirty" — acting on too many receptors — even though they were told to expect four distinct anti-addictive effects.[3]

[Ibogaine NMDA activity, according to Mash, is only responsible for down-regulating tolerance; the long-lived metabolite is necessary for the blockade of craving, by elevating serotonin.]

Frank Vocci says that on March 8th, the opponents of Ibogaine were simply stronger in their convictions... that its scientific supporters were too half-hearted. But when the showdown came, every single NIDA clinician was in favor of going ahead. The MDD Phase I/II Ibogaine trial was vetoed by the pharmacologists, the *industry reps.* The so-called "outside consultants" acted as little more than hired guns brought in to shoot down another Illegal

International Drug Strategy Institute
Eric Voth, MD, FACP, KS, Chairman
Bob Peterson, Esq. - MI, Vice-Chairman
Wm Bennett, MD, FACP - OR, Co-Chair, Scientific
Gabriel Nahas, MD, PhD - NY, Co-Chair, Scientific
Beverly Barron - TX
Joan Bellm - IL
Peter Bensinger - IL
Dan Brookoff, MD, PhD - TN
Guy Cabral, Ph D., - VA
Beverly Cox - TX
Lee Dogoloff, LCSW - MD
Robert DuPont, MD - MD
David Evans, Esq - NJ
Ron Gaetano, R Ph. - NJ
John F. Gilligan, PhD - IL
Mark Gold, MD - FL
Charles Graham, MD - KS
Franziska Haller, PhD, - Switzerland
Ed Jacobs, MD, FAAP - WA
John Lamp, Esq - WA
Janet Lapey, MD - MA
Ian MacDonald, MD - MD
Otto Moulton - MA
Adm. Paul Mulloy (Ret) - RI
Percival Pascua, MD - KS
Jill Pearman - England
Louise Perkins - Canada
Edwin Petrik, MD - KS
Tom Pool - WA
David Risley, Esq - IL
Wayne Roques - FL
Richard Schwartz, MD - VA
Alvera Stern, Ed D - VA
David Spencer, MD - MN
Donald Tashkin, MD - CA
Forest Tennant, MD, PhD - CA
Harold Voth, MD - KS
E. Joe Wiese - TX

1 Not to mention frivolous expenditure of research animals.

2 "100 Years of Ibogaine: Neurochemical and Pharmacological Actions of a Putative Anti-Addictive Drug," by Piotr Popik, Richard T. Layer, Phil Skolnick, *Pharmacological Reviews,* Vol. 47, No. 2, 1995.

3 See Chapter 10, p. 98.

DRUG WATCH INTERNATIONAL STATEMENT ON "HARM REDUCTION"

Prevention and the elimination of harm, not "Harm Reduction," has the best potential for effectively addressing the drug problem. "Harm Reduction" is a theory promoted by pro-drug advocates which holds that society must learn to accept levels of use of psychoactive or addictive drugs by adults and youth and teach them the "responsible use" of these drugs to reduce the harm. Drug Watch International opposes this theory of "harm reduction" and believes that no level of use of marijuana, cocaine and other harmful and illicit substances is acceptable.

Background:

The term "Harm Reduction" was "coined" in Great Britain by a group of individuals attempting to make the use of illicit drugs acceptable to society. The basic premise is that the personal use of illicit drugs should be legal, and can be made manageable and less harmful to the user. The goal or "harm reduction " according to proponents is to decrease the negative consequences of drug use rather than to decrease the prevalence of drug use. Abstinence, they say, may neither be a realistic or desired goal. Some have utilized this theory as a method attempting to "reduce" the spread of hepatitis among IV drug users. The onset of HIV infection has given major impetus to this flawed concept. The "harm reduction" concept has been incorporated into some treatment programs which allow for continued drug use rather than working towards no drug use. It has also made inroads into health programs and school curricula in Great Britain, Australia, and Canada.

Rationale:

"Harm Reduction" interpretations range from the legalization of some drugs to decriminalization to the legalization of all drugs. The fallacy of "Harm Reduction" is that dangerous and addictive drugs can safely be used if "properly" managed by the user or regulated by government.

"Harm Reduction" has no place in drug prevention. "Harm Reduction" includes educational strategies used to teach "responsible use" of drugs and which convey that drug use is tacitly if not openly acceptable regardless of the harmful effects of drugs.

The "responsible use" or "harm reduction" approach to drug use was attempted in the U.S. in the 1970's. The result was record levels of drug use by young people, many or whom became the middle-aged addicts of today.

"Harm Reduction" proponents falsely claim that education and prevention have failed. Prevention (no first drug use) programs, policies, and strategies have caused a positive change in public attitudes about illicit drugs and a significant decline in drug use, especially by youth. A social context in which drug use is not accepted is essential in decreasing drug use.

"Harm Reduction" ignores the proven physiological effects of drug use. "Harm Reduction" is counterproductive to individuals with addictive behavior. The most successful treatment programs are abstinence-based.

"Harm Reduction" policies in Europe resulted in a dramatic increase in the number of drug users in the United Kingdom, the Netherlands, Switzerland, Sweden and other countries. As a result, a number of European countries, returned to a restrictive drug policy when it became clear that lenient drug laws had a negative effect on society.

"Harm Reduction" proponents consider that legalizing drugs would be the ultimate "harm reduction" for the drug user. For them, the right to the personal use of psychoactive and addictive drugs supersedes what is beneficial and healthy for the rest of society.

Drug — couldn't even get their vasculitis theory together with the actual autopsy results. Long-time NIDA grantees who are expert on Ibogaine in human addicts, like Charles Kaplan, were never integrated into the process. MDD never notified the African American treatment professionals who had attended the May 16, '94 session about the March '95 conference with the outside consultants. At first, Vocci said there were only ten public seats.

Evidently it will take the entire time until the year 2,000 to get to a science-based drug policy. Decision-making at the highest level seems to have been hijacked by pressure groups dead set against any battle plan to get at addiction where the main attack doesn't center on marijuana —even if it involves a cure for addiction itself.

Yet if all it takes to split their consenus into furious controversy is one Ibogaine question, perhaps these people should not be so confident in claiming a monopoly on correctness. After all, many imagine that they speak for God, but as the child Sophia says just after the part about the minions of the Grim King lingering in the Pit —

> "What you teach is the word of man. Man is holy, and the true god, the living god, is man himself. You will have no other gods but yourselves; the days in which you believed in other gods end now, they end forever." (*VALIS,* p. 198)

Two thousand years ago, the Annointed One set out to civilize the pagan oppressors who destroyed and sowed cities with salt by enlightening them with the totality of Divine Disclosure.[1] Yet to this day, Western Civili-zation still reflexively tries to arrest, imprison, and kill its way through problems, instead of finding cures. To treat addiction, our society has opted for repression — drugs that perpetuate addiction — instead of treatments that maximize human autonomy and freedom. Whereas we know He came to free us from sin. Perhaps when enough Junkies take His place — die and are re-born, die and are re-born, each time returning more purified — He will finally be able to climb down off the Cross at last.

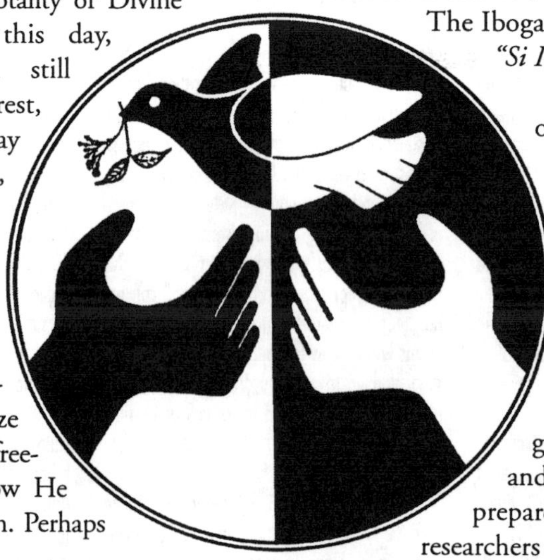

Ibogaine represents the next evolution of human life, in the sense that it introduces a new stage of development — the initiation — to the journey from birth to death. Ibogaine enables each person to go forward to the end of their life, see their life flash before their eyes, and come back to live out their life as they would have — if only they had known.

It is as if the Supreme Judge, in the Higher Interest of Justice, established the equivalent of a drug court, granting each person an appeal for extraordinary relief early on — in effect a pre-trial hearing which gives one's Advocate an additional opportunity to argue on your behalf — extending the reach of the due process, of the Advocate (*Yetzer ha tov)* and thereby the Court itself.

The sign and the seal of a Higher Jurisdiction is that afterwards, even the most reluctant addicts tend to concede that life after death is now a fact within their personal experience. They no longer fear it. They feel stronger, more optimistic; they no longer become so exasperated with things.

The miracle is that none of this contravenes any physical law. All of it happened, and happened according to the ordinary workings of nature. There are, of course, many other explanations for all of these things. But no other single explanation so elegantly explains everything. And even if everything else could be accounted for, one anomaly remains. The Ibogaine works.

"Si Il Mouve."

Underground use[2] of Ibogaine to treat addiction in the absence of FDA approval, and to get folks off of drugs in defiance of the DEA, is now being reported.

Ibogaine is not going away. This report and appendices have been prepared so that subsequent researchers know where to begin.

"ET SEPULTAS RESURREXIT. CERTUM EST QUIA IMPOSSIBILE EST."

[1] Re-enacting historically ancient Indo-European myths in order to "download" Torah into Western Civilization.

[2] One paraclinician operating out of Gainesville in the Bahamas, etc., reports the rapid interruption of full-blown delerium tremens. — Personal communication, Dana Beal.

Appendix 1

"Equatorial Excursions: The Quest for Revitalizing Dreams and Visions"

From *Bwiti: An Ethnography of the Religious Imagination in Africa*

James W. Fernandez

Za' kulu mbí awu.
(Come open the door of death.)

THE NEW LIFE OF OYANA NDUTUMU

When Oyana Ndutumu made up her mind that she wished to become a member of Bwiti the leaders of the chapel at Assok Ening asked why. She was a daughter of the village, the sister of a man who had long been a Banzie. She had just been sent back from her second marriage and her family was in turmoil trying to gather the bridepayment they were obliged to return. She replied that she hoped that Bwiti would enable her to make a successful marriage and to have children. In part her two divorces came, she said, because she was a nervous woman and infertile.

That evening the membership held a ceremony to "put the question," to find out from Bwiti whether the woman was a sorcerer and thus inadmissible or whether she had strength enough to eat eboga and to see Bwiti. Banzie only very occasionally died in initiation from an overdose of eboga but it was just such deaths that brought missionary reaction and administrative repression. So at midnight the membership filed out with candles in their hands to the forest to the spot where an *ôtunga* sapling had been located. It was pulled out of the ground without difficulty, a good sign that Bwiti was in favor of the initiation. Also that night the *nima na kômbô* ate large amounts of eboga in order to "talk" with the ancestors. He received no objections from them. So at the first hour, at dawn, after the engosie, the woman was brought to the chapel and admitted to initiation.

The first spoonful of eboga is given at 9 a.m. The initiate was seated in the front of the chapel close to the central pillar looking inward toward the altar. Before her on a mosingi skin (the skin of the wildcat *esinga*) was placed a basket full of eboga. Two members of the chapel, male and female, were assigned to be her father and mother of eboga (*essa ebôga, nyia ebôga*). Before midday they had urged upon her sixteen teaspoons of eboga. At midday the antelope horn is blown as a first alert to the ancestors that a descendant is coming among them. By 3 p.m. the initiate had consumed sixteen more teaspoons of eboga and was taken to the stream for initiation.

As Oyana was a slight woman I expressed concern to the kambo, the supervisor of ritual activity who was directing the initiation, about the possibility of an overdose. But Ona Pastor replied that no man or woman would *ku ebôga* (fall under the spell of eboga) in less than thirty teaspoons and it often took sixty teaspoons to swell the soul on the tendons and veins of the body so that it could break free and journey off to Bwiti. When the soul begins to expand, he said, the skin begins to feel like a silk shirt which will easily burst and allow the soul to escape. The father and mother of eboga were, in any case, keeping careful track of the initiate's condition in this respect.

Preceded by the *ngômbi,* the initiation procession made its way down to the stream. The initiate (*etema,* Popi, or *ebín,* Fang) was followed by her mother and father of eboga and by the director of initiation and his assistant. In final place came an old woman proffering a plate full of eboga. The procession made its way into the deep forest to a glade where the stream widened. The walking made the initiate sick from the eboga she had consumed and she had to be allowed to vomit before purification could proceed. This worried the Banzie present, for if she could not stomach eboga she would not "see" Bwiti. In any case it would simply lengthen the time before she would see it. The director of initiation ran his finger through the ejecta to see if there was any blood or evil substance, but none was found.

When she had recovered herself she was led into the stream and up beyond a bend by her mother and father of eboga to confess her sins. She was there stripped to the waist. Periodically the voice of the father of eboga would be raised beyond the intervening trees, remarking on a particular sin. Meanwhile the various leaves and powders of initiation were laid out on a leaf upon the bank. After the confession was over the father and mother of eboga waded back to get the plants of purification. The father took back a mixture of flowers and leaves of the plant called by Fang *myan* (*Costus lucanusianus*). In Bwiti it is called by the Pongwe term *ôkosakosa.* The mother took the leaves of the *abômenzan* plant (*Piper umbellatum*). Both of these plants give off a strong perfume. The father of eboga first chewed the myan and spat it out upon the initiate. He then washed her down with stream water. This was to purify her and open her eyes so that she would see Bwiti. Then the mother rubbed her down with abomenzan. The odor of this plant was attractive to the spirit of the dead and to Bwiti and would excite them to have pity and take interest in the plight of the initiate.

The father of eboga now returned downstream to obtain the final packet of powdered bark which he handed to the mother of eboga. The initiate, stripped entirely naked, was rubbed down with this bark powder. This powder was a mixture from the bark of twelve trees (one was actually a forest bush). They were named to the initiate one by one. They were described as good and pure trees, well regarded by the ancestors and all of important medicinal use. "Learn these trees !" the initiate was admonished, for they are the "forest of Bwiti" (*afan Bwiti*). Because of her infertility Oyana had once attempted to be cured in an MBiri ceremony, the curing cult collateral to Bwiti. The director of initiation therefore took the occasion to tell her, "Remember that Bwiti is a religion of trees (*nyiba bile*) while MBiri is a religion of herbs and plants (*nyiba bilawk*)." The twelve trees from which the barks were taken were: *asam (Kapaca guineensis),* the "palétuvier," *eyen (Distmananthus benthamianus), azap (Mimusops djave), ôvung (Guibourtia Tessmannii), azem (Psilanthemus manii), mfôl (Enantia chlorantha), eteng (Pycnanthus angolensis), aseng (Musanga acropioides),* the *ôtunga* umbrella tree *(Polyalthia suaveolens), mbel (Pterocarpus soyauxii), asas (Bridelia grandis),* and *adzam ntoma* called ele*galenga (Ocimum americanum),* the plant added to the mix to give it a perfume.

Though eight of these trees were those customarily sacred to Bwiti, four were unusual. But no special explanation was given. No one, said the kambo, knew the exact number of trees in the forest of Bwiti. In fact the membership had debated as to whether there were to be twelve or thirteen trees. They had settled on twelve barks as being the midnight number, the hour in which Bwiti would come to the initiate.

After being rubbed down with these barks the initiate donned her white dress of initiation and returned to the glade. Her father and mother of eboga stood spreadlegged in the stream. Oyana Ndutumu got down in the water and crawled through their legs. This represented her birth in Bwiti. The director of initiation then stepped into the stream and struck the initiate over the head with the large phallic-shaped flower of the parasol tree (*zôseng aseng*). There had been some joking about the phallic shape of this flower while descending to the stream. But the purpose of the action was to open the woman's head again, as it was when she was an infant, so that her soul might escape. Her mother and father of eboga followed suit in striking her head.

Finally, with only the initiate left in the water the director of initiation went 15 or 20 feet upstream and lit a cube of pitch on a manioc leaf. Gently placing the leaf in the water he floated it down through the woman's legs. All watched as, still alight, the "soul boat" (*byal nsisim*) disappeared around a bend on its way to the ancestors in the sea (*mang*). In a like manner, later in the initiation, the woman's soul would drift off to the ancestors, but in an opposite direction.

The initiate was brought to the bank and given eleven more teaspoonfuls of eboga. The procession back to the chapel reformed. The initiate, now quite rubber-legged, had to be helped up the hill. The procession circled the chapel once, the central pillar once, and then stopped just before the chapel. The otunga sapling that had been pulled up in the forest was now planted just in front of the chapel. All Banzie present aided in tamping down the earth around the plant. The otunga was to be the ladder by which the spirit of the initiate would mount to heaven. A chicken was then sacrificed at the otunga. The chicken would go to heaven and announce the coming of the spirit.

As it was still a long time until the commencement of the engosie, at 9 p.m., the initiate was taken off to a special chamber where she continued to eat eboga. At 10 p.m., now virtually comatose, she was brought out before the altar to face the harp. Propping her up, her father and mother of eboga listened carefully to her mumblings. It was apparent that she was having a visionary experience—that she was "seeing Bwiti." But the specifics of her vision could not be communicated or elaborated until the next morning when she had recovered from her narcotic inebriation to begin her "new life." At that time she claimed to have traveled up the path of birth and death and seen her dead grandmother who took her over a crossroads in which a red road intersected with a black one. Not far beyond she found herself in a great crowd of voices. One in particular repeated insistently what she took to be her new Banzie name, Nanga Misenge. She heard or saw nothing more.

THE EATING OF EBOGA

In important part the initiation experiences of Oyana Ndutumu (and of all Banzie) are stimulated by the large amounts of eboga ingested. "Eboga" or "eboka" is the Fang name for *Tabernanthe iboga.* The species name as well as the Fang name is taken from the Galwa-Mpongwe or Miene language term, *iboga.* The bush, which occurs in at least two varieties (*T. iboga* and *T. manii*—not always distinguished botanically and apparently of similar psychotropic qualities), is common in the equatorial underforest. Its psychotropic properties have long been known,[1*] particularly its capacity, in small quantities, to maintain wakefulness and confer resistance to fatigue. This may have induced German colonial authorities to allow the use of the drug by Africans building colonial roads and railroads in the Cameroons at the turn of the century.[2**] Indeed the capacity of the plant to suppress fatigue—quite apart from its capacity to produce visions—has been a principal attraction to Banzie. They must dance all night and hence they value the euphoric insomnia produced by the drug. So important is eboga that in some chapels the members are not called banzie but *nziebôga* (eaters of eboga). And the usual form of asking why a Banzie joined Bwiti is to ask him why he ate eboga. Indeed in some chapels there is a pervasive synecdoche in which eboga is taken for the whole—it is eboga that is prayed to and sung to and not Bwiti or any of the gods or ancestors.

The eboga bush, an apocynaceous shrub, grows to about four feet in height. It is cultivated in the open courtyards of Bwiti villages, usually at the sides of the chapel and the ancestral welcoming hut. It produces yellowish or pinkish-white flowers and a small orange fruit whose sweet pulp is edible though not narcotic. In Bwiti the fruit is sometimes used as a medicine for barrenness in women. The main alkaloid[3]—ibogaine—is contained in the roots and particularly in the root bark. The mode of consumption in Bwiti maximizes access to the alkaloid. The root bark is rasped and eaten directly as raspings or ground as a powder or left to soak in water to be drunk as an infusion.

Eboga was the psychotropic drug of choice in Metsogo Bwiti whereas in the Fang ancestral cult, Bieri, two *different* narcotics were employed: *malan (Alchornea floribunda)* and *ayang beyem*

* In his "Sketch of Gabon and Its Interior," Edward Bowditch mentions the "eboga" under fetish plants. It is a "favorite but violent medicine" which he took to be a charred fungus since he probably saw it in its powdered state (*Mission to Cape Coast Castle and Ashantee,* p. 445). French explorers knew it in mid-century and Griffon du Bellay brought specimens back from Cape Lopez ("Le Gabon"). The plant was investigated intensively after the turn of the century by the French. Raponda-Walker and Sillans give a bibliography of this French work (*Rites et croyances des peuples du Gabon,* pp. 89–91).

** The Germans became interested in the drug in the 1880s when references to it appear in the reports of District Officers from Kamerun in *Mitteilungen aus den Deutschen Schutzgebieten* (in particular, Vol. 1, 1888, p. 49). In Volume XI of this colonial journal (1898, p. 29) the instrumental value of the root is recognized: "Its exciting effect on the nervous system makes its use highly valued on long tiring marches, on lengthy canoe trips, and on difficult nightwatches." Old informants in northern Gabon, formerly German Kamerun, say that the use of eboga was permitted, if not encouraged, by the Germans in their work gangs and colonial projects such as the Douala-Yaounde railroad. See J. W. Fernandez, "Symbolic Consensus in a Fang Reformative Cult."

(Elaeophorbia drupifera).[4] We have seen how Bwiti origin legends credit the discovery of eboga either to the Pygmies (they may actually be the source of the drug for all equatorial peoples), or to the intervention of the ancestors, or the great gods. In point of fact the extensive use of eboga in Fang Bwiti diffused to them from the Metsogo.

The Metsogo claim to be surprised by the casual use of eboga by Fang and are not surprised to hear that death results. Before giving large amounts of eboga to initiates Metsogo test them out with small amounts first "to see if they can support the drug or if they have evil spirits which will use the drug as an excuse to kill their host." Metsogo also claim to watch over the initiate much more closely in the process of initiation. But in Fang Bwiti, the mother and father of eboga (roles, it appears, taken over from Metsogo) provide very close supervision.[5]

Eboga is taken in two ways. (1) At each engosie it is swallowed in small doses of two to three teaspoonfuls for women and three to five teaspoonfuls for men before and in the early hours of the ceremony. There may be an additional several grams eaten at mid-course, after midnight. This represents ingestion of between four and twenty grams of powdered eboga. (2) Once or twice in the career of a Banzie a massive dose of eboga is taken for purposes of initiation and to "break open the head" in order to effect contact with the ancestors through collapse and hallucination. One to three small basketfuls may be consumed at this time over an eight to twenty-four hour period. This represents an ingestion of between two hundred and one thousand grams, up to sixty times the threshold dose and, in the upper reaches, close to a fatal dose. Though the range between threshold and fatal toxicity in the alkaloids is great, it is not surprising that the death of initiates is commented upon in all chapels. In the past forty years a dozen charges of murder or manslaughter have been brought against Bwiti leaders who have lost initiates. The effect of such high dosages can last up to a week and for that reason Banzie say they can only tolerate this dosage once or twice in a lifetime.

The lighter regular dosage of two to five teaspoons does not produce hallucinations, though adepts of Bwiti claim that once a man has "met eboga" and been taken by "him" to the "other side," any subsequent amount will raise in his mind many of his former experiences. The regular dosage, therefore, may have that associative power, but it is taken primarily to enable the adepts to engage in the arduous all-night ceremonies without fatigue. Members often say that the eboga taken in this way also lightens their bodies so that they can float through their ritual dances. It enables them to mingle more effectively with the ancestors at the roof of the chapel. They do not report visions under the influence of such amounts, only modest change in body perception and some dissociation.

The massive doses taken at initiation produce both physical and perceptual changes—such things as a gross reduction in the initiate's ability to moderate or program motor activity, the appearance of chromatic spectrum on the margin of objects in the perceptual field, and a sense of "objectivity" or distancing from one's own body. This latter is a crucial sensation as far as Banzie are concerned. It is evidence of the beginning of the visionary excursion as well as of the rising to the ancestors at the roof of the chapel. But practically all physiological and perceptual consequences of eboga are given meaning in Bwiti.

Early in the day of initiation the initiates are allowed to rise and evacuate when they wish. Several hours into the initiation, as we have seen, they are taken down to a stream to be purified in preparation for their meeting with the ancestors. As ingestion of the drug proceeds the initiates rise no more. They sit upon their white cloth gazing expectantly toward the rear of the chapel and continuing to eat eboga heaped upon the civet-cat skin between their legs. They may gaze with fascination upon a mirror propped before them in those chapels which employ this device. In it their ancestors may seem to appear to them, though they are actually seeing their own faces perceived under the influence of eboga. Behind them sit their mothers or fathers of eboga, calming their anxieties and listening carefully to their excited mumblings as the eboga works upon them. They may already be experiencing a sense of departure from self and of visionary encounter. Their mumblings may convey important information to the entire membership.

Eventually the initiate will fall over and have to be supported and carried from the chapel to a special chamber within it or to a special hut or arena behind it. Being initiated and eating eboga is often called "sitting down" or "getting down" to the earth. All members of Bwiti have to "get down." The final stage of that process is collapse. The collapse is an indication that the initiate's soul has left him and in the company of the ancestors is wending its way through the forest to a final and confirming vision in the land beyond— the land of the dead.

The phrase "wending through the forest" describes the visionary experience of practically all initiates. For the forest is experienced first, whatever subsequent elements may appear. The visions thus confirm the fact frequently emphasized by Bwiti leaders that Bwiti is a religion of the forest (nyiba ye afan). It also explains why eboga, a plant of the forest, represents something beyond itself—it represents the forest and power over the forest. Banzie take the forest unto themselves in many ways, but most fundamentally and powerfully in the eating of eboga; it gives them both an identification with and mastery over the forest. Amidst the pressures upon Fang in the colonial world to leave the forest, to abandon their villages and launch themselves upon the arteries of commerce and wage labor, this powerful powder of the forest returns Banzie to that milieu in a meaningful way.[4]

EBOGA VISIONS

Dreams did not play a meaningful role in Fang life.[5] In initiation into the ancestral cult, however, visions were cultivated, and the dreams which took place after initiation as men slept close to the reliquary were studied carefully. In Bwiti the visions which accompany initiation and the eating of massive amounts of eboga are always elicited by leaders and interpreted for the adequacy of the experience, the acceptability of the initiate to the spirits and great gods, and the future role of the initiate in the religion. An eboga name is usually given in the vision as well as, very often, a religious specialty such as the playing of the harp or the guarding of the chapel. The eboga visions are an important part of the "breaking open of heads" (abwing nlo) and the opening up of the Banzie to the fuller possibilities of self and of universe which Bwiti promises.

More than sixty open-ended discussions were held with individual members of the religion concerning both their reasons for joining and the nature of their initiation. Fifty of these discussions contain reliable information on the initiation experience. Thirty-eight vision experiences or lack of experiences were reported. Twelve members of a particularly secretive chapel were reluctant to discuss the visions in any way.[6] Twenty-one vision experiences were noted in their entirety. Failure to see visions and refusal to tell them are frequent enough to be honestly reported. Before summarizing the reasons given for eating eboga and the contents of the visions it is instructive to give seven representative visions.

We begin with two visions which were refused. The particular chapel in which the following vision was refused had years before undergone severe repression by colonial authorities and by missionaries. This chapel tended to be wary of imparting any information to anyone. As far as the failure is concerned, our figures show it to be frequent enough in encounters with eboga. Not all initiates are as equable as this particular informant, however, and most would try the initiation again at a later time. Many who found nothing in the plant would leave Bwiti, since so much of its promise hinges upon "going down with eboga."

1. The vision (refused) of Engomo Obama (Zambi Evanga). Age 28, Clan Essabam. A younger brother, with one wife, no children. Has a small cocoa plantation but gets nothing from it. District of Medouneu, Bwiti Chapel at Efulan. Ate eboga two years before.

REASONS GIVEN: I danced and ate a bit of eboga when I was in Libreville years ago. But I saw very little. But now, recently, my brother became sick in the head. He began telling me to eat the eboga. I ate eboga because the beyim (witches) had put thunder (zalan) in the head of my brother, and he became a fool. He had already seen the road and was going to become a Banzie. But when the thunder came into his head he said he could no longer see in the eboga. He told me to take it because I should see what he had been looking for. The nima na kombo of our chapel said not to tell what we saw in our vision, because it belongs to us here. But I saw those whom my brother was seeking to see.

2. The failed vision of Nyimeh Ondo (Mendombo). Age 42, Clan Yebingwan. Five wives and four children. District of Mitzik, Bwiti Chapel at Ondondo. Ate eboga eight years ago.

REASONS GIVEN: I ate eboga at Ondondo. My father of eboga was Mba Ngwe, my mother's younger brother. He kept after me to eat eboga, but I could see no reason to eat it. But finally he convinced me to eat it because I would see something in it and perhaps my mother. I ate only because I wanted to see what was in it. He told me I would have to go to the ground to see. But then I ate the eboga several times and saw nothing. But I have continued to be a Banzie because my heart tells me it has been the right thing even though my head has not been opened. The heart of the Fang is more at home in the music and dance of Bwiti.

The following two visions have the incomplete quality of many that are collected in category 2 below (hearing voices) and particularly category 3 (seeing ancestors). The incompleteness may be a consequence of many factors—quality of the eboga taken, attitude set of the individual and the nature of the guidance he has received from the leaders of the chapel, and so on. But often it is a consequence of the initiate becoming so violently ill that he cannot complete the initiation, although he may still have visions. That is the case in these two accounts. The first account shows, incidentally, how similar delirium in sickness is to eboga hallucinations in the eyes of the Banzie. Their visionary component is essentially the same except that eboga has a therapeutic result.

3. The vision of Mebang Mbe (Ngondo Ekumu). Age 33. Last wife of a Banzie. No children. District of Oyem, Bwiti Chapel at Kwakum.

REASONS GIVEN AND VISION: For a long time I resisted eating eboga although my husband encouraged me. But when I became very sick and nearly died, my husband decided to transport me to the Chapel at Kwakum. I was in agony and saw a road going through a house. I followed this road a long way to a crossroads, where a man with a great lance stopped me and said, "Where are you going? You are not dead." And he pointed back. I found myself in bed in Kwakum. I remained sick for some weeks and my experience decided me to find the solution to this illness in eboga. But when I took it a year ago I saw only my father and a woman carrying a basin with various herbs. The woman was washed by my father, and my father turned to me and said, "You must return all the things that are in your stomach." I got up and with the help of my mother of eboga went to the river and threw up. I have not been sick since.

4. The vision of Abeso Mungeh (Nzambi Evanga). Age 54, Clan Nkojeng. Has a small coffee plantation. Has three wives and one child. District of Oyem, Bwiti Chapel at Kwakum.

REASONS GIVEN: I ate eboga here five years ago. I had seen Bwiti in Libreville but I had not danced it. I am a mimia (a person without a witch) and I have nothing to protect me, so I decided to eat eboga to see if that way our old people and God would listen to our prayers and grant them. Nothing was coming to me as a Christian.

VISION: I didn't see much. I traveled a red path and came to a village of one house with one door and one window. Two white men were sitting at either end of a table. They were writing. That was all. I returned then. But I was dissatisfied, so I took a big dose of eboga again and this time I saw my mother and she was surrounded by many people. She died when I was young and I didn't recognize her. But men surrounding her said it was my mother. She came and stood at my right. Another woman came with a child and stood at my left. I reached for the child but she held it away from me. Then I became sick and had to pass out to the edge of the forest to throw up. As I came back I saw a host of small babies laughing and playing together in the air. That was all I saw.

The following five visions, arranged by increasing length and showing some diversity within type, all have those stereotyped features characteristic of category 4 (walk down the long path) which comprises one-fifth of the visions collected. These visions are treated in more detail in our analysis below.

5. The vision of Biyogo Ondo (Zambi Evanga). Age 45, Clan Evon or Nkojeng. Two wives. A planter of four hectares of cocoa and coffee. District of Mimvoul, Bwiti Chapel at Engoen.

REASONS GIVEN: I worked at Libreville in a shop many years ago and I saw much Bwiti but I never ate eboga. When I returned to Mimvoul seven years ago I ate eboga. I was a man who ought to have been rich in the preparations my father gave to me (akomnge ening). But I have not become rich. Witches closed the path to me. The Banzie, whom I came to consult, told me to eat eboga. For if I ate eboga I would see my father again and he would give me counsel.

VISION: When I ate eboga I saw my elder brother. He didn't see me or speak to me. Then I next saw another brother, who was not dead, but I saw him there in the eboga. I saw his body on the ground beside the road I traveled. (Two weeks later, that brother died!) This road led to a great desert that had no limit. There my father descended before me in the form of a bird. He would accompany me back. On returning, I saw Christians dressed in animal skins—belts of antelope. They carried heavy crosses around their necks. They were to the left on a path that led off the path we followed. As we returned, my father gave me a ngombi, the harp, and he told me that would guarantee me in my life.

6. The vision of Mve Ndong (Mvanga Abena Mokuku Kanja). Age 36, Clan Efak. Two wives, no children. Coffee planter with four and a half hectares. District of Mitzik. Chapel at Amvan.

REASONS GIVEN: I have married many women, of whom I have only two now, but I got no children from them. One day after work I was asleep resting, and suddenly in my sleep my mother came from the left of the room and my father from the right. This was when I was working in Libreville some years ago. They asked me why I didn't eat eboga. I responded that it was mad medicine. My mother said no, and she showed me a small leaf package from which she ate eboga. She bid me go to a certain friend of mine who was a Banzie and have him give me eboga. Then I ate eboga these three days and three nights. [Interviewed just after initiation .]

VISION: I started up a red road and passed through a village full of people whom I heard in their huts crying and wailing. On each side was a hill with a fine house on each. Beyond the village I came to a river, and three women were there fishing bones out of that river and placing them on the bank. I floated across the river, at the other side of which was a crossroads with three roads: silver, gold, and red. Standing in the center there was my father. He said, "See where you have arrived with the power of eboga." I passed through his legs and started up the gold route, which became brighter and brighter. I came to another crossroads, where I found the otunga planted. There, under the otunga, the chicken that had been killed for me when I started eating eboga was alive and scratching. Beyond the otunga a man was shining on a cross. I knew him from his pictures. It was Eyen Zame. I passed beneath the cross to a house of glass on a hill. It was the house of Nyingwan Mebege. Within was my brother. He was secretary and writing for two men all in white, who sat at either end of a long table. He was writing my history and my name as a Banzie. Then my father of eboga called me back, for I should go no farther.

7. The vision of Mendame Nkogo (Ngadi). Age 32. Cocoa planter. One wife, two children. District of Oyem, Bwiti Chapel at Sougoudzap.

REASONS GIVEN: I was skeptical. The Banzie challenged me, so I decided to eat eboga. They actually convinced me by giving me three teaspoonfuls. I felt something. That was several years ago.

VISION: I saw in the mirror that they had set in front of me a great crowd of black men approach. They were then changed to a great crowd of white men. I found myself in a garden surrounded by a crowd of people whose color I do not know. I was surrounded by eboga bushes, and by two chapels of Bwiti. Then I saw my grandfather at the other end of the garden in a hollow in the rocks. And I saw myself as a child sitting between his legs. Then that child which was me changed into a ngombi (the cult harp), which my grandfather was playing. And now, whenever I play the ngombi I know it is my grandfather playing through me. My grandfather arose and took me in something like a plane to the land beyond. He took me to Nyingwan Mebege. She was a beautiful woman—just a glimpse I had. She was too beautiful to look at. Then my grandfather showed me again the ngombi and said that I must play. It would always lead me to another land and be the route of the Banzie. My grandfather then explained to me all the parts of the ngombi. At midnight the ngombi is no longer of wood. Nyingwan Mebege comes into it and it becomes her. Grandfather told me to look at the sun. It blinded me. I saw a path to Eyen Zame. I knocked against the door but Eyen Zame said I could not enter. This was because I still had black skin. All the dead are white. When I die I will become white like the ntangan. My father of eboga saw that I was already gone too long with eboga. He brought me back. He gave me sugar cane to eat. Now whenever I eat eboga, I see or hear my grandfather.

8. The vision of Ndong Asseko (Onwan Misengue). Age 22, Clan Essabam. Not married, he is an "aide-chauffeur" but also plants coffee in his father's village. District of Oyem, Bwiti Chapel at Kwakum. Taken several weeks after initiation.

REASONS GIVEN: Nzambi Evanga Beyogo Ondo mwan Evon gave me the eboga. I was a Christian but I found no truth in it. Christianity is the religion of the whites. It is the whites who have brought us the Cross and the Book. All the things in their religion one hears by the ears. But we Fang do not learn that way. We learn by the eyes, and eboga is the religion that enables us to actually see!

VISION: When I ate eboga I found myself taken by it up a long road in a deep forest until I came to a barrier of black iron. At that barrier, unable to pass, I saw a crowd of black persons also unable to pass. In the distance beyond the barrier it was very bright. I could see many colors in the air but the crowd of black people could not pass. Suddenly my father descended from above in the form of a bird. He gave to me then my eboga name, Onwan Misengue, and enabled me to fly up after him over the barrier of iron. As we proceeded, the bird who was my father changed from black to white—first his tail feathers, then all his plumage. We came then to a river the color of blood, in the midst of which was a great snake of three colors—blue, black, and red. It closed its gaping mouth so that we were able to pass over it. On the other side there was a crowd of people all in white. We passed through them and they shouted at us words of recognition until we arrived at another river, all white. This we crossed by means of a giant chain of gold. On the other side there were no trees but only a grassy upland. On the top of the hill was a round house made entirely of glass and built upon one post only. Within I saw a man. The hair on his head piled up in the form of a bishop's hat! He had a star on his breast, but on coming closer I saw that it was his heart in his chest beating. We moved around him, and on the back of his neck there was a red cross tattooed. He had a long beard. Just then I looked up and saw a woman in the moon—a bayonet was piercing her heart, from which a bright white fire was pouring forth. Then I felt a pain in my shoulder.[7] My father told me to return to earth. I had gone far enough. If I went farther I would not return.

9. The vision of Eman Ela (Misango ki Nanga). Age 30, Clan Essamenyang. One wife, who is a Banzie, and no children. He is the oldest of his brothers and a planter. District of Mitzik, Bwiti Chapel at Akuruzok.

REASONS GIVEN: A man of the Mvang Clan gave me the eboga. T ate the eboga for other black men. I am sorry for the other black men and their suffering. I also ate the eboga to be able to play the ngombi well. I also searched in it to have many children. Years ago my father, who was a Banzie for a time, gave me some eboga. But I saw nothing in it.

VISION: When I ate eboga, very quickly my father came to me. First he had black skin. Then he returned and he had white skin. My grandfather then appeared in the same way [i.e., in a white skin]. It was he that gave me my eboga name. Because my grandfather was dead before I was born, he asked me if I knew how I recognized him. It was through eboga. He then seized me by the hand and we found ourselves embarked on a grand route. I didn't have the sense of walking but just of floating along. We came to a table in that path. There we sat and my grandfather asked me all the reasons I had eaten eboga. A man there wrote all these down. He gave me others. Then my grandfather disappeared, and suddenly a white spirit appeared before me. He grasped me by the arm and we floated along. Then we came to a crossroads. The path on which we were traveling was red. The other two routes were black and white. We passed over. Finally we arrived at a large house on a hill. It was built on one post. Within, I found the wife of my mother's father. She gave me my eboga name a second time and also gave me the talent to play the ngombi harp. She told me to work it until eternity. We passed on and finally arrived, after passing over more crossroads, at a great desert. Nothing was there! There I saw descend from the sky—from the moon—a giant circle, which came down and encircled the earth, as a rainbow of three colors—blue, red, and white. There were two women in white at each side of that circle. I began playing the ngombi under the rainbow and I heard the applause of men. I returned. All the Banzie thought I had gone too far and was dead. Since then I have seen nothing in eboga. But each time I take it I hear the spirits who give the power to play the ngombi. I play what I hear from them. Only if I come into the chapel in a bad heart does eboga fail me.

In all the visions collected, not only the ones given here, we noted five different reasons given for eating eboga. In order of frequency the reasons given were: (1) because of the urging of a dead relative in a dream; (2) because of attacks by witches, causing impotence, sterility, pain, and sleeplessness; (3) because of discontent with the missionary religions; (4) because of a desire to know Zame; (5) because of a general malaise and sickliness. Inquiry was also made as to the content of what was seen. But this is a tricky question and subject to secondary elaboration. The visionary is likely to become a folk narrator, and standardized elements from Bwiti culture appear that were not part of the original vision. Also, the vision is more elaborated the further one is from the experience itself. Many Banzie solidify and embellish their visions the more they recount them. We shall not attempt the difficult task of sorting out secondary elaboration. Both primary and secondary vision experiences are an integral part of Bwiti culture.

CONTENT

1. Saw nothing and heard nothing.
2. Heard many voices, a great tumult, and recognized the voices of ancestors. Saw nothing.
3. Heard and saw various of my ancestors. They walked with me and instructed me on my life in Bwiti and elsewhere.
4. I walked or flew over a long multicolored road or over many rivers, which led me to my ancestors, who then took me to the great gods.

It was not clear from these discussions whether the high percentage who claimed to have no significant experience (24 percent) were those who, infrequently, became so nauseated as to vomit repeatedly and finally withdraw from the initiation. The last two categories of vision experience and particularly the fourth, the most detailed, show an instructive stereotyping. In general, women's accounts of their visions are much shorter than men's accounts though there is no belief in Bwiti that women have shorter excursions than men. It appears that women's primary objective is to make contact with a dead relative, very often a dead child, and when this is accomplished the vision experience is fulfilled. Men are more elaborative. They also confess to being, initially, more skeptical, and their visions tend as a consequence to be more exploratory, as if the very richness of what they discover overcomes their skepticism.

Looking directly at the twenty-one most fully reported visions we note four categories of experience, including the physical reactions to initiation. These reactions were seldom reported by the members except under prodding.

1. CONTACT WITH THE DEAD. All the visions involved visual contact with some dead relative or with a whole group of relatives. These could be children (7) or babies waiting to be born (2). In one vision a black baby Jesus (Emwan Mot) provided passage to the great gods. Other cases involved a paternal grandmother (5), a paternal grandfather (2), a mother (4), a father (7), an elder brother (2), unspecified brothers (3), or unspecified relatives (3). Sometimes these relatives appeared in exceptional manifestations. Father or grandfather descended in the form of a bird and took the initiate flying with him (3). In one case the grandfather took the initiate in a small airplane. On occasion the relatives changed from black to white (4). Or they might be all dressed in white. In one case the relatives wore brilliant uniforms. They might be sitting at a table, occasionally in a large house, doing paper work (3). The dead engaged in various actions besides escorting the visionary. They gave eboga names to initiates (8), gave ngombi (harp), or the power to play ngombi (5), taught initiates how to cure themselves (4), passed the initiate through their legs (1), or made the initiate eat eboga (1). Once, the father washed a woman.

2. EXPERIENCES OF THE VISIONARY EXCURSION. Fifteen of the visions involved a prolonged excursion up a long path usually in the company of a relative or with relatives along the way. Often the road was specified as red (8). In all cases, the mode of progress was unusual, sometimes being suggested as similar to floating or flying (6). The end of the road might offer a remarkably different landscape from that of the road itself, such as a large, grassy clearing, a grassy upland, or a grassy hill (6), or a desert (4). A house built on one post was sometimes found on this landscape (5), with entry either permitted (3) or denied (2). Descriptions of this house stated that it was built entirely out of glass (2), had one supporting pillar, one door, one window (2), or was simply a great house. In two cases eboga plants were seen on the grassy clearing. In one case a many-colored circle (full rainbow) descended from heaven on this clearing; in another case the otunga (sacred tree or post of origin) was reached. Rivers of various colors, but never more than three, were encountered as obstacles along the route (7). Twice a monster was discovered in a river—a giant snake or a giant crocodile who, however, enabled passage across. Once a giant gold chain spanned the river, and once women were seen fishing bones in the river. Crossroads were also encountered (11), but never more

than three times. The intersecting roads were varicolored. Sometimes white men or white Africans sat at a table in the crossroads checking identity, shuffling papers, and allowing passage (4). Once a man with a spear, and another time a white man, barred passage. Visionaries commented on various features experienced on the route: passing large crowds of black people (5), or white people (2), the whites once being a crowd of Christians in animal skins; passing a village taken to be the village of the dead (5), once having only one house, the chapel of Bwiti; and once seeing a Catholic and a Protestant church on hills on either side of the village.

3. EXPERIENCES WITH THE GREATER POWERS. In twelve instances the visionary encountered one of the greater supernatural powers, in particular Nyingwan Mebege, the Sister of Zame and the female principle of the universe. She was seen in various manifestations (9), as a beautiful woman (4), as the moon, which is her orb (2), once with a bayonet piercing her heart, as a ngombi (cult harp) that changed into herself and back again into the harp. Once she appeared inside the house of one post, and once she was doubly manifested, descending on either side of the many-colored circle.

The initiates viewed the personage of Eyen Zame Onyi Bot (5). He was seen three times as a person inside the one-pillared house, once as a bishop with a cap of hair and a star heart visible in his chest, and once as a black babe that retreated into the one-story house and locked the door against the visionary (his Mwan Mot aspect).

4. PHYSICAL REACTION TO THE EXPERIENCE. Visionaries infrequently volunteered any information about their physical reaction to the vision. They often described nausea, but not as a part of the visions. Three times they mentioned a floating, flying feeling, once a feeling that their body color was changing, and once a sensation of the heart burning and becoming pure as flame.

The Banzie consider the many diverse elements present in these visions as contained in the power of the root itself to reveal realities of the land beyond. But, of course, these visions have their source in previous experiences, the first of which is the experience of other Banzie who have taken the drug in initiation doses. Though there is no formal instruction preparing the initiate for his visions, the experiences of others are recounted to him. Since an occasional overdose, moreover, may lead to the death of an initiate, there is an air of expectancy to the whole experience, which is heightened by the hope of seeing a dead relative. These experiences together lead to an anxious search for preinformation on the part of many initiates. But afterwards there is remarkably little detailed recounting or anything approaching excited recall. The initiate soberly recounts his experience to the chapel leaders to confirm the power of eboga and to see whether an inspection of the vision will reveal any secret knowledge of value to the members. Otherwise a decorum of disinterest is shown toward the initiate. It is recognized that the eboga vision is an intimate affair which must be free from public prying.

EBOGA AND THE CONTINUITIES BETWEEN LIFE AND DEATH

It is clear that a fulfilled and satisfying eboga vision is an extension into the unseen, the death realm, of the path of birth and death which the all-night ceremonies evoke and follow. Most visions are a following of that path. What the liturgy can only suggest, the taking of eboga actualizes. The visionary experience of probing or passing out into unseen realms has long been a source of what Bot ba Njock calls "intellectual preeminence"[8] among Fang. Banzie do pride themselves on their "intellectual preeminence," at least in the cosmologic sense—and the visual intelligences brought to them by Bwiti confirms it. They repeatedly say of communion in the missionary churches, "There you take communion and only taste. In Bwiti you take communion with eboga and you see!"

It is eboga that fulfills the eschatological promise of Bwiti, the promise to pass members over to the realm of the dead. This coming to terms with death and the reestablishing of contact with the dead was fundamental in the ancestor cult as well. Indeed, mortality seems to have been of particular vexation to Fang. Early missionaries frequently found Fang asking them to explain death to them.[9] They were especially interested in Christian notions of resurrection. Correspondingly, commentators on Fang culture, beginning with Largeau, noted with surprise that Fang seemed to feel that a person who had fainted was dead. Alexandre, as well,[10] commented on differing Fang views of the definitiveness of the process and hence their different views of the possibilities and miraculousness of resurrection. Such diffused views of death were supported by Fang ideas of multiple souls. For while one soul was tied to the body as its animus, another could come and go until the disappearance of the body, and still another soul had permanent existence independent of the state of the body. " From such various views of death and such beliefs in multiple souls Bwiti could easily derive the belief that those inebriated, alienated, or comatose under the influence of eboga had passed over and explored the death side of things. They were as "dead men."

Beyond a notion of death which contained the possibility of experiencing death while still not dying definitively there was also an old notion of the struggle with death, the struggle to prevent its taking hold of mankind. Nassau says that among the Miene people of the coast there was an old salutation, "What evil law hath god made," which referred to death.[12] He interprets the Miene greeting "mbolo," widely adopted by Fang, as expressing the wish that the stranger should be free of the threat of death. The claim to have died, to have known and to have mastered death, and to have the power to resuscitate the dead, is a very old one among would-be religious leaders in western Equatorial Africa.[13]

Among the branches of Bwiti, Asumege Ening takes a particularly strong interest in the problem of death and frequently refers to the engosie as akomnge awu—the preparation for death. Accordingly, the chapels of Asumege Ening are often called Metsugu Etsenge (the last of the earth). The leaders of the chapel carry prestige in virtue of the number of times they have "died." Of any Banzie it is true to say, as they say themselves, that "he is accustomed to death," "he knows death because eboga has showed him death."

There are a variety of metaphors which Banzie, as Fang before them, escaped the discontinuity between life and death. These images suggest in fact that continuity is the more natural condition. There is the crossroads metaphor, which is an intermediate image between continuity and discontinuity, being both at the same time—a road that continues and yet a road that must be crossed over. The image even more suggestive of continuity is the umbilical cord, the cord that holds together life and death. The umbilical cord is ever-present in Bwiti and is represented in the braided red and white yarn. It is worn around the waist and held in the left hand as, during prayers, the genealogy is recited. For the genealogy is, figuratively, a long line of umbilical cords that attach a person directly to all those beings, ancestors and great gods, in the land of the dead. When a Banzie dies his genealogy is recited in order to alert all these ancestors whose names appear there of his coming. This "clears the path" in his genealogy. This recitation, said to "open the door of death" (kulu mbf awu), presents a motif which is recurrent in the song cycle. For Banzie feel that the door of death has been closed upon the African and that he or she has come to live in a state of pronounced discontinuity between life and death. A final image is the mirror employed in initiation (much more widely in MBiri than in Bwiti) in which the ancestor, actually the reflection of the initiate, appears during the final stages of the ingestion of eboga. This image implies not only a continuity but a unity of the living with the dead.[14]

Though the conditions of the colonial world have acted to exacerbate discontinuities between the living and the dead in the eyes of Banzie, such discontinuities were always a possibility for Fang. This is seen in the old custom of the lifting of the curse (ava meteng) on the deathbed. This was done in case any hostilities between generations had acted inadvertently to create discontinuity in the genealogical line and had thus blocked up the benevolence that should naturally flow down it. We recall as well that the elder generation might in the custom of showing naked (alere sheshe) abruptly cut off the younger generation from genealogical continuities.

THE DEAD AND THE DYING REDEEMED

The old Fang "lifting of the curse" was generally understood to proceed from elder generations to younger generations, and that is seen in its primary locale—the deathbed. It was initiated by the dying. But the lifting of the curse could also be initiated on the part of the younger generation about to embark upon some dangerous enterprise, hunting, or warfare. In Bwiti the lifting of the curse has entirely that emphasis. It is a redemptive act undertaken by a younger generation, the living, to restore the line of communication and the flow of benevolence from those older than they and particularly the dead.

There are two acts of ava meteng in Bwiti: the apongina and the ava meteng proper. The apongina is an act of respect and the Fang word for respect (eseme) is often used. It is an action performed by one younger to one elder. It removes bad feeling and assures blessing and benevolence from that person. The engosie itself is often called an act of respect to the dead. The younger person kneels in front of the older person, who takes the younger's two hands in his own, slides them against the sides of his chest under his arms, brings them forth, cups them, and blows into them. (In the old "lifting of the curse" the older blew on the head of the younger.) Then the younger person takes his hands, rubs them down his chest, and throws them wide in thanksgiving. Older Fang notions of the power and potential for enmity that resides in the chest (nkuk) appear to be involved here. That power is sought by rubbing from without and by blowing from within. The blessing is a passing down rather than a storing up of power.

An elder of the chapel does not need to be present as the agent for the passing of power. During prayer periods apongina may be made directly to the ancestors and the great gods. The kneeling membership taps three times upon the ground and then raises its cupped hands to the "above." Receiving the power they "pour" it over themselves. They rub the flats of their hands over their chests. Apongina is rarely given or taken unless under some influence of eboga. Eboga is felt by Banzie to be efficacious in all that concerns spiritual flow and in the passing of power.

Sometimes accompanying the apongina but usually independently of it and at appropriate moments in the path of birth and death, particularly in the path of the harp, a "lifting of the curse" will be recited in Popi Fang. This recitation is given together with the translation prevalent in the Kougouleu Kwakum Chapel of Asumege Ening.[15]

Ye ye kebwe Oh miwandzi etsenge. Oh miwandzi a kombi oh, nanga mi suo. Oh tita Zambi a Pongo oh! Me mana memboka o. Me mokaenya pasa bilondo ngadi ye duma ye nkumbe ye ngondo ye. Me pasama. Bebae'. Lube ye. Tsenge ye. Mepasama bebae'. Bazingo ye bama ye. Me pasama begae'. Naki, naki Ekoso. Kombi na mombango me. Yoki yoki, zaa ka, zua ka. Esumba na motina. Ngak, ngak, Angumba kambondo. Maga buti ye. Mikando miasiga. Vengo vengo. Mabondo musigo. Vengo vengo. Oh vengo vengo. Tsetsae tsae. Kubengi ngi, nzok ngi ngi. Adendang dang. Me yena nati, etuga medenga.

Banzie, nima na kombo, banganga bokaye!

Ye the beginning. Spirits of the earth. Spirits of the heaven. The place where we pass through. Father Zame who is the Gate Keeper. I come to a new country which is the cemetery. I strike out with the raffia streamers. Lightning and thunder. Sun and Moon, Sky and Earth. They are twins together. They are life and death. They are twins together. The yawning hole of the grave and the new life, they are twins together. Stamp stamp and no answer. The spirit is in the turbulent wind of the village of the dead. Joy, joy the ancestors give joyful welcome and hear the news. The troubled life of the born ones is finished, finished, finished. And now the disciplines of the dead. I go to the dead. All the misfortunes are shorn away! They leave, they leave. They leave. They leave. Everything clean, clean. All is new, new. All is bright, bright. I have seen the dead and I do not fear.

Banzie, leaders, priests, people of eboga!

The "lifting of the curse" in Bwiti, we see, makes a significant change from the traditional Fang recitation which was much shorter and more concentrated. The two forms are similar only at the end, in the cleaving away of the dirt of misfortune and unsuspected malevolence. The Bwiti lifting of the curse is otherwise a much more dramatic series of images portraying the voyage of the soul into the land of the dead. It is a lifting of the curse designed to facilitate that voyage and restore continuities between the living and the dead. But it is also integral to the whole dramatic celebration of the path of birth and death. The living who are to die are redeemed in relation to the dead who once lived. They are but "twins together."

There is a recondite and eliptical quality to this chant—a need for amplification that is also found in the midnight sermons. The effect produced is one of a succession of images which are not readily grasped without cultural context. For example, the phrase "stamp stamp and no answer": this refers to the Fang custom of the elders solemnly stamping down, in a kind of last farewell, the newly reshoveled dirt of the grave. In this stamping one is imagined to be knocking on this last earthly house of the departed. Because the chant is in Popi it is recondite and often inaccessible to Banzie.[16]

STAGES AND STEREOTYPES IN INITIATION

Initiation is expected to go through several stages and have a certain content. Both the mother and father of eboga watch the initiate and listen with this in mind. There are stages in both the mechanics of initiation and in the visionary experience itself. Though there is some variability in the Banzie sense of the divisions of initiation, six stages can be distinguished. First, Stage I, there is a period of probing the night before the day of initiation to see if the candidate is acceptable to Bwiti and to eboga. To test this a small amount of eboga may be given. The next day, Stage II, there is a long period from morning into the afternoon of quiet ingestion of substantial amounts of eboga (up to a hundred grams). With the initiate well under the influence of the narcotic he or she is taken, in Stage III, into the forest to be confessed, bathed, and purified as we have described. In Stage IV the candidate is returned to the chapel and continues to eat eboga amidst the activity of the engosie. Finally around midnight he or she will collapse—fall over in a stupified or comatose state. This is "eboga death" and it signifies arrival in the land of the dead. At this stage, V, the initiate is removed to a special chamber in the chapel or behind it in order to conclude in peace the visionary experience and to recover. No more eboga is given. The final stage, VI, is that of the morning return to the membership and the recounting of the experience. In a word, six stages: testing, ingesting, purifying, stupifaction, "dying" or excursion, and reintegration. This division accords well with the Banzie tendency to speak of stages or "sojourns" (azak) during the initiation: (1) "the stage of preparation" (azak akomnge); the stage of journeying (azak awulu); the stage of collapse and death (azak awu); the stage of wondrous reverence in the presence of the spirit (azak awume); and the stage of going to the above—to the ancestors and Zame (azak abet). Banzie do not consider the "return to the living" to be a stage in initiation, although it must be performed carefully as the reported experience of the returning initiate makes an important contribution to his own sense of membership as well as to the entire membership's sense of the surpassing reality with which they are dealing.

These stages of initiation constitute a set of expectations which are communicated to the initiate before he begins his narcotic journey.[17] His journey is adumbrated for him. It is not enough that he should merely pass out. In mild doses inebriation and uncoordinated physical behavior are condemned because they interfere with or confuse the proper treading of the path of birth and death. In the initiation, where stupefaction must inevitably take place there is, nevertheless, a certain orderliness that is expected. Thus the setting in which eboga is taken is controlled by chapel leaders; a set of attitudes and expectations about the experience is also conveyed. It is not surprising, therefore, that there is considerable stereotyping in the content of the visions.

The stereotyping is, in part, a consequence of the sequence of experiences the initiate undergoes. The experience of being moved out into the forest to a stream for purification and then being brought back into the tumult of the ongoing engosie in the chapel undoubtedly accounts for the frequency with which the crossing of streams and tumultuous encounters with a host of spirits are reported. There are other recurrent elements. It is very common in these visions to be met by a relative who guides one over the obstacles in the visionary landscape. Often these relatives are white of skin, clothed in white, or change to white, for white is the color of the dead and those entirely purified of the sin of birth. Crowds of black people may be seen at first. But they have not eaten eboga and are, therefore, not able to pass completely to the beyond.

In addition to the reasons already given, the frequent reference in visions to river crossings and a great snake in the waters is a motif taken directly from Fang migration legends, which involved difficulties in crossing various watercourses until aided by any of various giant chthonic animals: crocodiles, snakes, hippopotami, lizards. It is of interest that in crossing these rivers the visionary (as in number 8) comes finally to a grassy upland. This reverses the migration experience of the Fang, which began in a grassy upland (the savanna) and descended into the rainforest. We frequently note a correlation, in reverse then, between the eboga-induced visions and the events of Fang migration legends as shown in various collections and particularly in the literary version of Engutu, *Dulu Bon be Afri Kara* (1951). The visionary experience is very often represented as a journey down a long road that eventually leads to great powers. As the initiate pursues this route, other, older ancestors are presented to him. Various obstacles are encountered, including rivers of various colors. Finally the initiate passes out of the forest onto a bare hill, where he makes his confirming encounter with the great gods. Since Bwiti itself is, in important part, a ritual celebration of primordial Fang experiences, and since a key technique of worship is the recitation of long genealogies in which men ascend, ancestor by ancestor, to their clan origins and to the antecedent gods, it is not surprising that the eboga visions themselves follow a legendary genealogical framework, albeit in reverse. Eboga initiation is "miraculous," for it both takes the initiate forward to the other side of the sea and it takes him or her back to savanna origins.

This "going back" in the vision is true in another sense. Banzie also say that eboga enables a man or woman to return to infancy and to birth—to the life in the womb. All the sins of life cause people to forget their origins and particularly their ultimate origins in mang ayat, the land of the dead beyond the sea. This is the land from which all spirits come to be incarnated and to which they return. The two sins of early life which cause forgetfulness of this ancestral land are sins of violating one's mother's private parts. One sins in being born and one sins in eating at one' s mother' s breast. If this propensity to violate another's being is allowed to continue into adulthood it eventuates in witchcraft, the consuming of another's substance. But eboga, by returning initiates to the uterine condition, a condition in any case very close to life in the land of the dead, restores them to their own integrity—their pristine conditions. By carrying initiates forward to the land of the dead and backward both to savanna origins and the original uterine condition, eboga miraculously returns them to the same original and final place. It is another form of the "saving circularity."

Bwiti seeks in a variety of ways to attain to this "original and final" place—a spiritual Archimedean point, as it were, from which birth and death in all their contrarieties and complexities can be uniquely contemplated. This point is represented in several ways. The frequent reference in these visions to a one-stanchioned house—a glass or metal house built on a post—is an example. This visionary configuration seems to derive from Fang experience with a world globe seen in schools or colonial dwellings. Such a complete representation of the earth is more metaphysically impressive, Archimedean, than we might suspect. A similar ultimate place is obtained in the visions when the initiate arrives at the center of the rainbow. It is the spot from which he can see the entire circle of the rainbow as well as the entire circle of the earth. Even though the visionary may not have seen any spirits or gods in his journey this is a sign of the success of his vision.

The stereotyping of the visions reminds us of the fact, well recognized in the study of hallucinogens, that the content of the experience is more a function of the attitude set of the individual himself, of the social situation in which he takes the drug, and of the cultural setting of beliefs and values than of anything in the drug itself. The various chapels of Bwiti and the various branches of the cult differ, of course, in the sets they provoke in their initiates, the situation of initiation, and the Fang and Christian cultural setting they invoke.

When heavy doses of eboga are being taken, some chapels modify the ritual. Sometimes the initiate is surrounded by a vertiginous circle of members dancing, singing, and shouting. Drums may be beaten incessantly even in the initiate's ear, in representation of the sufferings of life pounding upon the spirit within the body until it is finally enabled to break through and fly. So fierce and insistent is the ritual turmoil that hardly any drug would be needed for the initiate to be astounded, mesmerized, and carried away in enthusiasm or ecstasis. Most chapels provide very careful supervision of the initiate. The eboga parentage, the mother of eboga and the father of eboga, watch over him solicitously and encourage him against anxiety while protecting him against overdosage. Initiates often begin to mumble or even shout incoherently under high dosage; the eboga mother and father listen intently to see if they can make out any message from eboga. It is their own soft voices whispering in the initiate's ear that he may take as the voices of the dead, while the turmoil of dancing and drumming is easily interpreted as the turbulent crowds of the dead. Some chapels provide none of this careful construction of set and situation, and these tend to be the houses afflicted with bad visions (ndem abe).

CONCLUSION: LIGHTENING THE BODY, RELEASING THE SPIRIT

Eboga is often described by Banzie as a "miraculous" plant. It amazes by opening up both the initiate (once in a lifetime by massive doses) and all the Banzie (regularly by smaller doses) to greater possibilities of the self. In the one case this is the possibility of knowing the land of the dead and the dead themselves, of reestablishing forgotten or obscured continuities between the living and the dead. In the other case it is the possibility of performing an arduous all-night ritual without faltering. In both cases the once clotted body is transformed (afwalen) into something it always had the potential to be, and the once benighted and bush bound mind is given privileged—preeminent— intelligence.

Eboga makes the body lighter so that it can dance beautifully and so that the spirit within can be released. Eboga also acts to purify the body—this is its capacity as a forest bush—so that the "sins" accumulated by the body, first and most notably the "sins" of birth and lactation but subsequently the sins that arise out of the angers and desires of village life, can be removed. For these "sins" sully and clot the body and make it "obscure" and unable either to recollect or hope for the continuity of the living and the dead. Eboga, in short, acts to make the part which is the individual body and the individual animus of everyday life aware of the whole, the surpassing genealogical body and encompassing spirit. It enables Banzie to act upon that awareness—to become the whole—in all-night dance and song and in those initiatory excursions energized by eboga among the dead.

Notes

1 Isolation of the crystalline Ibogaine from the dried roots shows a chemical structure typical of many alkaloids. Ibogaine, although the major one, is not the only alkaloid in *T. iboga*, and it may be the work of several alkaloids in combination rather than ibogaine alone that gives the effect. See H. Pope, "Tabernanthe iboga: An African Narcotic Plant of Social Importance," for the most recent compilation on iboga.

2 See also J. W. Fernandez, "Tabernanthe iboga: Narcotic Ecstasis and the Work of the Ancestors." There is some indication of earlier use of eboga by Fang, particularly in the *ngi* cult.

3 Indeed Banzie are quite cautious about giving eboga to people who otherwise seem susceptible to psychic disturbance such as Antoine the nightfool [discussed in Chapter 8]. It is said that eboga will carry such a person too far—to his death. It is also said that such a person will bring back a vision that is "difficult" (*njuk*). That is, it will be too idiosyncratic and a threat to the expected experience and its ready interpretation.

4 Indeed Banzie say of Bwiti that it is a "path of trees" (*zen bile*). They contrast it with their sister, curing-cult, MBiri, which is described as a path of plants, *zen bilok*. The reference is to the much greater therapeutic orientation in MBiri and hence the greater use of medicinal plants. For example, plants are used to provoke vomiting in MBiri while this is regarded as undesirable in Bwiti.

5 This fact about Fang was noted by Mary Kingsley (*Travels in West Africa*, p. 518) in arguing against the English anthropologist Tylor's notion of the origin of religion in dreams. Fang influenced by the coastal peoples, however, seem to have given more credence to the dreams, us the early American missionaries noted (R. H. Nassau, *Fetishism in West Africa*, p. 161). Later on missionaries throughout Gabon made use of troubling dreams as signs interpretable as the will of God. They could be used to effect conversion. This is recurrently discussed in the journal of the Paris Mission Society (*Journal des Missions Evangéliques [JME]*), for example, 33 (1908):376.

6 It is sometimes the case that the visions will contain some information that can be used against a person or a chapel. It may be for this reason that in most chapels the leaders wish to be the first to whom the vision is recounted so as to detect and suppress such information.

7 Several elements may be clarified. The bishop with the piled hair in the first vision may be Eyen Zame (Jesus), while the woman in the moon is Nyingwan Mebege. Their pierced and streaming hearts can probably be traced to Christian iconography which features the sacred heart of Mary in intrathoracic display.

8 Henri M. Bot ba Njock ("Preeminences sociales," pp. 155–156), points out the frequency with which intellectual preeminence had a visionary source.

9 Letters commenting on this persistent Fang question are frequent in the *JME*. See particularly the volume for 1893, p. 96.

10 Alexandre and Binet, "Le Groupe," pp. 104–106. Observations on Fang views of death are also found in Largeau, *Encyclopédie pahouine*, pp. 460–468. In *Fetishism*, Nassau comments on this problem among Gabonese coastal people (pp. 10, 53–54).

11 The existence and perdurance of multiple souls, the belief that souls could die and yet live, led to the curse of two deaths—wishing two deaths upon a person—a definitive death, as it were.

12 Nassau, *Fetishism*, p. 209.

13 This was essentially the promise made by the Antonian movement in the Kongo in the sixteenth century. Of course the suggestion that they can control death is frequently part of the attraction of religious movements.

14 Kopytoff has demonstrated linguistically that Western notions of the discontinuity between life and death falsify the understanding in a good many African societies of the continuities between the living and the dead and the perception of the dead as, essentially, more distant elders. (1. Kopytoff, "Ancestors as Elders in Africa.")

15 Once again the caution: since the words are in Popi the translation is not literal but a creative interpolation on the part of Bwiti informants. There is, however, a certain basic lexical knowledge of Tsogo on the part of most Banzie. *Mabasema* does mean twins in Tsogo, *duma* does mean thunder, etc.

16 The leader of the Asumege Ening chapel at Kougouleu who translated this chant says that Popi is the Tsogo name for the narrator of eboga visions. "He is the one," he said, "who relates to the ancestral cult house, *ebanja*, the miraculous experiences of those who have eaten eboga."

17 There are other ways of conceptualizing the stages of initiation. In chapels where other drugs are taken the stages are sometimes named after the drink or drug: the stage of eboga, the stage of "malamba," the stage of hemp, etc. Since Banzie believe that people occupy various earths (*esi'*) on their voyage from the below to the above, another way of conceiving of the stages is by reference to the four earths through which the spirits of men pass on their way to the land of the dead beyond the sea: the earth of birth (*esi abiale*), the earth of death (*esi awu*), the earth of the spirits (*esi minsisim*), and the earth of Zame (*esi Zame*).

Appendix 2

Pharmacodynamics and Therapeutic Applications Of Iboga And Ibogaine

Robert Goutarel, Honorary Research Director; Otto Gollnhofer and Roger Sillans, Ethnologists, C.N.R.S. (French National Scientific Research Center)

Translated from French by William J. Gladstone

Tabernanthe iboga H.Bn. is an apocynaceous shrub from Equatorial Africa whose roots are used in Gabon at low doses as a stimulant and at high doses during the ceremony for admission into the Gabonese initiation society, the Bwiti. Four periods are described: the first three relate to the pharmacodynamic studies conducted in France (1864–1905; and 1940–1950) and subsequently in the U.S.A., essentially CIBA's work (1950–1970). The low acute and chronic toxicity of ibogaine is established (Dhahir, 1971). Ibogaine *inhibits* the oxidation of serotonin and *catalyzes* that of catecholamines by a MAO (monoamine oxidase), ceruloplasmin (Barrass and Coult, 1972). Ibogaine is a type of hallucinogen (oneirophrenic) at high doses.

The present period began around 1960 and covers the applications of ibogaine in psychotherapy and psychoanalysis according to Naranjo (1969) and in combatting drug dependency according to Howard S. Lotsof. The role of iboga in Bwiti initiation ceremonies was studied by ethnologists in Gabon. The intoxication by iboga is characterized by four stages. The first three are essentially Freudian; while the fourth reflects the tribe's collective unconscious and has some similarities to the near death experience (NDE). The method of Naranjo reaches only the Freudian stages, while that of H.S. Lotsof attains a state comparable to the fourth stage (NDE).

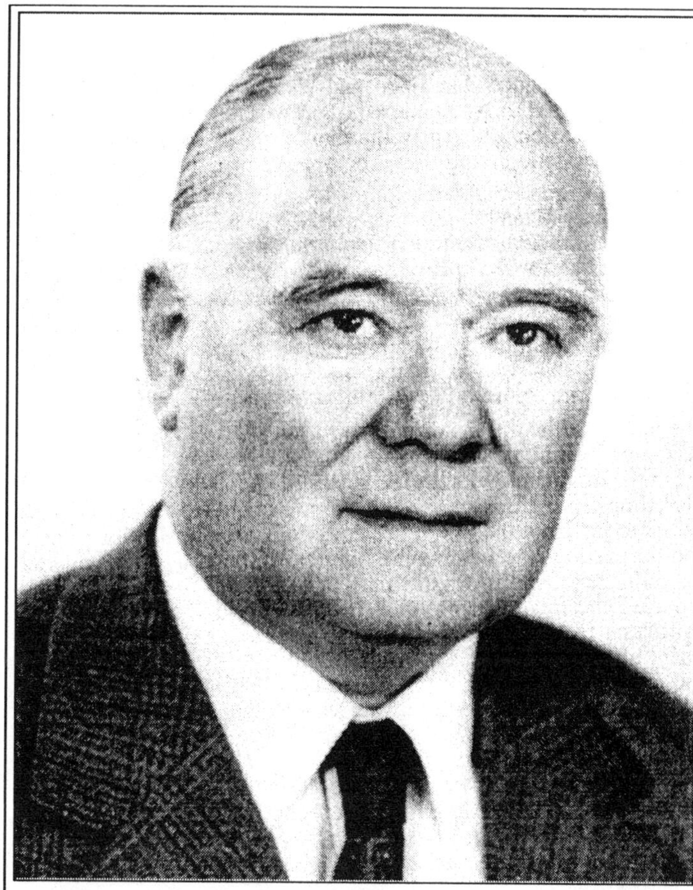

R. GOUTAREL, 1909–1994

BIOGRAPHICAL NOTE ON THE AUTHOR

Robert Goutarel was born on March 15, 1909 at Dôle, in the Jura department of France. He was a pharmacist, a doctor of medicine and doctor of sciences, and was a student of professor V. Prelog, Nobel prizewinner in chemistry, at the Federal Polytechnic School in Zurich, Switzerland.

A specialist in the chemical study of plants containing alkaloid, a research director at the French Scientific Research Center (C.N.R.R.), Goutarel was the co-founder with Prof. M.M. Janot of the alkaloid section at the C.N.R.S. Institute of Chemistry of Natural Substances at Gif-sur-Yvette. He is the author of numerous publications, particularly on steroidal alkaloids: *Les alcaloïdes steroïdiques des Apocynacea* Hermann Publ., Paris, 1964; *Steroidal alkaloids of the Apocynacea and Buxaceae, The Alkaloids Specialist Periodical Reports,* The Chemical Society, Burlington House, London, 1970 to 1976; and *On indole alkaloids: yohimbimes, indolo-quinuclidic alkaloids of the Rubiaceae* (Über China Alkaloids, über die Konstitution von Cinchonamin und Chinamin, R. Goutarel, M.M. Janot, V. Prelog und W.I. Taylor, *Helv. Chim. Acta,* 33, p.150, 1949); *Iboga and Voacanga alkaloids.*

R. Goutarel isolated several of the alkaloids of *T. iboga* and *Tsylessilis:* ibogamine (8), ibolutein, iboxygaine, ibophylline, etc., as well as alkaloids of the genus *Voacanga:* voacangine, voacamine, voacorine, vobtusine.

The observation of 3-methyl-5-ethylpyridine by alkaline fusion ibogaine *(Structure de l'ibogaïne,* R. Goutarel, M.M. Janot, F. Mathys and V. Prelog, *C.R. Acad. Sci* 237:1718,1953), led him to propose a partial formula comprising all of the structural elements and four ring structures of this alkaloid (1a). The definitive formula including a fifth closed chain formed by a C16–C17 bond was established in 1957 by W.I. Taylor.

Institute of Chemistry of Natural Substances of the National Scientific Research Center (C.N.R.S.) 91198 Gif-sur-Yvette Cedex, France.

Based on recent "neuroscientific" evidence concerning the mode of action of ibogaine, the National Institute on Drug Abuse (NIDA) has added ibogaine to the list of drugs whose activity in the treatment of drug dependency is to be evaluated. Ibogaine blocks the morphine and cocaine-induced stimulation of mesolimbic and striatal dopamine and reduces the intravenous self-administration of morphine in rats.

Note on the structure of ibogaine

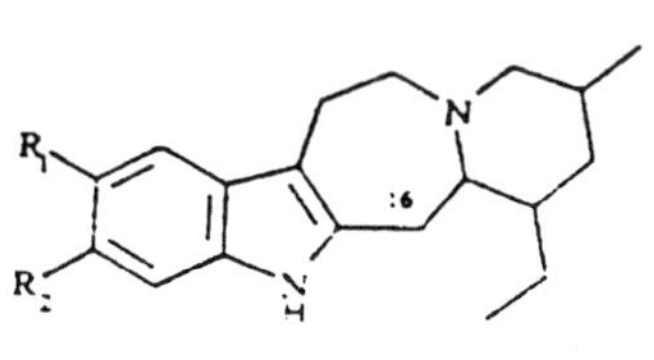

1A[25] Goutarel

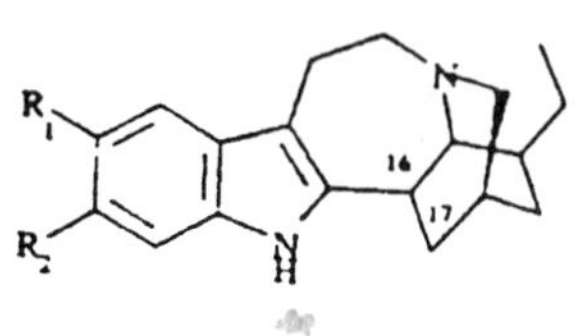

1B[3] Taylor

Chemical investigations for the purpose of establishing the structural formula of ibogaine were undertaken by two groups: a Swiss group headed by Professor E. Schlittler (Organisch chemische Anstalt der Universitat Basel), and a French–Swiss research group including Professor V. Prelog, Nobel laureate in chemistry (Zürich Federal Polytechnic School), Professor M.M. Janot (School of Pharmacy, Paris), and R. Goutarel.

The discovery of ibogamine, a nonoxygenated alkaloid, the basis of the other iboga alkaloids, was published jointly by C.A. Burckhardt, R. Goutarel, M.M. Janot and E. Schlittler *(Helv. chim. Acta,* 35, 1952, p. 642).[8]

Using the alkaline fusion of ibogaine, Schlittler's group isolated 1,2-dimethyl-3-ethyl-5-hydroxyindole (Schlittler, E., Burckhald, C.A., Gellert, E., Die Kalischmelze des Alkaloides Ibogain, *Helv. chim. Acta, 36,* 1337, 1953),[50] while the French–Swiss group (Structure de l'ibogaine, R Goutarel, M.M. Janot, F. Mathys and V. Prelog, *C.R Acad. Sci.*, 237, 1953, p. 1718)[26] characterized 3-methyl-5-ethylpyridine.

The combination of these results led R. Goutarel to propose, in 1954,[25] a formula that included all the elements of the structure of ibogaine; the definitive structure necessarily had to include a fifth ring formed by a bond between the C–17 or a carbon atom from the ethyl chain and another carbon atom of this molecule (most likely C–16).

The definitive structural formula was established by W.I. Taylor (Bartlett, *M. et al.*, 1958)[3] in which ibogaine has an ethyl chain, following the study of the seleniated dehydrogenation products of this alkaloid, (R_1=OM_2, R_2= H)[1b]

W.I. Taylor had belonged to the French–Swiss group before he joined Prof. Schlittler's staff at Ciba Laboratory in Summit, New Jersey, and contributed in particular to the study of cinchonamine and quinamine (R. Goutarel, M.M. Janot, V. Prelog and W.I. Taylor, *Helv. chim. Acta,* 33, 1950, p. 150, 164).[27]

"Clinical research, the one which is directly concerned with human illness, will be the bearer of great hopes." Philippe Lazar, Director General of INSERM (French National Institute of Health and Medical Research), Madame Figaro, No. 14110, 88 (1990)

History (1864–1905)

The pharmacodynamic and clinical research on iboga and ibogaine may be divided into four periods.

Henri Baillon, who established the genus Tabernanthe at the Muséum National d'Histoire Naturelle in Paris in 1889, and described under the name of *Tabernanthe iboga* the sample* brought back from Gabon in 1864 by Dr. Griffon du Bellay, a navy surgeon, wrote: "The root of this plant is the part that the Gabonese eat. They say that it is inebriating, aphrodisiac, and, with it, they claim that they feel no need for sleep."[1] However, as early as 1885, Father Henri Neu had written in a manuscript entitled "Le Gabon" (Neu 1885)[42]:

> Most Europeans (living in Gabon) have heard about this plant, used in fetishistic ceremonies. The natives use an infusion of iboga root scrapings as a potent philter that enables one to discover hidden things and to tell the future. The one who drinks it falls into a deep sleep during which he is obsessed by uninterrupted dreams which, until the time that he awakens, he takes to be actual events...

At the beginning of this century, Dybowsky and Landrin (1901)[17] isolated a crystallized alkaloid from the iboga roots and named it ibogaine.

Therapeutic applications

The first step in the pharmacodynamic studies began when Phisalix (1901)[43] showed that, in the dog, this alkaloid acts principally on the CNS and produces inebriation similar to alcoholic drunkenness (though this would be contradicted later).

This was the period of studies by the French pharmacologists, Lambert, 1901[30], 1902[31] Heckel, 1901[28] and Pouchet, 1905[44].

The results were that ibogaine, used clinically, was recommended as a stimulant in cardiac "atony" and neurasthenia by Pouchet and Chevalier (1905).[44]

This period ended in 1905 with the thesis for a medical degree, "De l'Iboga et de l'ibogaïne" (de Closmenil 1905)[9], defended in Paris by Mme de Closmenil, the daughter of Landrin, who advocated the use of ibogaine hydrochloride at doses of 10–30 mg/day in convalescence, neurasthenia and asthenia.

Thus, it was the "antifatigue" properties of ibogaine that particularly attracted the attention of investigators of this period, and another 40 years were to pass before the study of this alkaloid was resumed.

Pharmacodynamics (1939–1950)

In 1941, Raymond-Hamet[48] published a paper entitled "L'iboga, drogue défatigante mal connue" ("Iboga, a poorly known antifatigue drug"), in which he showed that ibogaine increases the responsiveness of animals to epinephrine and puts the organism in a state of hypersympathicotonus, and he would later refer to it as a "sympathicosthenic" agent, in contrast to yohimbines which, according to him, were "sympathicolytics".

During the same period, Delourme-Houde prepared a remarkable thesis for a doctorate of pharmacy which he defended after the war was over in France in 1944. In this thesis, he discussed the botany, chemistry, and pharmacodynamics of iboga. He also isolated a new alkaloid which he named *tabernanthine* (Delourme-Houde, 1944).[13] (R_1=H, R_2=OMe)[1b]

*This sample, along with the roots, was displayed at the Paris Exposition in 1867, and had been reported earlier by Aubrey-Lecomte ("Note sur quelques poisons de la cote occidental de l'Afrique," *Archives de Médecine navale,* 2, 1864, p. 264–265.) It was then given to the Paris Museum d'Histoire Naturelle.

Delourme-Houde determined the LD50 of ibogaine in the guinea pig intraperitoneally to be 82 mg/kg.

In 1941, Raymond-Hamet had demonstrated the "sympathicosthenic" activity of ibogaine and the fact that this alkaloid suppressed the hypertensive effects produced by carotid occlusion, that it increases tyramine-induced hypertension, and he further demonstrated its own hypotensive action, confirmed by Miss Sero (1944).[55] He showed that ibogaine acts as a true antagonist of "sympatholytics" (Raymond-Hamet 1939–1946).[47]

Vincent and Miss Sero, of Montpellier, demonstrated the inhibitory action of iboga on serum cholinesterase (Vincent, D. and Sero, I. 1942)[56].

Previously, in 1939, Wurman (1939)[57] had published a Doctorate of Medicine thesis in Palis, entitled "Contribution a l'étude experimentale et thérapeutique d'un extrait de *T. manii* (syn. *T. Sybsessilis)*, d'origine gabonaise" (Contribution to the experimental and therapeutic study of an extract of *T. manii* [syn. *T. sybsessilis*] from Gabon).

This extract reportedly contained about 6% total alkaloids including 4% ibogaine, as determined by the assays of Raymond-Hamet.

According to Wurman, this extract stimulates hematopoiesis in the mouse and has a hypotensive action.

Therapeutic application: Lambarène, (1939–1970)

It was during this period, in 1939, that a proprietary pharmaceutical preparation called **Lambarène** in honor of Dr. Schweitzer, was first marketed in France: it was based on a dry pharmaceutical extract of roots of *Tabernanthe manii,* with a drug content of 0.20 g of extract per tablet (about 8 mg of ibogaine), whose therapeutic action dosage regimen and effects were, according to package information, as follows: "a neuromuscular stimulant, promoting cell combustions and getting rid of fatigue, indicated in cases of depression, asthenia, in convalescence, infectious diseases, greater than normal physical or mental efforts by healthy individuals. 2–4 Tablets daily. Rapid and prolonged action, not followed by depression. May be administered to hypertensives."

The fact that it was recommended for physical or mental efforts by healthy individuals rapidly aroused the interest of post-war athletes (Paris–Strasbourg walking race competitors, mountain climbers, cyclists, cross-country runners, etc.).

Haroun Tazieff, celebrated French geologist and volcanologist, Honorary Research Director at the C.N.R.S., gave the following description of his experience with Lambarène in his book, *Le gouffre de la Pierre Saint-Martin* (Arnaud publ.).

> "Go ahead," said André (the expedition's doctor), "it will give you strength. And also swallow this, he added as he handed me a tablet.
>
> "Do you think we should already be taking this? Shouldn't we save it until we are completely exhausted?"
>
> It was Lambarène, a stimulant, a "doping" agent which was supposed to enable us to find the necessary strength in our exhausted bodies.
>
> "No, go ahead, what we have to do is to prevent fatigue. Later on, we'll be taking some more, regularly..."
>
> We had just swallowed our third tablet of Lambarène, and we could feel a tonic effect.
>
> I hastened, "doped up" on Lambarene, and jumped from one boulder to the next with renewed agility...
>
> Despite the Lambarène, I was really beginning to feel worn out and had trouble scaling the huge boulders which we immediately had to descend to start on the next one, while insidious cramps crept along the anterior portions of my thighs.
>
> I was hoping they wouldn't get worse...
>
> I took another Lambarène. While André climbed up the ladder, I massaged my legs. Within ten minutes, everything was in order and in turn I climbed up without any difficulty...
>
> In spite of the fact that I had swallowed a Lambarène, I really didn't feel talkative at all. Time flowed on, like a stream. One hour passed, and so did the effect of the Lambarène...
>
> And, on this last day, this frenzied race toward our discovery, these six hours of descent and climbing sustained by Lambarène, this day on top of all others, it was terrible...
>
> Only the stimulant enabled us to keep going. When the effect of the last tablet had passed and I had no more, I was nothing but a pitiful package of meat miserably dangling at the end of a wire.

Lambarène disappeared from the market around 1966 and the sale of ibogaine was prohibited.

Since 1969, this alkaloid has been on the list of doping substances banned by the International Olympic Committee, the International Union of Cyclists and the French State Secretariat for Youth and Sports.

Pharmacodynamics, 1950s–1970s

The 3rd period covers the time of the discovery of reserpine in the *Rauwolfias* by Schlittler (Mueller, J.M., Schlittler, E., Bein, H.J. 1952),[40] which prompted a new interest in plants containing indole alkaloids.

French chemists were outstanding in this field by virtue of their discovery of new indole alkaloids and by establishing their structures, but we must say that foreign pharmacologists were mainly responsible for the new research on the pharmacodynamics of Iboga.

A description of these investigations can be found in the Ph.D. thesis of Dhahir (1971),[12] and in an article by J. Delourme-Houdé which was published in *Fitoterapia* (Delourme-Houdé 1977).[19]

Structurally, ibogaine is a derivative of serotonin and an indole azepine.[25] It was this comparison with serotonin that was the main subject of Dhahir's thesis (1971).[14]

In this thesis at the Department of Pharmacology and Toxicology of the University of Indiana in 1971, Dhahir established the acute and chronic toxicities of ibogaine:

The intragastric LD50 in the rat is 327 mg/kg. The intraperitoneal LD50 in the rat is 145 mg/kg.

The mouse and the guinea pig are more sensitive than the rat. The toxicity is not changed by the ingestion of 1 g/kg of alcohol. Alcohol suppresses tremor in the animal as a result of its depressant effect on the CNS which attenuates the stimulant effects of ibogaine.

Therefore, the inebriation in the dog reported in 1901 by Phisalix is not comparable to alcoholic inebriation.

Larger quantities of alcohol (2 g/kg) slightly increase the toxicity of ibogaine.

Atropine sulfate at doses of 1–2 mg/kg does not affect the toxicity of ibogaine but does away with the ataxia, tremors and most of the external signs of intoxication.

The study of chronic toxicity shows that when ibogaine was administered for 30 days at a dose of 10 mg/kg i.p., it caused no liver, kidney, heart or brain damage.

The administration of 40 mg/kg for 12 days to 10 rats produced no pathological changes in the liver, kidneys, heart or brain.

This is in contrast with the toxicity of serotonin which, at doses four times lower, causes serious damage to the kidneys: tubular dilatation and degeneration and the presence of eosinophils.

Thus, ibogaine appears to be a relatively nontoxic alkaloid, particularly by oral administration, with a wide therapeutic index ranging from 10 to 50 mg as an antidepressant in humans and, as we shall see later, from 300 mg to 1 g when used for its oneiric action, the toxic doses being similar to those of aspirin and quinine.

Schneider and Reinehart (1957)[51] analyzed the cardiovascular effect of ibogaine hydrochloride in the dog and the cat and showed that at doses of 2 to 5 mg/kg, ibogaine exerts *negative chronotropic and inotropic* effects.

The slowing of the cardiac output is responsible for the drop in blood pressure. *These effects are suppressed by atropine.*

Gershon and Lang (1962)[16] suggested that the changes in the electrocardiogram of the unanesthetized dog indicate that ibogaine enhances sinus arrhythmia and potentiates the vagal effects. They confirmed what had been pointed out by Raymond-Hamet: ibogaine potentiates hypertension produced by epinephrine and norepinephrine.

They pointed out that the negative chronotropic activity of indole alkaloids is increased by the introduction of a methoxyl group on the indole ring.

Zetler and Lessau (1972)[58] synthesized two azepino-indoles and compared them with four indole alkaloids. These compounds have direct noncholinergic effects with negative chronotropic and inotropic actions.

Neuropharmacological studies were carried out by Schneider and Sigg (1957)[52] using isolated cat brain preparations, as well as curarized cats and dogs.

The electroencephalogram shows a *typical arousal* syndrome when 2 to 5 mg/kg of ibogaine hydrochloride are given intravenously. They suggested that the site of action of ibogaine must be in the ascending reticular formation.

Pretreatment with atropine (2 mg/kg) blocks this ibogaine-induced arousal. There is no effect on neuromuscular transmission.

Numerous researchers were interested in the tremor produced by certain indole alkaloids, particularly ibogaine. This tremor is of central origin and is suppressed by atropine.

In addition, Schneider explained the morphine-potentiating effect of ibogaine by its inhibiting action on cholinesterase.[53]

Finally, in 1972, in a study on the effects of some CNS-active drugs that can interact with ceruloplasmin, Barras and Coult (1972)[2] indicated that at a concentration equal to that of the substrate, ibogaine *inhibits* 50% of the oxidation of serotonin and *catalyzes* the oxidation of catecholamines (200%) by the copper-containing plasma globulin. *They classified ibogaine among the hallucinogens* and noted that LSD produces the same effects at a concentration 10 times lower.

It should be noted that Naranjo (1969)[41] explained the antifatigue and antidepressant properties of ibogaine by defining it as a monoamine oxidase inhibitor (MAOI).

We should add that more recently in France, Wepierre[45] studied the influence of tabernanthine, an isomer of ibogaine, on the kinetic parameters of the turnover of cardiac norepinephrine in the hypoxic rat. This hypoxia can serve as a model to assess the protective action of this substance against fatigue.

In addition, at Gif-sur-Yvette, in the CNRS Laboratory of Physiology of the Nervous System, Dr. Naquet demonstrated that in the cat, tabernanthine produces a calm and prolonged wakefulness, *very different from the one produced by amphetamines.* (Da Costa, L., Sulklaper, I., Naquet, R., *Rev. EEG Neurophysiol.* 1980, 10, 1, 105).[11] This wakefulness is followed by slow sleep without the anomalies that occur in REM sleep, the period of dreams (Da Costa, L. 1980).[11]

1970s–1990

This previous third period lasted about 25 years. It was not until the fourth period, which runs from the 1970s to the present, that knowledge was acquired, sometimes illegally, into the nature of the *oneiric effects in humans* of iboga and ibogaine, on the one hand through the remarkable studies in the field by the CNRS ethnologists O. Gollnhofer and R. Sillans and by the ORSTOM (Office of Overseas Scientific and Technical Research) ethnologist J. Binet, conceming the *Mitsogho Bwiti* and its extension to the different *Bwitis of the Fang* (Gollnhofer, O. and Sillans, R., 1985; Gollnhofer, O. and Sillans, R., 1983; Binet, J., Gollnhofer O., Sillans, R., 1972,)[23 24–4] and on the other hand through the researches conducted in Chile by Claudio Naranjo (1969),[41] and in North America by Howard Lotsof (1985, 1986, 1989, 1991).[32–37]

The Gabonese Rituals of Iboga: Bwiti of the Mitsogho[4–23.24]

The original Bwiti or Bwiti of the Mitsogho arose among the Mitsogho when they reached the territory that is now Gabon. In the remote period, the Bwiti itself was a product of a syncretism made up of ancestor worship enhanced by the discovery of iboga (perhaps imparted by the Pygmies of the equatorial forest) and of cultural elements acquired during the migrations of the Mitsogho.

Among the Mitsogho (and the Bapinzi), the Bwiti is *strictly for males,* and those who have been initiated are considered as Masters and sole custodians of the mystery of the *visual knowledge* of the beyond given to them by iboga, the "miraculous tree."

This initiation is indispensable for social promotion within the tribe and any individual who is unable to join the Bwiti is *strictly for* outcast and is considered by one and all as a girl.

Iboga brings about the *visual, tactile and auditory* certainty of the irrefutable existence of the beyond. Through his spiritually immutable substance, man belongs on two planes of existence with which he blends, knowing not where birth and death begin. Physical death loses all meaning because it is nothing but a new life, another existence. "It is Iboga that conditions the several existences."

Iboga does away with the notion of time, *the present, past and future blend into one,* as in the *supernouminous universe* of Regis and Brigitte Dutheill[6]: through the absorption of iboga, man returns to the birthplace whence he came.

In order to be admitted to the Bwiti Society, the candidates must submit to a series of trials or rites of passage that begin in an enclosure strictly reserved for the initiates.

Each candidate has a "mother," who is an old initiate; this is a *man* who sees to it that the initiatory ceremony is conducted properly.

This ceremony consists essentially of ingesting scrapings of iboga root *(Tabernanthe iboga* H.Bn. var. ñoke and mbassoka).This "chewing of iboga" is supervised by the "mother" who constantly checks the dosage of the drug according to the physiological reactions of his candidate who must take a very large quantity of root bark and stems of *T. iboga.*

This chewing is preceded by abstinence from sex and food the day before. The rite is very strict and each manifestation has great symbolic value.

Over a fire, the elders roast squash seeds. The sound they make as they pop symbolizes the release of the spirit — which supposedly leaves the body through the fontanelle — on its mystical joumey. The candidate's skull is *struck three times with a hammer* to help free his spirit.

The neophyte's tongue is pricked with a needle to give it the power to relate the visions to come.

Since the chewing can last *several days,* the *disincarnation* and the reincarnation of the neophyte are reenacted before the visions appear.

The candidate is led to the river, and a miniature dugout canoe made of a leaf, bearing a lit torch of okoume resin, is set upon the waters. This rite represents the journey of the spirit, downstream, toward the West, the setting sun, death, and symbolizes *disincarnation.*

A stake surmounted by a diamond-shaped wooden structure is planted in midstream: it represents the female sexual organ, which the candidate must go through (in a fetal state) *against the current,* thus swimming upstream, from the East, the rising sun, from *birth.*

For the enactment of this initiatory birth, the neophyte's head is shaved and is sprinkled with a red wood (padouk), as is done with the newborn.

Finally, as soon as the neophyte's psychological state after the chewing is considered satisfactory, he is led into the Temple where he is placed on the *left side,* symbolizing womanhood, darkness, death.

He remains in the Temple, on the left side, absorbing iboga leaves until the *normative perception of the visions* occurs.

During the chewing, the effects of the drug begin to be manifested twenty minutes after the first absorption of iboga by *violent and repeated vomiting:* "The belly of the neophyte (banzi) is emptied even of its mother's milk."

To go to the beyond, one has to die; the body remains on the ground with the elders, the soul departs.

The physiological manifestations begin with drowsiness, followed by motor incoordination, strong agitation, tremor, crying and laughter, partial anesthesia with intermittent hypothermia and hyperthermia, panting that may go as far as choking.

To assess the progress of the intoxication and to adjust the dosage, those in charge take the pulse, listen to the heartbeat, check the temperature simply by touching the body and evaluate sensibility by pricking with a needle at different times. According to the physiological state, the "mothers" regulate the dose of iboga up or down from time to time.

The oneiric effects do not begin to be manifested until after about ten hours, during which time the aforementioned rituals take place, partly in public with dances and music.

Among the Mitsogho, the subjects under the influence of iboga go through *four stages to* reach an image content corresponding to the required norms. The candidates are constantly questioned by the *initiated elders* as to the content of what they perceive. The elders are the ones who make a judgment as to the initiatory value of the vision described.

The first *vision* consists of hazy, incoherent, disordered images devoid of religious significance, whose authenticity is often questioned by the neophyte.

The *second stage* is characterized by a series of apparitions of menacing looking animals that sometimes break apart and at times form together again rapidly.

In the *third stage,* the oneiric vision clearly progresses toward the mythical stereotype. The neophyte grows more and more calm, a sign of a *pleasant, peaceful vision* that dispels his doubts as to the objectivity and factualness of the image perceived.

The neophyte feels himself enveloped by a wind that carries him off in the twinkling of an eye, to the sound of the *Ngombi harp,* to an immense village *without a beginning or end.*

We ought to say a word about the symbolic value of the musical bow whose melodious sounds accompany the ceremony. It represents a link between the village of the men here on earth and the village of the father in the beyond. The musical bow symbolizes the road of life and death.

On the way over, voices are heard: "Who is it that you seek, stranger?" And the traveler answers: "I seek the Bwiti." The voices suddenly take on human forms that ask the question again and then respond in a chorus: "You are looking for the Bwiti. The Bwiti is us, your ancestors, we constitute the Bwiti."

The vision tends more and more to become normative. The initiates then tell the candidate: "You are on the right path, the Bwiti will soon be here. Go further on. Look, and you will find it. You must not forsake the images; take up where you left off."

A voice gives the candidate his initiatory name. The neophyte is watched constantly by his "mother", who regulates his psychophysiological reactions to prevent him from letting *terrifying phantoms* interfere, for they would lead him down the wrong path, down the *road of death.*

The *fourth stage,* of vision (the one that ethnologists refer to as the stage of *normative visions)* is the one marked by the encounter with higher spiritual entities.

After a dialogue with his ancestors, the neophyte suddenly finds "his legs immobilized, before two Extraordinary Beings" who disclose that he is in the "Village of the Bwiti" (village of the dead). They ask him why he has come to this place.

After hearing the answer of the neophyte, the "Fantastic Beings" speak again. The first one says: "My name is Nzamba-Kana, the father of humankind, the first man on earth", and the one standing to his left says: "My name is Disumba, the mother of humankind (wife of Nzamba-Kana) and the first woman on earth."

Suddenly, the "Village of the Dead" is covered with increasingly intense sparks, a "ball of light" takes shape and becomes distinct (Kombe, the sun). This ball of light questions the visitor as to the reasons for his journey. "Do you know who I am? I am the Chief of the World, I am the *essential point!"* This is my wife Ngondi (the moon) and these are my children (Minanga) the stars. The Bwiti is everything you have seen with your own eyes."

After this dialogue, the sun and the moon change into a handsome boy and a beautiful girl.

Without any warning, the moon and the sun resume their original forms and disappear. The thunder (Ngadi) is heard and calm returns evelywhere.

The wind wraps around the neophyte for a second time and carries him to earth among the living.

The elders greet him with pride: "He has seen the Bwiti with his own eyes", and invite him to take his place on the right side of the Temple, the side of men and of life.

The candidate has become an initiate by discovering the Bwiti in another reality, that is, in *the other life stemning at once from physical death and initiatory death.*

Through the waking dream, he catches a glimpse, in the *present, past and future* of his own being, of man, immutable in his spiritual essence, and living on two planes of existence.

However, after the rites of passage, the new member will be isolated from the outside world for a period of one to three weeks. During this time, his meals will be prepared and served by a young woman who has recently given birth, because he is considered as a newborn.

The initiate has seen, he knows, he believes, but as a Mitsogho, he will only make this journey twice: *during the initiation and on the day of his death.* It is out of the question for him to take iboga again under the same conditions.

From then on, the sacred plant will only be used sparingly, to *"warm the heart"* and to help him *"in physical efforts or discussion."*

We can learn several things from this study of the Mitsogho Bwiti.

First of all, there are some striking similarities between the Bwiti initiation and the Freemasonry initiation rites. The end result is the same, the knowledge of the mysteries of the beyond, which the masons call the "sublime secret". Freemasonry initiation is preceded by the candidate's retreat during which he is assisted by one who has been previously initiated. The latter will convey to him, as he makes him pass through a narrow door, that the initiation is a *new birth.*

But most astonishing, in the Masonic ritual, are the three blows on the head with a mallet, in remembrance of the assassination of Hiram, the architect of the Temple of Solomon, by three of his companions to whom he refused to reveal the "sublime secret". The only difference between the Masons and the followers of the Bwiti is that the latter have the certainty of knowing this secret.

The Bwiti initiation, among the Mitsogho, concerns essentially the passage from adolescence to manhood, hence the necessity of eliminating the epigenetic elements of childhood and adolescence in order to reprogram in the young man a new ego corresponding to the cultural norms of the tribe.

To achieve this, the Mitsogho call on the *instrumental deprivation of sleep,* as the initiation lasts for days without sleep or food, as well as on *pharmacological deprivation* through the chewing of iboga.

The result is a *waking dream* without psychotic manifestations during which the subject remains perfectly conscious and can communicate with those around him, being at once an actor and a spectator of his visions.

What is remarkable is the fact that iboga intoxication is very gradual, which makes it possible to observe several stages during these visions.

Ethnologists were able to follow in the field the progression of this intoxication and to distinguish four characteristic stages during the initiation.

In the first three stages, the visions correspond essentially to what the psychoanalysts call the subterranean world of Freud.

The fourth stage is referred to by the ethnologists as the stage of *normative visions* corresponding to the *collective and cultural image* of the tribe (cf. Jung).

While, in the Bwiti *ritual,* we did not fail to bring out certain similarities between the Bwiti initiation and the Freemasonry initiation, we are compelled likewise to draw analogies between certain *aspects of the vision* resulting from the absorption of iboga and what certain persons see at the time of *clinical death.* We have discussed this topic in the conclusions.

The neophyte will have to face initiatory (or real) death that will enable him to gain access to the things of the beyond.

He can do so only if he has been properly prepared and, especially, if his *motivation* is sufficient.

For various reasons — poor preparation, inadequate motivation, fear, psychosis, neurosis — certain subjects are unable to get past this critical phase. They fall prey to evil genies who veer them off onto the road of death.

The elders will then decide to stop the initiation by means of an antidote whose composition is not known. We should note that the pharmacology of ibogaine has shown that atropine (an acetylcholine antagonist) suppresses all signs of ibogaine intoxication as well as ibogaine's arousal and inotropic activities.

The *Ombudi* (or Ombwiri, among the Fang) is an initiatory order reserved for women who belong to the therapists among the Mitsogho and the Fang.

The women take iboga in smaller quantities than the ones taken in the Bwiti initiation. In their case, the visions do not go beyond the *third (Freudian) stage* during which genies, good or evil, communicate to the women that they are in possession of the causes of the affliction or illness for which they were consulted.

Bwiti of the Fang

(Gollnhofer, O. & Sillans, R. 1985; Gollnhofer, O. & Sillans, R. 1983; Binet, J., Gollnhofer, O., Sillans, R. 1972)[23 24 4]

Along the coastal portions of Gabon, the Bwiti began to be known by the Fang at the time of the explorations of Savorgnan de Brazza, but according to a letter from Lucien Meyo, secretary of the Prophet Ekang Nwa, "it was in 1908 that the Mitsogho and Bapinzi arrived in Gabon, that is to say, in the Libréville estuary. That is where they taught the Fang how to eat iboga by the root." Prior to that time, the Fang used the leaves of iboga and of *alan (Alchornea floribunda,* an euphorbia from which Mrs. F. Khuong-Huu29 isolated a new alkaloid, alchorneine), but only the effects of iboga roots ultimately produce the visions of the Bwiti.

The Bwiti of the Fang, unlike that of the Mitsogho, accepts women as members, but all of them, regardless of sex, are admitted only after taking iboga.

The iboga root is absorbed not only in the form of fine scrapings but also in a preparation made of cane juice or sugar, palm wine or milk. While the extraction of iboga root is reserved for the men, the "galenic preparations" are made by the women and are referred to as "express" or "automatic".

Such preparations, which reduce the bitterness and partly prevent the vomiting, make it possible to achieve the phase of normative visions more rapidly.

During the rites of passage, the essential features of the Mitsogho rites are preserved and the ritual language is Mitsogho.

However, the "mother" is a woman, sometimes accompanied by her husband, who becomes the "father".

Great importance is given to the *retreat* and to the *confession* that precede the initiation.

The notion of purity is an obsession in the Fang mentality, and the chewing is perceived as a trial that serves to expiate (by vomiting) the wrongs that have been committed.

The Fang Bwiti is actually the result of an adaptation of the Original Bwiti of the Mitsogho to the traditional ancestor worship (Byeri), with the integration of Christian elements and concepts.

As a result, the Fang Bwiti is not uniform and is structured through many branches that are independent from each other, in the midst of which "prophetic and messianic movements" flourish.

According to Michel Fromaget (1986),[18] Chairman of the Department of Psychology of Libréville University from 1981 to 1983, there are two sorts of Bwiti in Gabon.

The Bwiti of the Mitsogho which has been preserved in a very sober, refined form close to the original model, the initial Bwiti or Disumba Bwiti, from the name of the first woman, which has two variants:

The Mitsogho Bwiti of the *nganga-a-misoko,* seers and divining sorcerers, eminent therapists who practice psychosomatic healing and a sort of psychoanalysis.

The N'dea Bwiti, a cult of sorcerers, a deviation from the Mitsogho Bwiti with human sacrifices and cannibalism, whose ultimate goal is magic, the securing of supernatural powers.

The Fang Bwiti, received mediately at a late period by the Fang, is an astonishing syncretism with a blend of Christianity and animism.

Bureau (1972)[7] mentions 12 subdivisions in the Fang Bwiti. Therefore, we must give up any thought of studying the Fang Bwiti as a uniform, homogeneous entity, and it would be illusory and inaccurate to try to look for a "normative Fang vision" comparable to the Mitsogho Bwiti.

Therefore, within a community in which the initiation is to take place, everything depends on the relationships that are accepted in that community between the worship of the ancestors (represented by their skulls), the original Bwiti, and Christianity.

If we compare, in broad terms, the Fang Bwiti and the original Bwiti, we find striking similarities between the contents of the vision. Only the setting and the figures or persons represented differ. The latter are entities derived from Christianity and may appear in unlimited numbers.

However, it would be a mistake to think that the Fang Bwiti has departed completely from the original Bwiti and from the ancestral culture of the Fang. The elements are in there, but are not very apparent. However, they can be if we know the connection between the figures that are recognized and those that are concealed behind them.

A Christian religious figure may incarnate at the same time several Fang spiritual entities, and vice versa.

During the rites of passage, we find the same psychophysiological effects as the ones observed among the Mitsogho.

After a long series of episodes, during his mystical ascension, the subject under the influence of iboga at its peak feels "as if transported by the wind" to the beyond before the house of Christ and of God. He is guided to that place by the ancestors, to the sound of the harp.

A voice gives him his initiatory name and tells him how much money he will have to pay to be initiated.

During his joumey, he sees many saints, Noah, priests in their cassock. Christ, dressed in gold galments, questions the stranger as to the reason for his visit. And the neophyte answers: "I am seeking, I want to see the Lord Jesus Christ". "I am the one you seek", Christ replies.

From one neophyte to the next, the content of the narratives describe encounters with Christ in some other setting.

The subject first goes through "purgatory, where men suffer", then on to heaven with its seven planes where angels glide. At the highest plane, the traveler sees a man bearing a cross, and further on the beard of God the Father.

In other visions, the Virgin Mary, Adam, and Lucifer appear.

The dialogue is practically identical in each vision with the dialogue reported among the Mitsogho.

In this syncretism, Nyingon (the female principle or the first woman, called Disumba among the Mitsogho) is assimilated both to Eve and to the Virgin Mary.

As for Nzame, the male principle, the first man, or Nzamba-Kana among the Mitsogho, he is represented by Jesus Christ.

To certain prophets, Adam and Christ personify Ngoroyo-Ama, that is to say, the *"Supreme Being",* who is never perceived in the Mitsogho vision.

Lucifer, the rainbow-serpent, is present in the Fang vision. He represents evil, that is, *Evus,* a well-known notion among the Fang.

In their lifetime, the Fang can make several journeys under the ritual conditions of the Bwiti, enabling them to confirm the reality of their visions. The initiates may also belong to the Ombwiri possession society (reserved for women and called ombudi among the Mitsogho). This society, which plays a great role in medical diagnosis, is characterized by the vision, under the influence of iboga, of genies who during the course of public divinatory sessions will reveal the nature of the affliction suffered by the patient who has come for consultation.

In the Ombwiri, we can note some similarity with Voodoo in the Caribbean and South America.

Among the Mitsogho, the *normative vision* is that of the whole tribe and collesponds in the initiate to the knowledge recorded *orally* since in his childhood within the tribe.

With the Fang, we observe many differences because of the changes and turnovers that may have taken place in the initiatory experience, the influence of Christianity and the competition among various more-or-less orthodox messianic and prophetic movements, and the loss of the tribal notion.

Some whites, most of them French, have voluntarily gone through the trial of chewing of iboga. A few of them were able to be interviewed. A study of the the interpretation of these interviews is in progress at this time (O. Gollnhofer and R. Sillans).

Ibogaine in psychotherapy: psychoanalysis according to Naranjo[41]

Claudio Naranjo is a Chilean psychotherapeutic physician who, while in training at the Institute of Personality and Research, University of California at Berkeley, in 1969, published a remarkable report entitled "Psychotherapeutic Possibilities of New Fantasy-Enhancing Drugs" in *Clinical Toxicology* (Naranjo, C. 1969)[41]

Naranjo, in this report, deals with the therapeutic action, at socalled *subtoxic doses,* of two alkaloids, harmaline and ibogaine.

C. Naranjo wrote: "Because of the lack of a systematic study of these drugs (harmaline and ibogaine), from the simple standpoint of chemotherapy they were considered as toxic at a certain dose.

The fact is that the phenomena of harmaline and ibogaine intoxication are the points of greatest interest insofar as psychological exploration and psychotherapy are concerned."

Harmaline was isolated in 1841 by Goebel[22] from the seeds of a plant of the family Malpighiaceae,* *Peganum harmala.* It has also been extracted from another South American Malpighia, *Banisteriopsis caapi* or yage.

Yage bark is the principal ingredient of the beverage used by the Indians of the region of the headwaters of the Amazon in connection, with certain divination rites and practices and it is known, according to research done at the University of Chile, that this drug was central to the

* Zygophilliaceae actually, according to David Flattery [personal communication]. Harmaline is found in eight completely distinct plant species. Editor's note.

culture of different Indian tribes as far back as the paleolithic period.

The effects of harmaline and of ibogaine are practically unique among the psychoactive drugs.

The best term to describe these effects is the one used by William Turner, a yage specialist, **oneirophrenia,** to refer to the states induced by drugs that differ from psychotomimetic states by the absence of any psychotic symptom while sharing with the psychotic or psychotomimetic experience the preeminence of a primary thought process.

Harmaline and ibogaine are characterized in their psychological effects by a state such that it involves a *dream phenomenon without loss of consciousness* or change in the perception of the environment or any illusions or formal deterioration of thought and without depersonalization.

In a word, we can say that there is an enhancement of fantasies which is remarkable in that it does not interfere with the ego. Such fantasies are more like *actual visions* than common everyday dreams.

In a study on the psychological effects of harmaline performed in Chile in 1963–64 together with other Chilean physicians and with Indian traditional therapists, Naranjo pointed out that one of the most remarkable aspects of the fantasy is its great consistency.

The themes or images that are evoked are mostly *archetypes* according to Jung's definition of the term, namely ancient memories, generally common to all humans, buried in their collective unconscious.

To cite Voltaire: "The world, according to Plato, was composed of archetypal ideas that always remained deep in the brain."

Naranjo distinguishes between two sorts of archetypes:

The *mythical style* similar to the dream of a lost treasure, a kind old man, an ideal woman, a saint, an ideal community and various socalled noble thoughts, and so on.

The *instinctive style* such as it may be expressed in a fantasy with aggression, sex, bloody scenes of all sorts, incest or other practices.

By their spontaneity, these *waking dream* sequences are more extreme than any other reported by patients from their usual dreams and *do not resemble* the visions on mescaline or LSD. In fact, the effects of the two types of drugs seem to be poles part, those of the common *hallucinogens* being a high and angelic domain of esthetic sensations, of a lack of union with anything else, while the domain of the *oneirophrenics* is that of Freud's subterranean world of animal impulse and regression.

Naranjo gives some examples of subjects treated successfully with harmaline at doses of 4–5 mg/kg orally (about 300 mg).

Concerning *ibogaine* Naranjo says that he knows less than about harmaline as regards the use of iboga by the Gabonese and Congolese. He is unacquainted with the *Bwiti* and apparently does not know the structure of ibogaine.

He knows that the drug has been used in the European pharmacopeia for its antifatigue properties at a low dose, which, according to him, is due to the fact that it is a MAOI.

As with harmaline, Naranjo uses ibogaine at doses of 4–5 mg/kg orally and one-quarter of it intravenously, and describes subjective reactions lasting about 6 hours.

Compared with the effects of harmaline, those of ibogaine appear less exotic. Even though the archetypal contents are common to both (visions of animals being frequent), the quality of the fantasy is generally more personal and concerns the subject himself, his parents and significant others.

At the same time, the fantasy evoked by ibogaine is easier for the subjects to manipulate, either on their own initiative or through the psychotherapist, so that, more often than with other drugs, they can stop to contemplate a scene, go back, explore an alternative in a given sequence, bring a previous scene back to life, etc.

This ease with which the events in a treatment with ibogaine can be manipulated and the fact that the experience can be directed to the desired area is probably one of the reasons for the success observed by many psychotherapists who have used this drug.

Naranjo was much more impressed by the effects obtained in an ibogaine session than with those observed with any other drug.

An example really shows the ease with which the psychotherapist is able to direct his analysis:

This is a young patient who, when treated with ibogaine, decides to lie down and close his eyes shortly after feeling the effects of the drug:

"First, he sees the face of his father, facing him as though they were playing a game, with a restrained smile. His comment at this point is that his father looks like a little boy to him. It was like someone unfamiliar and yet familiar, like something the patient had forgotten for many years.

Suddenly his father's features change, distorted by rage. The scene changes and the patient sees a naked woman hiding her face with her arm, afraid.

Close by, he sees his father, also naked, throwing himself on the woman in a sexual attack. He feels a controlled rage in the woman whom he now identifies as his mother."

At that moment, Naranjo asks the subject to have his father and mother engage in conversation, intending in this way to distance the latent content of these images. "What is she saying?" "Go away"; "what does he feel?" He cannot imagine. "I am perplexed", he suggests.

Naranjo then chooses another tack to make the subject's feelings more conscious and explicit.

"Now, you be your father: Become your father, to the best of your dramatic abilities, and listen to what he is telling you."

Then, personifying his father, the patient falls, not into perplexity, but into a great sadness, suffering and rejecting his anguish.

Shortly after this episode, a drastic change occurred in the way the subject viewed his parents and, consequently, in his feelings toward them.

The next day, he commented that only now did he know how much he identified with his mother, looking at things through her eyes, blaming his father, and more than that, a man, which had interfered with his own masculine aspirations.

In contrast to his usual idealization of his mother in a total love and his perception of his father as a selfish brute, he then had the feeling of knowing them as they are.

He wrote: "I have seen my mother as a hard person, without affection or fear, and I no longer look upon my father as an insensitive being who had hurt her in his love affairs, but as someone who wishes to open the door of his love, without succeeding. Now, I am full of compassion for my mother."

Compared to the dramatic quality of psychedelic experiences, this episode may appear insignificant or trivial, and yet it was the key to a radical change in the attitudes of the young patient.

That might be said of the experiences with ibogaine in general, when we compare its effects with those of LSD.

Here, the type of contact concerned by the unconscious material is symbolic (rather than assuming the form of a free-floating emotion, as with LSD), and may henceforth be assimilated in the form of lasting signs.

Such signs generally occur when a fantasy or a hypothesis that had been unconscious becomes conscious with such clarity *that the ego of a mature person is compelled to become aware of his or her deeprooted former error.*

Naranjo concludes as follows:

"I do not want to give the impression that I regard ibogaine as a psychiatric panacea that will bring changes by itself. I believe that many drugs may be used for psychological exploration, but that these drugs can only be an instrument.

I doubt that there is anything that can be achieved with a drug that cannot be done without it.

However, drugs can be psychological catalysts that make it possible to compress a very lengthy psychotherapeutic process into a shorter time and change its prognosis.

Although ibogaine cannot open a door by itself, it can be considered as the oil for its hinges".

At the time of the publication of his report on drugs that enhance fantasies, in June 1969, C. Naranjo, together with a Frenchman, D.P.M. Bocher, obtained a special drug patent in France pursuant to an application submitted on January 31, 1968 and issued on July 31, 1969, for:

"A new medication acting on the central nervous system that can be used in psychotherapeutic treatments and as an antidrug preparation". (Bocher, D.P. & Naranjo, C. 1969).[5]

The drug was composed of total alkaloids of *Tabernanthe iboga* roots combined with an amphetamine in a proportion varying according to the behavior of the patient.

Among the 50 cases studied in psychiatry, Naranjo described four in support of his application for a "nontoxic drug that clarifies thoughts and permits a very thorough introspection while preserving the patient's emotional character which is indispensable for the stimulation of thought and imagination."

However, in this same period, following the resolutions of the World Health Assembly of May 1967 and May 1968, the American federal government classified ibogaine, through the F.D.A., among the substances analogous to lysergides and to certain CNS stimulants.

"Whereas, in the interest of public health, certain regulatory provisions should be applied relating to the manufacture, transportation, possession, sale and distribution, delivery and acquisition for valuable consideration or free of charge of soporific and narcotic substances, and of certain substances likely to *produce drug dependency or endanger human health".*

These regulations are applicable to the following substances, to their isomers, unless *expressly exempted,* to their salts, ethers and esters, as well as to the salts of said ethers and esters in all cases where such salts may exist.

The list of these substances includes: amphetamines, ibogaine, compounds and derivatives of lysergic acid, amides of lysergic acids and other derivatives, peyotl and mescaline [harmaline is not mentioned], hallucinogenic mushrooms, psilocybin and derivatives of dimethyltryptamine, 4-OH-DMT and 5-OH-DMT".

We shall retum later to this decree which was applicable beginning in 1970 in several European countries, France and Belgium in particular.

The fact is that in France and in Belgium, nothing more was heard about ibogaine and the sale of Lambarene was prohibited.

Ibogaine for combatting drug dependencies, according to Howard Lotsof[32, 33, 34, 35, 36, 37]

In the early 1960s, a young American, Howard Lotsof, during the course of a drug party with some friends, offered six of them the trial of a single dose — about 500 mg — of ibogaine.

While interest in ibogaine may have started with this drug party, the unique effects of ibogaine became immediately evident in that it was not a substance conducive to such parties. There followed a period of six months of lay research which provided a dose-related response study ranging from 1 mg/kg to 19 mg/kg of ibogaine in both addict and non-addict human subjects.

Five of Lotsof's seven friends gave up the use of drugs during these six months. As for young Lotsof, he rebuilt his life, and although he was not a physician or a psychologist, he dreamed ("I had a dream", he told us the first time we met, paraphrasing the minister Dr. Martin Luther King), he dreamed that he would be the one who would contribute to curing drug addicts by providing them ibogaine.

H. Lotsof collected all the available documentation on iboga and ibogaine and, as a good American and businessman, founded a New York corporation, NDA International, Inc., whose purpose was partly a humanitarian mission and partly the marketing of a proprietary pharmaceutical preparation, *Endabuse,* composed of capsules of ibogaine hydrochloride.

In 1985, H. Lotsof took out a U.S. Patent on a *Rapid method for interrupting the narcotic addiction syndrome,*(Lotsof, H. 1985)[36], followed by another one in 1986 on a *Rapid method for interrupting the cocaine and amphetamine addiction syndrome* (Lotsof, H. 1986)[35] and subsequently yet another in 1989 for a *Rapid Method for attenuating the alcohol dependency syndrome.*(Lotsof, H. 1989)[34], and in 1991 for a *Rapid method for interrupting or attenuating the nicotine/tobacco* dependency syndrome.[37]

The heroin addiction syndrome had been interrupted in 5 of the 7 subjects described in the first patent.

A single treatment with ibogaine or ibogaine hydrochloride administered orally at a dosage ranging from 6 mg/kg to 19 mg/kg made it possible to interrupt the use of heroin for at least six months.

The duration of the treatment is about 30 hours, and ibogaine exerts a stimulant eflect during this period. An abreactive process takes place during the treatment but does not become evident until the patient awakens from a natural sleep that occurs after the primary and secondary efrects of ibogaine are diminished.

The drug addicts no longer desire to take heroin and show no perceptible signs of physical withdrawal. The subjects are relaxed and express themselves coherently. They demonstrate a *feeling of self-confidence.*

Lotsof describes the effects of the oral administration of ibogaine and divides these effects into three stages, comparable to the four stages of the *Bwiti of the Mitsogho.*

These three stages are described perfectly in the interview by the journalist Max Cantol[33] with a 44-year-old subject who had been a cocaine addict for more than eight years and was treatcd by the Lotsof procedure.

1st stage: 15 to 20 minutes after the start of the treatment, a numbing of the skin is accompanied by an auditory buzzing and an oscillating sound. Objects appear to vibrate intensely.

The first visions appear after an hour. Suddenly, on the walls, there appears a screen on which the subject views pictures that may be archetypes, more or less deformed animals, an abyss lit up by lightning, etc., or more personal episodes related either to childhood or to more recent events.

The subject may question the persons he sees, identify with one of them, be at the same time a spectator and an actor. He views a film of his subconscious and his repressed memories. He looks within himself.

2nd stage: 5 to 10 hours later, the visions cease and cutaneous sensitivity begins to retum. This stage is marked by an unusually high energy that lasts 5 to 8 hours, during which the subject see flashes of light around him. Then comes what the subject calls the question-and-answer period. He analyzes the visions that he remembers, seeks an interpretation and may communicate with the people around him.

Ibogaine *shows him where his problem is.* He has the impression that a reset button has been actuated. Everything is erased, everything becomes sharp and clear. He knows where his life took the wrong turn and what he must do to get back on the right path.

This question-and-answer period may last 20 hours, during which the subject remains under medical supervision.

3rd stage: the subject remains awake from a residual stimulation for up to 20 hours and then goes to sleep for as short a period as two hours and will wake up in top form, provided he is young and his general health had been good previously, *with a new self-confidence,* feeling no more need to take drugs. Mr. Lotsof, who knew of us, O. Gollnhofer, P. Potier (member of the French Academy of Sciences, Professor at the Museum of Natural History in Paris, Director of the Institute of Chemistry of Natural Substances, C.N.R.S., Gif-sur-Yvette, 91190 Essonne, France) and R. Goutarel, through his bibliographical documentation, came to France and contacted us. We were able to get some appointments, with Mr. Lotsof, at the Ministry of Health when Madame Barzach was Minister. We must say that we were received with courtesy and some skepticism. And then, Ministries change...

Our impression was that the people we met with, still impressed with the failures of LSD, were always afraid of making some mistake for which they would have been held accountable.

And yet, around the same time, in *Figaro Magazine* of February 14, 1987, there was a story on a shock treatment administered by the Buddhist monks of Tham-Krapok monastery in Thailand that resembles uncannily what is observed during the chewing of iboga.

A spectacular sequence presented to Madame Barzach and shown on television on the program *7/7* hosted by Madame Sinclair was the vomiting of the patients who, according to the commentator, had to get rid of the poisons in their system. Unfortunately, the drug was being kept secret, and it was said that Minister Chalandon had sent an observer over there to learn the secret. That secret seems obvious to us, and we know Apocynaceous plants from Asia containing ibogaine derivatives which, in all likelihood, have the same oneirophrenic properties as the latter.

At this time, Mr. Lotsof, who went to Gabon to collect a certain quantity of iboga, is having experiments pursued in several countries. Excellent results are being reported in the European and North American press. There have been several interviews with subjects successfully treated by the Lotsof procedure.

Pharmaceutical grade Ibogaine used in the treatment of addicts

Thanks to him, basic research is being conducted at Erasmus University of Rotterdam, at the Nathan Kline Institute at Orangeburg, N.Y., at Albany Medical College, N.Y., and through the Committee on Problems of Drug Dependence of the N.I.H., Bethesda, Maryland, for the purpose of investigating the different body systems, the CNS in particular, in which ibogaine is involved. Blockade of molphine-induced stimulation of mesolimbic and striatal dopamine by ibogaine has recently been demonstrated by the Albany Medical College researchers.[38]

The 1967–68 resolutions of the World Health Assembly classified ibogaine among the *drugs capable of producing dependency or impairing human health.*

When all is said and done, this alkaloid had been found guilty of the charge of being a hallucinogen similar to LSD, whose hazards for those who use it had recently come to light.

The fact is, however, that even though ibogaine is considered as a hallucinogen (oneirophrenic), it produces no drug dependency and it has proved to suppress dependency to opiates, amphetamines, cocaine, LSD and even alcohol and tobacco.

As for "impairing human health", the Gabonese experience shows that this is simply not true, quite the contrary.

The 1967–68 decree never did put an end to the illegal trade in amphetamines (the famous Ecstasy pill), nor to the trade in LSD. However, on that market, one never finds iboga or ibogaine.

According to Dhahir (1971)[14], the appearance of ibogaine on the illegal drug market was reported in 1967 by the police of Suffolk County, N.Y., on a single occasion, when it was used to dilute heroin, and after Haight Ashbury it was reportedly used by young addicts in San Francisco as a substitute for LSD.

Ibogaine suddenly disappeared from the market and it seems that the drug dealers rapidly became aware of the fact that its use would deprive them of part of their clientele.

Conclusions

What are we to conclude from this three-phase experience of the role of iboga (or ibogaine) at subtoxic doses, in the Bwiti, in psychotherapy according to Naranjo, and finally in combatting drug addiction?

1) In the Bwiti, and the Mitsogho Bwiti in particular in which we must emphasize the rigorous rites and the motivation inherent in it, the quantity of drug (scrapings of iboga root) is measured by the "mother", the initiate who accompanies and constantly watches over the initiate-to-be.

It is measured in the number of baskets and cannot be translated for us in weight of ibogaine. It is adjusted to the behavior of the subject and makes it possible to go past the first stage to reach the stage of so-called normative visions, corresponding to the *real motivation* of he who aspires to see and to know the things of the beyond.

The intoxication by iboga is slow and progressive, which makes it possible to observe four stages during the visions. The first three stages are essentially of the Freudian type and the fourth one, the so-called stage of normative visions, corresponds to the collective image of the tribe.

Finally, the initiation into the Bwiti among the Mitsogho concerns the passage from adolescence to adulthood. Hence the necessity of eliminating the epigenetic acquisitions from the period of childhood and adolescence in order to reprogram in the young man a new ego in keeping with the cultural norms of the tribe.

In the *Bwiti of the Fang,* the ceremony may be accelerated by substituting for the scrapings of iboga a galenic preparation flavored with milk, sugar or palm wine, known under the names of "express" or "automatic".

Women can be initiated in the Fang Bwiti, and many differences are observed due to the changes in the initiatory experience that may have occurred under the influence of Christianity and the competition among the various more or less orthodox messianic and prophetic movements and the loss of the tribal notion. Therefore, it is out of the question to speak of normative visions in the Fang Bwiti, which is a real syncretism between ancestor worship and Christianity. When all is said and done, the visions correspond to the culture of the future initiate: Christian and Western culture for whites who are initiated into the Fang Bwiti.

2) The doses of ibogaine used in *psychotherapy according to Naranjo* are relatively low, and the session does not last more than 6 hours. The dose of 300 mg orally appears to be the minimum required for triggering the visions analyzed by the psychotherapist who constantly guides the patients as he searches for the deep-seated causes of the neurosis for which the patient has consulted him. It appears that the sessions have to be repeated.

Naranjo's conclusion is that ibogaine cannot produce the changes just by itself, hence the need for a psychotherapist.

3) In the *treatment of drug addicts, H. Lotsof gives* a single dose of about 1 g of ibogaine hydrochloride orally.

The session is quite long, about 36 hours, which is comparable to what is observed during the initiation into the Bwiti, given that the slow chewing of iboga and the accompanying rites are dispensed with. We might note that in the Fang Bwiti, the session also lasts approximately 36 hours when the so-called "express" or "automatic" galenic preparation is substituted for the iboga sclapings.

Thus, the first visions appear two hours after the ingestion of ibogaine hydrochloride. The three phases described by Lotsof are comparable to the four phases of the Mitsogho Bwiti, the first phase being that of Freudian type visions, and the second phase ("questions and answers") being comparable to the phase of normative visions. Lotsof describes a third phase, one of residual stimulation followed by restorative sleep of short duration.

We should point out that in all likelihood, the success of the Lotsof method also depends on a *deep motivation* of the subject who is treated, which is the will to eliminate all drug dependency.

On November 17, 1989, the United States Senate Committee on the Judiciary published a Committee Report on Pharmacotherapy for Illicit Drug Use.

This report deals essentially with a research program, the Medication Development Program (MDP) entrusted to the National Institute on Drug Abuse (NIDA) in Rockville, Maryland.

Beginning in 1989, the Director of the MDP was given a subsidy of 30 million dollars. Starting at the beginning of 1990, the research budget was increased to 200 million dollars The research, at the time, was not oriented toward developing a chemical substance that might cure addicted persons, but toward substitution drugs like methadone that remove the need for hard drugs, particularly cocaine, while creating a less dangerous dependence

At the time, ibogaine had not been listed among the products of interest for combatting chemical dependency.

It was difficult to accept the fact that a chemical could, in a few days, suppress all dependency to opiates, cocaine or any other drug.

There were then and there are still two opposing schools of thought: the proponents of substitution chemical drugs and those of gentle, long-lasting psychotherapy that could somelimes result in a cure.

We can therefore understand that the method of H.S. Lotsof was initially met with disbelief and even hostility.

Before authorizing clinical trials for a new drug, the govemment agencies responsible still require, quite appropriately, that its activity be demonstrated in the animal.

In addition to proving that ibogaine has a low toxicity[14] and perhaps potentiates the analgesic action of morphine[32], the pharmacodynamic studies in animals had supplied few data demonstrating the incredible property of ibogaine to modify the behavior of an individual and result in a new individuation of the brain by eliminating certain tendencies detrimental to its full development.

However, new techniques developed by researchers in the neurosciences have recently provided some definite information as to the mechanism of action of ibogaine in the treatment of addicts (morphine and cocaine).

Using microdialysis, Di Chiara and Imperato (1988)[15] reported that acute administration of amphetamine, cocaine, morphine, nicotine and ethanol, all known to be addictive drugs increases the extracellular dopamine (DA) levels in the *nucleus accumbens* and to a lesser extent in the *striatum.*

I.M. Maisonneuve (1991)[38] showed that ibogaine blocks the morphine-induced stimulation of mesolimbic and striatal dopamine. Curiously, it appears that ibogaine affects brain DA systems for a period of time that exceeds its elimination from the body and during this time alters the responses of these systems to morphine. Furthermore, ibogaine alters cocaine-induced accumbens dopamine neurotransmission (Broderick, P.A., 1992).[6]

Ibogaine reduced the cocaine-induced locomotor stimulation when given two hours before an acute injection of cocaine to mice. This stimulation is also reduced when a second injection of cocaine is given 24 hours later (H. Sershen, 1992).[54]

Finally, S.D. Glick (1991)[21] demonstrated that ibogaine reduces the intravenous self-administration of morphine in rats, not only in the hour after ibogaine treatment (acute effect) but also one day or more later (after-effect). Since ibogaine is eliminated rapidly[14], the persistence of this after-effect suggests the formation of a metabolite of ibogaine with a long half-life.

Barrass, B.C. and Coult (1972)[2] had shown that ibogaine *inhibits* the oxidation of serotonin by a monoamine oxidase (MAO), ceruloplasmin, and *catalyzes* the oxidation of catecholamines by the same substrate.

Indeed, ibogaine is a potent serotoninergic that has ability to reduce the level of cerebral catecholamines. This decrease in the level of catecholamines, dopamine in particular, explains the results described recently on the blockade of the stimulation of mesolimbic and striatal dopamine induced by morphine or cocaine.

We should point out that ibogaine is not specific to morphine and cocaine but is active in the presence of all addictive drugs, which justifies the patent applications that followed the initial patent of H.S. Lotsof.

The decrease in the level of catecholamines and the joint increase in the cerebral serotonin level result in a suppression of REM sleep and the appearance of the hallucinatory phenomenon (C. Debru, 1990).[12]

LSD, like ibogaine,[2] is a potent serotoninergic that inhibits the oxidation of serotonin and catalyzes the oxidation of catecholamines by MAO.

However, there is an enormous difference between these two alkaloids: LSD is active at doses of less than a milligram. Its activity is difficult to control and the hallucinatory phenomena produced belong to a high and angelic domain of esthetic sensations, whereas ibogaine is hallucinogenic only at doses in excess of 100 mg, and the domain of this oneirophrenic substance is that of the subterranean world of Freud, of animal impulse and of regression.

The toxicity of ibogaine is very low, lower than that of aspirin, which makes this alkaloid easy to use.

The initiated masters in the Bwiti have an *antidote* that enables them to interrupt at any time the course of the visions if, for any reason, the absorption of iboga were to be actually life-threatening for the neophyte.

Let us note that serotonin is the neurotransmitter of the cerebral parasympathetic system, catecholamines being neurotransmitters in the cerebral orthosympathetic system, and that the negative chronotropic and inotropic effects as well as the arousal-producing action of ibogaine are nullified by atropine, an acetylcholine antagonist, acetylcholine being the neurotransmitter of the autonomic nervous system.

The long waking-dream period that follows the absorption of iboga or ibogaine at a subtoxic dose (or oneirophrenic dose according to Naranjo) appears to be responsible for a temporary destructuring of the ego, followed by its restructuring.

This hypothesis is consistent with the observations made by the ethnologists in their studies of the Mitsogho Bwiti, and may be compared to the hypotheses of Michel Jouvet and Sir Francis Crick (C. Debru, 1990)[12] on the role of dreams in the programming and deprogramming of basic behavior pattems, resulting in a new individuation of the human brain.

Normally, the stages of wakefulness of the human brain are: waking, NREM (slow wave or deep) sleep, PGO (pontogeniculo-occipital) waves, and REM (rapid eye movement or paradoxical) sleep. REM sleep is the period of dreams.

Michel Jouvet and Sir Francis Crick consider PGO waves to be the ***principal coding tool*** that acts at the cortical level in recording the genetic and epigenetic acquisitions necessary for the individuation of the human brain.

In addition, through random activation mechanisms, the PGO waves eliminate from certain types of neuronal networks an informational overload linked to pathological behavior: This is what C. Debru calls "cleaning out the neuronal circuitry."

REM sleep apparently undertakes a sorting out process among the "residues" stirred up by the PGO wave sleep pattern and disposes of these residues during dreaming.

Michel Jouvet (letter of November 7, 1990) wrote: "The oneiric effects observed in humans and which are produced by hallucinogens do not enable us to approach the dream mechanisms directly, because it does appear that these two phenomena cannot be linked together as one.

We know, however, that the principal difference between dreams and hallucinations resides in the way in which the stages of wakefulness are organized, with the suppression of REM sleep and the intrusion of PGO waves in the arousal (waking) stage and in NREM (or slow) sleep.

The new organization becomes: waking (arousal) stage, stage of PGO waves, hallucination stage, sleep stage, and it appears possible that hallucinatory manifestations, the waking dream, eliminate "residues" stirred up by the PGO wave pattern in the absence of REM sleep.

Near Death Experiences

According to the Mitsogho, the initiate will see the Bwiti only twice in his life: on the day of his initiation and on the day of his death.

This means that the visions at the approach of death, what are called *near death experiences* (NDE), are the same as those termed normative visions.

We know that at the time of dying, some individuals see their whole life pass before them. In those who are "rescued from death", a spectacular transformation is observed. They no longer fear death, they feel stronger, more optimistic, calmer, and contemplate their life more positively.

Two Americans, the psychiatrist Raymond Moody[39] and the cardiologist Michael B. Sabom[49] have been particularly interested in the oneiric manifestations of NDE.

After a statistical study of 150 people "rescued from death", M.B. Sabom established a chart of these manifestations.

SABOM CHART

Autoscopic phase
1. Subjective feeling of being dead
2. Peace and well-being
3. Disembodiment
4. Visions of material objects and events

Transcendental phase
5. Tunnel or dark zone
6. Evaluation of past life
7. Light
8. Access to a transcendental world - Entering in light
9. Encounter with other beings
10. Return to life

Most of these manifestations are to be found in the Mitsogho Bwiti. Starting at the 3rd stage, a peaceful and agreeable vision, disembodiment; the neophyte feels himself wrapped up by a wind that carries him off to an unknown village without beginning or end; a vision of two extraordinary Beings, Nzamba-Kana, the first man and Disumba, the first woman on earth. The village is covered by sparks, then a brilliant ball of light appears, the sun, and the moon and the stars. The sun is transformed into a handsome youth, the Master of the World, and the moon into a beautiful woman, his wife, the mother of his children, the stars. The wind carries the initiate back to earth where he is rebom and is greeted with joy and pride by the elders.

In the Fang Bwiti, where we have a syncretism between the religion of the ancestors and Christianity, it is difficult, because of many divergent forms, to describe a coherent whole corresponding to the normative visions of the Mitsoghos.

Interviews with young Frenchmen

However, interviews with young whites from France who were willing to go through the Fang Bwiti initiation trial show a set of visions characteristic of their Western and generally Christian culture, which for the most part fit in with Sabom's chart.

Thus, in the narration of a young man named Christophe, after some personal Freudian type visions and a few visions influenced by the Fang Bwiti, there is the following description: an absolute white, an indescribable luminous blue, the joy and perfection of blue, a cave and a cavernous sound, bright light entering through the forehead like a third eye, things seen in the astral, the sight of the spiritual world that cannot be seen with the body, a large sun fueled by our particles, the light of which we are a part. Paradise that can be reached only through the spirit. The awareness of an envelope preventing him from joining the spiritual world, etc.

The visions, both in the Mitsogho Bwiti and in the Fang Bwiti, seem to be dominated by this impression of shining lights that we find at the second stage described by H.S. Lotsof in his first patent [36] (H.S. Lotsof, U.S. Patent 4,499,096, Feb. 12, 1985).

After a first stage characterized by Freudian type visions, the second stage is marked by a high energy during which the subject sees lightning or brief flashes of light that dance about him. During this period, thoughts continue that seem to amplify the meaning of the vision seen during the primary phase. This is the question-and-answer period described by one of the subjects treated according to H.S. Lotsof.

What is important is that this luminous phase of questions and answers is followed by a restorative sleep from which the subject awakens in great form and with a new self-confidence.

Lotsof notes that the first two stages together last 24 to 48 hours or longer, followed by only 3 to 4 hours of sleep. This reduced need for sleep may continue for 1 to 4 months.

The persistence of this long-term effect is consistent with the hypothesis (I.M. Maisonneuve, 1991; S.D. Glick, 1991) of a metabolite of ibogaine with a long half-life.

Some subjects treated according to Lotsof retain for a fairly long time the impression of being under the influence of ibogaine.

A young Dutch woman wrote: "I lost a great deal of interest in drugs in general, because the effect of ibogaine goes far beyond their effect, though not necessarily in a pleasant way", and "Up until four months after the treatment, I kept experiencing colors and light very intensely."

The conclusion of the report that was written recently by this 28-year-old woman six months after a treatment with ibogaine shows that this alkaloid produced a real change in what she calls her "addictive ego", and also shows the necessity of having a strong motivation.

"Ibogaine was a mental process for me, a form of spiritual purification and a truth serum in which I had to experience its results through time. It's only now, after six months, that I can say I am not addicted anymore. It takes time to admit that there is no way back. Ibogaine is not a solution in itself, although it takes away withdrawal completely. Ibogaine helps you to realize that all knowledge is available to cure yourself through will power. It's up to you if you are ready to give up your addictive ego."[1]

The recent decision of the National Institute on Drug Abuse (NIDA) to add ibogaine to the list of drugs whose activity in the treatment of drug dependency is to be evaluated should prompt the competent authorities in European countries to engage rapidly along the same lines. This applies to France in particular, where research on iboga and its alkaloids began at the end of the 19th century and has continued well beyond the second half of the 20th century.

If we consider all the pharmacodynamic and therapeutic investigations conducted on iboga and ibogaine, we may conclude that this alkaloid, unjustly condemned as a hallucinogen, is a key that opens the door of the fascinating realm of today's neurosciences, and we should like to see the creation of a *multidisciplinary organization* including ethnologists, medical doctors, psychiatrists and psychologists, chemists, pharmacists and pharmacologists, and even technical writers, so that we can get a definite opinion on the psychotherapeutic properties of iboga and ibogaine, whose use must now take place under the norms of pharmaceutical development and medical ethical review.

ADDITIONAL POST-PUBLICATION NOTES, GOUTAREL TO LOTSOF

CAN IBOGAINE SUBSTITUTE FOR DREAMS IN REPROGRAMMING THE BRAIN?

The question is: can oneiric or oneirophrenic hallucination replace dream in the repeated deprogramming and reprogramming of the subject treated with ibogaine.

The concept of the role of dreams in the process of forgetting has been developed in particular by Crick F. and Mitchison G., 1983 ("On the Function of Dream Sleep", *Nature* 304, 111–114): "We dream in order to forget".

This notion has been completed by that of *iterative* (or repeated) *programming,* developed in particular by Jouvet M. (Michel Jouvet, *Le Sommeil et le Rêve,* Ed. Odile Jacob, Paris, 1992). This iterative programming of the circuits (PGO, cortical neurons) responsible for hereditary idiosyncrasy does not require the production of new neurons by neurogenesis.

Since this neurogenesis is absent in man (neurons die but are not renewed), it is accepted that certain genetically programmed neurons can be deprogrammed and then reprogrammed for the purpose of constant, ongoing individuation of the human brain.

This iterative programming involves PGO waves, cortical activation and REM activity, which is the outwardly visible sign of dreaming: "The neuronal orchestras play the oneiric score under the guidance of the invisible conductor of PGO activity" (Jouvet M., 1992).

The *REM sleep rebound* phenomenon was studied in 1960 by Dement W. (1960, "The Effect of Dream Deprivation", *Science* 131, 1705–1707).

"Instrumental deprivation" of dreaming (swimming pool method in the rat or the cat; arousal of a human subject as soon as the first REM signs appear) is followed, on the one hand, by an increasing *need to dream,* manifested by the appearance of increasingly frequent REM episodes (nearly every minute following a 24–h deprivation in the cat), and on the other hand by *REM sleep rebound,* a relative increase in the amount of REM sleep after deprivation has been discontinued.

Jouvet acknowledges that experimental situations that are able to produce a particular form of stress that could be called "strain" are responsible for this rebound which appears to be a cerebrostatic mechanism intended to restore the cortical circuitry adversely affected by situations of constraint imposed upon the organism and are *non-gratifying.*

In contradistinction to this, Jouvet indicates (Valatz, personal communication) that when a rat is himself allowed to choose *arousing* (and *gratifying*) *central stimulations* through self-stimulation of the lateral hypothalamus, continuous wakefulness of 10 hours (stimulation effectuated at the rate of several tens of times per minute) *is not followed by an increase in REM sleep.* We may therefore presume that, in this case, self-stimulation involves only genetically programmed individuation circuits. *Self-stimulation* (*gratifying*) *could then replace the iterative programming of dreams.* This self-stimulation presumably sets into action the genetic circuits of individuation by assuming the functions of dream and *apparently does not trigger the rebound mechanisms* (Jouvet M. 1992).

Under *conditions of security,* it is believed that *oneiric hallucinations* are more gratifying than frightening (Snyder F.M.D., "Towards an Evolutionary Theory of Dreaming", *Amer.J.Psychiat.* 123, 2 Aug. 1966).

Naquet (Da Costa L. 1980)[11] has shown that tabernanthine, an isomer of ibogaine, produces calm and prolonged waking in the cat, very different from the one produced by amphetamines. This wakefulness is followed by slow, deep sleep without the abnormalities of REM sleep, the period of dreams. *Therefore, there is no rebound.*

The same is true of ibogaine, not only in the animal but in man.

If we examine the three stages of the treatment described by Lotsof in his first patent (Lotsof H.S. 1985), we can concede that the forgetting of epigenetic acquisitions begins during the 1st stage with Freudian visions. This process of forgetting prepares the neurons (genetically programmed) for a new individuation.

Iterative reprogramming may begin in the 2nd stage (period of luminous visions) and continues after it (question and answer period).

The 3rd stage is characterized by a slow, deep sleep lasting a few hours, *without the rebound phenomenon* of REM sleep.

Therefore, we may consider oneirophrenia (a hallucinary phenomenon peculiar to ibogaine) as particularly gratifying and capable of assuming the same functions as REM sleep in a new individuation of the human brain. "The invisible conductor of PGO activities has left the dream for a more 'rock' and *gratifying* score: oneirophrenia".

Finally, since the ratio between wakefulness (36–48 h) and NREM sleep (2–4 h) continues for several months following the treatment, we can concede that iterative reprogramming goes on throughout this period and will not be over until REM sleep returns.

LE SOMMELL ET LE RÊVE, MICHEL JOUVET, ODILE JACOB PUBLLSHERS, 1992

Paradoxical sleep: State characterized by external signs: postural atony, REM, erection of sexual organ in the male; and internal signs: cortical activation and PGO activity.

To refer to this state merely as REM — and some go so far as to use REM to mean dreaming — is to take the part for the whole.

The role of paradoxical sleep (PS) in the brain's iterative *deprogramming* and *programming.*

This notion of the role of dreams in forgetting (deprogramming) has to be completed by that of *iterative programming,* developed in particular by Jouvet.

This iterative programming of the *circuits responsible* (PGO, cortical neurons) for hereditary idlosyncrasy does not require the development of new neurons by neurogenesis.

Since such neurogenesis is absent in homeotherms ("warm-blooded" creatures), man in particular (neurons die but are not renewed), we accept the idea that certain genetically programmed neurons can be deprogrammed and then reprogrammed for purposes of a constant individuation of the human brain.

This iterative programming involves PGO waves and dreaming (cortical activation: "The neuronal orchestras play the oneiric score under the guidance of the invisible conductor of PGO activity" — Jouvet, p. 20C).

PS (PARADOXICAL SLEEP) REBOUND, Dement W. (1960), "The Effects of Dream Deprivation, *Science* 131, 1705–1707.

Dement was the first to demonstrate the PS (REM sleep) rebound phenomenon that follows after its "selective" deprivation.

The "instrumental" deprivation of PS (the swimming pool method in the rat or the cat, and waking up the human subject as soon as the first REM signs appear) is followed, on the one hand, by the *need for PS* which is reflected by the appearance of ever more frequent episodes of PS (nearly each minute after a deprivation of 24–h in the cat), and on the other hand by *PS rebound,* which is a relative increase in the quantity of PS after deprivation has ceased.

It is recognized today that experimental situations that are able to give rise to a particular form of stress that could be called "strain" are responsible for this rebound, and it appears that this PS rebound is a cerebrostatic mechanism designed to *restablish the cortical circuits that have been impaired by situations of constraint imposed upon the organism that are nongratifying.*

At the opposite end, when a rat is able to choose for himself arousal-producing central stimulations (and at the same time gratifying ones) through *lateral hypothalamus self-stimulation,* continuous arousals of 10 hours (stimulations performed at the rate of several tens of times per minute) *are not followed by an increase in PS.* Therefore, we can suppose that, in this case, the self-stimulation involves only genetically programmed individuation circuits. *The self-stimulation could then replace the iterative programming of PS.* This self-stimulation would appear to bring into play the genetic circuits of individuation of PS and not set off rebound mechanisms. Naquet (Da Costa L., 1980[11] showed that tabernanthine produces a calm, prolonged wakefulness, very different from the one produced by amphetamines). This waking is followed by slow sleep without the abnormalities of REM sleep, the period of dreams. Therefore, there is no rebound.

It is likely that the same is true with ibogaine, where the hallucinatory phenomenon is accompanied by the intrusion of PGO into the waking phase and the suppression of REM (PS).

Arousal, PGO, hallucinations, slow sleep

The combination PGO/hallucinations could then be gratifying and have the same value as the combination PGO/PS and replace the iterative programming of PS.

Bibliography

1. Baillon, H. 1889. "Sur l'oubouele du Gabon" ("The Oubwele of Gabon"). *Bulletin mensuel de la Socie'te' Lineenne de Paris* vol. 1(98):782–783.
2. Barras, B.C. and Coult, D.B. 1972. "Effects of some centrally-acting drugs on caeruloplasmin." *Progress in Brain Res.* 36, 97–104 (1972).
3. Bartlett, M.; Dickel, D.F.; Taylor, W.I. 1958. *J. Amer. Chem. Soc.* Vol. 80:126.
4. Binet, J.; Gollnhofer, O.; Sillans, R. 1972. *Cahiers d'Etudes africaines* vol. 46(Xii/195):253.
5. Bocher, D.P. and Naranjo, C. 1969. "Nouveau medicament agissant au niveau du SNC, antidrogue" ("A New CNS-active Medication for Use Against Drugs"). *Bulletin Officiel de la Propriété Industrielle,* No. 35, September 1, 1969 (Special Drug Patent P.V. No. 138.081, No. 7131M, Int. Class. A 61k)
6. Broderick, P. A., Phelan, F. T. and Berger, S. P., "Ibogaine alters cocaine-induced biogenic amine and psychostimulant dysfunction but not [3H]GBR-12935 binding to the dopamine transporter protein". *Problems of Drug Dependence 1991: Proceedings of the 53rd Annual Scientific*

Meeting, The Committee on Problems of Drug Dependence, INC., NIDA Research Monograph Series, 119.285, 1992.

7. Bureau, R., "La religion d'Eboga. Essai sur le Bwiti fang" ("The Religion of Eboga. Essay on the Fang Bwiti"). Thesis, Paris V, 317 pp., 1972.
8. Burckhardt, C.A., Goutarel, R., Janot, M.M., and Schlittler, E., 1952. *Helv. chim. Acta 35,* 642.
9. Closmenil, A. de. 1905. "De l'iboga et de l'ibogaine" ("Iboga and Ibogaine"). Thesis for the Degree of Doctor of Medicine, Paris.
10. Crick, F. 1979. "Reflexions sur le cerveau" ("Reflections on the Brain") *Pour la science* Vol. 25(Nov.): 168.
11. Dacosta, L.; Sulklaper, I; Naquet, R. 1980. *Rev. E.E.G. Neuro physiol.* Vol. 10(1):105.
12. Debru, C., 1990. *Neurophysiologie du reve* (*The Neurophysiology of Dreams*), Paris, Hermann, Edition des Sciences et des Arts.
13. Delourme-Houde, J. 1944. "Contribution a l'etude de l'iboga" ("Contribution to the study of iboga"). Thesis for Doctor's Degree (Pharmacy) Paris University; Ann. Pharm. Fr. Vol. 430,1946.
14. Dhahir, H.I. 1971. "A comparative study on the toxicity of ibol and serotonin." Thesis, Ph.D. (Toxicology), Indiana University, University Microfilms International, Ann Arbor, MI (71-25, 341)
15. Di Chiara, G. and Imperato, A. 1988. "Drugs abused by humans preferentially increase synaptic dopamine concentrations in the mesolimbic system of freely moving rats." *Proc. Nat. Acad. Sci.* Vol. 85:5274.
16. Dutheil, R. and Dutheil, B., *L'homme superlumineux* (*The Superluminous Man*), Sand Publ., 1990.
17. Dybowski, J. and Landrin, E. 1901. *C.R. Acad. Sci.* Vol. 133:748.
18. Fromaget, M., 1986. "Contribution of the Mitsogho Bwiti to the Anthropology of the Imaginary: A Case of Divinatory Diagnosis in Gabon" *Anthropos* 81, 87–107.
19. Gaignault, J.C. & Delourme-Houde, J. 1977. "Les alcaloides de l'iboga" ("Iboga alkaloids"). *Fitolerapia* Vol. 48(6):243.
20. Gershon, S. and Lang, W.J. 1962. *Arch. Inlt. Pharmacodyn.* Vol. 135:31.
21. Glick, S.D.; Rossman, K.; Steindorf, S.; Maisonneuve, I.M.;Carlson, J.M. 1991. "Effects and after-effects of ibogaine on morphine self administration in rats." *European J. Pharmacol.* 195 (1991):341–345.
22. Goebel, F. 1841. *Ann.* Vol. 38:363.
23. Gollnhofer, O. & Sillans, R. 1985. "Usages rituels de l'iboga au Gabon" ("Ritual Uses of Iboga in Gabon"). *Psychotropes* Vol. 2(3):95–108.
24. Gollnhofer, O. & Sillans, R. 1983. "L'iboga, psychotrope africain" ("Iboga, an African Psychotropic Agent"). *Psychotropes* Vol. 1(1):21
25. Goutarel, R. 1954. "Recherches sur quelques alcaloides indoliques, leurs relations avec le metabolisme du tryptophane et de la dihydroxyphenal alanine" ("Research on some indole alkaloids and their relations with the metabolism of tryptophan and dihydroxyphenylalanine"). Thesis, Doctor of Science Degree, Paris.
26. Goutarel, R., Janot, M.M., Mathys, F., and Prelog, V., 1953. 9,1 "Structure de l'ibogaïne" ("The structure of ibogaine"), *C.R. Acad. Sci.* 237,178.
27. Goutarel, R., Janot, M.M., Prelog, V., and Taylor, W.I., 1950. *Helv. chim. Acta* 33, 150, 164.
28. Haller, A., and Heckel, E., 1901. "Sur l'ibogaïne, principe actif d'une plante du genre Tabernaemontana, originaire du Congo" ("Concerning ibogaine, the active principle of a plant of the genus Tabernaemontana, native to the Congo") *C.R. Acad. Sci.* 133:850–853.
29. Khuong-Huu, F., J.P. Leforestier, G. Maillard and R. Goutarel. *C.R. Acad. Sci.* 270, 2070, 2072.
30. Lambert, M., 1901. "Sur l'action physiologique de l'iboga" ("On the Physiological Action of Iboga"), *C.R. Soc. Biol.,* 53:1096–1097.
31. Lambert, M., 1902. "Sur les propriétés physiologiques de l'ibogaïne" ("On the Physiological Properties of Ibogaine"), *Arch. int. Pharmacodynamie et Therapie,* 10:101–120).
32. Lotsof, H.S. 1990. Personal communication.
33. Lotsof, H.S. 1990. Personal communication. [The Max Cantor interviews have since been published in the San Diego-based journal *The Truth Seeker:* 1990, Vol. 117(5):23-26].
34. Lotsof, H.S. 1989. U.S. Patent No. 4,857,523.
35. Lotsof, H.S. 1986. U.S. Patent No. 4,587,243.
36. Lotsof, H.S. 1985. U.S. Patent No. 4,499,096.
37. Lotsof, H.S. 1991. U.S. Patent No. 5,026,697.
38. Maisonneuve, I.M., Keller. R.W. Jr., and Glick, S.D. 1991. "Interactions between ibogaine, a potential anti-addictive agent, and morphine: an in vivo microdialysis study." *European J. Pharmacol.* 199:35–42.
39. Moody, R.A.: *Life After Life: The Investigation of a Phenomenon, Survival of Bodily Death,* Walker & Co., 1988. *The Light Beyond,* Bantam, 1989.
40. Mueller, J.M.; Schlittler, E.; Bein, H.J. 1952. *Experientiua* Vol. 8:338.
41. Naranjo, C. 1969. "Psychotherapeutic possibilities of new fantasy enhancing drugs." *Clinical Toxicology* Vol. 2(2):209.
42. Neu, Henri (Father). 1885. *Archives génévales des Peres du Saint Esprit,* Vol. 148-B-i.
43. Phisalix, M.C. 1901. "Action physiologique de l'ibogaïne" ("Physiological action of ibogaine"). *C.R. Acad. Sci* Vol. 53:1077.
44. Pouchet, G. and Chevalier, J. 1905. "Note sur l'action pharmacologique de l'ibogaïne. Sur l'action pharmacodynamique de l'ibogaïne" ("Note on the pharmacological action of ibogaine. On the pharmacodynamiec action of ibogaine"), *Bull. Genl. de Thérapeutique.*
45. Prioux-Guyonneau, M.; Rapin, J.R.; Wepierre, J. 1977. *J. Pharmacol. Paris,* Vol. 8(3):383.
46. Raymond-Hamet & Vincent, D. 1960. *C.R. Soc. Biol.* Vol. 154:2223, Raymond-Hamet; Vincent, D.; Parant, M. 1956. *C.R. Soc. Biol.* Vol. 150:1384; Vincent, D. & Sero, I. 1942. Traumax Membres *Soc. Chim. Biol.,* Vol. 24: 1352.
47. Raymond-Hamet 1946. *C.R. Acad. Sci.* Vol. 223:757;1943. *Bull. Soc. Chim. Biol.,* Vol. 25:200;1942. *Bull. Soc. Chim. Fr.,* Vol. 9:620;1941. *C.R. Acad. Sci.,* Vol. 212:768; 1940. *C.R. Soc. Biol.,* Vol. 134:541; 1940. *C.R. Soc. Biol.,* Vol. 133:426;1939. *Arch. Immunocology,* Vok 63:27.
48. Raymond-Hamet 1941. "L'iboga, drogue défatigante mal connue" ("Iboga, a poorly known antifatigue drug"). *Bull. Acad. Med.,* Vol. 124:243.
49. Sabom, M.B. *Recollections of Death,* Harper & Row, 1982.
50. Sehlitler, E., Burckhard, C.A., Gellert, E. 1953. "Die Kalischmelze des Alkaloides Ibogain," *Helv. Chim. Acta,* 36:1337.
51. Schneider, J.A. and Rinehart, R.K. 1957. *Arch. Int. Pharmacodn.* Vol. 110(1):92.
52. Schneider, J.A. and Sigg, E.G. 1957. *Ann. N.Y. Acad. Sci.,* Vol. 66:765.
53. Schneider, J.A. 1956. *Experientia,* Vol. 12:323.
54. Sershen, H., Hashim, A., Harsing, L., Lajtha, A. "Ibogaine antagonizes cocaine-induced locomotor stimulation in mice." (In press, *J. Life Sciences.*)
55. Sero, I. 1944. "Une apocynacée d'Afrique équatoriale" ("An Apocynacea from Equatorial Africa"). Thesis, Doctor of Pharmacy, Toulouse.
56. Vincent, D. and Sero, I, 1942. "Action inhibitrice de Tabernanthe iboga sur la cholinesterase du serum" ("The inhibitory action of Tabernanthe iboga on serum cholinesterase"), *C.R. Soc. Biol.,* 136:612–614.
57. Wurman, M. 1939. "Contribution a l'étude experimentale et therapeutique d'un extrait de Tabernanthe manii d'origine gabonaise" ("Contribution to the experimental and therapeutic study of an extract of T. manii from Gabon"), Thesis, Doctor of Medicine Degree, Paris.
58. Zetler, G. & Lessau, W. 1972. *Pharmacology,*Vol. 8:235.

Appendix 3

"Quantum Coherence in Microtubules: A Neural Basis for Emergent Consciousness?"[1]

Stuart Hameroff[2]

Abstract: The paper begins with a general introduction to the nature of human consciousness and outlines several different philosophical approaches. A critique of traditional reductionist and dualist positions is offered and it is suggested that consciousness should be viewed as an emergent property of physical systems. However, although consciousness has its origin in distributed brain processes it has macroscopic properties—most notably the 'unitary sense of self, non-deterministic free will, and non-algorithmic 'intuitive' processing—which can best be described by quantum-mechanical principles.

There have been many attempts by physicists and philosophers to apply quantum mechanical principles to the realm of consciousness, but they have been primarily speculative and analogical as there has been little supportive evidence from the neurosciences. This paper postulates that cytoskeletal microtubules within neurons could be a possible site for quantum effects.

Although the supportive evidence for such a thesis is, of necessity, highly technical, the article has been structured in such a way that the general arguments are accessible to the general reader. For those more technically minded, full supportive evidence is available in footnotes and appendices.

Introduction: Emergence of Consciousness

The nature of human consciousness is the greatest frontier facing science and mankind and is being approached by many disciplines—including neuroscience, cognitive science, computer science, physics, mathematics, medicine, pharmacology, philosophy and religion. Within this diverse approach exists a spectrum which, at one extreme, considers consciousness as simply the sum total of brain activities. This *reductionist* view is best exemplified by functionalist philosophers (e.g. Dennett, 1991) and proponents of "strong artificial intelligence" or "strong AI" (e.g. Minsky, 1986) who contend that all mental events may be reduced to an algorithm and that all brain functions, including consciousness, may eventually occur in computers. On the other end of the spectrum is a *dualist* view which considers the brain and mind as distinct, separate entities and consciousness as existing in a separate reality (e.g. Popper and Eccles, 1977). This reductionism/dualism dichotomy may potentially be resolved by views which contend that consciousness has a distinct quality, but one which *emerges* from brain processes which can be accounted for by natural science.

One aspect of natural science, quantum theory, may be especially relevant. In particular, the concept of *quantum coherence* leading to macroscopic quantum states may help explain several of the qualities of consciousness which are difficult to explain by conventional neuroscience. These properties, and their possible quantum correlates (in parentheses) are:

- The "binding problem" or "unitary sense of self" (quantum coherence, non-locality).
- Randomness, non-deterministic free will (quantum indeterminacy).
- Non-algorithmic "intuitive" processing (computing via quantum superposition).
- Reversible ablation by general anaesthesia (prevention of quantum coherence by anaesthetic inhibition of quantum mobility in protein hydrophobic regions).
- Difference (and transition) between pre-, sub- and non-conscious processes and consciousness (collapse of the wave function).

This paper describes a potential "bottom-level" mechanism in the brain's recursive, hierarchical organization driven or selected by (and also driving and selecting) higherlevel mechanisms (e.g. neural networks, attentional scanning circuits, coherent firing of distributed neurons). At this "bottom" level, quantum events can couple directly to conformational states of cell proteins. Quantum coherence in cytoskeletal microtubules and associated water within each of the brain's neurons may be a bottom level from which consciousness can emerge.

Emergence implies a qualitatively new property or phenomenon which appears at a hierarchical level above the level at which rules of interaction are implemented. Emergent properties (including chaos) occur in many complex systems including networks, vortices, lasers, chemical oscillations, genetic networks, weather and developmental patterns. Numerous authors have described consciousness as an emergent phenomenon arising from a hierarchy of lower-level brain processes.[3] Emergent phenomena can exert downward modulation on

[1] Reprinted in part in the proceedings from the Abisko (Sweden) Conference on *Matter Matters — On the Material Basis of the Cognitive Acrivity of the Mind*, ed. Rolf Wasen, Peter Arhem, and Uno Svedin.

[2] I am indebted to Alwyn Scott for guidance and suggestions, to Roger Penrose for validation and inspiration, to Richard Hofstad for patience and clerical talent, and to Gordon Globus, Jane Clark, Keith Sutherland and the journal's referees for review, criticism and restructuring. Supported in part by NSF Grant No. DMS-9 1 14503. Summer 1994 support from MIDIT, Danish Technical University is also appreciated.

Reprinted with permission from the *Journal of Consciousness Studies*, 1, No. I, Summer 1994, pp. 91–118.

[3] Atkin (1992) has defincd consciousness as emergent *information itself* at the moment of its generation—ongoing, self-organizing change in a self/world model. Baas (1994) has mathematically described "hyperstructures" with intrinsic observer functions which emerge from hierarchies, and hierarchical schemes of brain organization leading to consciousness have been proposed (e.g. Scott, 1978, 1994; Somjen, 1983). Globus (1992)describes thebrain as "fractal-like", with recursive levels, each using "edge of chaos" non-linear dynamic processing with ongoing tuning/detuning.

lower-level interactions to provide reverberation, feedback, error correction and reward. In the brain's hierarchy, consciousness (and subconscious factors) can regulate, by downward control, volitional actions and bodily functions.

Consciousness also appears to have emerged at some point in evolution. Perhaps occurring initially as a 'helpless-spectator' epiphenomenon, consciousness then assumed control of its biological environment (Jaynes, 1976). The emergence of consciousness in our brains (during each conscious moment, during evolution and during the development of each human being) may be likened to new properties of materials which develop from microscopic or quantum-level events. For example, the distinct properties of superconductivity and superfluidity emerge from materials as their individual atoms reach a high level of coherence. In these cases, ordered alignment or coherence is due to lowering temperature to near absolute zero to reduce thermal oscillations. Consequently, at a critical degree of coherence, totally new macroscopic properties (superconductivity, superfluidity) emerge (Leggett, 1989)

This paper suggests that consciousness may emerge as a macroscopic quantum state from a critical level of coherence of quantum-level events in and around a specific class of neurobiological microstructure: cytoskeletal microtubules within neurons throughout the brain.

Microtubules (MTs) are cylindrical protein polymers interconnected by cross-bridging proteins (MAPs), which structurally and dynamically organize functional activities in living cells (*see Figure 1,* page 202), including synaptic regulation inside the brain's neurons (*see Figure 2,* page 202). In Sections II and III, we look at some of the current models of cognitive processes and make a case for the relevance of sub-neuronal structures. The basic thesis is that brain-wide microtubule-based quantum states, when coupled to synaptic events and neuronal firing, can help account for the five properties of consciousness highlighted on page 244, and can provide a quantum/classical (mind/brain) interface.

II

Organization of Consciousness within the Brain

The organization of consciousness has been approached along three general lines: 1) neural networks, 2) attentional scanning circuits, and 3) coherent activity of distributed neurons.

Neural networks

Neural networks originated from the work of McCulloch and Pitts (1943) describing threshold logic neurons and from Hebb's (1949; 1980) concept of the "cell assembly": a three-dimensional array of interconnected neurons whose firing was predicted to correlate with a specific mental state.[4]

The neuronal cell assembly concept helped to lead the way to "artificial neural networks" ("ANNs")—parallel, distributed computer systems designed to implement aspects of brain function (e.g. Hopfield, 1982). Weighted connections ("synapses") among processing elements ("neurons") provide ANNs with "brain-like" learning, pattern recognition and self-organization. Churchland and Sejnowski (1992) have reviewed how "ANN-like" parallel distributed processing can operate in the brain, and ANNs are clearly more similar to brain function than are conventional algorithmic-based AI schemes.

However, the brain/ANN analogy falters in at least two major areas. First, rather than being simple threshold logic switches as depicted in ANNs, neuronal synapses are complex, dynamic connections ("plasticity"). "In living nets everything is continually fluctuating: connection weights, transfer functions, parameters, input, and even the very connectivity, without leaving any traces of the fluctuation" (Globus,1992). Many of these fluctuating functions depend on the intra-neuronal cytoskeleton; for example Friedrich (1990) has shown that learning by increased synaptic efficacy requires cytoskeletal restructuring in the sub-synaptic region.

It has been claimed that the second major difference between ANNs and brain structure is that many types of ANNs (e.g. back-propagation, adaptive resonance, RCE, sigma pi, etc.) use internal processing within each "neural element". For example in ANNs such as the useful back-propagation type, resulting outputs are compared to expected outputs and the difference, or error, is conveyed back to an input layer. Werbos (1974) originated ANN back-propagation algorithms based loosely on Freud's notion of retrograde flow of "psychic energy" serving feedback/reward functions. Because the back-propagation of error is counter to unidirectional membrane depolarization and synaptic transmission, these types of ANNs have been considered biologically irrelevant. However retrograde signalling is now known to occur across synapses [dendrite to axon via nitric oxide and other mediators (e.g. Barinaga, 1991)], and retrograde information flow *within* neurons could be conveyed within microtubules and other cytoskeletal structures (Dayhoff et al. 1994; Rasmussen et al., 1990). Thus cognitive processes may extend below the level of synaptic connectionism and include molecular-level processing in the cytoskeleton.

Attentional scanning circuits and the problem of qualia

Where in the brain does consciousness occur? Early theories of consciousness invoked a single brain location of *self, observation and control,* now characterized as the search for the "grandmother neuron." This focalized concept is often generalized to a "homunculus" —the "little man" inside the brain which observes, controls and represents the "self". But where in the brain does the homunculus reside? Descartes proposed the pineal gland as a unitary focus of self (although acting as a channel for a dualistic mind entity) partly because it was the only single, midline brain structure. In his functionalist argument, Dennett (1991) criticizes such a "Cartesian theater" within the brain whose "audience" observes and controls.

Contrary to these focal models, the evidence gathered from many avenues of research —stemming from Lashley's (1950) demonstration of the non-localized distribution of memory—suggests that aspects of consciousness are *distributed* throughout wide areas of the brain. Somehow, parallel-arrayed, distributed neuronal groups—perhaps analogous to Hebb's assemblies of assemblies (e.g. "modules", "cartels", etc. (Freeman, 1975; Gazzaniga, 1985; Minsky, 1986))—give rise to a serial, integrated stream of consciousness (Baars, 1993). Certain brain and brainstem areas appear to be involved in the regulation, control and focusing of attention and consciousness.[5] Baars

[4] Hebb estimated that simple assemblies fire for 1 to 5 milliseconds, more complex "assemblies of assemblies" for a half-second, and a "phase cycle" (a series of assemblies of assemblies) for ten seconds or more (Freeman 1975; Scott 1994). Repeated firing of any assembly would lower its threshold and result in learning or recognition as the assembly adapts to become more sensitive (by lowering of synaptic threshold — synaptic plasticity) to a given input.

5 These include the reticular activating system which regulates wakefulness, the nucleus reticularis of the thalamus which directs attention to different regions of the brain (Scheibel, 1980; Crick, 1984), and the superior colliculus of the tectum which integrates sensory infor-

(1988; 1993) has formalized a "global workspace" model in which multiple brain "processors" compete for access to a broadcasting capability which disseminates the "winner's" information globally throughout the brain.[6] Adding the brain stem/limbic "hedonic" system and language centres to the external thalamo-cortical system, Edelman (1989) describes re-entrant circuitry from which global mappings of neuronal populations are 'selected' to reach consciousness by a Darwinian-like survival mechanism.

Mappings of neuronal activity which correlate with a specific mental event still fail to describe the content, meaning or subjective sense of self and observer/controller inherent in consciousness. These issues are addressed in Searle's (1980) famous "Chinese Room" thought experiment (a man sorting Chinese characters) which distinguishes syntactic (logical, algorithmic, computer-like) from semantic interpretation (meaning, understanding, human consciousness-like). Taylor (1992) observes that content may only be relevant when compared to previous memory: "the meaning of an input... is given by the degree of overlap such an input has to past inputs." But how do past inputs have meaning? What is the substance of *qualia:* "the phenomenal qualities of the things of which we are conscious, the raw feels and sensations that make up much of our conscious lives" (Korb, 1993).

Functionalists like Dennett (1991) argue that qualia are illusory, while dualists believe they are "ineffable" and cannot be understood. Can the redness of a red object be explained by a given pattern of neuronal firing, perhaps accented by a neurochemical bathing of a particular transmitter concoction? Do two people experiencing red have the same sense of redness in their minds? Are we little better than Searle's uncomprehending man (or Dennett's "zombies") with only the illusion of sentient consciousness? Or do our senses of beauty, oneness, joy and despair come from another realm? Is there a middle ground between reductionism and dualism? Once again quantum coherence at the molecular level of the cytoskeleton offers a possibility. Consider the *quale* of redness; red is "merely" a specific frequency of the electromagnetic spectrum, a brand of photon. As will be described, the theory of quantum coherence in the cytoskeleton implies excitations of a ground state yielding a condensed field of coherent bosons (phonons, photons, etc.) with specific frequency characteristics. Red of the electromagnetic spectrum can then correlate with a specific frequency boson-condensed field excitation in the brain. If true, and when technologically possible, the frequency of boson-field excitations corresponding to red in two people could be compared. More complex qualia (e.g. love, a pepperoni pizza, etc.) can then be viewed as complex mixtures of coherent boson fields, which as macroscopic quantum states, may also have suitable properties for a unitary sense of self.

These quantum features, unlike neural firing correlates, convey more than a reductionist representation of sentience; quantum boson fields are unitary, though non-local states. Their components are indistinguishable from one another by any measuring technique and they can exist in superposition of many states, collapsing to a single one. To which state a superpositioned quantum wave function collapses can be seemingly random and "non-deterministic". Thus macroscopic quantum states, unlike neural firing-level correlates, can have non-deterministic properties suggestive of "free will".

Coherent activity of distributed neurons—the "binding" problem

Current neurobiological approaches to explain how brain-wide activities result in a singular perceptual entity involve coherent firing of widely distributed neurons. Based on Hebb's cell assembly theory, Milner (1974) proposed that different neurons responding to a common "figure" fire *synchronously.* Using multi-unit recording in awake monkeys, Abeles (1982) found that temporal correlation among groups of neurons were related to high-level perceptual tasks and formalized a "synfire chain" model of cortex. Von der Marlsburg and Schneider (1986) showed how temporal synchronization of subsets of simultaneously active neurons could "segment" different mental objects (e.g. two different speakers at a noisy cocktail party) by a postulated fast (ten to hundreds of milliseconds) Hebbian synaptic modulation mechanism. (Such rapid synaptic modulation requires cooperative activities of the intra-neuronal cytoskeleton.) Following Freeman's (1978) suggestive findings in olfactory cortex, Eckhorn *et al.* (1988) and Gray and Singer (1989) found rapid oscillations above EEG frequencies (40 Hz) in cat visual cortex and Gray *et al.* (1989) then showed that these oscillatory responses can become synchronized in a stimulus-dependent manner. Based on these findings, Crick and Koch (1990) formalized a theory of consciousness in which coherent firing of widely-distributed neurons in the range of 40 Hz "bind" them together in mental representation and a unitary sense of self (see also, Koch, 1993). Studies of auditory-evoked responses in humans have shown inhibition of 40 Hz coherence with loss of consciousness due to induction of general anaesthesia (Madler and Poppel, 1987; Plourde and Picton, 1990).

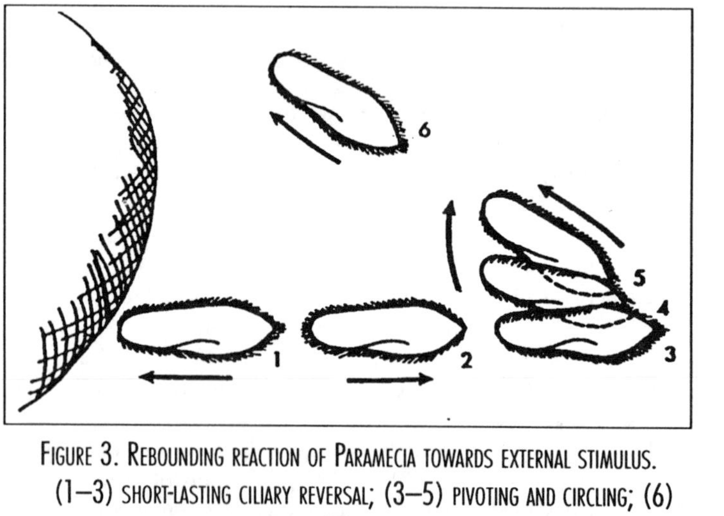

FIGURE 3. REBOUNDING REACTION OF PARAMECIA TOWARDS EXTERNAL STIMULUS. (1–3) SHORT-LASTING CILIARY REVERSAL; (3–5) PIVOTING AND CIRCLING; (6) SWIMMING IN NEW DIRECTION. (WITH PERMISSION FROM DRYL, 1974).

Coherent neural activity raises the possibility of a holographic paradigm. Pribram (1971) proposed that interference of coherent electromagnetic fields at the level of dendritic-dendritic interactions results in a holographic mechanism of cognitive representation. The holographic paradigm is appealing because memory can be recalled by a "reference" signal, and vast amounts of information can be stored in a distributed rather than localized manner. Quantum coherence, as proposed to

mation (Strehler, 1991). Thalamo-cortical projections, along with reciprocal cortico-thalarnic feedback have been implicated in directing attention to specific brain regions by "reentrant feedback loops" (Edelman, 1989). Thalamo-cortico-thalarnic feedback loops have been observed which sweep from frontal to occipital cortex approximately every 12.5 msec. and indicate brain-wide scanning at a frequency of about 80 Hz. (Ribary et al., 1991).

6 For example, a cortical focus which by thalamo-cortical feedback is suf~lciently self-sustaining may be broadcast "brain-wide" by associative pathways.

occur in cytoskeletal microtubules, can provide a mechanism for intracellular quantum holography (Hameroff, 1987; Schempp, 1993).

Neurobiological approaches (neural networks, attentional mechanisms and/or coherent activity) generally describe patterns of neural firing which may correlate with mental states, including consciousness. However, even if the exact patterns of neuronal firing correlating with specific mental activities become known, would consciousness be better understood? The reductionist view would be *yes* and strong AI advocates would be validated. To manifest consciousness, computers would merely need to reach the connectionist complexity of the brain's neurons and synapses—a feat strong AI advocates believe attainable within decades. The view of dualists would be emphatically *no;* the firing pattern *is* the brain's activity, but it is clearly not equivalent to consciousness. Emergence partially resolves this question; consciousness may indeed be a phenomenon derived from, but not equivalent to the brain's activity. But what exactly is consciousness? How are distributed neural activities, even coherently synchronized activities, bound into a unitary sense of self? Macroscopic quantum states offer one solution; but how could they be supported? Where and how could they exist?

III
Cognition within Living Cells

One possible path to solving this question is by examining the complexity of neurons and their synaptic connections. Reductionists tend to overlook the fact that neurons are alive and most views of the hierarchical organization of the brain stop at the synapse as the fundamental switch, analogous to states or bits in computers. The complexity of neurons and their synapses, however, are closer to entire computers than individual switches. This implies the mechanism of consciousness may depend on an understanding of the organization of adaptive ("cognitive") functions within living cells.

Like the rest of our cells, neurons are eukaryotic cells which, unlike prokaryotic bacteria, have a true nucleus and cytoskeleton and exhibit mitotic cell division.[7] Single eukaryotic cell organisms (protozoa) such as paramecia show remarkable, seemingly intelligent abilities without the benefit of a single synapse (*Figure 3*)! Observation of amoebae hunting food and paramecia avoiding obstacles led Charles Darwin and other 19th century biologists to project human psychology and aspects of consciousness onto protozoa. Popular books of that era included *The Psychic Life of Microorganisms* by Alfred Binet and *The Animal Mind* by M.F. Washburn. Darwin viewed adaptive activities of single-cell organisms as rudimentary consciousness related to man through evolution. Others (e.g. Jaynes, 1976) objected to this linkage, stating that protozoari behaviour "depended entirely on physical chemistry rather than introspective psychology". However it now seems introspective psychology itself may be an emergent function of physical chemistry (and quantum mechanics) at some level. The famous neuroscientist C.S. Sherrington (1951) wrote:

> Many forms of motile single cells lead their own independent lives. They swim and crawl, they secure food, they conjugate, they multiply. The observer at once says "they are alive"; the amoeba, paramecium, vorticella, and so on. They have specialized parts for movement, hair-like, whip-like, spiral and spring-like. Sense organs, beyond a pigment spot, seem to inspection wanting. Of nerve there is no trace. But the cell framework, the cyto-skeleton, might serve. There is therefore, for such mind as might be there, no need for our imagination to call halt and say "the apparatus for it is wanting".

As Sherrington observed, the cytoskeleton may act as the nervous system of single-cell organisms. Paramecia, for example, can apparently learn (Gelber, 1958), remember (Applewhite, 1979) and exhibit adaptive responses such as avoidance and habituation which involve movement performed by coordinated actions ("metachronal waves") of hundreds of hair-like appendages called cilia (See Figure 4, p. 121).[8]

External events which initiate adaptive responses via ciliary and/or membrane perturbation in paramecium are similar to receptor binding of neurotransmitter molecules in neuronal synapses.[9] In paramecia, adaptive behavioural responses to external stimuli involve motor activities performed by complex activities of cilia; in neurons they include regulation of synaptic strengths, and cognitive functions related to learning, memory, and aspects of consciousness.

Is consciousness a property of protoplasm in general? Do single-cell organisms, such as paramecium, exhibit consciousness? If not, at what point in the evolutionary hierarchy does consciousness *emerge?* These distinctions may be somewhat arbitrary, but the *fabric* of consciousness may be present within all eukaryotic cells. If so, how low in the organizational hierarchy of single cells do the rudiments of consciousness extend? An extreme view ("panpsychism") is that consciousness is a quality of all matter: atoms and their subatomic components having elements of consciousness (Spinoza, 1677; Rensch, 1960). But then what distinguishes non-living material from living,

7 According to Margulis (1975), eukaryotic life is the result of a symbiotic merger of prokaryotes (immobile chemical factories) and spirochetal invaders (highly motile flagellates with minimal chemistry). The motile spirochetes are thought to have invaded prokaryotes and found shelter and biochemical energy. The filamentous proteins which comprised the spirochetal flagellae and provided movement became the eukaryotic cytoskeleton and offered the new type of cell abilities to 1) divide chromosomes and thus mutate and evolve, 2) compartmentalize, leading to specialization, 3) move around, explore and avoid predators, 4) grow asymmetrically (e.g. neurons), and 5) generally adapt.

8 Comprised of nine microtubule doublets arranged in a ring around a central microtubule pair, cilia are membrane-bound extensions of the cytoskeleton in cells ranging from protozoa to human epithelium. In addition to several types of motor movement, cilia have sensory function in that their perturbation is transmitted to the cell. Lund (1933) showed that microtubules within paramecia were "conductile" and transmitted information, and Atema (1974) proposed that signal transduction in sensory cilia involved propagating conformational changes along ciliary microtubule subunits. Complex action of paramecium ciliary '"metachronal waves" are coordinated by a peripheral cytoskeletal network to which the cilia are anchored; this network is in turn connected to internal microtubules and other cytoskeletal structures. Several authors (e.g. Lund, 1933; 1941) identified a central confluence of cytoskeletal structures (the "neuromotorium") characterized as the paramecium "brain". Metachronal waves of ciliary beating in paramecia are reversibly inhibited by the general anaesthetic chloroform (Parducz, 1962), suggesting some link to consciousness in higher organisms.

9 Each triggers "second messenger" transduction cascades (G proteins, calcium ion flux, adenyl cyclase, phosphatidylinositol, cyclic AMP, etc) which in turn activate enzymes [e.g. dynein AT-Pases, cytoplasmic phosphatases and kinases such as calcium-calmodulin protein kinase, MAP kinase, calcineurin, protein kinases A and C (Eriksson et al., 1992; Montoro et aL, 1993)]. Among the responses of the enzymes (kinases in particular) are phosphorylation/dephosphorylation of cytoskeletal structures including microtubule-associated-proteins ("MAPs") and intermediate (neuro) filaments which can initiate cytoskeletal signalling and structural reconfiguration (Johnson and Pope, 1992) In addition, external events acting through membrane proteins can directly connect to the internal cytoskeleton by linking proteins such as fodrin, ankyrin and actin.

and how are all the atomic and sub-atomic consciousness entities unified (the binding problem taken to extreme)?

Many contemporary thinkers feel that quantum mechanics may provide answers to at least some of these questions and that consciousness may emerge at a critical amount of non-local quantum processing linked to some neural structure. It is the particular proposal of this paper, developed in the next section, that cytoskeletal microtubules are the most likely location for such an effect. Preliminary technical arguments are developed in Appendices 1–3. Appendix 1 discusses the structure of microtubules in detail and reviews recent evidence for their role in cognition; Appendix 2 outlines Fröhlich's work on protein dynamics, whilst Appendix 3 outlines the mechanisms by which proteins may act as complex information processors and "quantum computers". The arguments are, of necessity, somewhat technical. Readers with a scientific background should read the appendices in full at this stage, while others may prefer to proceed to the next section.

IV

Quantum Physics and Consciousness

Quantum theory describes fundamental properties of matter and energy which comprise our universe. Seemingly bizarre and counter-intuitive, quantum properties—including wave/particle duality, the (Heisenberg) "uncertainty principle", randomness or acausality, and quantum inseparability or non-locality (quantum coherence)—have been repeatedly verified by experimentation over much of this century. These strange properties may help explain the mysterious nature of consciousness. "Perhaps our minds are qualities rooted in some strange and wonderful feature of those physical laws which actually govern the world we inhabit" (Penrose, 1989).

At the base of quantum theory is the wave/particle duality of atoms and their components. When *unobserved,* an atom or sub-atomic particle behaves as a "wave of possibilities"; *observation* in effect "collapses the wave function" and a particle appears. The Heisenberg uncertainty principle dictates that either the position or momentum of a particle (but not both) can be known with arbitrary precision. Beginning over four decades ago, these properties prompted very general comparisons to mental processes. As observation of a quantum particle alters its state, Bohm (1952) observed that thoughts and mental processes, when focused upon, become altered and might therefore have some basis in quantum mechanics. Szent-Gyorgyi (1960) and Pullman and Pullman (1963) made broad analogies between wave/particle and mind/brain dualities.

Quantum randomness stems from the superposition of an unobserved atom or particle in many possible states; which particular state will be observed is apparently random. Einstein objected to this quantum randomness or acausality: "I cannot believe that God would play dice with the Universe". However as Pagels pointed out "if things at base are utterly random, nothing can make them more disordered. Complete randomness at the heart of things is the most stable situation imaginable" (Herbert, 1993). Noting that the "material" world consists of nothing but "relentlessly unrealized vibratory possibilities", von Neumann proposed and Wigner and others elaborated (Wheeler and Zurek, 1983) that by observing (measuring) the real world, the conscious mind collapses wave functions and confers solidity, single-valueness and dependable constancy. Globus (1987) argues that

> possible worlds are superposed *within the brain*—the "holoworld", and perception, both waking and dreaming, selects a world for unfolding from the holoworld. The collapse of the wave function is a selection process from *a priori* implicate worlds.

These ideas are comparable to Bohm's (1980) "implicate order", and Everett's (1957) many universe view. But then what is it about the conscious mind which causes this collapse?

Another view is that matter consists of fleeting vibratory patterns in a vast field of consciousness: a universal mentality interpenetrates the physical world. This concept ("quantum animism") suggests that every quantum wave contains consciousness and vice versa: "where there's a will, there's a wave" (Herbert, 1993). This view is a quantum version of dualist and idealist concepts such as Cartesian mental substance or Hegelian world spirit (Searle, 1980); the quantum/mental realm interacts with the physical realm in the structures of our brain Several approaches to elucidate the site and mechanism of this quantum interaction have focused on the synapse.

Beck and Eccles (1992) proposed that quantum randomness results in what appears to be probabilistic, acausal synaptic function. Noting that in an apparently random fashion only one of approximately six axonal action potentials results in synaptic release of neurotransmitter vesicles, they pinpoint the quantum effect as the "movement of a hydrogen bridge by electronic rearrangement" acting on vesicle release through the pre-synaptic vesicular grid. A hexagonal lattice on the inner surface of the presynaptic region, the vesicular grid was chosen by Beck and Eccles as the site for quantum influence because of its "paracrystalline structure" which "makes it possible to have long-range interactions between the constituents". (A similar argument can be made for more ubiquitous paracrystalline microtubule arrays.) Other candidates for mediation of quantum randomness effects include ion channels (Bass, 1975; Donald, 1990) and ions (e.g. calcium ions) themselves (Stapp, 1993).

Quantum coherence

The greatest surprise to emerge from quantum theory is quantum inseparability or non-locality which implies that all objects that have once interacted are in some sense still connected! Schrödinger observed in 1935 that when two quantum systems interact, their wave functions become "phase entangled". Consequently, when one system's wave function is collapsed, the other system's wave function, no matter how far away, instantly collapses too (Herbert, 1993). The non-local connection (quantum coherence) is not only instantaneous and independent of distance but impervious to shielding. Einstein, Podolsky and Rosen (1935) proposed an experimental method for testing inseparability involving observation of polarization states of two photons emitted in different directions from a common source. J.S. Bell in 1964 (e.g. Bell, 1987) formulated the notion that, if quantum inseparability were false, then changing the measurement context of one photon would not affect the other photon's behaviour ("Bell's theorem"). Amazingly, experiments by Clauser *et al.* (1969) and Aspect and Grangier (1986) disproved Bell's theorem by showing that choice of context of measurement of one photon instantly affects outcome of measurement of a distant photon. The quantum world is truly interconnected; *quantum entities are "aware" of the states of their spatially separated relatives!*

Such "knowing" has prompted linkage of non-local quantum coherence to mental processes. Bohm (1951) described the quantum world as an "undivided wholeness" or "implicate order" and related it to a holographic model of consciousness which accents the wave nature of experience. Pribram (1971) has proposed that mental representation occurs holographically by interference of coherent waves (e.g. dendritic field potentials). Non-local quantum effects among different individuals have been related to "Jungian synchronicity" ("meaningful coincidence") originating from what the famous psychoanalyst C.G. Jung termed the "collective unconscious" (Peat, 1992; Insinna, 1992).

Quantum coherence has also been linked to more specific biological function and computation. Conrad (1992) has argued that superposition of spatially-separated electron states facilitates common biomolecular interactions such as antigen-antibody, neurotransmitter-receptor, enzyme-substrate, protein self-assembly and other functions. Conrad further suggests that quantum coherence and parallelism inherent in the quantummechanical wave function can enhance the speed, reliability, and energy dissipation of elementary switches such as those involved in molecular computation (including, perhaps, tubulins within microtubules) Theoretical descriptions of quantum computers propose utilizing quantum coherence, superposition and parallelism for technological purposes.[10] Penrose (1989; 1994) sees such quantum computing in the brain as a mechanism for "non-algorithmic" processing intrinsic to human consciousness. He speculates that conscious thinking involves resolution of alternatives that were previously in linear superposition.

Coherent quantum phenomena cannot perform computation if the system undergoes significant "measurement-like interactions" with the outside world; only well-isolated quantum computers are possible. Inherent isolation implies a "subjectivity", or internal information inaccessible to external observation within quantum computers, a property suggestive of consciousness (Deutsch, 1992). An appropriate "classical" interface for quantum computers could be "selective driving of resonances" (Haddon and Stillinger, 1982). Lloyd (1993) proposes an array of weakly-coupled quantum systems which would be subjected to sequences of electromagnetic pulses of well-defined frequency and length, permitting loading, processing and unloading of information. Cytoskeletal polymers subjected to neuronal firing might constitute such a system.

Penrose (1989) has also invoked the possibility of quantum superposition in synaptic plasticity. Non-periodic tiling patterns of quasicrystals ("Penrose tiles") require "nonlocal" effects; it appears necessary to "know" the state of the pattern many tiles away from the point of assembly. Rather than classical crystal growth in which individual units attach themselves at a continually moving growth line, Penrose considers this to occur as an "evolving quantum linear superposition of many different altemative arrangements" and likens this situation to learning and memory by synaptic plasticity in which neuronal connections are rapidly formed, activated or deactivated. "Thus not just one of the possible altemative arrangements is tried out, but vast numbers, all superposed in complex linear superposition" (Penrose, 1989). Synaptic connections are formed and regulated by cytoskeletal polymers, including microtubules. Complex linear superposition of many cytoskeletal configurations corresponding to synaptic connection pattems collapsing to a single one could account for the extremely rapid synaptic plasticity required for cognition. Penrose (1989; 1994) also considers that collapse of superpositioned states and conversion from quantum to classical behaviour depends on a threshold related to quantum gravity. He predicts that gravity, although an extremely weak force, influences the quantum realm because it acts on the spacetime structure itself. Objects that become larger than a crucial size spontaneously actualize one of their possibilities; spacetime curvature causes the system's wave function to collapse "under its own weight". Herbert (1993) has used a "quantum realm" approach to estimate a mass value for "quantumness" and obtains a rough estimate of 10^6 daltons. This is the size of Eccles' pre-synaptic "microsite" and also of about ten tubulin subunits within a microtubule. Penrose calculates a higher number of tubulins whose coherence for a critical time will self-collapse, and result in a single conscious event. According to Penrose, the manner in which quantum gravity can act as a bridge between the quantum world and the classical world will await new discoveries in quantum physics.[11]

[10] For example Deutsch (1985; 1992) and Lloyd (1993) forsee quantum-level bit states (e.g. 1,0) which can be in quantum superposition of both I and 0. If the bit state sites (in an array or polymer) are locally interactive as in a cellular automaton (e.g. from overlap among unit-unit electron wave functions, van der Waals forces, conformational changes of subunits, dipole coupling, etc.), then parallel logic and quantum coherence can result in quantum computation; multiple computations collapse into a macroscopic quantum state.

Bose-Einstein condensates

Concluding that quantum effects are necessary to explain the "unity of conscious experience", Marshall (1989) has searched for a quantum mechanism that is extended in space (non-local, long-range order), capable of many states, and has a "shared identity" unanalyzable into parts ("diversity in unity"). Marshall concludes these properties are unique to systems known as "Bose-Einstein condensates" (see Appendix 2). Usually, each particle/wave in a quantum system possesses its own wave function. However, under certain circumstances, many quantum particle/waves move coherently, described by the same wave function. Arising in quantum field theory, Bose-Einstein condensates are collective, macroscopic quantum states named after Indian physicist Satyandra Nath Bose and Albert Einstein who independently predicted the types of particle/waves ("bosons") and conditions necessary for realization of such states (Zohar and Marshall, 1994).

Quantum field theory describes the underlying reality of everything in the universe (including consciousness) as consisting of three components: the *vacuum*, space and time. A "field of fields" which contains no particles, the vacuum gives rise to quantum wave/particles as excitations or energy fluctuations within it (like "sound from a drum skin" (Zohar, 1990)). A *ground state* is a component field of the vacuum whose excitation can yield the two types of wave/particles: fermions and bosons. Fermions are the ingredients of matter (electrons, protons, and neutrons) which tend to be individual; their wave functions cannot overlap entirely (although fermion *pair* wave functions have bosonic properties and *can* overlap as in superconductors, supermagnets and superfluids). Bosons are wave/particles of relationship which convey forces and which can *merge* as their wave functions overlap; they can coherently share identities. Bosons include photons, virtual photons, phonons and other entities including possibly gravitons; the forces they convey include electromagnetic, weak and strong nuclear and possibly gravity. In concert with the uncertainty principle, a set of boson ground-state excitations can act coherently by entry into the lowest momentum state so that position becomes undefined (Tilley and Tilley, 1986). Consequently, a large set of bosons is described by a single wave function and coherent, collective macro-

[11] See also Nunn *et al.*(1994).

scopic quantum states result (Herbert, 1993).

Quantum field theory was initially linked to consciousness by Ricciardi and Umezawa (1967) who proposed that each brain cell contains a spatially distributed system with a full complement of quantum-mechanical degrees of freedom. Without specifying the intraneuronal structural correlate, they suggested that memory of an external stimulus is imprinted as a perturbation of the vacuum ground state of the unspecified intraneuronal system. By violating the system's original dynamical symmetry, long-range correlation waves (bosons) condense and correlate with mental processes.

Examples of known Bose-Einstein condensates include the laser, in which many photons occupy exactly the same optical state, superconductors, in which numerous linked electrons ("Cooper pairs") take on identical quantum possibilities, supermagnets in which micro-dipoles align, and superfluids like helium, in which quantum synchronized atoms create a friction-free fluid. In each case the overlapping of position gives a shared identity and the ground state has a long-range order (coherence).

Superconductors, supermagnets and superfluids require temperatures near absolute zero to reduce thermal oscillations and bring the particles into coherence. Lasers require high energy to drive crystals into coherent excited states. Of known systems akin to Bose-Einstein condensates, only Fröhlich's proposed pumped phonon system (see Appendix 2) can operate at body temperature (Marshall, 1989). Fröhlich predicted that a set of proteins in a common electromagnetic field (e.g. proteins within a polarized membrane, subunits within an electret polymer like microtubules) undergo coherent conformational excitations if biochemical energy were supplied ("pumped phonons").

Using a set of assumptions for a layered sheet of dipoles, Clarke (1994) has questioned the feasibility of Fröhlich's biological Bose-Einstein condensates. However cooperative effects of coupled, ordered water and non-planar geometries (in particular cylindrical protein lattices like microtubules) make Fröhlich's biological Bose-Einstein condensates more likely (e.g. Sataric *et al.,* 1993; Jibu *et al.*,1994).

Citing Fröhlich's pumped phonons in unspecified "neural proteins" as a Bose-Einstein condensate, Marshall predicted that conscious phenomena (thoughts, images, etc.) would occur as excitations of the ground state, like waves in superfluid helium or holograms in laser light. He reasoned that such a condensate could suffice even as only a minor facet of brain dynamics (in a superconductor only one material part in ten thousand participates in the phase change, but the macroscopic properties are dramatically altered). Cytoskeletal microtubules have suitable qualifications to act as a brain substrate for Bose Einstein condensates related to consciousness.[12] Consciousness may then be seen as a dynamic macroscopic quantum state originating from a mixture of coherent states originating in microtubules.

Super-radiance

Quantum coherence has been theoretically applied not only to membranes and cytoskeletal structures, but to water molecules ordered at their surfaces (*Figure 5*).[13] Using quantum field theory, Jibu *et al.* (1994) have proposed that ordering of water molecules and the quantized electromagnetic field confined inside the hollow microtubule core manifest a specific collective dynamics called ***super-radiance.*** Accordingly, each microtubule can transform incoherent, disordered energy (molecular, thermal, or electromagnetic) into coherent photons within its hollow core. Furthermore, coherent photons created by super-radiance may penetrate without loss along the microtubule as if the optical medium were made "transparent" by the propagating photons themselves. This is a quantum phenomenon called ***self-induced transparency*** (McCull and Hahn, 1987) (*Figure 6*). Some evidence suggests weak photoemission from living cells, and Popp (1986) has proposed a regulatory role for "coherent biophotons". Thus Jibu *et al.* suggest that microtubules can behave as optical waveguides which result in coherent photons; they estimate that this quantum coherence is capable of superposition of states among microtubules spatially distributed over hundreds of microns. These in turn are in superposition with other microtubules hundreds of microns away in other directions and so on. Consequently microtubule quantum dynamics may be coupled over brain-wide areas, a superposition which could solve the "binding problem" and account for unity of thought and consciousness.

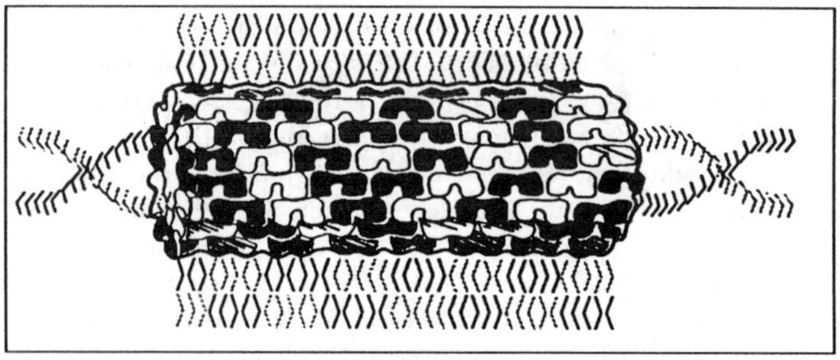

FIGURE 5. MICROTUBULE AUTOMATA (MTA) WITH ORDERED WATER.

To summarize, cytoskeletal microtubules are likely candidates for quantum coherence relevant to consciousness because:

- Microtubule individual subunit (tubulin) conformation may be coupled to quantum-level events (electron movement, dipole, phonon) in hydrophobic protein regions.
- Microtubule paracrystalline lattice structure, symmetry, cylindrical configuration and parallel alignment promote long-range cooperativity and order.
- Hollow microtubule interiors appear capable of water-ordering, waveguide super-radiance and self-induced transparency.

12 Fröhlich pumped phonons have already been considered in microtubules as a basis for information processing via spin-glass behaviour and as a clocking mechanism for cellular automata functions. The cooperative coupling resulting in coherence has been assumed to be phonons (bosons) coupled to dipoles or electrons "trapped" in hydrophobic regions (e.g. aromatic amino acid residues with resonant orbitals). Microtubules' paracrystalline periodic lanice and cylindrical configuration provide an ideal coherent structure, and the functions of microtubules are crucial to intracellular cognition.Thus spin-glass and aulomata models, similar if not equivalent to Bose Einstein condensates, may manifest quantum computing by interactive pattems of coherent sets of pumped phonons (bosons).

13 Fröhlich theorized that energy could be stored without thermal loss in coherent dipolar propagating proteins or in a thin layer of water and ions just beneath the cell membrane Watterson (1987) has shown how organized, dynamic water clusters ('pixels') can represent information at membrane and cytoskeletal surfaces. Considering the layer of ordered water outside and inside microtubules Del Giudice *et al.* (1983) proposed that microtubules' cylindrical structure may be understood by quantum-vacuum symmetry breaking and boson self-focusing by ordered water. Like the Meissner effect for superconducting media, electromagnetic energy would be confined inside filamentous regions around which the microtubule subunits gather. Del Giudice's group (1983) showed that this self-focusing should result in filamentous beams of radius 15 nanometers, precisely the inner diameter of microtubules!

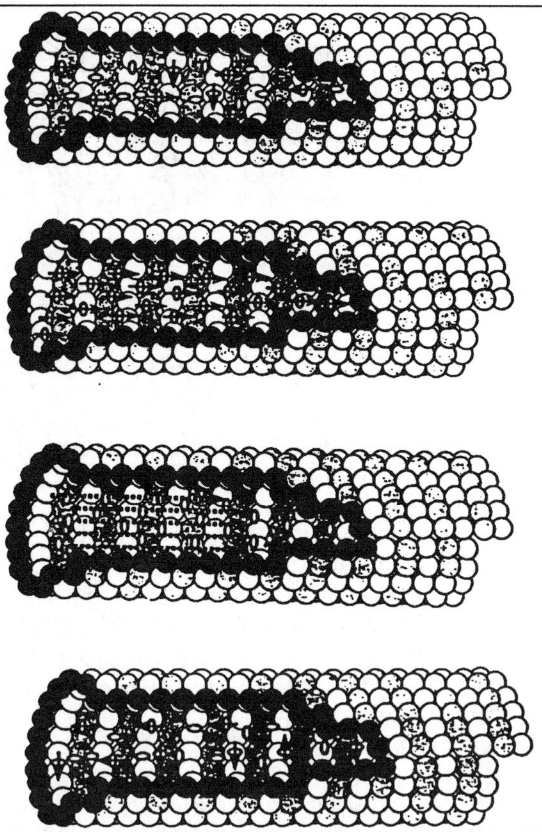

FIGURE 6.

A SCHEMATIC REPRESENTATION OF THE PROCESS OF SUPER-RADIANCE IN A MICROTUBULE

Each oval within an arrow stands for a water molecule in the lowest rotational energy state. Each oval with an arrow stands for a water molelcule in the first excited rotational energy state. The process is cyclic (a), (b), (c), (d), (a), (b), and so on.

(a) Initial state of the system of water molecules in a microtubule: energy gain due to the thermal fluctuations of tubulins increases the number of water molecules in the first excited rotational energy state.

(b) A collective mode of the system of water molecules in rotationally excited states: a long-range coherence is achieved inside a microtubule by means of spontaneous symmetry breaking.

(c) A collective mode of the system of water rmolecules in rotationally excited states loses its energy collectively, and creates coherent photons in the quantized electromagnetic field inside a microtubule.

(d) Water molecules, having lost their first excited rotational energies by super-radiance, start again to gain energy from the thermal fluctuation of tubulins, and the system of water molecules recovers the initial state (a), With permission from Jibu *et al.*, 1994).

It is proposed, therefore, that microtubules' ubiquitous presence and crucial involvement in regulatory and cognitive functions in neurons and other eukaryotic cells can mediate quantum effects in a wide range of significant biological functions. In particular, quantum coherence (Fröhlich pumped phonons, Bose-Einstein condensation, ordering of water) in cytoskeletal microtubules and related structures can lead to quantum computing and emergence of macroscopic quantum states suitable for a unitary sense of consciousness.

V
Anaesthesia, Quantum Coherence and Consciousness

As a putative mechanism for consciousness, microtubule-based quantum coherence should be sensitive to general anaesthesia. Brains of patients under general anaesthesia are commonly quite active: EEG, evoked potentials, respiratory and autonomic drives and other brain functions persist despite a lack of consciousness. Thus, at just the right level, general anaesthesia *is* the ***absence*** of consciousness.[14]

If quantum coherence in microtubules is essential for consciousness, anaesthetics must somehow inhibit or prevent it, either indirectly or directly.[15] At concentrations of anaesthesia just sufficient for ablation of consciousness, anaesthetic action at hydrophobic regions of membrane receptors and channels, tubulins and other proteins could have profound effects by retarding mobility of dipoles/electrons in those hydrophobic regions, thereby inhibiting conformational dynamics, coherent phonons and Bose-Einstein condensation. Wulf and Featherstone (1957) showed that anaesthetic-protein binding within hydrophobic regions alters protein-water binding at the protein surface. Thus anaesthetic-tubulin interaction would alter cooperative water-binding and ordering, with consequent effects on quantum vacuum symmetry breaking and attendant "superradiance" and "self-induced transparency". By having such effects in hydrophobic regions of tubulin and other proteins, anaesthetics can reduce and prevent quantum superposition and coherence. This is consistent with the quantum realm interacting with the brain via a collection of quantum-level events in hydrophobic regions of brain proteins—in particular tubulin subunits within microtubules.

VI
Summary

Consciousness is described as an emergent macroscopic quantum state driven or selected by neurobiological mechanisms (neural networks, attentional scanning circuits, coherent firing of distributed neurons) with origins in quantum coherence in cytoskeletal microtubules within the brain's neurons. Microtubule quantum coherence is thought to derive from two possibly inter-related mechanisms:

- Bose-Einstein condensates stemming from a "Fröhlich pumped photon" mechanism of dipoles in hydrophobic pockets of microtubule subunits.
- A quantum-dynamical system of water molecules and the quantized electromagnetic field confined inside the hollow microtubule core. The latter induces a specific collective dynamics called superradiance by which coherent photons are created and penetrate without dissipation in the microtubule core in a quantum effect called self-induced transparency (Jibu *et al.*, 1994).

[14] A variety of different types of gas molecules constitute general anaesthetics; they range from halogenated hydrocarbons to ethers to inert gases such as xenon. What they share in common are 1) solubility in a specific "hydrophobic" environment, and 2) binding by weak van der Waals forces (e.g. Halsey, 1983) After many years of investigating effects in hydrophobic *lipid* regions of membranes, anaesthetic gas molecules are now recognized to reversibly inhibit consciousness by weak, van der Waals binding in hydrophobic regions of some set of neural (presumably synaptic membrane) *proteins* (Franks and Lieb, 1982). As previously described, quantum-level events (dipole/electron oscillations, phonons) in protein hydrophobic regions are thought to couple to functional dynamic protein conformational states. Anaesthetics are known to retard mobility of electrons (Hameroff and Wan, 1983), and by doing so in hydrophobic regions anaesthetics may prevent protein conformational responsiveness.

[15] Possible indirect ways includc inhibition of activities of membrane, second messenger or membrane-cytoskeletal linking proteins which could disconnect and isolate cytoskeletal dynamics from the external milieu. Anaesthetics may also disrupt hydrophobic links among microtubule-associated-proteins (MAPs) which interconnect microtubules into functional networks (Lewis *et al.*, 1989). Alternatively, anaesthetics may directly alter cytoskeletal quantum coherence. General anaesthetics are known to bind to microtubules and at high enough concentrations cause their depolymerization (Allison and Nunn 1968.

A macroscopic quantum state approaching brain-wide dimension can provide properties which define consciousness. These include: 1) a unitary sense of self, 2) randomness or non-deterministic 'free will', 3) non-algorithmic "quantum" computing. Coupling of this quantum state to microtubule subunit conformational states can account for cellular control, adaptive behaviour, synaptic regulation and cognition by propagating signals through cytoskeletal networks and information processing via mechanisms including molecular ("cellular") automata, spin-glass and holography. Microtubules are appropriate candidates for quantum coherence leading to consciousness because their subunit conformation (and consequent function) can couple to quantum events in hydrophobic regions, their paracrystalline lattice structure and symmetry promote long-range order and their hollow cylindrical core can lead to water ordering with waveguide super-radiance and self-induced transparency. The essential and ubiquitous roles microtubules play in cellular control and regulation and their communication and proximity with membrane proteins, cell nucleus and other biomolecular structures can link microtubule-based quantum events to basic biological functions.

General anaesthetic gas molecules, which selectively inhibit consciousness at appropriate concentrations, act at hydrophobic protein regions and are known to inhibit electron mobility. Thus anaesthetics, whether acting directly on microtubules or indirectly via membrane proteins or membrane-cytoskeletal connections, can reversibly erase consciousness by inhibiting quantum-level events in protein hydrophobic regions and thus disrupting quantum coherence.

As a model of consciousness, quantum coherence in microtubules is reductionist in that a specific molecular structure is featured as a site for consciousness. It is seemingly dualist in that the quantum realm (which is actually intrinsic to all of nature) is seen to act through microtubules. General anaesthesia is viewed as reducing and preventing quantum superposition and coherence in protein hydrophobic regions, a view which also speaks to an intrinsic quantum nature of consciousness.

APPENDIX

1

Microtubules and the Cytoskeleton

Interiors of living eukaryotic cells are structurally and dynamically organized by networks of interconnected protein polymers. Originally termed the cytoskeleton because of their "bone-like" structural support, these networks also orchestrate and control dynamic cellular activities and may be considered as the cell's nervous system. The cytoskeleton consists of microtubules ("MTs"), actin microfilaments, intermediate filaments and an organizing complex called the centrosome whose main components are MT supercylinders called centrioles (Dustin, 1984). Parallel-arrayed MTs are interconnected by cross-bridging proteins (MT-associated proteins: "MAPs") to other MTs, organelles, filaments and membranes to form dynamic networks. Contractile MAPs such as dynein and kinesin participate in cell movement as well as intra-neuronal ("axoplasmic") transport which moves material and plays a major role in maintaining and regulating synapses. MAPs which form structural bridges stabilize MTs, prevent their disassembly and may be phosphorylated and impart energy into the cytoskeleton. Thus MAP–MT cytoskeletal networks determine cell architecture and dynamic functions (e.g. mitosis, growth, differentiation, movement, synapse formation and function, etc.) essential to the living state.

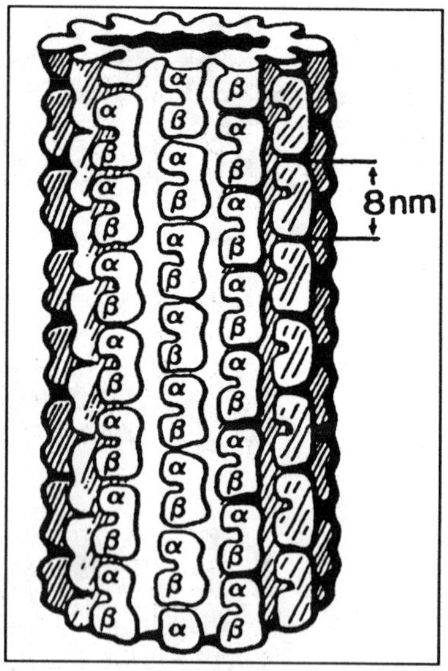

FIGURE 7
MICROTUBULE (MT) STRUCTURE FROM X-RAY CRYSTALLOGRAPHY (AMOS AND KLUG, 1974). TUBULIN SUBUNITS ARE 8 NM DIMERS COMPRISED OF A AND B MONOMERS.

Of the filamentous structures which comprise the cytoskeleton, MTs are the best characterized. MTs are hollow cylinders 25 nanometers ("nm": 10^{-9} meters) in diameter whose walls are 13 chains of subunit proteins known as tubulin. Each tubulin subunit is a polar, 8 nm dimer which consists of two slightly different classes of 4 nm monomers (molecular weight 55,000 daltons) known as α and β tubulin (*Figure 7*). Each dimer (as well as whole MTs) has a dipole with negative charges localized towards α monomers (DeBrabander, 1982). Thus MTs are "electrets": oriented assemblies of dipoles with piezoelectric properties (Athenstaedt, 1974; Mascarenhas, 1974). Dimers self-assemble into MTs, apparently in an entropy-driven process which can quickly change by MT disassembly and reassembly in another orientation ("dynamic instability" [Kirschner and Mitchison, 1986]). The tubulin dimer subunits within MTs are arranged in a slightly twisted hexagonal lattice, resulting in differing neighbour relationships among each subunit and its six nearest neighbours. Tubulin undergoes conformational changes induced by hydrolysis of bound GTP to GDP (high energy phosphate molecules analogous to ATP and ADP (Engelborghs 1992; Melki *et al.*, 1989)) and biochemical energy can also be pumped into MTs by phosphorylation/dephosphorylation of MAPs (Theurkauf and Vallee, 1983). Genes for α and β tubulin are complex and give rise to varying tubulin primary structure. For example, at least 17 different β tubulins can exist in mammalian brain MTs (Lee *et al.*, 1986). Tubulin in MTs can also be modified by binding various ligands, MAPs, enzymatic addition or removal of amino acids ("post-translational modification") and conformational state changes. Thus, the number of different possible combinations of tubulin states (and information capacity) within MTs is extremely large.

In addition to providing structural support and transport, a role as the cell's nervous system is suggested by evidence that links the cytoskeleton with cognitive function. For example, production of tubulin and MT activities correlate with peak learning, memory and experience in baby chick brains (Mileusnic *et al.*, 1980). When baby rats first open their eyes, neurons in their visual cortex begin producing vast quantities of tubulin (Cronley-Dillon *et al.*, 1974). Selective destruction of animal brain MTs by the drug colchicine causes defects in learning and memory which mimic the symptoms of Alzheimer's disease (in which neuronal cytoskeleton becomes tangled and dysfunctional [Bensimon and Chernat, 1991]).[16]

[16] Other evidence for cytoskeletal involvement in cognition comes from studies of long term potentiation ('LTP'), a form of synaptic plasticity that serves as a model for learning and memory in mammalian hippocampal cortex MAP2 (found only in dendrites) is linked to membrane receptors and their activities by 'second messengers' (G proteins, cyclic AMP,

The cytoskeleton could serve cognitive functions by propagation, storage and processing of information within neurons and other cells. Tubulin subunits in closely arrayed MTs have a density of about 10^{17} per cm^3, close to the theoretical limit for charge separation and thus have maximal density for information representation by charge. In general, proteins function by coupling their conformational state to a variety of factors; in essence each protein is a computer element with multiple inputs determining a specific conformational state as output.

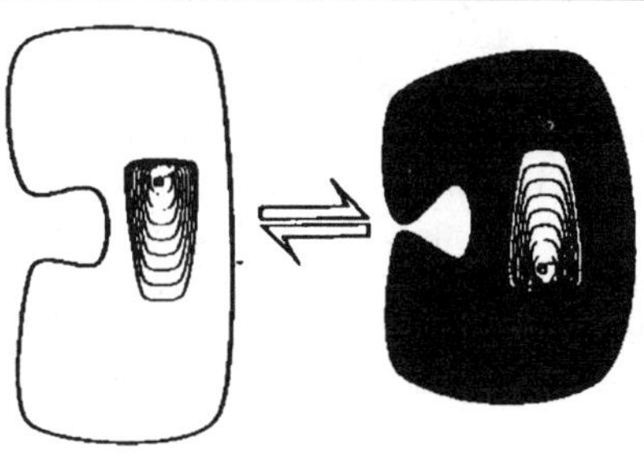

Two states of protein (e.g. tubulin) in which quantum event within hydrophobic region couples to conformatiogal change with 10^{-9} to 10^{-11} sec transitions. Quantum event shown within hydrophobic region as electron (e^- density probability topography. General anaesthetics bind within these hydrophobic regions and prevent conformational transitions by van der Waals forces acting on quantum event.

Figure 8

II
Protein Conformational Dynamics

Proteins undergo conformational motions over a wide range of time and energy scales. However significant conformational changes related to protein function generally occur in the nanosecond (10^{-9} sec) to 10 picosecond (10^{-11} sec) time scale (Karplus and McCammon, 1983). Related to cooperative movements of protein sub-regions and charge redistributions, these changes are linked to protein function (signal transduction, ion channel opening, enzyme action etc.) and may be triggered by factors including phosphorylation, ATP or GTP hydrolysis, ion fluxes, electric fields, ligand binding, and neighbouring protein conformational changes. In the case of tubulin within MTs, such programmable and adaptable states can represent and propagate information.

Fröhlich (1968, 1970, 1975) proposed that protein conformational changes are coupled to charge redistributions such as dipole oscillations or electron movements within specific *hydrophobic* protein regions (*Figure 8*). Hydrophobic regions within proteins are comprised of non-polar side chains of amino acids which exclude water; general anaesthetic gas molecules apparently act there to prevent protein conformational responsiveness. Fröhlich predicted that quantum-level events such as the movement of an electron within these hydrophobic regions (for example among resonant bond orbitals of amino acid side chains like the aromatic rings of tyrosine, tryptophan or phenylalanine) act as a trigger or switch for the conformational state of the entire protein. Fröhlich further proposed that a set of proteins connected in a common electromagnetic field such as within a polarized membrane (or polar polymer electret like a microtubule) would be excited coherently if biochemical energy such as protein phosphorylation or ATP or GTP hydrolysis were supplied. Coherent excitation times on the order of 10^{-9} to 10^{-11} sec (the time domain for functional protein conformational changes, and in the microwave or gigaHz (GHz) spectral region) were deduced by Fröhlich, who termed them acoustoconformational transitions, or coherent "pumped" phonons. Such a system of coherent excitations in quantum-mechanical terms is called a "Bose-Einstein condensate" (Wu and Austin, 1978). Fröhlich also predicted metastable states (longer-lived conformational state patterns stabilized by local factors) and polarization waves (travelling regions of dipole-coupled conformations).

Experimental evidence for Fröhlich excitations in biological systems includes observation of GHz-range phonons in proteins (Genberg *et al.*, 1991), sharp-resonant nonthermal effects of microwave (GHz) irradiation on living cells (Grundler and Keilmann, 1983), GHz-induced activation of microtubule pinocytosis in rat brain (Neubauer *et al.*, 1990) and Raman detection of Fröhlich frequency energy (Genzel *et al.*, 1983). Vassilev *et al.* (1985) demonstrated propagating signals in microtubules.

III
Models of Microtubule Information Processing

Consideration of MTs as lattice arrays of coupled (tubulin) dipoles which cooperatively interact with their immediate neighbours leads to two types of systems suitable for information processing: spin glasses and cellular automata.

In general, three types of arrangements of dipoles in lattices may occur: a) random, b) ferroelectric (parallel-aligned) and c) spin-glass (regions of locally frozen orientations). Tuszynski *et al.* (1994) have examined behaviour of MTs in this context; depending on the values of assumed parameters, MT dipole lattices may exhibit "frustration", conflict in satisfying all dipole couplings. This phase structure is defined as a spin-glass which exists close to the edge of chaos and has properties suitable for efficient information processing and computation. By slightly altering temperature and external field (both within physiological conditions), MT dipole coupling lattices may assume a ferroelectric phase with long-range order and alignment with capabilities to propagate kink-like excitations or solitons The ferroelectric phase appears to be optimal for propagation of signals and regulation of assembly/disassembly.

Coupling among tubulin dipoles within MTs in the context of coherent Fröhlich excitations has been proposed as a basis for information processing, signalling and cognition in a paradigm of *cellular automata,* a universal system of computation in a lattice structure. Von Neumann described cellular automata (which include computers as special cases) as systems that consist of a large number of identical "cells" connected in a uniform pattern. The essential features of cellular automata are: 1) at a given time, each cell is in one of a number of finite states (usually two for simplicity). 2) The cells are organized according to a fixed geometry. 3) Each cell communicates only with other cells in its neighbourhood; the size and shape of the neighbourhood are the same for all cells. 4) There is a universal clock. Each cell may change to a new state at each tick of the clock (or "generation")

phosphatidylinositol, calcium ions, and protein kinases and phosphatases). MAP2 crosslinks MTs, is essential for LTP and consumes a large proportion of brain biochemical energy by phosphorylation/dephosphorylation (e.g. Theurkauf and Vallee, 1983; Wang and Resnick, 1991; Surridge and Burns, 1992). Excitatory neurotransmitter activation of LTP post-synaptic receptors induces rapid dephosphorylation of dendritic MAP2 (Halpain and Greengard, 1990), causes rearrangement of MAP2 connections on MTs (Bigot and Hunt, 1990) and potentiates excitatory synaptic pathways in rat hippocampus (Montoro *et al.*, 1993). In cat visual cortex MAP2 is dephosphorylated when visual stimulation occurs (Aoki and Siekevitz, 1985). In animals whose brains are temporarily deprived of oxygen, the degree of cognitive damage correlates with reduction in dendritic MAP2 (Kudo *et al.*, 1990).Studies of protein kinase C suggest learning and memory are structurally represented in a more complex and interconnected sub-synaptic cytoskeleton (Friedrich,1990).

depending on its present state and those of its neighbours. The neighbour 'transition' rules for changing states, though simple, can lead to complex, dynamic patterns manifesting chaos, fractal dimensions, partial differential equations and computation. Patterns which move through the lattice unchanged are called "gliders"; Von Neumann proved mathematically that with sufficient time and cellular automaton space, gliders can solve virtually any problem. One popular example of cellular automata is Conway's the "Game of Life" in which each "cell" in a rectangular grid is alive ("on") or dead ("off"). Each cell's state at a given time depends on the state of its eight neighbours in the previous time step. Cells with 0–1 (too few) or 4–8 (too many) live neighbours will be "dead"; cells with 2 or 3 live neighbours

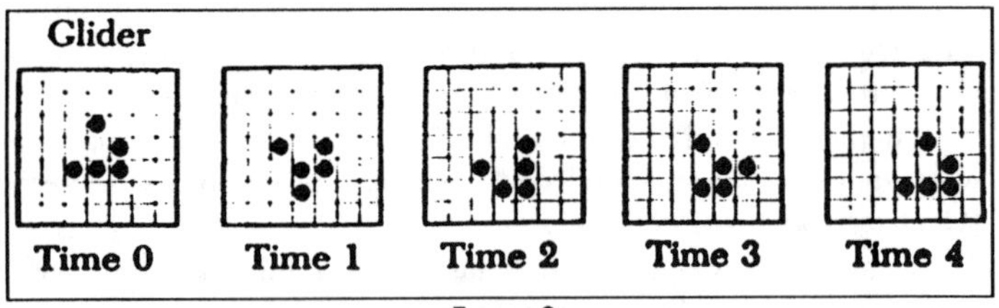

Figure 9

Five time steps from Conway's "Garne of Life" cellular automaton. Black dot: "alive", white space: "dead". Squares ("cells") with two or three live neighbours are "born" in the next generation; cells with zero or one (insufficient nourishment) or four to eight (overcrowding) die. After four time steps, the unchanged glider has moved rightward and downward.

("parents") will be "alive". Despite these simple rules, complex "lifelike" behaviours can ensue (*Figure 9*).

Cellular automata are theoretically advantageous for molecular computing because the internal connections are intrinsic to the material, external connections need only occur in one limited region, and computation can occur by local interactions with speed dependent on the clocking frequency. Quantum automata, in which each state can exist in 1,0 or alive/dead superposition (like Schrödinger's cat) have been proposed (e.g. Albert, 1983). An extreme view has been taken by Fredkin (e.g. Wright, 1985) who contends that the universe is a cellular automaton—a lattice of interacting sub-atomic logic units, each one deciding billions of times per second whether it will be "off" or "on" at the next instant. Conrad (1974) used the concept of "molecular" automata within neurons as an information processing system subserving the brain's synaptic connectionism. In a series of papers (e.g. Hameroff *et al.*, 1982; 1984; 1986; 1987; 1989; 1992; Rasmussen *et al.*, 1990) cellular ("molecular") automata principles were applied to the dynamic conformational states of tubulin within cytoskeletal microtubules ("microtubule automata"; MTA). A rough estimate for the time steps, assuming one coherent phonon or "sound" wave across the MT diameter ≈25nm and Vsound $\approx 10^3$ meters/second, yields a clocking frequency of approximately 4×10^{11} Hz and a time step of 2.5×10^{-11} second. Thus Fröhlich's coherent excitations can provide a "clocking frequency" for MT automata. Transition rules were derived for each tubulin using electrostatic coupling forces from each of its six neighbours (*Figure 10*).

The net force

$$f_{net} = \frac{e^2}{4\pi\varepsilon} \sum_{i=1}^{6} \frac{y_i}{r_i^3}$$

where *y* and *r* are defined as illustrated in *Figure 10, e* is the electron charge and *£* is the average protein permitivity, yields forces of +1.5 picoNewtons. Energy per tubulin state change is estimated as 10^{-21} Joules, an order of magnitude greater than random thermal fluctuations without considering cooperative, shielding effects from MT-ordering or surrounding water.

Using these transition rules, simulations of MT automata reveal gliders (including bidirectional gliders), travelling and standing wave patterns, oscillators, linearly growing patterns, and frozen pattems (*Figure 11*). What functions could such gliders and pattems have? They could represent information being transmitted through the cell; glider numerical quantities and pattems may manifest signals, binding sites for ligands, MAPs or material to be transported. By determining MAP binding sites, MT-assembly/ disassembly, cytoskeletal network architecture and thus cell structure and function could be regulated. Frozen pattems may store information in a memory context, information may become "hardened" in MT by post-translational modifications, and/or MT automata patterns could transfer and retrieve stored information to and from neurofilaments via MAPs.

MT automata gliders travel one dimer length (8 nm) per time step (10^{-9} to 10^{-11} sec) for a velocity range of 8 to 800 meters per second, consistent with the speed of travelling nerve-membrane potentials. Thus travelling MT automata patterns or gliders (equivalent to phonons, Fröhlich depolarization waves, kink-like excitations or solitons) may propagate in the cytoskeleton in concert with membrane depolarizations and ion fluxes. Membrane-related voltages, ion fluxes or direct structural links could induce transient waves of conformational switching along parallel-arrayed MT. Consequently, extemal inputs and activity of a particular cell could directly elaborate pattems within that cell's MT automata—phenomena important in cognitive and behavioural functions ranging from simple organisms to human brains. Long-range cooperativity, resonances and phase transitions emerging from locally-determined microtubule automata pattems may occur among spatially-distributed microtubules as quantum coherence phenomena and correlate with some aspect of consciousness.

Viewing the cytoskeleton as the cell's nervous system, with microtubules serving as processors or signal carriers and MAPs as molecular

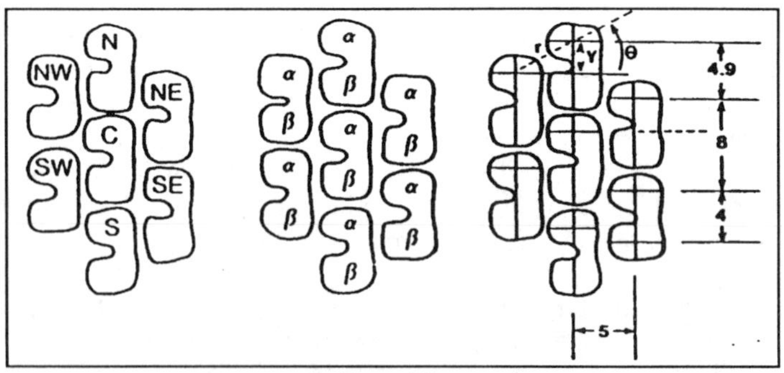

Figure 10

Microtubule automata (MTA) neighbourhood: left, definition of neighbourhood dimers; centre, a and b monomers within each dimer; right, distances in nm and orientation among lattice neighbours. Transition rules for MTA are based on net electrostatic coupling forces on each tubulin from its surrounding six tubulin neighbours. Coupling force values (described in text) are given in Hameroff *et al.*, 1989 and Rasmussen *et al.*, 1990.

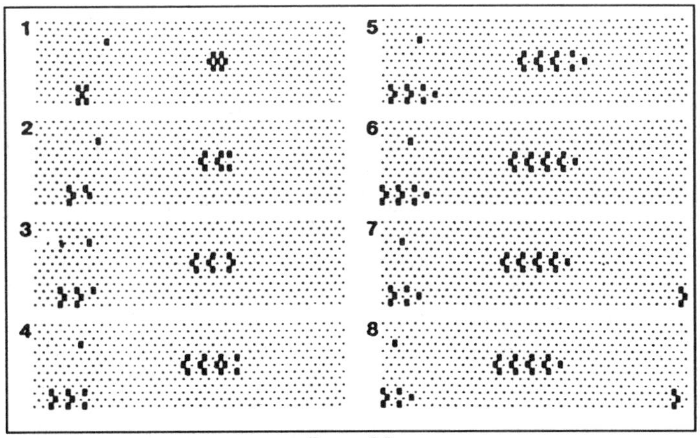

FIGURE 11

EIGHT TIME STEPS OF A MICROTUBULE AUTOMATA (MTA) COMPUTER SIMULATION. MT IS SHOWN AS HORIZONTAL OPEN RECTANGLE. INITIAL PATTERN IS BLACK 'SEEDS' (BETA STATE CONFORRNATIONS OF TUBULIN) ON WHITE BACKGROUND (ALPHA STATE CONFORMATIONS). SEEDS 'WIGGLE', EXPAND BIDIRECTIONALLY AND ORGANIZE INTO 'BUS' GLIDERS WHICH MOVE LEFTWARD AT A VELOCITY OF 8 TO 800 METERS PER SECOND (FROM HAMEROFF *ET AL.*, 1989).

cross-bridge connections ('synapses') suggests that the cytoskeleton within each ofthe brain's neurons could be viewed as a 'fractal-like' sub-dimension in a hierarchy of adaptive networks. This is consistent with Globus's (1992) observation that 'nervous tissue has fractal geometric, statistical, and dynamic properties and that there are fractal correlates of cognitive activity'. Exploring only a few facets of the possible parameter space for cytoskeletal automata, an enormous information-processing capacity is implied. For example, the 'strong AI' information-processing capacity of a human brain based on consideration of conventional neural synaptic transmissions as fundamental switches has been estimated as 100 billion neurons, each with over 1000 synapses 'switching' 100 times per second to yield approximately 1016 'bits' per second (Moravec, 1987). Considering the simplest case of microtubule automata (two conformational states per microtubule subunit switching at 10^{-9} sec. intervals, 10^4 microtubule subunits per neuron) yields about 1023 brain 'bits' per second.

Whether computer-like information processing and molecular automata in the cytoskeleton can help explain consciousness remains questionable. Considering only local interactions, the concept takes the reductionist argument to a molecular level, increasing the complexity of the brain (and goal for strong AI) about 7 orders of magnitude, but does not address emergent properties of consciousness. For this, quantum coherence provides a possible resolution.

REFERENCES

Abeles, M. (1982), *Local Cortical Circuits* (Berlin: Springer Verlag).

Albert, D.Z. (1983), 'On quantum mechanical automata', *Physics Letters*, 98A (5,6), pp. 249–52.

Allison, A.C., & Nunn, J.E. (1968), 'Effects of general anaesthetics on microtubules: a possible mechanism of anaesthesia', *The Lancet*, 2 pp. 1326–29.

Aoki, C., & Siekevitz, P. (1985), 'Ontogenic changes in the cyclic adenosine 31, 51 monophosphate-stimulatable phosphorylation of cat visual cortex proteins, particularly of microtubule-associate protein 2 (MAP2): effects of normal and dark rearing and of the exposure to light', *J. Neurosci.*, 5, pp. 2465-83.

Aspect, A. and Grangier, P. (1986), 'Experiments on Einstein-Podolsky-Rosen-type correlations with pairs of visible photons', In: *Quantum Theory and Measurement* eds. Wheeler, J.A., Zurek, W.H., (Princeton University Press).

Atema, J. (1973 t74]), 'Microtubule theory of sensory transduction', *J. Theor. Biol.*, 38, pp. 181–90.

Athenstaedt, H. (1974), 'Pyroelectric and piezoelectric properties of vertebrates', *Ann. NY. Acad Sci*, 238, pp. 68–93.

Atkin, A. (1992), 'On consciousness: what is the role of emergence?', *Medical Hypotheses*, 38, pp. 311–14.

Baars, B.J. (1988), *A cognilive theory of consciousness* (Cambridge University Press)

Baars, B.J. (1993), 'How does a serial, integrated and very limited stream of consciousness emerge from a nervous system that is mostly unconscious, distributed, parallel and of enormous capacity?', In: *Experimental and Theoretical Studies of Consciousness*, Ciba Foundation Symposium, 174, pp 282–303. (Chichester: Wiley).

Baas, N.A. (1994), 'Hyperstructures as tools in nanotechnology and nanobiology', In: *Nanobiology* eds. S. Rasmussen, S. Hameroff, J. Tuszynski, P.A. Hansson, (Cambridge, MA: MIT Press), in press.

Barinaga, M. (1991), 'Is nitric oxide the retrograde messenger', *Science*, 254, pp. 1296–7.

Bass, L. (1975), 'A quantum-mechanical mindbody interaction', *Foundations of Physics*, 5, pp. 159–72.

Beck, F., Eccles, J.C. (1992), 'Quantum aspects of brain activity and the role of consciousness', *Proc. Nat. Acad Sci. USA*, 89, pp. 11357–61.

Bensimon, G. & Chemat R. (1991), 'Microtubule disruption and cognitive defects: effect of colchicine on learning behavior in rats', *Pharmacol. Biochem. Behavior*, 38, pp. 141–5.

Bigot, D. & Hunt, S.P. (1990), 'Effectofexcitatory amino acids on microtubule-associated proteins in cultured cortical and spinal neurons', *Neurosci. Lett.*, 111, pp. 275–80.

Bohm, David (1952), 'A suggested interpretation of the quantum theory in terms of 'hidden' variables, I and 11,' *Phys. Rev.*, 85, pp. 166–93.

Bohm, David (1980), *Wholeness and the Implicate Order*, (London, Boston and Henley, UK: Routledge and Kegan Paul).

Churchland, P., Sejnowski, T. (1992), *The Computational Brain*, (Cambridge, MA: MIT Press).

Clarke, C.J.S. (1994), 'Coupled Molecular Oscillators Do Not Admit True Bose Condensations', To appear in *Journal of Physics A*.

Clauser, J.F., Horne, A.H., Shimony, A. and Holt, RA. (1969), 'Proposed experiment to test local hidden variable theories', *Phys. Rev. Lett.*, 23 pp. 880–4.

Conrad M (1974) 'Molecular automata', in *Lecture Notes in Biomathematics, Vol.4: Physics and Mathematics oJ the Nervous System*, ed. M. Conrad, W. Guninger and M. Dal Cin pp. 419–30 (Heidelberg: Springer–Verlag).

Conrad, M. (1992), 'Quantum molecular computing: the self-assembly model', *Int. J. Quantum Chemistry: Quantum Biology Symposium*, 19, pp. 125–43.

Crick, F.H.C. (1984), 'Function of the thalamic reticular complex: the searchlight hypothesis', *Proc. Natl Acad. Sci. USA*, 81, pp. 4586–93.

Crick, F., Koch, C. (1990), 'Towards a neurobiological theory of consciousness', *Seminars in the Neurosciences*, 2, pp. 263–75.

Cronly-Dillon, J., Carden, D. & Birks, C. (1974), 'The possible involvement of brain microtubules in memory fixation', *J. Exp. Biol.*, 61, pp. 443–54.

Dayhoff, J.E., Hameroff, S., Lahoz-Beltra, R., Swenberg, C.E., (1994), 'Cytoskeletal involvement in neuronal learning: a review', *Eur. Biophys. J.*, 23, pp. 79–93.

DeBrabander, M. (1982), 'A model for the microtubule organizing activity of the centrosomes and kinetochores in mammalian cells', *Cell Biol. Intern. Rep.*, 6, pp. 901–15.

Del Giudice, E., Doglia, S., Milani, M. (1983), 'Self focusing and ponderomotive forces of coherent electric waves: a mechanism for cytoskeleton formation and dynamics', in *Coherent Excitations in Biological Systems*, ed. H. Fröhlich and F. Kremer (Berlin: Springer Verlag).

Dennen, D. (1991), *Consciousness Explained* (Boston: Little Brown).

Deutsch, D. (1985), 'Quantum theory, the Church-Turing principle and the universal quantum computer', *Proc. R. Soc. London*, A400, pp. 97–117.

Deutsch, D. (1992), 'Quantum computation', *Physics World*, pp. 57–61.

Donald, M.J. (1990), 'Quantum theory and the brain', *Proceedings of the Royal Societyy of London,* 427A, pp. 43–93.

Dustin, P. (1984), *Microlubules 2nd Revised Ed.,* Berlin: Springcr.

Eckhorn, R, Bauer, R., Jordan, W., Brosch, M. Kruse, W., Munk, M., Reitbock, H.J. (1988), 'Coherent oscillations: a mechanism of feature linking in the visual cortex?', *Biol Cybern.,* 60, pp. 121–30.

Edelman, G. (1989), *The remembered present: a biological theory of consciousness* (New York: Basic Books).

Eistei4 A., Podolsky, B., Rosen, N. (1935), 'Can quantum-mechanical description of physical reality be considered complete?', In: *Quantum Theory and Measurement,* ed. Wheeler, J.A., Zurek, W.H. (Princeton University Press).

Engelborghs, Y. (1992), 'Dynamic sspects of the conformational states of tubulin and microtubules', *Nanobiology,* 1, pp. 97–105.

Eriksson, J.E., Brautigan, D.L., Vallee, R, Olmsted, J., Fujiki, H. & Goldman, R.D. (1992), 'Cytoskeletal integrity in interphase cells requires protein phosphatase activity', *Proc. Natl. Acad. Sci.,* 89, pp. 11093–97.

Everett, H. (1957), 'Relative state formulation of quantum mechanics', *Reviews of Modern Physics,* 29, p. 454.

Franks, N.P., Lieb, W.R. (1982), 'Molecular mechanisms of general anesthesia', *Nature,* 300, pp. 487–93.

Freeman, W.J. (1978), 'Spatial properties of an EEG event in the olfactory bulb and cortex', *Electroencephalogr. and Clin. Neurophysiol.,* 44, pp. 586–605.

Freeman,W.J.(1975), *Mass Action in the Nervous System* (New York: Academic Press).

Friedric4 P. (1990), 'Protein structure: the primary substrate for memory', *Neurosci.,* 35, pp. 1–7.

Fröhlich, H. (1968), 'Long-range coherence and energy storage in biological systems', *Intern. J Quantum Chem.,* 2, pp. 641–9.

Fröhlich, H. (1970), 'Long range coherence and the actions of enzymes', Nature, 228, p. 1093.

Fröhlich, H. (1975), 'The extraordinary dielectric properties of biological materials and the action of enzymes', *Proc. Natl. Acad. Sci.,* 72 pp. 4211–15.

Gazzaniga, M S. (1985), *The Social Brain Discovering the Networks of the Mind* (New York: Basic Books).

Gelber, B. (1958), 'Retention in Paramecium aurelia', *J. Comp. Physiol. Psych,* 51, pp. 110–15.

Genberg, L., Richard, L., McLendon, G., Dwayne-Miller, R.V. (1991), 'Direct observation of global protein motion in hemoglobin and myoglobin on picosecond time scales', *Science,* 251, pp. 1051–54..

Genzel, L., Kremer, F., Poglitsch, A., Bechtold, G. (1983), 'Relaxation processes on a picosecond time scale in hemoglobin and poly observed by millimeter-wave spectroscopy', *Biopolymers,* 22, pp. 1715–29.

Globus, G.G. (1992), 'Toward a noncomputational cognitive neuroscience', *J. Cog. Neurosci.,* 4 (4), pp 299–310.

Globus, G.G. (19Y7), *Dream Life, Wake Life,* (Albany, NY: Slate IJniversity of New York Press).

Gray, C.M., Konig, P., Engel, A.K., Singer, W. (1989), 'Oscillatory responses in cat visual cortex exhibit inter-columnar synchronization which reflects global stimulus properties', *Nature,* 338, pp. 334–7.

Gray, C.M., Singer, W. (1989), 'Stimulus-specific neuronal oscillations in orientation columns of cat visual cortex', *Proc. Natl. Acad. Sci. USA,* 86, pp. 1698–1702.

Grundler, W., Keilmann, F. (1983), 'Sharp resonances in yeast grovlth nonthermal sensitivity to microwaves', *Phys. Rev. Lett.,* 51, pp. 12–46.

Haddon, RC., Stillinger, F.H. (1982), 'Molecular, memory and hydrogen bonding', pp. 19–30, in *Molecular Electronic Devices* ed. F.L. Carter, New York: Marcel Dekker.

Halpain, S. & Greengard, P. (1990), 'Activation of NMDA receptors induces rapid dephosphorylation of the cytoskeletal protein MAP2', *Neuron,* 5, pp. 237–46.

Halsey, M.J. (1983), 'Mechanisms of general anesthesia', in *Anesthesia Uptake and Action,* ed. El Eger, (Baltimore: Williams and Wllkins).

Hameroff, S.R., Smith, S.A., Watt, R.C. (1984), 'Nonlinear electrodynamics in cytoskeletal proteir. lattices', in *Nonlinear Electrodynamics in Biological Systems,* eds. W.R. Adey, A.F. Lav.wrence (New York: Plenum Press).

Hameroff, S.R, Rasmussen, S. & Mansson, B. (1989), 'Molecular automata in microtubules: basic computational logic for the living state?', in *Artificial Life, the Santa Fe Institute Studies in the Sciences of Complexity, VoL VI,* pp. 521–53, ed. C. Langton, Reading, MA: Addison–Wesley.

Hameroff, S.R., Watt, R.C. (1983), 'Do anesthetics act by altering electron mobility?', *Anesth. Analg,* pp. 936–40.

Hameroff, S.R., Watt, R.C. (1982), 'Information processing in microtubules', *J. Theor. Biol.,* 98, pp 549–61.

Hameroff, S.R., Dayhoff, J.E., Lahoz-Beltra, R., Samsonovich, A., Rasmussen, S. (1992), 'Models for molecular computation: conformational automata in the cytoskeleton', *IEEE Computer* (Special Issue on Molecular Computing), pp. 30–9.

Hameroff, S.R., Smith, S.A., Watt, R.C. (1986), 'Automaton model of dynamic organization in microtubules', *Ann. NY. Acad. Sci.,* 466, pp. 949–52.

Hameroff, S.R. (1987), *Ultimate Computing: Biomolecular Consciousness and Nanotechnology* (Amsterdam, Elsevier North Holland).

Hebb, D.O. (1949), *The Organization of Behavior* (New York: Wiley).

Hebb, D.O. (1980), *Essay on Mind* (Hillsdale, NJ: Lawrence Erlbaum Associates).

Herbert, N. (1993), *Elemental Mind: Human Consciousness and the New Physics* (New York: Dutton/Penguin).

Hopfield, J J (1982), 'Neural networks and physical systems with emergent collective computational abilities', *Proc. Natl. Acad. Sci. IJSA,* 79 pp. 2554–8.

Insinna, E.M. (1992), 'Synchronicity and coherent excitations in mierotubules', *Nanobiology,* 1, pp. 191–208.

Jaynes, I. (1976), *The Origin of Consciousness and the Breakdown of the Bicameral Mind* (London: Alan Layne, Penguin Books).

Jibu, M., Hagan, S., Hameroff, S.R., Pribram, K.H., Yasue, K. (1994), 'Quantum optical coherenee in cytoskeletal microtubules: implications for brain function', *BioSystems,* 32, pp. 95–209.

Johnson, G.V.W., Jope, R.S. (1992), 'The role of microtubule-associated protein 2 (MAP-2) in neuronal growth, plasticity, and degeneration', *Neurosci. Res.,* 35, pp. 505–12.

Karplus, M. & McCammon, J.A. (1983), 'Protein ion channels, gates, receptors'. In: 'Dynamics of Proteins: Elements and Function', *Ann. Rev. Biochem,* ed. J. King, pp. 263–300, Benjamin/Cummings, Menlo Park.

Kirschner, M. & Mitchison, T. (1986), 'Beyond self assembly: from microtubules to morphogenesis', *Cell,* 45, pp. 329–42.

Koch, C. (1993), 'Computational approaches to cognition: the bottom-up view', *Current Opinion in Neurobiology,* 3, pp. 203–8.

Korb, K.B. (1993), 'Stage effects in the Cartesian theater: a review of Daniel Dennett's "Consciousness Explained" ', *Psyche,* 1(1), December, (electronic).

Kudo, T., Tada, K., Takeda, M. & Nishimura, T. (1990), 'Learning impairment and microtubuleassociated protein 2 (MAP-2) decrease in gerbils under chronic cerebral hypoperfusion', *Stroke,* 21, pp. 1205–9.

Lashley, K. (1950), 'In search of the engram', in *Symposium of the Society for Experimental Biology* No. 4, (Cambridge: Cambridge University Press).

Lechleiter, J., Girard, S., Peralta, E., Clapham, D. (1991), 'Spiral waves: spiral calcium wave propagation and annihilation in Xenopus laevis oocytes', *Science,* 252, pp. 123–6.

Lee, J.C., Field, D.J., George, H.I. & Head, J. (1986), 'Biochemical and chemical properties of tubulin subspecies', *Ann. NY. Acad. Sci,* 466, pp 111–28.

Leggett, A. (1989), 'Low temperature physics, superconductivity and superfluidity', In: *The New Physics,* ed. P. Davies, pp. 268–88.

Lewis, S.A., Ivanov, I.E., Lee, G.H., Cowan, N.J. (1989), 'Organization of microtubules in dendrites and axons is deterrnined by a short hydrophobic zipper in microtubule-associated proteins MAP2 and tau', *Nature,* 342, pp. 498–505.

Lloyd, S. (1993), 'A potentially realizable quantum computer', *Science,* 261, pp. 1569–71.

Lund,E.E. (1933), 'A correlation of the silverline and neuromotor systems of Paramecium'. *University of California Publication in Zoology,* 39 (2), pp. 35–6.

Madler, C., Poppel, E. (1987), 'Auditory evoked potentials indieate the loss of neuronal oseillations during general anesthesia', *Naturwissenschaften,* 74, pp. 42–3.

Margulis, L. (1975), Origin of EYkaryotic Cells (New Haven: Yale University Press).

Marshall, I.N. (19X9), 'Consciousness and Bose-Einstein condensates', *New Ideas in Psychology,* 7, pp. 73–83.

Masearenhas, S. (1974), 'The electret effect in bone and biopolymers and the bound water problem', *Ann. NY. Acad. Sci,* 238, pp. 36–52.

McCall, S.L., Hahn, E.L. (1967), 'Self- indueed transparency by pulsed coherent light', *Phys. Rev. Lett.,* 18, pp. 908–11.

McCulloch, W.S., Pitts, W.S. (1943), 'A logieal calculus of the ideas immanent in nervous activity', *Bull. Math. Biophys.,* 5, pp. 115–33.

Melki, R., Carlier, M.F., Pantaloni, D., Timasheff, S.N. (1989), 'Cold depolymerization of microtubules to double rings: geometric stabilization of assemblies', *Biochemistry,* 28, pp. 9143–52.

Mileusnic, R., Rose, S.P. & Tillson, P. (1980), 'Passive avoidance learning results in region specific changes in concentration of, and incorporation into, cochicine binding proteins in the chick forebrain', *Neur. Chem.,* 34, pp. 1007–15.

Milner, P.M. (1974), 'A model for visual shape recognition', *Psychol. Rev.,* 81, pp. 521–35.

Minsky, M. (i986), *The Society of Mind* (New York: Simon and Schuster).

Montoro, R.J., Diaz-Nido, J., Avila, J., LopezBarneo, J. (1993), 'N-metnyl-d-aspartate stimulates the dephosphorylation of the microtubule-associated protein 2 and potentiates excitatory synaptic pathways in the rat hippocampus', *Neuroscience,* 54 (4), pp. 859–71.

Moravec, H. (1987), *Mind Children* (San Francisco: University Press).

Neubauer, C., Phelan, A.M., Keus, H., Lange, D.G. (1990), 'Microwave irradiation of rats at 2.45 GHz activates pinocytotic-like uptake of tracer by capillary endothelial cells of cerebral cortex', *Bioelectromagnetics,* 11, pp. 261–8.

Nunn. C M.H., Clarke, C.J.S., Blott, B.H. (1994), 'Collapse of a quantum field may affect brain function', *Journal of Consciousness Studies,* pp. 127–139.

Parducz, B. (1962), 'On a new concept of cortical organization in Paramecium', *Acta. Biol. Acad. Sci. Hung.,* 13, pp. 299–322

Peat, F O. (1992), 'Non-locality in nature and cognition', In: *Nature, Cognition and Systems II,* ed. M.E. Carvallo (Netherlands: Kluwer Academic Publishers).

Penrose, R. (1989), *The Emperor's New Mind* (London: Oxford University Press).

Penrose R. (1994), *Shadows of the Mind* (London: Oxford University Press).

Plourde, G, Picton, I.W. (1990), 'Human auditory steady-state response during general anesthcsia', *Anesth. Analg.,* 71, pp. 460–8.

Popp, F.A.. (1986), 'On thc cohercnce of ultraweak photoemission from living tissue', In: *Disequilibrium and self- organization,* ed. C.W. Kilmister, (Dordrecht and Boston: A. Reidel Publishing).

Popper, K.R, Eccles, J.C. (1977), *The Self and Its Brain* (Berlin: Springer).

Pribram, K. (1971), *Languages of the Brain: Experimental Paradoxes and Principles in Neurophysiology* (New York: Brandon House).

Pullman, B., Pullman, A. (1963), *Quantum Biochemistry* (New York: Interscience).

Rasmussen, S., Karampurwala, H., Vaidyanath, R., Jensen, K.S., Hameroff, S.R., (1990), 'Computational connectionism within neurons: a model of cytoskeletal automata subserving neural networks", *Physica,* D42, pp. 428–49.

Rensch, B. (1960), *Evolution Above the Species Level* (New York: Columbia University Press).

Ribary, I., Ioannides, A.A., Singh, K.D., Hasson R., Bolton I.P., Lado, F., Mogilner, A., Llinas R. (199l), 'Magnetic field tomography of coherent thalamocortical 40 Hz oscillations in humans', *Proc. Natl. Acad. Sci. USA,* 88, pp. 11037–41.

Ricciardi, L.M., Umezawa, H. (1967), 'Brain and physics of many-body problems', *Kybernetik,* 4, pp. 44–8.

Sataric, M.V., Tuszynski, J.A., Zakula, R.B. (1993), 'Kinklike excitations as an energy transfer mechanism in microtubules', *Phys. Rev. E.,* 48 (1), pp. 589–97.

Scheibel, A.B. (1980), 'Anatomical and physio1ogical substrates of arousal', In: *The Reticular Formation Revisited,* eds. Hobson, J.A., Brazier, M.A. (New York: Raven Press).

Schempp, W. (1993), 'Bohr's indeterminacy principle in quantum holography, self-adaptive neural network architectures, cortical self-organization, molecular computers, magnetic resonance imaging and solitonic nanotechnology', *Nanobiology,* 2 (2), pp. 109–64.

Scott, A.C. (1994), *Stairway to the Mind* (Berlin: Springer-Verlag), in press.

Scott, A.C. (1978), 'Brain theory from a hierarchical perspective', *Brain Theory Newsletter,* 3, pp. 66–9.

Searle, J.R. (1980), 'Minds, brains, and programs', *Behavioral and Brain Sciences,* 3, pp. 417–24.

Sherrington, C.S. (1951), *Man on His Nature, Second Edition* (Cambridge: Cambridge University Press).

Somjen, G.C. (1983), *Neurophysiology, the essentials* (Baltimore: Williams and Wilkins).

Spinoza, B. (1677), *Ethica in Opera quotque reperta sunt. 3rd edition,* eds. J. van Vloten and J.P.N. Land (Netherlands: Den Haag).

Stapp, H.P. (1993), *Mind, Matter and Quantum Mechanics* (Berlin: Springer-Verlag).

Strehler, B.L. (1991), 'Where is the self? A neuroanatomical theory of consciousncss', *Synapse,* A7, pp. 44–91.

Surridge, C.D., Burns, R.G (1992), 'Phosphatidyinositol inhibits microtubule assemhly by binding to microtubule-associated protein 2 at a single, specific, high affinity site', *Biochemistry,* 31, pp. 6140–04.

Szent-Gyorgyi, A. (1960), *Introduction to a Sub-Molecular Biology* (New York: Academic Press).

Taylor, J.G. (1992), 'Towards a neural network model of the mind', *Neural Network World,* 6, pp. 797–812.

Theurkauf, W.E., Vallee, R.B. (1983), 'Extensive cAMP-dependent and cAMP-independent phosphorylation of microtubule associated protein 2', *J. Biol. Chem.,* 258, pp. 7883–86.

Tilley, D.R., Tilley, J. (1986), *Superfluidity and Superconductivity, 2nd Edition,* Bristol, England: Adam Hilger.

Tuszynski, J.A., Hameroff, S., Sataric, M.V., Trpisova, B., Nip, M.L.A. (1994), 'Spin-glass and ferroelectric behavior in microtubule dipole lattices; implications for information processing, signaling and assembly/disassembly', submitted.

Vassilev, P., Kanazirska, M., Tien, H.T. (1985), 'Intermembrane linkage mediated by tubulin', *Biochem. Biophys. Res. Comm.,* 126 (1), pp.559–65.

Von der Marlsburg, C., Schneider, W. (1986) 'A neural cocktail party processor', *Biol. Cybern.,* 54, pp. 29–40.

Wang, N., Rasenick, M.M. (1991),'Tubulin-G protein interactions involve microtubule polymerization domains', *Biochemistry,* 30, pp. 10957–65.

Wanerson, J.G. (1987), 'A role for water in cell structure', *Biochem. J.,* 248, pp. 615–7.

Werbos, P. (1974), 'Beyond Regression: New Tools for Prediction and Analysis in the Behavorial Sciences', Ph.D. Thesis, Harvard University.

Wheeler, J.A., Zurek, W.H. (1983), 'Quantum Theory and Measurement', Princeton, New Jersey: Princeton University Press,

Wright, R. (1985), 'The on/off universe. Thc information age', *The Sciences,* May/June 7–9.

Wu, T.M., Austin, S. (1978), 'Bose-Einstein condensation in biological systems', *J. Theorel. Biol,* 71, pp. 200–14.

Wulf, R.I, Featherstone, R.M. (1957), 'A correlation of Van der Waals constants with anesthetic potency', *Anesthesiology,* 18, pp. 97–105.

Zohar, D., Marshall, I. (1994), *The Quantum Society: Mind, Physics, and a New Social Vision* (New York: William Morrow).

Zohar, D. (1990), *The Quantum Self: Human Nature and Consciousness Defined by the New Physics* (New York: Quill /William Morrow).

Appendix 4

"Haoma and Harmaline: The Botanical Identity of the Indo-Iranian Sacred Hallucinogen 'Soma' and its Legacy in Religion, Language, and Middle Eastern Folklore"

David Stophlet Flattery and Martin Schwartz

CONTENTS

List of Tables and Figures

Part I
By David Stophlet Flattery[1]

INTRODUCTION

§1 In this monograph I intend to demonstrate that harmel or wild rue, *Peganum harmala* L. (Zygophyllaceae), a common weed of the Central Asian Steppes, the Iranian Plateau, and adjacent areas, was the original intoxicant plant represented in the Iranian religious tradition by the term *haoma* and in the religious tradition of India by the etymologically identical term *soma.* I also intend to show that this identification of the plant improves our understanding of the origin and nature of certain rituals that were central to Indic and Iranian religions, and of the nature of the religions themselves.[1]

§2 Both in the ancient Vedic rites of India, which are partially recorded in post-Vedic literature and to some extent are still practiced, and in the rites preserved by the surviving representatives of the ancient Iranian religion, the Zoroastrians, *soma/haoma* appear as the central and most important elements. The modern day rituals of the two traditions are accompanied by recitation of liturgies whose highly formulaic language preserves the most archaic forms of Indic and Iranian. These liturgies were memorized and transmitted orally and written down only much later. The attested texts speak of *soma/haoma* as intoxicating, yet the plants used in the present ceremonies associated with these texts are not intoxicating, nor is intoxication reflected in the conduct of the ceremonies. The plants now called *soma* and *haoma* lack the distinctive properties or cultural importance that could account for their being the focus of such ancient and elaborate practices.

§3 Despite the apparent conservation of minute details, these contemporary ceremonies are based on earlier practices which involved the drinking of an extract of an *intoxicating* plant. In neither tradition is the ceremony conducted with an open acknowledgment that the plant regularly used as *soma* or *haoma* is not the one originally used, or that the character of the rite was ever markedly different from what it is now.[2] The respective secondary literatures of commentary and interpretation virtually ignore the absence of the intoxication indicated by the liturgical texts.

§4 The terms *soma* and *haoma* (pronounced *hauma*) are applied to the nonintoxicating plants used in modern ceremonies. In this connection it should be noted that **sauma-*, the form which must be reconstructed for the Proto-Indo-Iranian ancestral language, merely denoted a 'pressed out (liquid or plant)', without reference to any more specific properties of the substance. Thus, rather than exclusively designating the primary intoxicant plant, the term **sauma* could have referred to either nonintoxicating or intoxicating plants extracted in ceremonies, and early on came to be used as a common name for a secondary plant (namely *Ephedra*, see below, §106). Nevertheless, because of the narrowly Indian or Iranian sense of *soma* or *haoma*, the term sauma (without italics or asterisk to distinguish it from the hypothetical word **sauma-* as it may have been historically used in Proto-Indo-Iranian) will be adopted here with restricted reference to the original intoxicant plant.

§5 Numerous scholars have attempted to find evidence for the identification of sauma in the numerous references to *soma* in the ṚgVeda, enigmatic though these may be. The most important of these studies is R. Gordon Wasson's *Soma: Divine Mushroom of Immortality* (1968) and his subsequent publications, where it is argued that *soma* was the fly-agaric or *Amanita muscaria*, a hallucinogenic mushroom consumed until recently for intoxication by peoples in Siberia.[3]

§6 Wasson (1971:171) states that the following four points respecting the ṚgVeda lead him to equate *soma* with *Amanita muscaria*: (1) there is no mention of the roots or branches or blossoms or seed of *soma*; (2) the poets locate the plant high in the mountains (and *A. muscaria* may be the one psychotropic plant which can *only* be found at high elevations in the Indo-Iranian area); (3) there appears in the hymns "a succession of tropes each appropriate for the fly-agaric, indeed fitting it like a glove"; and (4) "no word in the ṚgVeda is inconsistent with this plant." The last of these points touches on a major difficulty of using the ṚgVeda to resolve the botanical identity of sauma, for the descriptions in the ṚgVeda are so general that they may be applied to any psychotropic plant and not just to *Amanita muscaria.* Hence, the Vedic evidence cannot be used as positive support for a specific identification of the plant; its value is merely corroborative. While Wasson's first three points would seem to make *A. muscaria* a reasonable candidate, the actual significance of each is not beyond doubt, as may be noted: (1) A major reason why there is so little mention of the constituent elements of the *soma* plant is not that they were absent from the plant, but rather that, except in a very few cases (see Geldner 1951: 241), the *soma* referred to in the ṚgVeda and adduced by Wasson as pertaining to the mushroom is the liquid extract (*soma pavamāna*) or the deity Soma, and hence not the *soma* plant at all. Moreover, one cannot make too much of what the poets omit: all living things that appear in the ṚgVeda have parts of some kind which the text fails to mention, but one cannot on that account claim that a given part did not exist. (2) While *soma* in the ṚgVeda (and *haoma* in the Avesta) is indeed repeatedly said to grow in the mountains, it may be questioned whether these passages were intended to locate the plant physiographically, to indicate that it grew wild, or merely to assert its lofty origins (see below, §83). (3) Many allusions to *soma* could suit *A. muscaria*, albeit as it is seen in the field and not as it would appear in the circumstances of *soma* ceremonies, but each such allusion can be interpreted quite as appropriately in other ways. Ambiguity pervades virtually all of the complex metaphors and similes associated with *soma* in the ṚgVeda. There is,

1 The synonyms harmel and *Peganum harmala* will be used interchangeably here. It may be claimed that harmel was implicitly the plant first identified with *soma* in Western scholarship. In 1794 Sir William Jones translated the only occurrence of *soma* in the *Laws of Manu* as "a species of mountain rue" (1796: 72). The reasons for Jones's identification are unclear, but the plant growing in India which he could have most accurately characterized as "a species of mountain rue" is *Peganum harmala*. Neither the mountain rue known in Europe, *Ruta montana* L., nor any other species of the genus *Ruta*, occurs as a wild plant east of the Euphrates (see below, §127). The only genuine rue (i.e. *Ruta* species) known in India (or in Iran) is the cultivated garden herb *Ruta graveolens* L. Traditional Persian botany, however, regards *Peganum harmala* and *Ruta graveolens* as, respectively, the wild and cultivated species of the same genus, and since both plants have become widely known in India largely through their introduction by way of Iran, this taxonomy prevails in India as well. Since there is no uncultivated species of *Ruta* to which "rue" could refer in India, "mountain rue" must represent the Persian *sudāb-i kūhī* which is defined in Indo-Persian lexicons and botanical works as, in effect, *Peganum harmala*.

"*Soma*" was therefore virtually identified at the outset of the comparative study of Indo-Iranian cultures. This book may be regarded as the vindication of Jones's original proposition. The probability that harmel was the source of *soma* has also been apparent to others since Jones, e.g. to Paul Lagarde (1866), the zoologist Wilkins (see Roth 1884: 136n.), and Claudio Naranjo (Efron 1967: 445-446).

2 Indian Brahmans know the plant now used as *soma* in south Indian rituals, *Sarcostemma brevistigma*, to be a substitute for an earlier "*soma*". The "*soma*" which *Sarcostemma* has directly replaced, however, seems not to have been the original plant but an *Ephedra*, a nonintoxicating plant which was itself a secondary constituent of rituals. See §§107-114.

3 For a summary of the history of scholarship on the botanical identification of sauma, discussing over 140 publications, see O'Flaherty (1968).

moreover, little reason to attribute to the Vedic poets any intention to describe the appearance of the *soma* plant.

§7 Although direct links between *soma* and *Amanita muscaria* have not been established, this mushroom has a remarkable property which may allow its presence to be determined indirectly. The urine of a person intoxicated by *A. muscaria* may itself be drunk for intoxication, and such urine drinking is actually attested in Siberia. Since such practices are not known for any other plant, if evidence could be found that the urine of *soma* drinkers was itself drunk, this would strongly support Wasson's identification. No evidence for this, however, has come to light. According to Wasson (1970: 28): "there is only one overt passage in the ṚgVeda that refers to the *soma-urine*," namely, "the swollen men piss the flowing (*soma*) [9.48.4]." Even interpreting this literally (and supposing the "men" to refer to priests, which is not at all certain), there is still nothing to suggest the *drinking* of such urine. Wasson's reason for suspecting that the urine of *soma* drinkers was consumed comes from an ostensible reference to this practice not in the ṚgVeda but in an Iranian source, namely in the Gathas of Zarathushtra, where, in *Yasna* 48.10, a passage occurs whose contents are summarized by Wasson as "[Zoroaster] excoriates the priests who evilly delude the people with the urine of drunkenness" (Wasson 1968: 32). If this were what was actually said in the Gathas, Wasson's proposal would justify continued investigation. However, close examination of the text by Schwartz (1985a and 1987:4; see below, §158) reveals that such a translation is based on an erroneous reading; the alleged word "drunkenness", *madahyā,* did not originally occur in this passage and appears in manuscripts as a scribal error for *magahyā.* In addition, the word translated as 'urine', *mūθrəm,* more likely means 'feces, filth'. In reality, the passage has no connection with drinking at all, either of urine or of anything else, and has nothing remotely to do with sauma. Apart from the illusory support of this passage, none of the data presented by Wasson on the subject of urine drinking has any relevance for *soma.*[4]

§8 The limits of the possibilities of determining the botanical identity of sauma from the ṚgVeda have been made clear in Wasson's work. As already mentioned, the Vedic descriptions of *soma* are so general that they cannot be used to prove or disprove his or any other hypothesis. Since no effective criteria have been established from the ṚgVeda, any probative evidence for the botanical identification of sauma must have its basis outside of that text.[5]

§9 Wasson attempted to find a plant that would provide a material basis for a widely assumed theory, namely, that the *soma* hymns of the Ninth Book of the ṚgVeda reflect direct experience of the drug, and that, as the hymns imply, *soma* was consumed in order to experience ecstasy, but that not long after the hymns were composed, the original plant ceased to be available, for which reason it was replaced in the ceremonies by nonintoxicating substitutes.[6] Rather than dwell upon the uncertainties of his conclusions,[7] it is important here to examine whether the underlying assumptions are adequately founded.

§10 One need not suppose that all the poets of the ṚgVeda had direct experience of sauma intoxication, for it appears that "*soma* intoxication" had become a fixed literary theme, a subject for elaboration by poets in verbal contests for many generations before the fixation of the Vedic texts. In the ṚgVeda *soma* is represented as an offering, made above all to Indra, who is said to depend upon it for his strength. The concept of the extract as an offering to be drunk by the gods, however, is not found in Iranian texts, and must have emerged in India at a time when the extract no longer had the purpose of intoxicating the priests who consumed it. Because an extensive mythology associated with this apparent rationalization of the ritual presence of *soma* had already developed, it may be supposed that the use of the intoxicating plant had vanished from the usual ceremonies long before the final fixation of the *Ṛksaṁhitā* as we have it.

§11 The ṚgVeda indicates *soma* regularly induced a state of ecstasy, which, again, is not verifiable from the Iranian materials for *haoma.* Even if we could be sure that the Vedic poets had personal experience of the effects of the drug, there is good reason to hesitate before assuming that those effects would be accurately described in hymns. If one were going to drink *soma* anyway, he might well pray that the result be beneficial, but simply because beneficial effects are alone mentioned in the Vedas does not establish that they were always or ever actually experienced. The *soma* hymns could be expected to extol sauma intoxication regardless of how it was usually experienced or the purpose for which the drug was taken.[8] As will be noted (§87), the effects attributed to *haoma* in the Avesta may have been intended to influence the outcome of consuming the drug and to encourage results which were not expected as a matter of course, and the same perspective may be applicable to the Vedic panegyrics to *soma.*

§12 It is also a ṚgVedic cliché that *soma* induced battle fury in Indra, so that it has been supposed (Bergaigne 1878:150; Lincoln 1981) that it must have been consumed for that effect by warriors. Without denying that sauma drinking may have had such potentialities, it may be said that if sauma reliably produced a state either of battle fury or of ecstasy, or of any subjective state valued *for its own sake,* then the ceremonies would have been essentially superfluous for achieving these objectives and the ceremonies would not likely have been everywhere the form chosen to represent the use of the drug. Moreover, if one assumes that sauma was drunk for these results, it cannot be expected that its consumption would have been confined to such ceremonies; it would surely have been drunk by many more people than only priests. Since such results would have remained valuable in later times as well, the consumption of the drug outside of, as well as within, the ceremonies should have continued to the present day. Because there is no clear evidence from India of sauma consumption outside of the ceremonies at any time and because, instead of sauma, nonintoxicating plants appear in present day rituals, it has been generally concluded that sauma must have become unavailable. Although

4 The recycling of ones own urine for therapeutic purposes in modern India, to which Wasson (1978: 222; 1979: 104) draws attention, appears to reflect the influence of the popular book *Human Urine, An Elixir of Life,* by Rajivbhai Manibhai Patel (1963), the precedent for whose self experiments with urine drinking came not from Indian tradition but from 20th century Arkansas.

5 Some association of Indian vernacular plant names with sauma are considered below (§§109 and 140). The significance of such names is generally ignored by Wasson, probably because Indo-Iranian vernacular names for species of mushrooms are without links to sauma. Even if the Santal name *putka,* which Wasson found to be the name for a puffball in Orissa, could derive from a Sanskrit word *pūtika,* meaning "stinking" (as Kramrisch [1975] proposes), this could be explained by the puffball's cadaverous stench and there would still be no grounds for believing that a plant called in Sanskrit *pūtika* 2000 years earlier was a mushroom (and that, therefore, the *soma* which the *pūtika* replaced [as an additive to the clay of a ritual pot] was a mushroom). At all events, Kuiper (1984) has now shown that the Santal term *putka* has no etymological connection with Sanskrit *pūtika,* and is thus irrelevant.

6 This theory seems to be an elaboration of the historically uncritical view of pious Brahmans that the Vedas reflect a golden age which ended when the gods withdrew from this wicked world, taking with them the source of divine ecstasy, the *soma* plant. There is no genuine evidence that the absence of the original *intoxicant* from the ceremonies necessarily results from a shortage of it.

7 For the various views, see Brough [1971a and 1971b] and the other articles and reviews listed in R. G. Wasson [1978 and 1979].

8 A further motive for priests claiming to find the experience agreeable may have been to show themselves as enjoying the approval of the gods (see below, §150). The "ecstasy" of *soma* may be an exaggeration, for in the Atharvaveda the remains of the sacrificial offering (4 34, 35) (and perhaps [at 11.1.25] the porridge [*odana*]) are said to produce ecstasy (Keith 1925: I, 275).

no reference to a shortage of the plant appears in the ṚgVeda or in Iranian sources of any date, it has been alleged as a criterion for its identification that sauma must be a plant not now obtainable in India or Iran. The question of how such a useful plant utterly vanished from the botanical repertory of whole nations who literally worshipped it has added considerably to the mystery of this subject.

§13 If the purpose of the ceremonial use of the plant was ecstasy, the natural response to an unavailability of sauma would have been to abandon the ceremonies rather than to reenact them using nonintoxicating substitutes. It cannot be supposed that a universal, spontaneous transition from using sauma to using substitute plants occurred as soon as the plant completely disappeared, nor can it be supposed, alternatively, that there was a unanimous and universal conspiracy of priests in both India and Iran to replace the missing sauma and, saying nothing publicly about the change, proceed as before. Considering only the geographical and linguistic problems this would entail, it is clear that nothing of this sort could have happened.

§14 Previous attempts to explain the absence of sauma seem not to have noted that its "replacement" in ceremonies with nonintoxicating plants should be of Proto-Indo-Iranian date. The mere simulation of drinking sauma extract is a common feature of all the relevant Indic and Iranian ceremonies. This continuation of ceremonies without the intoxicant essential to their ostensible purpose is too extraordinary an occurrance to have developed independently, rather ceremonies omitting the intoxicant must have already been practiced before the two peoples became separated. Consequently, if these merely imitative ceremonies came about because sauma was unavailable, it must have become unavailable at a time even antedating the earliest parts of the ṚgVeda, so that the ṚgVeda would be of no value as evidence for the unavailability of the plant. Iranian evidence for the continued use of the intoxicant into historic times (see next chapter) shows that the plant remained available and hence that its displacement from the ceremonies cannot have been caused by difficulties in its supply. Rather, it must be the case that from the earliest times ceremonies merely imitating the drinking of sauma existed side by side with ceremonies in which sauma was actually consumed.

§15 The Indian sources have not only failed to yield the botanical identity of sauma, but also have not provided satisfactory explanations for why the consumption of sauma took place in ceremonial contexts, nor for specific features of the sauma ceremonies such as the intimate association of sauma drinking with animal sacrifice. Nor has any hypothesis based on Indic materials plausibly accounted for the displacement of sauma in the rituals by other plants, for the particular plant species chosen to represent sauma, nor for why in the two distinct religious traditions, sauma rituals lacking the intoxicant became the central organizing principle.

§16 The present work differs from all previous studies in focusing not on Indian but on Iranian sources, which have hitherto received little or no attention in this connection. The Iranian testimony on sauma is by any reckoning at least as cogent as the Indian, and in light of the failure of the Indic materials to provide acceptable solutions, an investigation of the Iranian situation is the only viable alternative. The value of this approach will ultimately be judged on the merits of the solutions proposed below, but it is strongly supported by the considerations now to be detailed.

§17 Iranian data have precedence over those of India because sauma is to be placed in an Iranian, not Indian, geographical perspective. The use of sauma has been ascribed above to the Proto-Indo-Iranians, that is, the speakers of the reconstructable prehistoric ancestor of the Indic and Iranian languages. During the period of linguistic unity the Proto-Indo-Iranians clearly lived northwest of India. The disintegration of the Proto-Indo-Iranian unity culminated in the emigration of those groups that eventually became the Indo-Aryans. The vacuum left by their departure resulted in the expansion, in Central Asia and eventually Western Asia, of the people known in history as the Iranians.[9]

§18 There is every reason to believe that the use of sauma was developed by the speakers of Proto-Indo-Iranian while they were living somewhere within that area of Central Asia which from the beginning of recorded history has been predominantly Iranian in culture and, until the arrival of the Turks from the fifth century C. E. onwards, also Iranian in speech. The Greater Iranian cultural area (which should be understood wherever the term *Iran* is used geographically here) should therefore include the environment where sauma grew; thus sauma must have remained available at least to those Iranians who continued to occupy the lands of their ancestors. This cultural area is relatively homogeneous in climate and flora. Regardless of whether the same species of plant continued to be available also to the groups who migrated toward India, the social and economic adaptations required in the radically different environments to the south are likely to have had some effect on the ethnobotany of the migrating tribes. These factors will not have affected the environmental relationships of those people who remained in the Iranian area. Hence it is probable that there has been a continuity of Proto-Indo-Iranian and Iranian ethnobotanical traditions absent in India.

§19 It must not be assumed that because of its early date the ṚgVeda, as against the Avesta, more closely reflects the Proto-Indo-Iranian situation and therefore bears more directly on the problem of sauma. There is scholarly consensus that in general the Avesta is the more conservative text, that is, it more faithfully reflects archaic realia than does the ṚgVeda, which is prone to extensive poetic elaboration. The Vedas and the Avesta are products of a Proto-Indo-Iranian oral literature connected with sauma rites. Only when that tradition of oral composition began to decline in India and Iran did the hymns become fixed. In the case of the ṚgVedic hymns this occurred soon after the arrival of Aryan-speaking peoples in India (*c.* 1200 B.C.E.). In Iran the formation of that portion of the Avesta in the Gathic dialect spoken by Zarathushtra also dates from around the end of the second millinum B.C.E., the bulk of the Avesta, however, results from processes of oral transmission and composition that continued far longer and allowed for textual reflections of the actual ethnobotanic situation of sauma, as against the Indian situation of a long-ossified corpus, which is, moreover, largely poetic in its "recollection" of the plant. The Iranian *haoma* texts probably became fixed in their present form little earlier than the time of the Achaemenian Empire (i.e. sixth to fourth centuries B.C.E.).[10] The lateness of the Iranian materials indicates that productive oral composition persisted in Iran for perhaps a thousand years longer than it did in India and is evidence for the continuity of ancient traditions into historical times.

§20 This is the working definition of sauma used in the arguments

[9] While the precise location of the homeland of the Proto-Indo-Iranian-speaking peoples remains undetermined, it can confidently be surmised to have been somewhere within an area well defined by the topography of interior Eurasia. Given that their language was the southeasternmost branch of the Indo-European family and that their descendents occupy India and Iran, they must have lived in an area west of China, north of India, east of the civilizations of Mesopotamia (whose annals do not record their existence until marked linguistic differentiation had occurred), and south of the subarctic forests of Siberia. (Although it has sometimes been argued that at one time the speakers of Proto-Indo-Iranian occupied areas to the far north, it is certain that they were cattle-rearing herdsmen, and they could not have evolved such an economy living in Siberia.) These limits demarcate the Greater Iranian Area. (On the Indo-Iranian homeland, see further §112 n.6).

[10] The Iranian *haoma* hymns are in the Younger Avestan language, in which texts continued to be composed in the Hellenistic period, and perhaps even later. The *haoma* hymns do not show the grammatical degeneration of the latest Avestan texts and linguistically and stylistically give the impression of belonging to the older stratum of the later Avesta, but cannot be strictly dated.

which follow: a plant (1) regarded as intoxicating by the early Indo-Iranians and (2) available over the area occupied by Indo-Iranian peoples, which (3) was revered by these peoples as sacred and (4) was consumed in the central rites of their priests. The four parts of this definition serve as an organizing principle for the data presented below; they provide parameters which increasingly restrict the range of botanical alternatives to *Peganum harmala* as sauma.

2

PHARMACOLOGICAL CORRESPONDENCES

SAUMA INTOXICATION IN IRANIAN ACCOUNTS

§21 That the Avestan term *maδa-* (root *mad-*) meant 'intoxication' has been established on the basis of cognate words in Indic and in later Iranian languages, and the term's use in the Avesta to refer to both the effects of *haoma* and those of wine (see Spiegel 1883; Harlez 1883; Bartholomae 1883). In the surviving Avesta, however, elaboration of the experience to which *haoma* intoxication referred is limited to the following passages from *Yasna* 9-11 (i.e. the *Hōm Yasht*, see below, §78):[1]

***Yasna* 9.17:**

ni.tē zāire maδəm mruyē	O, Yellowish One, I call down thy intoxication.

***Y.* 10.8** (partially repeated in *Yasht* 17.5):

vīspe zī anyē maiδåŋhō	Indeed all other intoxications
aēšma hacinte xrvīm.drvō	are accompanied by Violence of the Bloody Club,
āaṯ hō yō haomahe maδō	but the intoxication of *Haoma*
aša hacaite urvāsmana	is accompanied by bliss-bringing Rightness.
rənjaiti haomahe maδō	The intoxication of *Haoma* goes lightly.

***Y.* 10.14:**

mā mē yaθa gaoš drafšō	May (thy intoxications), besetting me at their own
āsitō vārəma caire	impulse, not move me about as a cow's trembling.
fraša frayantu tē maδō	May thy intoxications come forth clear(ly).
vərəzyaŋuhåŋhō jasəntu	May they arrive bringing straightness of mind.
pairi.tē haoma ašāum ašavāzō	To thee, *Haoma*, righteous, promoting Rightness,
daδāmi imąm tanūm	do I give this body,
mē vaēnaite huraoδa	which seems to me well formed.

***Y.* 10.19:**

måsə tūmciṯ māvōya	May thee thyself, and may these
fraša frayantu tē maδō	thy intoxications come forth to me clear(ly).
raoxšna frayantu tē maδō	May thy intoxications come forth bright(ly).
*rənjyō +vazåinte *tē maδō*	May thy intoxications move lightly.

***Y.* 11.10:**

pairi.tē haoma ašāum ašavāzō	To thee, *Haoma*, righteous, driving forth Truth,
daδāmi īmąm tanūm	do I give this body,
yā mē vaēnaite huraoδa	which seems to me well-formed,
θwaxšāi +haomahe maδāi	for the active intoxication *of *Haoma*,
havaŋuhāi ašavastāi	for well being, for Rightness.
pairi.mē tūmciṯ dayå	May thou give me, righteous *dūraoša Haoma*,
haoma ašava dūraoša	the Best Existence of the righteous,
vahištəm ahūm ašaonąm	full of light, and having every comfort.
raocaŋhəm vīspō.x^{v}*āθrəm*	

[1] Avestan translations are by Schwartz and are discussed by him below, §§162–182.

§22 The sources for ancient Iranian religion preserved in Zoroastrianism include as well as the Avestan texts from the first millennium B.C.E., a literature in Middle Persian (Pahlavi) which reflects the Zoroastrianism of Sasanian Persia (*c.* 230-630 C.E.). By the time that the Sasanian clergy translated the Avesta into Pahlavi, the meaning the *haoma* texts seems to have become for them a matter of speculation, and the *Yasna* rite at which these texts were recited had come to be so exclusively performed using as *haoma,* not sauma, but a nonintoxicating plant, that the priests seem no longer to have been aware that the *haoma* (Middle Persian *hōm*) consumed in that ceremony had ever been an intoxicating drug. Their ignorance of this is revealed by the fact that the Avestan term *maδ(a)-* 'intoxication' is never correctly rendered in the Pahlavi translation of the above Avestan passages.[2]

§23 Most of the Sasanian Avesta is now lost. Pahlavi translations of much of it still existed in the ninth century, however, and served as the basis for a number of books then composed in Pahlavi by Zoroastrian priests in Fars. These Pahlavi books appear to contain descriptions of the effects of sauma; in these descriptions, however, sauma is not referred to by the name *hōm/haoma.* It seems that at the time these accounts were composed the term *hōm/haoma,* rather than continuing its original reference to sauma, had come simply to designate the *nonintoxicating* plant consumed in daily *Yasna* rites. Consequently, in order to refer to sauma in the Pahlavi texts recourse would have been necessary to terms other than *hōm/haoma.*

§24 The most explicit and detailed Iranian account of intoxication for religious purposes is the *Ardā Wīrāz Nāmag.* The prologue (Chapters 1-3) of this Pahlavi text says that in order to dispel doubts about the claims of the Iranian priests to religious knowledge, Wīrāz, having been selected as the most righteous of men, is given a drug before a public assembly, whereupon, lying tranquilly before the people, he has a vision of the fate of souls after death, which he afterwards dictates to a scribe. This prologue demonstrates the belief that pharmacologically induced visions were the means to religious knowledge and that they were at the basis of the religion that the Magi claimed to have received from Zoroaster. It has previously been supposed that the event described in this text was outside the tradition of the sauma ceremonies; its possible relevance to the question of sauma has therefore never been explored. It will consequently be necessary to show that, although the drug administered to Wīrāz is termed *mang,* it is the same substance as sauma. Here follows an abridgement of the opening chapters of the *Ardā Wīrāz Nāmag* as translated by W. Belardi (1979: 89-92):

> (I.2) And after that (there) were sedition and contention among people of the Iranian kingdom, and thus they had no king, no ruler, no chieftain, no theologian aware of the Religion, and concerning matter(s) of God they were doubtful. And doctrines of many kinds and different manners of faith, and skepticism and different legislations appeared in the world . . . . And several decisions and judgments were made (in conformity) with diverging doctrines and diverging faiths, and this Religion was in confusion and people in doubt.
>
> And afterwards (besides those) (there) were other Magians and theologians of the Religion; compared with those scoundrels (these) were submissive and sorrowful. And an assembly of them was summoned to the

[2] Avestan *maδa-* would have been correctly translated by Middle Persian *mastīh* 'intoxication' (e.g. in *Pahlavi Vendidad* 19.41). Instead, for the above cited Avestan passages the Pahlavi has *m'dšn'* (i.e. *māyišn* 'copulation', which gives little sense here), except in two cases: in *Yasna* 10.14 Avestan *maδō* is translated *mēnišn* 'thinking', and in *Yasna* 11.10 Avestan *maδāi* is not translated at all. See J. M. Unvala (1924: 28–29, 60), J. Darmesteter (1892–1893: I, 100, n.22), and B. N. Dhabhar (1949: Glossary 125). These Pahlavi forms are discussed below §§183–185.

temple of the victorious Farrbag Fire; and (there) were speeches and considerations of many kinds on this (subject). (They said) that "it is necessary for us to seek means in order that someone of us goes and brings information from the spirits, so that people who exist in this time will know whether these *yazišn* and *drōn* and *āfrīnagān* and *nērang* and ablution(s) and purification(s), which we bring (to God) according to (our) rite, attain to God or to the Devs, and come to help of our souls or not."

And afterwards, with the consent (coming) from the theologians of the Religion, they called all the people to the temple of the Farrbag Fire. And from the whole they separated seven men who were most undoubtful about God and the Religion and whose own thought(s) and speech(es) and deed(s) (were) most fit and righteous. And they said: "Sit down in your turn, and from (among) you choose one who (is) good for this enterprise, and most sinless and most renowned."

And afterwards these seven men sat down, and from (these) seven three (men) were chosen, and from (these) three one, named Wīrāz [was chosen] . . . .

And then this Wīrāz, as he heard that speech, stood upon (his) feet, and joined (his) hands on (his) breast and said: "If you please, then don't give me the *mang*[3] which I don't desire, until you, Mazdayasnians, cast lots for the trial. And if the lot comes to me, I'll willingly go to that place of the pious and the wicked (souls); and I'll exactly refer and truly bring this message."

And then the trial lots of these Mazdayasnians were drawn . . . [and] each of the three lots came to Wīrāz.

[II.1] And seven sisters were of this Wīrāz and all these seven sisters were as wives of Wīrāz . . . [they said]: "Don't make this thing, you Mazdayasnians . . . (if) you send (him) from this realm of the living to that of the dead before (the natural) time, a fulfillment of violence is made upon us without reason."

And afterwards the Mazdayasnians, when they heard these words, gave satisfaction to the seven sisters, and said: "We shall deliver Wīrāz to you within seven days, perfect in (his) body; and the glory of this journey will remain on this man." And then they became agreeing.

And afterwards this Wīrāz, before the Mazdayasnians, joined (his) hands on (his) breast and said to them: "It is of (our) custom that first I (have to) worship (the departed) souls, and eat food, and accomplish the prescription(s), then you will give me wine and *mang*." The theologians ordered: "Do it accordingly."

And afterwards these theologians of the Religion in the abode of the Spirit selected, for that good (man); a thirty-step (wide) place. And this Wīrāz washed (his) head and (his) body, and put on a new garment; perfumed (himself) with an agreeable perfume, spread a new, clean blanket on some appropriate boards. At a (given) moment (he) sat down on the clean blanket, and performed the (rite of the) *drōn,* and remembered (the departed) souls, and ate food. And afterwards the theologians of the Religion filled three golden cups with wine and with the Wishtāspian *mang,* and they gave one cup over to Wīrāz . . . and the second cup . . . and the third cup . . . . And he drank that wine and *mang* and consciously said grace and fell asleep on the blanket.

The theologians of the Religion and the seven sisters . . . chanted the Gathas and kept watch in the dark. . . . The seven sisters together with all theologians and herbads and mobads of the Religion of the Mazdayasnians did not in any manner neglect protection (to the body of Wīrāz).

[III] [The third chapter relates how Wīrāz arises, asks for and receives a meal as his due, and dictates his vision to a scribe.]

§25 In Wīrāz's vision, he arrives in the spirit world at the bridge over which the dead must pass, and because of his extraordinary righteousness is welcomed across it by two spirit guides who remain with him and interpret what he sees. For a while he beholds multitudes in splendor and enters into the presence of beings whom he is told are Ohrmazd and his entourage. Then there begins the spectacle of horror and violence that occupies the largest part of the narration. He perceives a vast territory filled with writhing bodies and sees in fine detail the terrifying circumstances of each: some ceaselessly being torn apart by demons, some crushed by snakes, and so forth. In each case his guides relate their torment to an infraction of the moral or ritual injunctions propounded by the Magi.

§26 It is not possible to determine the date of this text with much confidence. Although the extant version is not older than the ninth century C.E., there are reasons to believe it was originally composed somewhat before the third century establishment of the Sasanian state (Belardi 1979: 121). At all events, it was written at a time when it had apparently ceased to be understood that the Iranian ceremonies had once included the consumption of the drug sauma. Since one did not then think of *hōm/haoma* as a plant which produced visions, that term would not have been used for the drug in this text even if that drug was sauma. There is, however, little reason to expect that the Middle Persian word *mang* identified more precisely the substance given Wīrāz than as a "psychoactive drug." In the contexts in which *mang* occurs its sense is primarily pharmacological, not botanical, and there is no warrant to assume it to have named a specific plant.[4] The drug given Wīrāz was clearly an extract, and its identification by the term *mang* does not disqualify it as the sauma drug, which must surely have been included in the same pharmaceutical class as the extract which Wīrāz consumed.

§27 That this *mang* was indeed sauma can also be inferred from the circumstances of its administration to Wīrāz. This occurs at just that point in the recital of the *Yasna* liturgy appropriate for consuming sauma, that is, where the *Hōm Yasht* is now recited (see below, §133). Wīrāz sits before the fire, performs the *drōn* rite (see below, §§133 and 152), and has the *mang* handed him in three cups (corresponding to the three swallows of *haoma* in the *Yasna* preceeding recitation of the Gathas).

§28 The drug given Wīrāz is, moreover, not simply called *mang* but specifically the "*mang* of Wishtāsp". The latter is clearly linked with sauma in a ninth-century Pahlavi text, the *Dēnkird* (Book VII, 4.84-86), itself from a lost Avestan source, which tells how Kay Wishtāsp (Avestan Kavi Vištāspa) accepted Zoroaster's (i.e. Zarathushtra's) teaching. Here it

3 Belardi translates *mang* as 'narcotic'.

4 The fact that *bang,* while being the Pahlavi gloss of *mang,* also appears as a Persian name for henbane (*Hyoscamus*) in early Islamic pharmacognosy, does not necessarily mean that *mang* specified henbane in the context of Zoroastrian literature. As a loan word into Arabic, *banj* (with verbal forms) has been used of intoxicating plants in general and not exclusively of henbane (see Rosenthal 1971), while the use of Persian *bang* since at least the 13th century for both henbane and hashish implies its earlier reference to a general class of substances (as does also al-Bīrūnī's 11th-century use of *banj* for datura). Schwartz (below, §§198-222) shows that Avestan *banga-*, long supposed to be the etymon of Middle Persian *mang* and to have an extensive history as a Eurasian *"Wanderwört"* (see, e.g. Eliade 1972: 399-402; Crevatin 1983) was, in fact, never a name of a specific drug or plant.
Henning's (1951: 32-34) claim that the story indicates the *mang* given Wīrāz was a deadly poison and hence must have been henbane seems (as Belardi notes) directly opposed by the text itself, for Wīrāz's sisters *ask* if the drug will harm him and are assured it will have no ill effects. Wīrāz's behavior does not particularly suggest that he thought he was risking his life, and no motive is supplied for why he would have been willing to do so. It would certainly have won few converts to the cause of the Magi if Wīrāz had never regained consciousness, and the danger of a mishap would not have been lessened by selecting the most righteous of men to take the chance. If *mang* was thought to be potentially lethal to the righteous, it would have been disadvantageous to suggest that religious knowledge depended on its use, for this would discourage belief that the Magi easily and frequently put themselves in contact with the spiritual world.

is said Wishtāsp was given *hōm* and *mang*.[5] This was regarded as the most important single event in the legendary history of the Zoroastrian religion. In order to influence Kay Wishtāsp, Ohrmazd (Avestan Ahura Mazdah) sends three spirit beings to promise that ruler a life of 150 years and an immortal son, on condition that he accept Zoroaster into his court, and, if he refuses to do so, to tell him that he will be immediately destroyed (through being devoured in midair by birds). Although Wishtāsp still declines, the threat is not carried out. Instead, Ohrmazd decides to cause him to see displayed for him in the spiritual world the future benefits he can realize by accepting Zoroaster:

> . . . Also to visibly show Wishtāsp victory over Arjāsp and the Hyōnians, his own higher place and imperishable dominion, health and glory, Ohrmazd the creator sent at the same time to the residence of Wishtāsp the divinity Nērōsang as a messenger to the Ameshaspand Ashawahisht [Avestan *Aša- Vahišta* - 'Best Truth'] to cause Wishtāsp to consume the illuminating nourishment which would give his soul eye vision over the spiritual (*mēnōg*) existence, by reason of which Wishtāsp saw great mystery and glory. As it says in the Avesta: "Ohrmazd the creator said to the divinity Nērōsang: 'Go, fly on, notable member of the community Nērōsang, to the residence of Wishtāsp, rich in cattle, of wide renoun, and say this to Ashawahisht: "Powerful Ashawahisht, take the excellent bowl, more excellent than the other bowls which are well made (that is, that cup so excellent should be made in lordliness) for conveying for our sake *hōm* and *mang* to Wishtāsp and cause the lofty ruler Kay Wishtāsp to drink it."' Agreeing to these words, Ashawahisht took the excellent bowl and caused the lofty ruler Kay Wishtāsp to drink it and the lofty ruler Kay Wishtāsp lay down. When the lofty ruler Kay Wishtāsp came forth from (being) *stard*, he said to Hutōs [his wife and sister]: 'Let it be, Hutōs, that Zoroaster Spitāma come swiftly to me with zeal. (Let) Zoroaster Spitāma quickly expound to me the Religion (*dēn*) of Ohrmazd and Zoroaster.' "[6]

§29 In this account the drink causes Wishtāsp to see into *mēnōg* existence and to become *stard* (or *stird*). The parallel account in *Pahlavi Rivāyat* 140.6-10 relates: "When [Wishtāsp] drank, he became *stard* immediately, and they led his soul to paradise and showed him the value of accepting the Religion. When he emerged from *stard*-ness he called for Zoroaster . . . " (*ka-š xward būd pad gyāg stard būd u-šān ruwān be ō garōdmān nīd u-šān arzōmandīh ī dēn padīrift ān be nimūd ka az stardīh frāz būd a-š . . . wāng kard . . . Zarduxšt*). Etymologically *stard* or *stird* means 'spread out, sprawled'. It is used in Pahlavi to indicate the result of being stunned or dazed from a blow and, with few exceptions, is experienced by evil creatures; for example, demons become *stard* upon hearing Zoroaster recite the *Ahuna Vairya* prayer. Confirmation that the *Yasna* rite in which sauma was drunk was known to induce the *stard* condition is provided by a simile in *Yōišt ī Fryān* 2, 7-8: "As soon as the sorcerer Axt heard these words, he became as *stard* as when a man who performs a *Yasna* becomes *stard* (*ud Axt ī jādūg čiyōn ka-š ān az-iš āšnūd stard be būd čand ka mard ī yašt-ē be kunēd stard būd ēstēd* [Haug and West 1892: 212]).

§30 Fundamental to ancient Iranian religion was a belief in two existences, the material, tangible, visible existence (Avestan *gaēiθya-*, Middle Persian *gētīg* or *astōmand*) and the intangible, invisible, spirit existence (Avestan *mainyava-*, Middle Persian *mēnōg*), as was glimpsed by Wīrāz and Wishtāsp by means of sauma. This "spiritual" existence (for which see especially Shaked 1971) differs from the conception of the spiritual realm in other Near Eastern religions in being neither morally superior nor necessarily more sacred than the material world. Ohrmazd created the material world to assist him in defeating the Evil One in the spiritual world. He does not, however, create material existence directly, but first creates it in spiritual form. All material things and creatures exist simultaneously in spirit form. These spirit forms include the double or *frawahr* (Avestan *fravaši-*) of each person, living, dead and unborn. The overall appearance of this intangible, *mēnōg*, world may in many respects resemble the material world but in addition to the forms of all past present and future creatures of Ohrmazd, it encompases the pandemonium generated by the Evil Spirit. The creations of the Evil Spirit are not generally to be observed in the tangible world of ordinary experience but in essence have only *mēnōg* existence, although they may "borrow" material forms (such as reptiles and invertebrates, for all matter is the creation of Ohrmazd. Evil spirits pervade the intangible world (except of course within the confines of the "Best Existence" or heaven).[7]

§31 The consumption of sauma may have been the only means recognized in Iranian religion of seeing into *mēnōg* existence before death; at all events, it is the *only* means acknowledged in Zoroastrian literature and, as we have seen, is the means used by Ohrmazd when he wishes to to make the *mēnōg* existence visible to living persons. In ancient Iranian religion there is little evidence of concern with meditative practices which might foster development of alternative, nonpharmacological means to

5 Although this *Dēnkird* account (Madan 1911: 642.13f.; Nyberg 1964: 60.16) of the episode seems to have been directly translated from Avestan, the fact that Avestan *haoma-* could refer to the nonintoxicating routinely administered ritual drink may have motivated the addition of the word *mang* to indicate a drug with the capability of causing Wishtāsp to have an experience of the sort indicated. Somewhat later versions of the episode later texts omit the original word *haoma* altogether and describe the drink as "*mang* and wine" or "(*drōn*) wine". Thus, in the *Pahlavi Rivāyat* narration of the same incident (*Pahlavi Rivāyat* 140.6-10; see below, §29), Wishtāsp drinks *mang* in wine. In the account of the Persian *Zarādušt-Nāma* (ed. F. Rosenberg 1904) written in the 10th century C.E. (so dated by Rempis 1963:341) and in *Wizīrgird-ī Dēnīg* 19 (as transcribed by Molé 1967: 132-135), it is the wine of the *drōn* ceremony which is given to Wishtāsp: "On the day Māraspand [<Avestan *Mąθra- Spənta-* 'Sacred Mantra'] of the month Spandarmad [<Avestan *Spənta- Armaiti-* 'Sacred Obedience'] Zoroaster, with the help of the Lord Ohrmazd, spread *barsom* and performed the *drōn* rite. On [the occasion] of that *drōn* were placed things such as milk, a flower, wine, and pomegranate [*abār ān drōn čiyōn sir ud gul ud bādag ud anār nihād*]. He gave the wine to Wishtāsp so that he slept and saw the Best Existence". This provides an additional example of the practice, seen in the *Ardā Wirāz Nāmag*, of administering sauma at the *drōn* ceremony (i.e. after the recital of *Yasna* 8.4), rather than after the recital of the *Hōm Yasht* as in the full *Yasna* (see below, §133).

6 [*Dēnkird* VII 4.84; Madan 1911:642f.] . . . *wēnābdāg ī nimudan ī ō Wištāsp pērōzīh abar Arjāsp ud Hyōnān xwad-iš abardar gāh ud ašāzīsnīg xwadāyīh ud rāy ud xwarrah rāy frēstēd ī andar ham zamān Dādār Ohrmazd Nērōsang yazad ō mān ī Wištāsp pad aštagīh ō Ašawahišt Amahraspand xwārēnd ān ī ō Wištāsp pad ān gyān čašm pad abar wēnišnīh ī ō mēnōgān axwān rōšngar xwarišn kē rāy-iš dīd Wištāsp wazurg xwarrah ud rāz. 85. čiyōn ēd ī dēn gōwēd ku u-š ō Nērōsang yazad guft ku kē dādār Ohrmazd ku be raw, waz, Nērōsang hanjamanīg abar ō mān ī Wištāsp ī abzār gōspand dūr frāz nāmīg ud ēn gōwē ō Ašawahišt ku Ašawahišt +pādixšāy stānē tašt ī nēk ī abar nēktar az ān hutaštagān ī kard (ku jām ēdōn nēk pad xadāyīh sāyēd kardan) abar hōm ud mang amāh rāy barē ō Wištāsp u-š pad ān abar frāz xwārēn dahibed burzāwand Kay Wištāsp ī-š ī ōy gōwišn padīrift Ašawahišt ī pādixšāy u-š stān tašt ī nēk u-š pad ān frāz xwarēnēd dahibed burzāwand Kay Wištāsp ud nibast* [Widengren 1979: 348-350, following Nyberg 1974: 184b, in place of *nibast*, reads *šast nasāi* 'lay down, a corpse.' However, a corpse being a locus of evil according to Magian conventions, it is highly unlikely that Wishtāsp's body would have been abandoned to that state so casually, for in the very next sentence he is indicated not to have died but only become *stard*. As Molé saw, the letters *dyh* which appear before *dahibed* are dittography.] *dahibed burzāwand Kay Wištāsp ka +az stard frāz būd u-š ō Hutōs ē guft ku bawēd Hutōs kē Spitāmān Zarduxšt tēz ō man be ēd rasēd pad tuxšāgīh Spitāmān Zarduxšt tēz ō man ē nigēzēd dēn ī Ohrmazd ud Zarduxšt.*

7 Confusion could presumably result among such multitudinous forms, for instance, when Zoroaster first beheld the divine beings (*Ameshaspands*) he thought they were demons (*Epistles of Manuščihr* I. 10.9; West 1882: 319; Kanga 1985).

such vision. In Iran, vision into the spirit world was not thought to come about simply by divine grace nor as a reward for saintliness. From the apparent role of sauma in initiation rites (see Chapter 6), experience of the effects of sauma, which is to say vision of *mēnōg* existence, must have at one time been required of all priests (or the shamans antecedent to them). Since sauma was the means by which Ohrmazd brought such vision to Zoroaster's champion, Wishtāsp, there is no reason to doubt that sauma would also have been the means whereby Zoroaster (who as a *zaotar* consumed sauma in *Yasna* rites) also saw into *mēnōg* existence and drew from it his knowledge of Ohrmazd and his revelation.

§32 The Pahlavi epitomes of the lost Avestan biography of Zoroaster include allusions to *hōm* (*haoma*) which suggest that that substance was of great importance in the Avestan account of his prophetic mission. For instance, Zoroaster is reported in Pahlavi books to have been created within a twig of *hōm* (see below, §54 n.13) and to have been born as a result of his parents' consumption of an extract of that twig (*Dēnkird* VII 2.25-31; see below, §93).[8] Elsewhere (*Zātsparam* 4.14-16), the *frawahr* 'spirit form' of Zoroaster is said to reside in *hōm*. In the Avestan *Yasna* liturgy Zoroaster is said to come to the drinker of *haoma* (*Yasna* 8.1) and Zoroaster is also said to have been granted as a son to Pourushāspa as a reward for the latter's preparation of *haoma* (*Yasna* 9.13, see below, §92). The Pahlavi biographies say Zoroaster's initial revelation occurred in connection with his entering a river for (or of) *hōm* water (*Zātsparam* 21; *Dēnkird* VII, 3.51), but do not further elaborate the means by which he came to see the other world. The Pahlavi texts, however, were completed only in the predominantly Muslim setting of ninth century Fars, and at that time, because of the vulnerability of the Zoroastrians to criticism by Muslims and their tenuous status as a "People of the Book," the Zoroastrian priests who wrote them may have deemed it imprudent for canonical works to explicitly stress intoxication by sauma as a source of religious belief. A similar defensiveness may be the reason for the entire absence from the Pahlavi sources of explicit acknowledgement that intoxication was *ever* involved in Zoroastrian ceremonies and that it was intoxication to which the ritual consumption of *hōm* referred, though it is also likely that by the ninth century few Zoroastrian priests themselves could still have been aware of the intoxicating property characterizing the Avestan *haoma*.

§33 One Pahlavi account, however, exists which describes how Zoroaster came to confer with Ohrmazd and indicates that in the original Avestan his revelation was indeed said to have occurred through *haoma*. The account is part of an introduction to the *Zand ī Wahman Yasht*, a ninth-century apocalypse. This introduction seems to have been a secondary addition to the text because it describes Ohrmazd interpreting Zoroaster's dream of a tree with branches of seven metals, a role which is rather uncharacteristic for Ohrmazd and has evidently been derived from the Biblical Book of Daniel.[9] Before the episode of this dream, the introduction describes a situation (very similar to the events in the *Ardā Wīrāz Nāmag*) in which Zoroaster, during a sleep of seven days brought about by Ohrmazd's administration to him of "liquid omniscient wisdom," sees the condition of the righteous and the unrighteous in the other world. Since, according to the Pahlavi summary of the lost Avestan *Waršt-mānsr Nask*, "omniscient wisdom was produced for Zoroaster through *hōm*,"[10] the "liquid omniscient wisdom" here apparently refers to sauma. There seems to be no plausible explanation for the attachment of this introduction to the *Zand ī Wahman Yasht* except as an attempt to give to that text the appearance of having come from an Avestan source. The formal feature adopted, namely, the sequence of having Ohrmazd administer sauma to Zoroaster, who then perceives the state of things in *mēnōg* existence, indicates that texts of Avestan origin must have existed at the time this introduction was created which presented a similar origin for the revelation of Zoroaster. The passage in question (*Zand ī Wahman Yasht* III, 6-22) reads:[11]

> (6) Ohrmazd the Sacred [*abzōnīg*= Avestan *spəṇta-*] Spirit, creator of the righteous corporeal existence, took the hand of Zoroaster and put liquid omniscient wisdom into it, and said "drink it." (7) And Zoroaster drank it and omniscient wisdom was mixed into Zoroaster. (8) Zoroaster was within the wisdom of Ohrmazd for seven days and nights. (9) Zoroaster saw in the seven earthly continents men and useful animals: how many individual hairs, one by one, which they had from the back to the head. (10) He saw shrubs and trees—how many were the roots of plants in Spandarmad the earth, that is, how many had grown, had become mixed (therein). (11) On the seventh day omniscient wisdom was taken back from Zoroaster. (12) Zoroaster reflected: "I saw (something) in the pleasant Ohrmazd-created dream; I have not yet recovered from the dream." (13) He raised both hands and repeatedly rubbed his own form. "From the end of the time I slept I have not (yet) recovered from this pleasant Ohrmazd-created dream." (14) Ohrmazd said to Zoroaster Spitāma: "What did you see in the pleasant Ohrmazd created-dream?" (15) Zoroaster said: "Sacred Spirit Ohrmazd, creator of the corporeal world, I have seen a wealthy (person) of much property who was notorious in body and of contemptible *soul-form and he was in hell; (he) did not seem exalted to me. (16) I saw a poor (person) who, out of necessity, had not property but a fat soul in heaven; (he) seemed exalted to me. (17)

8 According to the *Dādistān-ī Dēnīg* (48.14 [*K35* 165*v*.15-17]) 'Through *haoma* the world is occupied by creatures. By means of *haoma* Zoroaster was created': *hōm ān-iš gēhān dāmānōmand hōm kē-š dahišn ī Zarduxšt abar būd.*

9 The "mixed iron" of the seventh branch of Zoroaster's tree is parallel with the iron mixed with clay at the foot of the statue in Nebuchadnezzar's dream, which, through Daniel, God interprets as representing the Ages to Come. As Jacques Duchesne-Guillemin (1982) has brought to light, "mixed iron" must have arrived in the Iranian text from *Daniel* 4, for the technique of casting large statues in second century B.C.E. Mesopotamia resulted in the mixing of iron and clay as a permanent part of the base of the statue, whereas from the perspective of the Iranian tradition there is no explanation for the presence of "mixed iron" in the prophecy at all (the parallel is not explained by Boyce's [1984] suggestion that the mixed iron could have referred to iron ore, which, at all events, is without metallic properties).

10 *Dēnkird* IX.36 (Madan 1911: 851.1) *u-š mad ān ī hōm urwāhmanīh nimāyišn ud sagrīh u-š mad xrad ī harwisp āgāhīh* 'and to [Zoroaster] came the *haoma* joy-revelation and satiation of *haoma* and omniscient wisdom came to him'.

11 *Zand ī Wahman Yasht* III, 6-22: *u-š ān ī Zarduxšt dast frāz grift u-š Ohrmazd mēnōg abzōnīg dādār ī gēhān astōmandīh ahlaw u-š xrad ī harwisp āgāhīh pad āb kirb abar dast ī Zarduxšt kard (7) u-š frāz xward u-š xrad ī harwisp āgāhīh pad Zarduxšt andar gumēxt. (8) 7 rōz šabān Zarduxšt andar Ohrmazd xradīh būd. (9) u-š be dīd Zarduxšt pad haft kišwar zamīg mardōmān gōspandān ku harw yak mōy čand pad pušt tāg tāg sar ō ku dārēd. (10) u-š be dīd ud dar ud draxt kē čē čand rēšag ī urwarān pad Spandārmad zamīg ku čand rust ēstēd ku gumēxt ēstēd. (11) u-š haftom rōz šabān xrad ī harwisp +āgāhīh az Zarduxšt abāz stad. (12) Zarduxšt pad ēd dast ku pad xwamn ī xwaš ī Ohrmazd dād dīd az xwamn nē winnārd hōm. (13) u-š harw 2 dast burd ān ī xwēš kirb abāz mālīd ku sar zamān xuft ēstōm nē winnārd hōm az ēn xwāb ī xwaš ī Ohrmazd dād. (14) guft-aš Ohrmazd ō Spitāmān Zarduxšt ku-t čē dīd pad xwāb ī xwaš ī Ohrmazd dād. (15) guft-aš Zarduxšt ku Ohrmazd mēnōg ī abzōnīg dādār ī gēhān ī astōmandān dīd hom hangad ī was xwāstag kē pad tan dušraw ud +ruwān-kirb* [In MS DH. »σ̆, in K20. »σ♀ for ̑σ̆, cf. *ruwān kirb* at Madan 1911: 647.16] *nizār ud pad dušōx būd a-m nē burzišnīg sahist. (16) a-m dīd driyōš ī nēst xīr ī ačārag u-š ruwān frabīh pad wahišt a-m burzišnīg sahist. (17) a-m dīd tuwānīg nēst frazand a-m nē burzišnīg sahist. (18) a-m dīd skōh ī was frazand a-m burzišnīg sahist. (19) a-m dīd draxt-ē kē 7 azg padiš būd yak zarrēn yak asēm yak rōyēn ud yak brinjēn yak arzīzēn yak pōlāwadēn yak āhan čē gumixt ēstēd. (20) guft-iš Ohrmazd ku Spitāmān Zarduxšt ēn ān ī ō pēš gōwam. (21) draxt ī bun ī tō dīd ān gētīg hast ī man Ohrmazd dād. (22) ān 7 azg ī tō dīd ān 7 āwām hast ī rasīd.*

I saw a childless, powerful person and he did not seem exalted to me. (18) I saw a humble (person) with many offspring; (he) seemed exalted to me. (19) I saw a tree with seven branches on it, one gold, one silver, one copper, one brass, one lead, one steel and one mixed iron". (20) Ohrmazd said to Zoroaster Spitāma: "This is what I prophesy: (21) The archetypal tree which you saw is the material existence which I, Ohrmazd, created. (22) Those seven branches which you saw are the seven ages which have come."

§34 To summarize, the three Pahlavi accounts are consistent in showing that sauma brought about a condition outwardly resembling sleep (i.e, *stard*) in which targeted visions of what is believed to be a spirit existence were seen. Essentially consistent with these accounts is a passage found in two stone inscriptions written in Fars about 300 C.E. by Kirdīr, the founder of the Sasanian Zoroastrian ecclesiastical establishment. In the analyses of Back (1978), Brunner (1974), Gignoux (1979; 1981; 1984), and Skjærvə (1985), Kirdīr's inscription asserts in this passage, as a basis of his claim to religious authority, that his spirit double visited the other world and was shown heaven and hell. The account thus parallels the *Ardā Wīrāz Nāmag* in reaffirming the reliance placed on a vision of *mēnōg* existence as the means to religious truth. Kirdīr does not say how his vision came about, perhaps because it would have been unsuitable to the political purposes of his inscription, but the precedents we have examined point to the possibility that he would have resorted to the same means used by Zoroaster and Wishtāsp; that is, sauma.

Harmel Intoxication

§35 As is well known to researchers, there are significant differences in the patterns of effects of psychotropic ("hallucinogenic") drugs of different composition. The salient features of the ancient Iranian religio-metaphysical outlook which cannot clearly be attributed to the Indo-European background may be regarded as conditioned by the particular effects of sauma upon a tradition developed over many generations of Iranian priests in the greater Iranian area. The Pahlavi accounts show that sauma brought about a condition outwardly resembling sleep (i.e. *stard*) in which visions of what was believed to be a spirit existence were seen. They also show that the experience of sauma was the source of revelation in Iranian religion. In order to decide if sauma could have been harmel it is necessary to examine what evidence there is that the consumption of harmel could have led to the experiences reflected for sauma in the Iranian religious data.

§36 To directly compare the psychopharmacology of *Peganum harmala* with that of sauma, however, involves a methodological difficulty. Our data for the experience for which sauma was valued in Iran are extrapolated from Zoroastrian Middle Persian texts which, although only compiled in the ninth century C.E., reproduce demonstrably older material, much of it taken directly from lost Avestan soures. These texts reveal aspects of a cultural-religious matrix which gave shape and content to the subjective effects of sauma and took shape and content from those effects, and which prevailed when sauma was in actual use. This matrix seems to have altogether disintegrated with the Islamic conquest of Iran in the seventh century C.E. As a result of the collapse of this matrix, one cannot expect to find significant use of sauma as an intoxicant in Iran today, and indeed one does not find *Peganum harmala,* nor any psychotropic plant, regarded as a source of authentic knowledge in Iran during Islamic times. The subjective experiences of modern Westerners who would consume the drugs of harmel can have but limited relevance, in lack of a traditional context giving form and meaning to the experience. Zoroastrians of today, far from the ancient mythological world of their ancestors, after centuries of influence of Islam, Christianity, and finally modernism, not at all associating their faith with intoxication, would hardly yield suitable testimony or be willing to undergo the frequently harrowing effects of drugs such as these.

§37 What is called for is evidence from another people, one whose culture has arisen, like that of archaic Iran, alongside the same psychoactive drug. Here would be sought parallels to what has been found for ancient Iran as regards the way the drug is used and the belief system it helped shape. Precisely such a situation exists in the upper Amazon and contiguous areas of northwestern South America, where native peoples extract the same psychoactive alkaloids as contained in *Peganum harmala*, the β-carbolines harmine, harmaline, and tetrahydroharmine, from *Banisteriopsis caapi,* a malpighiaceous vine found throughout this region.

§38 *Banisteriopsis caapi* is consumed by perhaps fifty tribes and groups (Friedberg 1965) under the name *yagé* (or *caapi, ayahuasca, natemä, xuma, jauma,* etc.).[12] The *Banisteriopsis caapi* is usually not consumed alone but with the addition of other plants. Frequently these additives, which are said to intensify the *yagé*'s effects (Rivier and Lindgren 1972; Schultes 1957 and 1982; Pinkley 1969), are plants containing another alkaloid, N,N,dimethyltryptamine. The degree to which the presence of these and perhaps other additive plants alters the effect of *yagé* has not yet been established, but may be considerable (McKenna *et al.* 1984a and 1984b). Nevertheless, because *yagé* seems always to be based on an infusion of *Banisteriopsis caapi,* and in some cases apparently consists only of that species, it seems justifiable to regard the psycho-pharmacological data on *yagé* as chiefly reflecting the properties of the harmala alkaloids.

§39 Close relationship has also been reported by Dr. Claudio Naranjo between the effects of *yagé* on shamans in Amazonia and the effects of pure harmaline, which he administered to urban volunteers in Chile. The following are some of his observations on the subjective effects of *yagé* and of harmaline, drawn from notes which he has kindly made available to me.

> The "visions" are frequently called "dreams," and rightly so, for these do not constitute true hallucinations, but vivid imagery contemplated with closed eyes. Usually the "dreaming" individual lies still—so much that among the Jivaro, for instance, the special individual huts where the person who has taken *yagé* goes are called "*sonaderos*" 'dreaming places.' There are exceptions to the immobility of the "dreamer," however. The effect of *yagé* is that of making oneiric activity possible while awake, so that the person may choose to move or engage in specific actions and still contemplate his visions. The typical instance is that of the shaman, who may sing of his visions while still in contact with a reality other than that of wakeful consciousness.
>
> *Yagé* is used chiefly by shamans, even in the case of tribes where it is also used by nonshamans, the individual's initiation to the drug is under a shaman's direction. Shamans are persons generally distinguished by exceptional capacity for experiencing the supernatural, which they do through *yagé.* The experiences for which the drug is valued are not, however, immediately available even to those who eventually become shamans. Shamans assert they must learn to use *yagé* and that initially their visions may be incoherent or of threatening monsters. During initiation as a shaman the novice may drink *yagé* for many consecutive days until he is able to learn from nature and the spirits and see the visions his guide considers necessary and meet and ally himself with at least one spirit guide. The power of shamans is dependent on such guides.

12 *(Oni) xuma* in Amahuaca means '(visionary) extract' (Lamb 1975 [who does not clarify the phonetic value of "*x*"]); *jauma* (pronounced "hauma") designates the *Banisteriopsis* preparation among Guarani Indians of Amazonas medio (P. Naranjo 1983: 97; R. Karsten 1964:95). An etymological connection with Iranian **hauma-* is, of course, impossible. Luna (1986: 171-173) lists these and over 40 additional local names.

While the common man experiences terror, the shaman is at home with the beings *yagé* reveals to him. It may have taken him months or years to reach the depths of hell or the heights of heaven, but once he has done so, these doors are open to him, he will need only a short time now, with the help of *yagé* to travel from one world to another there to meet the spirits he must contact and summon to his aid. Fully initiated shamans continue to take *yagé* for healing, initiations, presiding over festivities, prophesying and making decisions and before hunting and battle. In the latter connection, *yagé* is taken for a function that transcends mere practicality: that of ascertaining that men are acting in accordance with cosmic laws, the will of the gods, or the balance of nature. In a situation as delicate as that of taking the life of other beings, it is quite understandable that men should seek supernatural confirmation for the rightness of their action.

A second use, in small quantities, seems to be that of a stimulant. Hunter and warrior alike may chew stems of *Banisteriopsis* on their way to the site of action in order to see better.

It has sometimes been reported that the drinking of *yagé* is immediately followed by a frenzy of aggressive behavior. Since, however, about half an hour is required for the absorption of the drug, the exhibition of frenzy may manifest the individuals summoning up a feeling that his tradition prescribes as the desirable attitude in which to place oneself before the onset of the drug's effect. This is an attitude of courage in confrontation with the demonic presences by which he may see himself surrounded. Beyond this there lurks in the experience of the drinker the confrontation of destiny as a psychological, rather than physical, reality. Sometimes death itself is personified. At others, the agents of death—the spirits of disease—threaten the initiate; still, at other times he may feel that he is about to be devoured by fierce animals. In all such instances he must not be afraid. If he can do this, he will be transformed by his experience. I have little doubt that the confrontation of death, or an intensified awareness of mortality, is a salient trait of the typical *yagé* experience. If this is so, we should think of *yagé* as an ordeal in itself.

Among non-Indians to whom I have administered the *Banisteriopsis* alkaloids, the almost universal reaction is that of lying flat with eyes closed. Only a few subjects have felt enough energy to sit up or move, or have had enough interest in contacting their environment. Yet there appears to be a relationship between the individual's physical well being, the amount of movement displayed, and the quality of his visionary experience. The same individuals who felt at ease in this reality—being able to walk, write or talk with comfort—were those who felt at ease in their visions, these not being nightmares but beautiful scenes. More specifically, the difference between the two lies not in the content of visions, but in the affective component in them, and the role played in them by the beings imagined. The individual who lies in a drowsy state and feels the most physical discomfort and nausea is the same one who visualizes the tiger as an attacker or the snake as a repulsive creature. The person who feels physical comfort and enjoys movement is generally the same one who visualizes the tiger as a friend or the snake as a guide.

I think that the most pervasive "harmaline themes" may be regarded as abstract emotion in the same sense that the content of music is. Specific images contribute different combinations of these abstract emotions or elemental experimental ingredients in the same manner that musical chords are formed by musical notes.

§40 *Yagé* seems generally to be taken in a formal ceremony, such as is described below by G. Reichel-Dolmatoff (1978:11–14), who has studied the use of *Banisteriopsis caapi* by the Tukano Indians of Colombia over a period of many years:

The amount and quality of light are said to influence the sensitiveness of the participants who occasionally should stare for a while into the red glow of the torch or of a hearth fire . . . . Finally, acoustical stimulation is said to be of importance. The sudden sounds . . . are said to release or to modify the luminous images that appear in the field of view after a few drinks of the narcotic potion. As a matter of fact, the entire ritual is orchestrated, so to say, in a very complex fashion, and no sounds, movements, or light effects are quite arbitrary occurences, but obey an overall plan of well-defined and predetermined sensory signals.

Shamans and elders play an important part in these rituals, serving as guides and commentators once the participants begin to feel bewildered by the maze of disquieting visions. They explain and exhort, reciting fragments of myths or of songs, and thus constitute an ever present and most reassuring element of guidance and council in the midsts of, what can be celestial, or nightmarish, visions.

According to the Indians the drug experience can be divided into three stages. In the first stage, after some violent bodily reactions such as vomiting, diarrhea, and profuse perspiration, the person will feel like flying upward through the air toward the Milky Way, and will perceive, with half-closed or completely closed eyes, an increasing number of luminous sensations. After a series of brilliant yellow flashes dancing dots will appear, soon to be replaced by a multitude of small luminous images that seem to float in space and now begin to change their shapes and colors in kaleidoscopic fashion.

The onset of the second stage is marked by the gradual disappearance of the symmetric light patterns and by the slow formation of larger images of irregular shapes. Now the ecstatic flight takes the person beyond the Milky Way and before him begin to unfold dimensions that offer visions of dreamlike scenes that overwhelm the beholder. Three-dimensional forms, like rolling clouds, begin to fill the visual field and slowly turn into multicolored, recognizable shapes of people, animals, and monsters. In visualizing these figures the explanations of the shamans or the old men are of importance because they constitute an element of imprinting which stabilizes similar visions on future occasions. The Indians see in these visions mythological scenes full of profound significance to the viewer who watches them with apprehension while becoming more and more emotionally involved in trying to interpret the changing images. People say that they can see the Sun-Father and his daughter, the Snake-Canoe of the Creation Myth, the Master of Animals, Thunder-Person, jaguar-spirits and other supernatural beings and that these appear to reenact the Creation. Thus the beholder is present at the construction of the first *maloca* [cult lodge], the execution of the first dance, or the introduction of the musical instruments. But there also appear monstrous animals and menacing shadows in weird shapes. The game animals crowd the scene and—speaking a language that can be understood by humans—clamor for justice and accuse the hunters of killing too many of them.

It is said that the individual "dies" when he drinks the potion and that now his spirit returns to the uterine regions of the Beyond, only to be reborn there and to return to his ordinary existence on this earth when the trance is over . . . . Once inside the womb and, as the Tukano say, "beyond the Milky Way," the person believes he is able to see all the preternatural entities of Creation, to hear their voices, see their brilliant regalia, and what is more, witness them act out the principal scenes of the Creation of the Universe. They will reenact the Creation, or, rather, the beholder will have returned in time to witness the original creation, and so he will be able to see the birth of plant and animal life, the beginning of the institution of the *yarupari* ritual, the establishment of the *yagé* trance, and any other event mentioned in myth and tradition.

But not all the visions are as rewarding as these; sometimes the images are blurred and the person perceives only huge shapeless masses of color moving vaguely in space. And sometimes these shapes will turn into terrifying monsters, into jaguars and serpents that approach and threaten to devour the person, who, terror stricken, will call out in anguish. The beatific vision of the beyond is not achieved by all, but those who have had a glimpse of its peaceful radiance, will tell of its wonders and will yearn to see it again and again. But others will be horrified by the dangers that seem to threaten them, and will be deeply disturbed by the visions.

> There are many other occasions when a man might drink *yagé* for some personal reason and shamans are, of course, frequent consumers of narcotic drugs in various forms. The main objective of entering in a trance is, after all, the acquisition of knowledge, a knowledge that is expected to exist in the Otherworld and that people try to obtain from the supernatural beings.

This knowledge includes, according to Reichel-Dolmatoff (1975: 191–192), awareness of spirit beings who are:

> in every aspect, the exact doubles of every man and woman . . . . The idea of the double is fundamental to many Tukano concepts . . . . There is . . ."another world" matching in detail our world of empirical reality, and between these two "worlds" there is thought to exist a thin shell, an invisible wall which can be penetrated only in a hallucinatory trance. Under the influence of *viho* or *yagé* people say they have visited this other dimension and have seen its inhabitants . . . behaving just like ordinary people in this world.

§41 The use of *yagé* among the more aggressive and individualistic Jivaro of eastern Peru is somewhat differently oriented in Harner's (1968) description:

> The Jivaro Indians of the Ecuadorian Amazon believe that witchcraft is the cause of the vast majority of illness and nonviolent deaths. The normal waking life, for the Jivaro, is simply a "lie," or illusion, while the true forces that determine daily events are supernatural and can only be seen and manipulated with the aid of hallucinogenic drugs. A reality view of this kind creates a particularly strong demand for specialists who can cross over into the supernatural world at will to deal with the forces that influence and even determine the events of the waking life.
>
> The specialists, called "shamans" by anthropologists, are recognized by the Jivaro as being of two types: bewitching shamans and curing shamans. Both kinds take a hallucinogenic drink, whose Jivaro name is *natemä*, in order to enter the supernatural world . . . . When I first undertook research among the Jivaro in 1956-1957, I did not fully appreciate the psychological impact of the *Banisteriopsis* drink upon the native view of reality, but in 1961 I had occasion to drink the hallucinogen in the course of field work with another Upper Amazon Basin tribe. For several hours after drinking the brew, I found myself, although awake, in a world literally beyond my wildest dreams. I met bird-headed people, as well as dragon-like creatures who explained that they were the true gods of this world. I enlisted the services of other spirit helpers in attempting to fly through the far reaches of the Galaxy. Transported into a trance where the supernatural seemed natural, I realized that anthropologists, including myself, had profoundly underestimated the importance of the drug in affecting native ideology. Therefore, in 1964 I returned to the Jivaro to give particular attention to the drug's use by the Jivaro shaman . . . .
>
> The use of the hallucinogenic [*yagé*] among the Jivaro makes it possible for almost anyone to achieve the trance state essential for the practice of shamanism. Given the presence of the drug and the felt need to contact the "real," or supernatural, world, it is not surprising that approximately one out of every four Jivaro men is a shaman.

§42 There are parallels in the intoxicant use of sauma in ancient Iran and of *Banisteriopsis* by the Amazonian Indians which show the alkaloids of *Banis-teriopsis*/harmel to be suited to purposes similar to those for which sauma was used. In both cases the plant is consumed under the supervison of specialists (who are the shamans/priests) in ceremonies performed for initiations and in connection with the killing of animals for food, and characterized by the chanting of selected songs before a fire. There is also to be considered, however, the more unusual parallelism in beliefs about the spiritual world with which the use of sauma and *Banisteriopsis* are associated. In both ancient Iran and among the Amazonians the plants consumed in their respective ceremonies are thought to reveal spiritual worlds containing mythological and historical events, heaven and hell, and the precise counterparts of past, present and future entities and events known in the empirical world. The conception of the spiritual world in ancient Iran seems to have been of a superior reality occupied by good and evil spirits and also by spirit forms of all material entities. These relatively unusual ideas are similar to Tukano Indian conceptions, although there is no possibility of a transmission of beliefs between Iran and the Colombian Amazon. These parallel constellations of views of the supernatural must therefore be independent developments, and explanation must be sought in some factor common to both societies. For the Tukano, these conceptions of the spiritual world can be regarded as an outcome of numerous generations of study and interpretation of experiences of the psychopharmacology of the harmala alkaloids, visions induced by which may have the quality of dreams experienced in the waking state (C. Naranjo 1967). Like the dreams of sleep, the visions are experienced as real, but when the eyes are opened, there is no distortion of ordinary vision and, though the visions are sometimes superimposed, there is little confusion between what is visionary and what is tangible reality. It is apparent from the description of the Tukano's "going beyond the Milky Way" that the visions not only seem real, but that those seeing them believe that their content is witnessed by many people, thus giving consensual validity to their reality, while witnessing the simultaneous existence of forms identical to those encountered in ordinary reality inspires a concept of spirit doubles. Since these specific aspects of Tukano beliefs have their basis in the subjective effects of the harmala alkaloids, it follows that the development of parallel beliefs in ancient Iran could have resulted from consumption as sauma of these same alkaloids, obtained from *Peganum harmala.*

3

HISTORICAL AND GEOGRAPHICAL AVAILABILITY OF HARMEL

IRANIAN AWARENESS OF THE PROPERTIES OF HARMEL

§43 Since the ancient Iranians believed in the reality of a spirit world and the need to obtain information regarding it, the fact that harmaline offers a means to see such a world suggests that if they had been aware of the pharmacological potential of *Peganum harmala* they would have made use of it for that purpose. In this chapter we shall see that the availability and conspicuousness of *Peganum harmala* as a drug make it unlikely that it escaped the attention of the ancient Iranians. In Iranian folk medicine today harmel is recognized as having psychotropic properties; to swallow an infusion of the seeds is believed to produce madness.[1] The intoxicating

[1] An extract made by boiling harmel in vinegar is still used for toothache in central Iran. Dr. Mahmoud Omidsalar tells me that his great aunt related to him that once in her childhood she was administered this medication and accidentally swallowed it despite warnings that doing so would lead to madness. She recalled that she "saw everything moving in front of her and beheld wells in the earth." Though she could understand, she was herself unable to

properties of the plant are recognized in its vernacular names among neighboring peoples, such as Arabic *mogannana* (Ducros 1930) 'that which makes mad' and Turkish *mahmur çiç[egi]* (Bedevian 1936) 'dreamy flower'. Evidence for what plants were anciently classed as intoxicants is not directly available because no pre-Islamic Iranian writings on pharmacognosy survive. Early Iranian ethnopharmacology was apparently well developed, however, and contributed much to Islamic knowledge of drugs. Intoxication is recognized as an effect of harmel by some of the earliest Islamic pharmacological writers, for example, Abū Jurayj (*c.* 900 C.E.) in Abū Bakr M. ibn Zakariyā' al-Rāzī's *Kitāb al-Ḥāwī fī al-ṭibb* (*Rhazes' Liber Continens*) (Hyderabad 1967:20, 326), and authorities quoted by Ibn Bayṭār (see below) say *Peganum harmala* "intoxicates like wine" (cf. Avestan *maδa-* used for the intoxication of both *haoma* and wine). This may reflect ancient Iranian views about the plant, since the power to intoxicate is not mentioned for harmel by Dioscurides (*c.* 78 C.E.) or Galen (*c.* 180 C.E.), the Greek authors whose works, translated into Arabic about 850 C.E., provided the core of systematic Islamic pharmacology.

§44 The most extensive compendium of Islamic pharmacological knowledge is the *Kitāb al-Jāmiʿ li-mufradāt al-adwiya wa al-aγδiya*, written by Ibn Bayṭār in the mid-thirteenth century. The following is the entry on *ḥarmal* (with some rearrangement of subsections) from this work (ed. Cairo 1967; cf. Leclerc 1877-1883: I, 423; Sontheimer 1842: I, 217-219):

[A. The *Ḥarmal* Plant]

[The Arabic translation of] **Dioscurides** [states] "This plant grows in Cappadocia and Galatia in Asia and they name it *mūly*; some call it wild rue (*saδāb γayr bustānī*). This is a shrub which has many stalks extending from one base. Its leaves are longer, softer and more strongly scented than the leaves of garden rue, and the flower is white and the head is a little larger than the head of garden rue and is triangular and contains the seeds, reddish in color, with three angles and of intense bitterness. The seeds are what is used. They ripen in autumn. Mixed with honey, wine, chicken gall, saffron and fennel juice it is useful for weak vision. Some call it *ḥarmalā* and the Syrians call it *basāsā* and the people of Cappadocia call it *mūly* because it is similar in having a black root and white flowers. It grows on hills and in fertile places.

Abū Ḥanīfa al-Dīnawarī [Arab philologist who wrote *The Book of Plants* (*Kitāb al-Nabāt*) about 895 C.E.]: "*Ḥarmal* is of two kinds. One is a kind with leaves like the Egyptian willow and flowers which in being white and fragrant are like jasmine flowers. Sesame oil and moringa seed oil become fragrant with this blossom. Its odor is not like the odor of olives. Its seed is in a capsule like the capsule of *Cassia*. The other kind is that which is called in Persian *isfand*. The capsule of this is round and that of the other is long. The capsule is the vessel containing the seeds."

Ibn Samajūn [d. 1001 C.E.]: "There are two: a white and a red. The white is the Arabic *ḥarmal*, called in Greek *mūly*, and the red is known as common *ḥarmal* and is called *isfand* in Persian."[2]

[B. Pharmacological Properties]

Galen: "It is warm and dry in the third degree. It loosens thick viscid humors and removes them through the urine."

Masīḥ al-Dimashqī [c. 850 C.E.]: "The seed expels tapeworms from the intestines. It is used against colic, sciatica and coxalgia in a pubic compress. It purifies the chest and lungs of viscid mucus and dissipates visceral flatulence."

ʿĪsā ibn Māssa [9th century C.E.]: "We at the Marw hospital use the seed to expel black bile and various kinds of mucus by means of diarrhea. It is of the greatest use in treating epilepsy."

Al-Rāzī [d. 925 C.E.]: "*Ḥarmal* obstructs and breaks up pain. It induces the flow of menstruation and urine. Some physicians say an infusion undoes the black bile, purifies the blood and softens the womb."

Ibn Wāfid [d. 1074 C.E.]: "It is useful to those possessed by love (*asḥāb al-ʿišq*) because of inducing intoxication and sleep."

ʿAlī ibn Rizayn: "It is useful for colds of the brain or the body."

Anonymous: "It clarifies the complexion. It inclines one to coitus. It fattens and stimulates menstruation and urination."

Another: "One and a half mithqal of pulverized seed taken over 12 nights is effective against sciatica. When not available cardamum seed of equal amount may be used."

[C. Preparation]

Ḥubaysh ibn al-Ḥasan [d. 880 C.E.]: "It causes vomiting and intoxicates like wine or nearly so. This is how to employ it as a vomitive: Wash five drachmas of seeds in gentle water several times and dry them, then pound them in a mortar with a wooden pestle and sift through a coarse linen weave. Pour four ounces of boiling water over [the pulverized seeds]. Pound in a wooden mortar and pass through a coarse linen weave and discard the residue. To this infusion add three ounces of honey and two ounces of sesame oil. It is then ready for use and induces strong vomiting."

Isḥāq ibn ʿImrān [d. 901 C.E.]: "One puts two parts of it into a vessel with 30 parts of wine and heats this until one quarter of it evaporates. Ten drachmas may then be successively administered daily to epileptics. It may also be administered for three consecutive days to a woman who has conceived at least once but is unable to conceive again. The proof that the medicine works is that it induces vomiting."

§45 Since the constituents, harmaline and harmine, that are the chief cause of vomiting are also responsible for the intoxicating effects of harmel, the preparation of the drug as an emetic or as an intoxicant would be the same.[3] The first of the two methods of preparation above includes the crushing in a mortar (and filtering) characteristic of the preparation of sauma. Crushing of harmel materials is essential for all their drug uses and can therefore be assumed to precede the boiling of *Peganam harmala* seed in wine as well.[4] This process of crushing must have been important for the preparation of sauma because it is attested in the very name **sauma-/soma-/haoma* - '(plant) submitted to pressing [in mortar] or drink obtained from it'.[5] It is unlikely that the drug would be named from its extraction by pressing if the equivalent results could be obtained by simply chewing the plant materials, as is the case with psychotropic mushrooms.

§46 *Peganum harmala*, shown in Figure 1 [*see page 177*], is a bushy shrub with numerous 1-2 foot stems extending radially from the apex of a woody tap root. The stems are much branched and curve upwards towards their ends, bearing alternate multi-lobed leaves and white, five-petaled, half-inch terminal flowers. From these develop pea-sized, 3-

speak during the entire day, most of which she spent asleep. Ivanov *et al.* (1965) report that dilute acetic acid extracted 98% of harmel seed alkaloids.

2 The red and white *ḥarmal* are distinguished by the color of the seed capsules. Neither the color nor the roundness of the capsules appears to have genuine taxonomic significance, however, and in Islamic materia medica no practical distinction is made either between red and white *ḥarmal* or between "common" or "Arabic" *ḥarmel*.

3 Vomiting is a frequent but not an invariable effect of harmaline ingestion. C. Naranjo reported 18 out of 30 of his subjects responded to harmaline by vomiting (see his comments §39).

4 In R. N. Chopra *et al.* (1965: 221) one reads: "the seeds . . . in an elephant are said to bring about a condition of tremendous excitement whereby the animal loses control over himself, i.e. becomes '*mast*.'" These animals are able to adequately crush the seeds with their teeth. Harmel seeds are also said to produce excitement in horses.

5 From a root **sau* 'to extract'; the formation of Proto-Indo-Iranian **sauma-* is reexamined below, §§187-197.

TABLE 1: SOME NAMES FOR *PEGANUM HARMALA* L.

* = designates seed of *Peganum harmala*

PORTUGUESE: *harmale* (44). SPANISH: *harma* (44), *harmaga* (44), *alharma* (44), *alfarma* (44), *armage* (44), *alhargama* (44), *amargaza* (44). CATALAN: *armala* (44), *ruda borda* (50). FRENCH: *rue savauge* (62), *erimola* (62). GERMAN: *Harmel* (49), *Harmelstaude* (49), *Harmelkraute* (49), *Harmelraute* (49), *wilde Raute* (49), *Steppenraute* (49). YIDDISH: *bibek* (41). ITALIAN: *armora* (44), *ruta selvatica* (61), *pegano* (61). UKRAINIAN: *ruta-dyka* (46), *rebrik-sobačj* (46), *rebryk* (46), *sobače-zillja* (46), *sobača-loboda* (46), *sobakarne* (46), *smerdioxa* (46), *vonyučka* (46). RUSSIAN: *mogil'nik* (63). BULGARIAN: *zarniš* (32). GREEK (Modern) *βρφμοýρταρο*(28), *ἡριο-π῀ηανο(ν)* (30), κολλιἄά(30), χῖαχια(30), ωενδον (16α); π῀ανο (30). TURKISH: *üzerlik* (15), *ilezik* (15), *mahmur-çiçeĕi* (65); UZBEK: *isiriq* (67a); UC: *ildrük* (15); AZARI: *uzerrik* (24a); OGUZ: *yidiĕ* (15); KIRGHIZ: *adraspan* (25), *adrašman* (25); SART, CHAT: *abdaraspani* (47), CHINESE TURKISTAN: *ädräsmān* (53). MONGOLIAN: *mkhī-övös* (Classical *ömekei-ebüsü)* (11a). ARMENIAN: *aspand* (35), *sbant* (24), *šan-p'in* (29), *sanam* (7), *khowniv* (7), *vahri-esbant* (7), *vahri-pegenay* (7), *p'egenay* (29). BERBER: *bender-tīfré/tāfré* (27). ARABIC: *ḥarmal* (42), *zariʿat-al-harer* (18), *ɣalqa* (36), *δafrā* (36), *mogannanna* (20), *saδāb-šamī* (20), *saδāb-barī* (20), *ɣalqat-al-δiʾb* (26), *saδāb-al-jibalī* (45), *šagarat-al-xanīzīr* (57), *xinīza* (54), *xanaize* (17), *xabīza* (72), *xāīs* (54), *xyais* (17), *xayyāsa* (54), *qays* (54), *ḥaramlan* (69a), *ḥarmelun* (69), *ḥurremlan* (11), *ḥaremlān* (1), *ḥuraymilān* (3), *nigti** (13), *xarjal* (11), *xarguel* (64), *harjal* (3). PERSIAN: *spand* (38), *spend* (38), *sifand* (68), *sipand* (68), *sipandīn* (68), *asbatān* (68), *istabān* (68), *isfanj* (60), *sepanj* (60), *šīrsādū* (34), *šaqrdāna* (34), *fātarālstīn* (34), *fāšarsīn* (68), *nīl** (51), *navand* (16), *navan* (60), *nīwandī-maryam* (56), *hazār-isfand* (16), *ṣandal-dāna** (16). LARI: *sandolos* (23), *sondoros** (6); KERMANI: *svon* (66), *seben* (66), *espend* (66), *daštī* (5). SEMNANI / SANGESARI *espan* (67), *esban* (67), *espond* (67), *esbond* (67), *esbund(i)* (67). TABARI: *espan* (56). GILAKI: *span-dāna** (56). SISTANI: *dudnī* (75), *dudnuk* (43a), *bidnik* (43a). KURDISH: *aspand* (37). LURI: *dī* (40), *espan* (40), *esvan* (40), *dēništ* (43). BALUCHI: *spand* (74), *spanj* (74), *hurmul* (74), *ispanthān* (74), *spandā* (2), *spinguli* (2), *spanguli* (2), *spangaoli* (2), *espantān** (4), *spanyānān** [plural](4), *gandāxo* (53), *gandhiyo* (10), *sadāp-i-kōhī* (58a). PASHTO: *spilanai* (52), *spalanaey* (52), *spandah* (52), *ašdun-buta* (73). WAZIRI: *spēlanai ** (55), *spōnda* (55). WAKHI: *spandr* (33), *spand* (33), *spanddoná** (33). S HUGNI: *ispandur* (33). OROSHORI: *səpăn* (21). ISHKASHMI: *spondana* (33). YAZGULAMI: *spāndān* (22), *s(ə)pánt* (22), *s(ə)pantā(g)* (22). BRAHUI: *kisánkúr* (8). BURUSHASKI: *supándur* (9). BALTI: *isman* (70). URDU: *hurmur* (48). PUNJABI: *karnal* (71), *hurmul* (14). SINDI: *spelani* (74), *hurmur* (74). HINDI: *fijal* (34), *harmul* (74), *isbund-lahouri* (74), *hurmol* (74), *kaladana* (74), *lahouri-hurmul* (74). GUJARATI: *ispun* (74), *hurmaro* (74). BENGALI: *ispand* (14). MARATHI: *sarmala* (74). TAMIL: *šimai-arvandi-virati* (74), *simaai-zhavandi-virai/vittula* (14), *simaiyaravandi* (14). DECCAN: *vilayati-isband* (58), *vilayati-mhendi* "foreign henna" (58). KANARESE: *sime-goranti* (58). TELUGU: *sima-goronti-vittulu* (58). Chinese: *luòtuo péng* (11a).

1. Ascherson & Schweinfurth 1887. 2. Aitchison 1891. 3. Bailey & Danin 1981. 4. Bailey 1953. 5. Baqāʿī 1959. 6. Bastakī 1980. 7. Bedevian 1936. 8. Bellew 1874. 9. Berger 1956. 10. Bhandari 1978. 11. Blatter 1919-1936. 11a. James Bolson, letter of 5/88. 12. Brockelmann 1928. 13. Burtt & Lewis 1954. 14. Chopra *et al.* 1965. 15. Clauson 1972. 16. Dehkhudā 1947-1973. 16a. Delatte 1939. 17. Dickson 1955. 18. Dozy 1881-1927. 19. Drower & Macuch 1963. 20. Ducros 1930. 21. Edel'man 1966. 22. Edel'man 1971. 23. Eqtedārī 1955. 24. *Flora Armenij* 1954-1966. 24a. *Flora Azerbaidzhan SSR* 1950. 25. *Flora Kirgizskoj SSR* 1957-1967. 26. Förskål 1775. 27. Foucauld 1951. 28. Frass 1845. 29. Gabikean 1968. 30. Gennadiou 1914. 32. Gilliat-Smith & Turrill 1930. 33. Grjunberg & Steblin Kamenskij 1976. 34. Hādī Khān al-ʿAlawī 1824. 36. Hava 1915. 37. Hooper 1937. 38. Horn 1893. 39. Hübschmann 1897. 40. Izadpanāh 1964. 41. Kaganoff 1977. 42. Lane 1863-1893. 43. Läffler *et al.* 1974. 43a. Leonard 1984. 44. Lokotsch 1927. 45. Löw 1924. 46. Makowiecki 1936. 47. Maksimovich 1889. 48. Mallik & Mohajir 1958. 49. Marzell 1943-1958. 50. Masclans i Grivés 1954. 51. Massé 1938. 52. Mayer 1909. 53. Menges 1933. 54. Migahid 1978. 55. Morgenstierne 1927. 56. Muʿin 1951-1956. 57. Musil 1927. 58. Nadkarni 1954. 58a. Nāṣerī 1971. 59. Osadča 1930. 60. Parsa 1960. 61. Pedrotti & Bertordi 1930. 62. Rolland 1903. 63. Safina *et al.* 1970. 64. Schweinfurth 1912. 65. Redhouse 1974. 66. Soroushian 1956. 67. Sotoudeh 1963. 67a. Steblin-Kamenskij 1982. 68. Steingass 1894. 69. Steinschneider 1897. 69a. Täckholm 1969.

lobed seed capsules, the color of which changes from green to reddish brown to dull white as they mature. Each compartment of these capsules contains 11-15 angular dark red-brown seeds.

§47 The total amount of the psychoactive constituents of *Peganum harmala*, harmaline and harmine, is greatest (2-7%) in the mature seeds (Kutlu and Amal 1967: 135; al-Shamma and Abdul-Ghany 1977) and in the roots (1.4 - 3.2%; *ibid.*), but the ratio of these two alkaloids as well as the total amount contained vary seasonally, geographically, and possibly with other factors.[6] Harmaline and harmine are qualitatively similar pharmacologically but differ in potency. Similar subjective effects are reported after oral doses of 4mg./kg. harmaline or 8mg./kg. harmine (C. Naranjo 1967).[7] Much larger doses in mammals (from 20 to 300 mg./kg. harmine [Gunn 1937]) bring tremor, lowering of blood pressure and of body temperature, and ultimately cardiovascular disturbances resulting in death. For a person of average size the characteristic subjective effects of these alkaloids is usually obtained by consuming 5–10 grams of seeds, 10–30 grams of root, or slightly larger quantities

[6] The quantity of harmaline may be twice that of harmine in seeds collected in January, with the ratio between the two alkaloids reversed in June (Kamel *et al.* 1970). The total content of harmaline and harmine of roots is greatest in the thicker root parts (Safina *et al.* 1970: 230) and varies from 1.5 to over 3 percent. Root alkaloid content varies significantly seasonally; it is highest in winter and declines after the appearance of flowers and with the maturing of the seeds. From October to February roots reportedly averaged 0.4% harmaline and 1.8% harmine, whereas during August they contained 0.6% harmine and 0.8% harmaline (*ibid.* see also Khashimov *et al.* 1971:382), but specimens collected in Iraq assayed by al-Shamma and Abdul-Ghany (1977) contained nearly twice these amounts.

[7] Pennes and Hoch (1959) report oral administration of up to 960 mg. harmine failed to produce hallucinatory effects in their subjects, who were, however, institutionalized schizophrenics.

TABLE 2: SOME NAMES FOR SPECIES OF *RUTA*

(Exclusive of European Forms Derived from Greek/Latin *ruta*)

Ruta graveolens except where marked by *=*Ruta chalepensis* L. or **=*Ruta montana* L.

ARABIC: *faijal (12), faijan (12), galec (12), galega (12), fiyal (13), fayyal (13), fayyan (13) saδāb* (3), sidāb (18), ḥarmal* (17), sadāb (23), šadāb (23);* MOROCCO: *sadāb* (37), fiīel* (37), fijla* (37), issin* (37), bou-ranes* (37), rūṭa (12), ārūta (13), rūta (13);* TLEMCEN: *sadāb-al-jibalī* (37), fijela-al-jibalī** (37), jell (39), zenn (39), figeen (39), fijel (39), fizol (38);* TUNIS: *ḥašiš-al-jinn (20);* EGYPT: *sandāb (27), sandāb* (35), sendāb (15), xuft (1);* ARABIA: *sakab* (28), sazāb* (21a);* PALESTINE: *begām (23), sabād (23), sadābie (23), ḥarmal* (1a);* YEMEN: *xuft (11), xīl (11), šadābah (6), sadāb* (35).* BERBER: *iwármi (38), iurmi (22), iwermi (22) awerma (34), awram (12), ʾuʾrmi (12).* COPTIC: *bašouš (10), kanon (7a).* GALLA: *dscharte (31).* TIGRINA: *dhen (31).* AMHARIC: *tal-addam (31), tena-addem (31).* GREEK: π̓ηανι (16), π̓ηανια (16), π̓ανι (16), π̓ανο (16), π̓ηανον (16), ὦπ̓ηυŸ (16), π̓ηανυŸ (16). BULGARIAN: *sedefče (17).* HUNGARIAN: *virnanc (4).* ROUMANIAN: *virnani (4).* UKRAINIAN: *zymozelen (25).* ARMENIAN: *halebi-sbant* (2), sadaf-khod (2), sadab (2), sazsaz (2), garan (2), vahri-pegenay** (2), vahri-sazab** (2).* TURKISH: *sedef (17), sadaf (29).* PERSIAN: *sudāb (23), saped (23), sadāb (23), payjan (40), payɣan (40), sapandān-i-ganda (40).* DAILAM: *bīm (19).* KERMAN: sedōw (5). BALUCHI: *zirag (26).* SANSKRIT: *brahmakanyaka (30), brāhmaṇī (30), brāhmī (30), chandrávallarī (30). guchhapatra (9), kapōtavegā (30), maṇḍūka (30), pitapuṣpa (9), sárasvatī (30), sarpadaṃṣtra (9), saumyā (30), somalatā (9), somavallarī (30), viṣap (9).* PUNJABI: *katmal (9).* URDU: *sudah (9).* HINDI: *pisamarum (9), sadab (9), satari (9), saturi (33), allooda (33), sānūl (19), sātrī (19).* BENGALI: *ermul (32), ermal (32), isband (32), ispund (9), tatlī (19).* KANARESE: *hāvananju (9), nāgaldāli (9), sadābu (9), sudabugida (32).* MALAYAM: *somarayam (24), arūta (24), naagadhali (36), sādsā (1).* TAMIL: *aruvadam (9), arvada (9), pambuko (9), tirumuti-patchi (8), arroda (33), aruvadān (24), pāmbugolli (24), aruvadaamchedi (36).* TELUGU: *aruda (9), sadapa (9), suddapo-akoo (33), sudapaha (32).* URIYA: *maruā (41)*

1. Anisle 1826. 1a. Ascherson *apud* Löw 1924. 2. Bedevian 1936. 3. Blatter 1919-1936. 4. Borza 1968. 5. Boyce 1966b. 6. Brauer 1934. 7. Budge 1913. 7a. Ibn Kabr (d. 1368) in Budge 1927. 8. Chandrasena 1935. 9. Chopra *et al* 1965. 10. Crum 1939. 11. al-Dimyaṭī 1965. 12. Dozy 1881-1927. 13. Dubler & Teres 1952-1957. 14. Fleurentin *et al.* 1983. 15. Förskål 1775. 16. Gennadiou 1914. 17. Gilliat-Smith & Turrill 1930. 18. Guigues 1905. 19. Hadi Khān al-ʿAlawī 1824. 20. al-Ḥayla 1968. 21 Khattab & Nabil el-Hadidi 1971. 22. Laoust 1920. 23. Löw 1924. 24. Lushington 1915. 25. Makowiecki 1936. 26. Mayer 1909. 27. Meyerhof 1918. 28. Migahid 1978. 29. Monchi-Zadeh 1969. 30. Monier-Williams 1899. 31. Mooney

of entire fruiting stems of harmel. These are amounts which may easily be prepared for consumption in a hand mortar of moderate size.

§48 As well as these alkaloids, harmal seeds also contain an edible oil (14–17%); nevertheless, the commercial value of the plant has never been great. *Peganum harmala* is the source of a red dye which in early nineteenth-century Anatolia was used in dying the Turkish fez. The substance was obtained by a complex process involving the treatment of harmel seeds for six months with a mixture of saltpeter and sal ammoniac dissolved in brandy. This red dye, which is apparently an oxidation product of the alkaloids (Schutzenberger 1867: 2, 61–67), was later rapidly produced by treatment of seeds with alcohol and sulfuric acid (Goebel 1838). A yellow pigment (and also brown and greenish ones, see Kasumov 1983) can be obtained merely by water extraction of the seeds (Dollfus and Schlumberger 1842). Because of supplying this yellow dye, harmel is sometimes referred to in India as a kind of henna (i.e. as *mhendi* or *goranti*, see Table 1). Investigation of the possible industrial value of these dyes indirectly lead to the isolation and identification of the alkaloids harmaline (Goebel 1841) and harmine (Fritzsche 1847).

Geographical Distribution of Harmel

§49 One may expect that sauma was sufficiently abundant throughout Greater Iran for its use among the various Indo-Iranian groups there to have long continued. In the absence of any indication of the cultivation of sauma or, in the Iranian materials, of any suggestion of either scarcity or local advantages in its supply at any time, sauma should have been easily obtained as a wild plant within the Greater Iranian area. Among the few uncultivated indigenous plants known to contain psychoactive drugs, *Peganum harmala* is uniquely abundant over this territory.

§50 A possible limit to the geographical range of sauma is provided by the fact that no equivalent intoxicant plant seems to have been known to other Indo-European groups. Sauma could well have been unique to the Indo-Iranian peoples because the plant grew where they alone encountered it, and was not available to the kindred peoples occupying lands to the northwest until after the fixation of distinctly different religious practices.

§51 The historical distribution of *Peganum harmala* corresponds to the area which may thus be assumed *a priori* for sauma. In some late Greek writings, *Peganum harmala* is called περςᾶια βοτᾶνθ 'the Persian plant' (Thomson 1955: texts D.11 and T.10), and the center of its distribution seems indeed to have been the Iranian area, where it occupies vast areas of the hinterland.[8] The antiquity of *Peganum harmala* among the Iranian people is reflected by the fact that far-flung later Iranian languages have names for the plant which evolved independently from a single Proto-Iranian form (see below, §61), indicating that the Iranian peoples were acquainted with it from the earliest period. *Peganum harmala* was early known elsewhere in Western Asia; its Akkadian name was

[8] A. Engler (1931: 19a, 154) supposed *Peganum harmala* to have originated in Persia. According to M. Zohary (1973: 391): "The center of its distribution range lies within the Irano-Turanian region."

apparently *šibburratu* (Von Soden 1978:13,1226; Thompson 1949: 74), cf. Aramaic *šabbārā* (Mandaic *šambra*) '*Peganum harmala*' (Löw 1881: 321). Its dispersal has been as a weed, thriving on the nitrogenous wastes accompanying human settlement and invading disturbed ground. West of Khorasan the plant is increasingly encountered only as a weed on overgrazed, abandoned fields (Thalen 1979: 301 *seq.*) and most typically beside roads. In Iraq, harmel is described as "the ruderial plant *par excellence* of the desert; it is invariably found along caravan routes, in the vicinity of wells, etc." (Guest and al-Rawi 1966: 93).

§52 In the earliest description of *Peganum harmala*, which is that of the first century C.E. herbal of Dioscurides (III, 45-46; the Arabic translation of which was quoted in §44A), it is described as a variety of rue, namely *π῾ηανον ἤριον* 'wild rue' (Wellmann 1907-1914:2, 57–60). From Dioscurides we learn that among the "Syrians" it had the names *βθςαςᾶ* and *αρμαλᾶ* (i.e. *baššāšā* and *ḥarmalā*), among the "Africans" *γουρμᾶ* in Egypt *π̆νουβοε̆*[9] (for these names see below, §§265-268), and in parts of Anatolia (Cappadocia and Galatia) *μλ̑υ*.[10] *Peganum harmala* does not appear to have become established in Greece, Italy, or elsewhere in Europe much before Dioscurides' time, for Theophrastus (*Enquiry into Plants* 7.4.1; Hort 1916) was ignorant of it. It is now a circum-Mediterranean weed and is found in Eastern Europe as far north as Budapest (Löw 1924). Expansion of the plant into southern Europe seems largely to have occurred after the advent of Islam, for its European names are predominantly derived from the Arabic *ḥarmal* (e.g. Spanish *garmarza, harmaga, alhargame, alfarma, armage, alharma, amargaza,* etc. [Lokotsch 1927]). *Peganum harmala* has apparently been present longer in the southern parts of the European U.S.S.R., where is is known as a weed especially characterized by its association with sites of human occupation (for instance in cemeteries, reflected by its Russian name *mogil'nik* 'tomb' [see Osadca 1930; Ossadcha-Janata 1952]). In the east of the Iranian area *Peganum harmala* is gradually replaced by a second species, *P. nigellastrum* Bunge, which extends into Mongolia and north China.[11]

§53 Harmel is universally associated with the cultivated garden rue, *Ruta graveolens* L., and the two other Mediterranean *Ruta* species, *Ruta chalepensis* L. and *Ruta montana* L. (*see Figure 2*). These *Ruta* species are small evergreen herbs similar in size, leaf form and in the shape and size of seeds and seed capsules to harmel, which they resemble also in being strongly scented. The association of harmel with species of *Ruta* is manifest in the frequent interchange of their vernacular names, as may be seen in Tables 1 and 2. Where harmel has been introduced into areas where *Ruta* species are already known, it is described as a kind of *Ruta* (thus many European names for harmel such as *Syrian wild rue, African rue, rue sauvage, Harmelraute,* and so forth; exemplified by the botanical name *Peganum* which is from the Greek *π῾ηανον*, the usual ancient Greek name for *Ruta* species). Likewise where harmel is the older plant, *Ruta* has been named from harmel (e.g. Coptic *bašouš* ['*Ruta*'] < Syrian *baššūšā* ['harmel']; Bengali *ermal* ['*Ruta*'] and Berber *iurmi* ['*Ruta*'] < Arabic *ḥarmal* or **ḥurma* [see below, §265]; Armenian "*sbant* of Aleppo", Bengali *ispund* and Persian *sepandān-i ganda* [all '*Ruta*'] < Old Iranian **svanta-* ['harmel']). In many other cases, however, forms of the Greek name *π῾ηανον* or the Latin name *Ruta* (also originally a Greek word [André 1956]), have been adopted for *Ruta graveolens* at the same time as its cultivation. The most widespread name for *Ruta graveolens* throughout the Muslim world, *sudāb/sadāb* (the etymology of which is discussed below, §§274-286) was probably also originally a name for harmel (still known locally as 'wild-' *sadāb* or 'mountain-' *sadāb*) which was transferred when the cultivation of *Ruta graveolens* was introduced into Iran.[12]

§54 In the Indian area *Peganum harmala* has also become established as a ruderial and, because it is generally known by forms of the Arabic *ḥarmal* or Persian *isfand*, is usually presumed to have been introduced by the Muslims (e.g. Burkill 1935), who import its seeds from the Iranian Plateau for medicinal and apotropaic purposes. It appears, however, already to have had an Indian name in the time of al-Bīrūnī (*c.* 1030 C.E.),[13] which suggests (as do other factors discussed in §141) that

9 The names *χουρμᾶ* and *π̆νουβοε̆* are absent from the Arabic version of Dioscurides (see Dubler and Teres 1952-1957).

10 Paul Anton de Lagarde (1866: 173 *seq.*) claimed the name *"moly" (Greek μλ̑υ)* links *Peganum harmala* with *haoma*. Lagarde's remarks concerned a passage in Plutarch's *De Iside et Osiride 46* on Persian religious practices in Cappadocia in the second century B.C.E. Here it is said that a herb *ἤμφμι* was pounded in a mortar and mixed with the blood of a wolf as an offering to the devil, Areimanos. This herb *ἤμφμι* must be ultimately connected in some way with Iranian *hauma-* (although its use with wolf's blood in offerings to Ahriman is hardly orthodox). Lagarde argued that *ἤμφμι* was a Greek reflex of Cappadocian *μλ̑υ* and hence that *Peganum harmala* must have been used in Cappadocia as a substitute for *haoma* (why it would not itself have been *haoma* he does not explain clearly). As was shown by E. Benveniste (1929), Lagarde's effort to derive phonologically *ἤμφμι* from *μλ̑υ* is not possible. (Dübner may have independently come to the same conclusion as did Lagarde, however, in emending *ἤμφμι* to *μλ̑υ* in his 1867 edition of the Plutarch text [see further Griffiths 1970]). Despite Lagarde's sound intuition into the botanical origins of *haoma*, his discussion of the matter has seemed obscure (e.g. even while professing to corroborate Lagarde's arguments, Brunnhofer [1910] misunderstood him to have identified *haoma* with *Ruta graveolens*). For the forms *ἤμφμι* and *μλ̑υ*, see below, §§269–271.

Moly is the name of the magical plant which in *Odyssey* X, 304–306, Hermes provides to Odyssus as antidote to Circe's pottage (Rieu 1946:163). Whether Dioscurides' report that *moly* was an Anatolian name for harmel establishes the botanical identity of Hermes' *moly* is a matter of some controversy (for which see J. Stannard [1967], K. Raehner [1969], and J. Clay [1970]). That harmel was *moly* is made increasingly plausable by the data linking harmel with sauma, for parallels between the mythology of *soma* and that of *moly* have been noted by J.-F. Cerquand (1873:55–58) and analyzed by him as having a common origin. There are also parallels to certain elements of *soma* rituals in the ingredients of the drug prepared by Circe (involving barley, cheese, honey, and Pramnian wine and identical to mixtures attested elsewhere in Greek literature), which have been brought to light by C. Watkins (1978).

11 Whether species of *Peganum*, or varieties of *P. harmala* (of which Nabil el-Hadidi [1972] distinguishes three in Iran) differ significantly in their content of harmaline or other drugs awaits investigation. A third species, *P. Mexicanum* Gray (*P. Texicanum* [M. E. Jones 1933–1935: 47]) is indigenous to remote parts of Texas and northern Mexico. Around 1920 *Peganum harmala* was introduced into the American Southwest (Dayton 1937; Cory 1949; Correll and Johnstone 1970) where it has swiftly colonized roadsides; it now flourishes along much of Interstate-10 between Pecos, Texas, and Phoenix, Arizona.

12 The close connection of *Ruta graveolens* with *Peganum harmala* (Arabic *ḥarmal*) is evident in perhaps the earliest attestation in Arabic of the name *saδāb* for *Ruta graveolens*, found in the *'Uyūn al-axbār* of Ibn Quṭayba (*c.* 850 C.E.), where a popular belief is reported: "upon standing, the seeds of *saδāb* become those of *ḥarmal*" (Brockelmann 1908: 489.10).

13 In Abū Bakr ibn ʿAlī ibn ʿUṯmān al-Kāsānī's Persian translation of the *Kitāb al-Ṣaydana fī ṭibb* made in 1228 C.E. (Sotoudeh and Afshar 1973: 225; British Library Or. 5849, f.56.16) that name is *dwpw*; in the Arabic text (Said and Elakie 1973: 155) it is given as *hmlw*. These names are discussed below, §272.

A link between *Peganum harmala* and the plant known in Islamic materia medica as *hawm al majūs* is provided by al-Bīrūnī's remark that some people apply the name *ḥarmal* to *buxūr maryam*, for *buxūr maryam* is identified as *hawm al-majūs* in some later Persian materia medica (e.g. the *Tuḥfat al-Muʾminīn* [*c.* 1669]). Al-Bīrūnī speculates that both plants might be called *ḥarmal* because, like *Peganum harmala*, *"buxūr maryam"* induces menstruation, but this property does not in fact seem to provide sufficient explanation for referring to *buxūr maryam* as *"ḥarmal"*. In Arabic *buxūr maryam* is usually *Cyclamen europaeum* L. (Primulaceae) (Schmucker 1969:105). This *Cyclamen* species is in no way associated with Zoroastrian rituals (although the intriguing name *Zoroastris* is given by Dioscurides as a name for it [Gunther 1934:202; Kühn 1829:25,303]). The name *buxūr maryam* is, however,

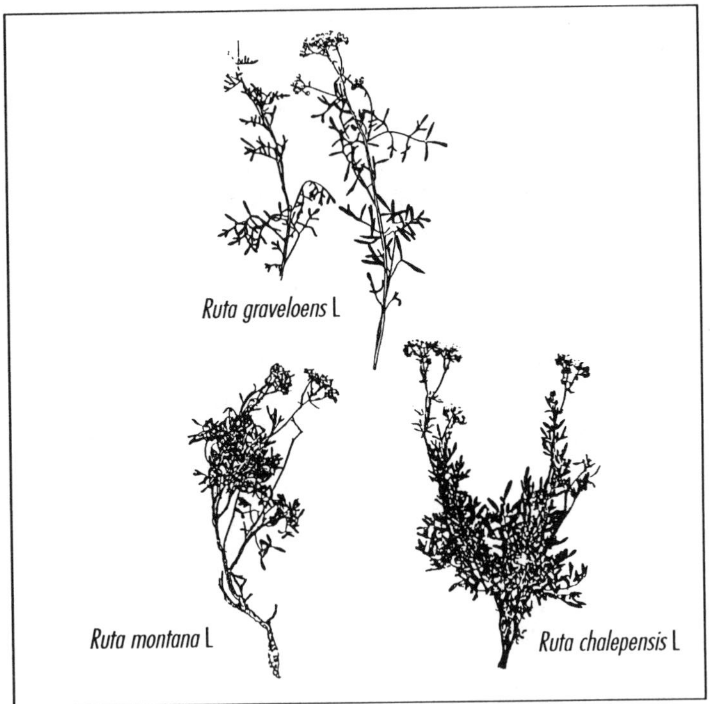

FIGURE 2

it had reached India earlier.

§55 *Peganum harmala* is characterized by a strong, peculiar odor,[14] which issues from the leaves when they are disturbed. The plant is made especially noticeable to herdsmen, such as the Indo-Iranians were, by the fact that grazing animals (camels, goats, and some donkeys excepted [Bailey and Danin 1981]) will not eat of its fresh stems and leaves even in the face of starvation (Black and Parker 1936: 12). Its foliage is not actually toxic to large animals, and when it is cut and allowed to sit a few days, the upper part of the plant may be used as fodder (*ibid.*). The avoidance of the living herb by livestock may make it seem strangely protected (Vonderheyden 1937:457). It appears that the property of being shunned by animals may have been regarded in Iran as a mark of plants that were powerful drugs.[15] But doubtless of greater importance in drawing attention to *Peganum harmala* is the fact that because of this avoidance by grazing animals, stands of the plant are left isolated as the surrounding vegetation is consumed. Thereby harmel becomes one of the most available materials for fires, for which purpose, despite its relatively poor quality, it must always have been exploited in the severe winters of interior Asia.[16] When harmel is gathered in this season, the whitish seed capsules crowning the ends of branches, from which the leaves have largely disappeared, are mature and contain numerous small seeds. These seeds have an unusual tendency to snap dramatically when placed in contact with fire, and they then emit volumes of richly scented smoke, describable as having "a heavy, narcotic odor" (Dymock 1889:255). In Iran the scent of this smoke has traditionally been regarded as incense. The smoke contains appreciable amounts of volatilized harmine and harmaline, the psychoactive potential of which must be considered in evaluating the historical origins of the tradition of burning harmel seeds. The smoke is valued as an analgesic for toothache (Boulos 1973: 195) or headache (Venzlaff 1977:65)[17] and may be effective as an antiseptic for wounds (Ghafoor 1974) and as an insecticide (Volk 1955), but, with respect to psychoactive properties, the amount of harmaline that might be absorbed by inhalation of this smoke would not ordinarily be significant, except perhaps in the case of young children.[18] After having consumed a threshhold dose of harmaline, however, the rapid absorption of additional quantities of the drug from inhaling this smoke could have immediate and marked subjective effects. If this pharmacological potential of the smoke has indeed contributed to the importance in Iran of burning harmel seeds (examined in the next chapter), then originally the plant must have been consumed as well as burned.

§56 Given that the Proto-Indo-Iranians were sufficiently interested in the intoxicating properties of plants to evolve a ritual based on the consumption of sauma, it is difficult to believe that they would have remained unaware that an extract of the seeds of *Peganum harmala* prepared in the same way as sauma produces the very effects for which sauma was valued.

4
ETHNOBOTANIC CONTINUITY OF SAUMA IN IRAN
THE IRANIAN NAMES FOR HARMEL IDENTIFY IT AS SAUMA

§57 The texts of the ceremonial tradition refer to sauma by terms such as *haoma*, pertaining to its ritual preparation as a drug, and not by

also sometimes applied to *Calendula officinalis* L. (Compositae) (Meyerhof and Sobhy 1932-1940:148). *Hawm al-majūs* would from its name '*haoma* of the Magi' have reference to a plant used by the Zoroastrian priests. From all indications, the plants used by Zoroastrian priests (i.e. the Magi) to which *hawm al-majūs* could have referred (see below, §123) were pomegranate, tamarisk, *Ephedra, Ruta graveolens*, or *Peganum harmala*, and none of these much resembles either *Cyclamen europaeum* ("sow bread") or *Calendula officinalis* ("marigold"). While sometimes Arabic *buxūr maryam* names *Calendula officinalis*, the usual Persian name for *Calendula officinalis* is *āftāb parast* 'sun worshipper', and this term is given by al-Bīrūnī himself as a synonym for *hawm al-majūs*. Thus, by way of al-Bīrūnī, Arabic *ḥarmal* (= *Peganum harmala* and *buxūr maryam*) is linked with Arabic *hawm al-majūs* (= *buxūr maryam* = *āftāb parast*). It is unclear, however, whether a real plant was intended by his entry *hawm al-majūs* (translated below); because there he does not record his own observations, but instead presents a partial version of the account, found in the Pahlavi *Dēnkird* VII (2.25-31 [Madan 1911: 605f.]), of how *haoma* brought about the birth of Zoroaster. Bīrūnī's entry is found only in the Arabic text of the *Kitāb al-Ṣaydana* [Togan 1941: 141; Said and Elakie 1973; cf. Habib 1979: 462]; it is missing from Persian MSS of the work:

"*Hawm al-majūs*: In Sogdian (it is called) *xwm* and in Syriac *ʿrzʾd mɣwšy* and in Persian *āftāb parast* and *hwyɣwr* [?]. The Magi claim that it is a tree without branches *(šaqq)* that grows where no one can reach it, in Azarbaijan. (There) snakes would eat the young of two birds, and an angel came with a twig (*ɣuṣn*) of *hawm* and threw it in their nest and the snakes stopped their attack and their mouths were closed and the twig hung in that tree and it remains there yet."

14 The odor is reflected in the Ukrainian name *vonyučka*, Baluchi *gandhiyo, gandāxo*, and perhaps also in Armenian *šan-pʿin* 'dog dung' (Gabikean 1968; pointed out to me by Professor James Russell).

15 The aversion by animals may have been a characteristic traditionally imputed to sauma. Zakariyāʾ ibn M. al-Qazwīnī (d. 1283) (*Kitāb ʿAjāyib al-maxlūqāt* ed. Saad 1973: 210) mentions a plant growing on Mt. Savalān in Azerbaijan, remarkable for being shunned by animals. From the context it is clear that Qazwīnī's account derives from the very same legend as does al-Bīrūnī's *hawm al-majūs* (see n.13 above) and that the plant referred to is the same *hōm* that conveyed Zoroaster to his father. It is of interest that Pseudo-Democritus (in Pliny, see below, §149) gives *hippophobas* 'that which puts horses to flight' as a synonym for *achaemenis* (=sauma?).

16 Abū Ḥanīfa al-Dīnawarī's (d. 895 C.E.) *Kitāb al-Nabāt* (ed. Lewin 1953) notes the use of harmel as a fuel by Arabian bedouins. See Jackson (1911:118) for a photograph of bundles of harmel collected for fuel.

17 Harmine is the basis of a patented analgesic (*Chemical Abstracts* 61, 15942).

18 An exception would be the case of a Moroccan exorcism reported by Vonderheyden (1937: 459) to consist of remaining in a tent of harmel vapor until demons are heard to cry out and depart. According to Ossadcha-Janata (1952: 7), "village fools" ("*douvans*") in Bukhara used to inhale the smoke of harmel seeds.

its common name as a plant. However, the ceremonial imitation of consuming sauma, which seems to be of Proto-Indo-Iranian origin, could have been efficacious only if there was wide general understanding of what was being imitated. This implies that the intoxicating power of sauma was originally well known; however, use of the common name of the plant in the texts recited in the ceremony would have ultimately resulted in acknowledgement that some performances only imitated the act of drinking the drug. It was thus necessary for the plant to be so designated in the liturgy as to make it possible for other plants to be used as ceremonial equivalents.

§58 Reference to the plant as *haoma* 'extract' was well suited to this situation. This seeming obscurantism should not be taken to mean that the identity of the intoxicating plant was secret; on the contrary, the institution of the ceremony must have depended on the reputation of that plant. What would appear to have been secret was whether the plant used on a given occasion was actually sauma (see below, §153). The ambiguity of the term *haoma* has served to permit the continuation of the ceremonies using only nonintoxicating plants. As we shall next consider, there appears to be only one instance in surviving Avestan texts where *haoma* is linked with the real name of an intoxicating plant, and that plant is *Peganum harmala.*

§59 The usual names for *Peganum harmala* in Iranian languages are forms such as *isfand, sepand, sven,* etc. (see Table 1) deriving from Proto-Iranian **svanta-* (Avestan *spənta-*) which meant in effect 'possessing productive numinous power' (see Bailey 1934; Gonda 1949); it may be conveniently translated 'sacred'. This fact provides two arguments for the identity of harmel with sauma.

§60 First, at the time when Avestan was a commonly understood (if not commonly spoken) language, *spənta-* and its cognates already named *Peganum harmala.* This is shown by the fact that the precise forms of the name in modern Iranian languages[1] could not phonologically have resulted from borrowing from one modern language into another.

§61 Second, *spənta-* occurs in the Avesta (*Vīsperad* 9.3) as an epithet of *haoma* in the phrase *haoma sūra spənta* 'the *haomas*, powerful, sacred', and is the only adjective associating sauma with the name of any Iranian plant.[2] Moreover, the apposition of *spənta* to *haoma* in this phrase could have been understood in Old Iranian as an allusion to *Peganum harmala.*

§62 The connection of *Peganum harmala* with sauma through the name **svanta-, spənta-* and the like, to which Paul Lagarde (1866:173; see §55 n.10 above) pointed over a century ago, is unassailable. The only objections to a simple and straightforward conclusion from the name arise from W. B. Henning's (1965: 39) remarks:

> The proper place of wild rue *Peganum harmala* is in witchcraft, which the Zoroastrian church ever combated; its seeds are thrown into the fire to excite fat black smoke—a truly Ahrimanian practice. That a seal of approval was set on this sorcerer's favorite in the Avesta itself by the attribution of semi-divine origin, should not be assumed so readily.
>
> That is not to say that we need reject the common derivation of *sipand* "wild rue" from *spənta-*, for which "sacred" is a broad equivalent; for to a *daēvayasna* or devil-worshipper the plant was indeed "sacred".

§63 It is impossible to accept the implication that throughout the various Iranian languages so common a plant as *Peganum harmala* could owe its name, 'sacred', to a predominant influence of the jargon of devil-worshippers. Henning implicitly affirms by his argument that the use of *spənta-* as a name for *Peganum harmala* existed while the word still meant 'sacred'. Moreover, the plant most *daēvayasnas* considered sacred was surely sauma. Even if Henning's effort to relegate the use of harmel exclusively to devil-worshippers were supported by the evidence, the connection of its Iranian names with *spənta-* would still be best explained by identifying harmel with sauma.

§64 It is less likely that in nonritual contexts sauma would be usually known by a term such as *haoma* referring to *how* the plant was prepared for a ceremony than by a name reflecting some inherent property related to *why* the plant was significant in ceremonies and elsewhere. The use of the term *haoma* in the Avesta is explicable because of the relevance of the preparation of the plant to that textual tradition, but "(plant) pressed out with mortar" seems to be a means of referring to a plant without naming it rather than to be itself a phytonym. Nothing is more certain about sauma than that it had the property of possessing numinous supernatural power, that is, what in Old Iranian was *spənta.* More relevant, unambiguous, and conclusive linguistic evidence than the fact that the Old Iranian name of harmel, *spənta* etc., is the single most descriptive Old Iranian word for what distinguished sauma from other plants in ancient Iran, can scarcely be imagined.[3]

CORRESPONDENCE OF HARMEL TO SAUMA IN APOTROPAIC FUNCTION

§65 Throughout the history of Islamic Iran to the present day, *isfand,* that is, *Peganum harmala,* has been esteemed chiefly for its apotropaic power and has been the chief plant regarded as having such power. Allusions to it in the very earliest New Persian literature show this is a continuation of pre-Islamic belief.

§66 In particular, the burning of the seeds of *Peganum harmala* is mentioned frequently in Classical Persian poetry and is found in the works of Nāṣir-i Khusraw, ʿAṭṭār, Khāqānī, Saʿdī, Jāmī, and many less famous writers.[4] In modern ethnographic and geographical literature it is regularly recorded as a practice still encountered throughout the Iranian area. The purpose of burning these seeds is not witchcraft, as Henning thought: the seeds are thrown onto braziers not primarily to elicit smoke, fat, black, or otherwise (a purpose for which other oil-rich seeds will do at least as well), but for the snapping sound and the pungent fumes released, results intended not to invoke demons but, on the contrary, to be rid of them.[5] The seeds are burned apotropaically on all occasions where there are special

[1] For the independent derivation of the modern forms, as well as for other aspects of the history of the term, see below, §§259-264.

[2] By contrast, the possibility of deriving a name for rhubarb in Khowar, Kati and Prasun from an unimportant Vedic epithet of *soma, śvātrá-* 'strengthening, invigoration', is the only objective argument adduced by G. Morgenstierne (1954) for his proposed identification of rhubarb as sauma. The situation of *haoma* as a name for *Ephedra* is discussed below, §106.

[3] Another epithet of *haoma* may be reflected by the Persian term *naivand/nīvand,* etc., 'swift', used only of horses and (in Fars) of *Peganum harmala,* and thus parallel to Avestan *aurvan-/aurvant-,* also meaning 'swift' and used in the Avesta precisely of horses and of *haoma* (*Yasna* 10.10; 11.2). The Iranian association of *Peganum harmala* with swiftness is also indicated by the Persian expression *sipand-āsā* 'like harmel, quick'. *Naivand/nīvand* is given as a name for *Peganum harmala* in lexicons (where a verse of Sanāʾī is usually cited [but the attribution of this verse is questioned by R. ʿAfīfī 1972, *s.v.*]) and is actually attested as *navan 'Peganum harmala'* in the Fars dialect of Jahrom (Parsa 1960: 68).

[4] See the verses quoted by I. Shokurzade (1974: 366-367) and in ʿA.-A. Dehkhudā (1947-1973: II, 2075-2076, 2327).

[5] Cf. hatred ironically expressed as "the love of the jinn for *ḥarmal*" in the North African Arabic data of Vonderheyden (1937: 360). The latter also reports (without citing his apparent source: Legey 1926:14, 93) that women of Tlemcen throw *ḥarmal* on their doorsteps and over their shoulders saying: "The harmel is sacred, O Prophet of God, protect (us) from male *jinn* and female *jinn*" ("*Lḥarmel ḥarma, ia rasoul Allah, T'ahdina men djenn ou djennia*". This assertion that *Peganum harmala* is sacred expresses the same notion as the Old Iranian name **svanta-* (which indeed underlies the Arabic name *ḥarmal,* as Schwartz shows below, §265) and suggests that the importance of the plant in Islamic North African folk-religion (for which see, e.g. Westermarck [1926]; Vries [1985]) may ultimately be of Iranian origin.

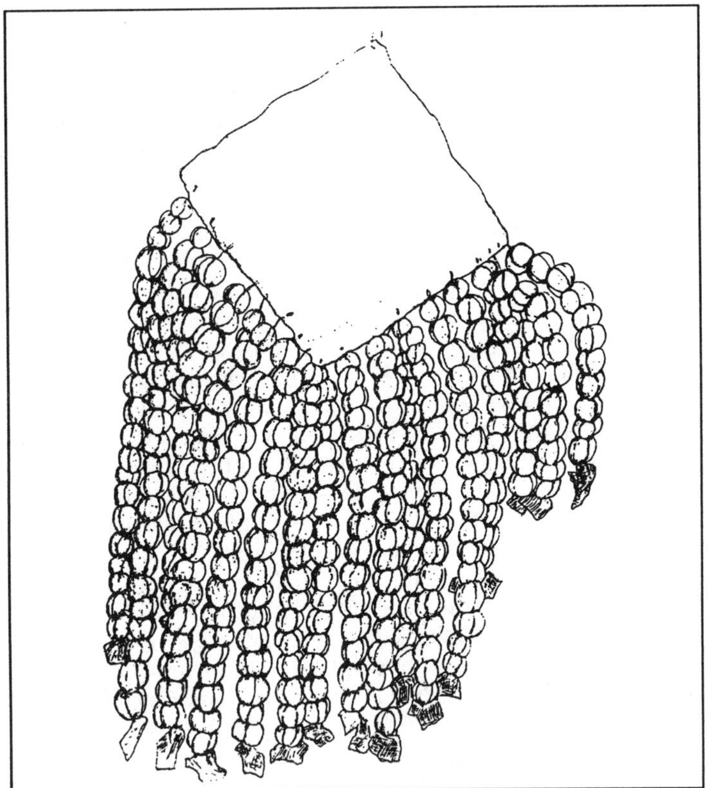

FIGURE 3.
PANJA, CONSISTING OF HARMEL CAPSULES STRUNG FROM A CLOTH SQUARE.

dangers of malign influences: at marriages, births, sicknesses, and circumcisions, as well as when one feels vigorous and joyful, and whenever there is suspicion of the evil eye. Harmel seeds figure also as the critical elements in numerous amulets and the capsules containing the seeds are strung together to make the *panja* (see Figure 3) frequently displayed in conservative Iranian households (cf. Watson 1979: 248).

§67 Since the apotropaic use of *Peganum harmala* in Iran antedates Islam, we may ask what the earlier significance of the practice of burning the seeds may have been. From the usual Islamic viewpoint, as a consequence of the strict monotheism which was absent from earlier Iranian culture, the capacity to ward off demons, customarily imputed to *Peganum harmala* in Iran, would lack any inherent relevance to religious concerns. In the dualistic conceptual world of pre-Islamic Iran as expressed in Zoroastrianism, however, the power to repel evil appears to be the very *essence* of religion. It is difficult to believe that any long-standing practice credited with accomplishing this end would not have been made use of within Zoroastrianism. As the purpose of the customary use of harmel is identical with the apotropaic aim of the Zoroastrian religion itself, the burning of the seeds of harmel would have been regarded as a religious activity in pre-Islamic Iran.

§68 The present-day apotropaic burning of harmel is accompanied by the recitation of formulaic verses, whose content reveals the essentially religious attitude shown toward the plant. These verses assert that the use of harmel is sanctioned by the most revered sources of religious authority in Islamic Iran.

> *Esfand* and *sepand:*
> Our Prophet chose it,
> ʿAlī planted it, Fāṭima collected it
> For Ḥusayn and Ḥasan.
> Saturday born, Sunday born,
> Monday born, Tuesday born,
> Wednesday born, Thursday born, Friday born.
> Under the earth, on the ground,
> Black-eyed, azure-eyed, blue-eyed, ewe-eyed;
> Whoever is seen, whoever is unseen,
> Neighbor to the left, neighbor to the right;
> Before the face, behind the head.
> —May the eye of the envious and of envy burst.[6]
>
> *Esfand* and *esfand* seed, *esfand* of thirty-three seeds,
> For relatives and friends and strangers,
> All who go out by the door, all who come in by the door,
> May the eye of the envious and of envy be blind!
> Saturday-born, Sunday-born, Monday-born, Tuesday-born,
> Wednesday-born, Thursday-born, Friday-born.
> Who planted it? The Prophet. Who gathered it? Fāṭima.
> For whom do they make it smoke? For the Imam Ḥasan and the Imam Ḥusayn.
> By the grace of the King of Men, turn away misfortune and pain.[7]

§69 Similar verses are addressed to the harmel plant itself. An apt example of these are the following Azari Turkish verses addressed to *Üzerlik* (the chief Turkish name for the plant):

[6] Alluding to the bursting of the seeds as they are thrown onto the fire of a brazier.

[7] These verses are translated from Ṣ. Hedāyat (1933:43-44). Similar verses are seen in E. W. Lindquist (1936:174 n.36), B. Donaldson (1938:21), H. Massé (1938), H. Īzadpanāh (1964:5), J. Ṣafīnažād (1966:414), I. Shokurzade (1967:241; 1974:77), and N. A. Kisljakov and A. K. Pisarchik (1970:268). Some previously unpublished examples, very kindly collected for me by Dr. Mahmoud Omidsalar in central Iran during 1976, are the following:
(1) From Lenjān-e Tāt, 300 km. southeast of Isfahan: *esmand-o seband sī o se dūne esmand / peiɣambar-i mā ferestāde bar šahr-i yaman / hamsāye-ye das-i rās, hamsāye-ye das-i čap / hamsāye-ye rūberū, hamsāye-ye pošt-i sar / betereked čašm-i hasūd o hasad.* "*Esmand* and *seband*, three and thirty seeds of *esmand*, / Our Prophet sent (you) for the sake of the land of Yemen. / Neighbor to the right, neighbor to the left, / Neighbor in front, neighbor behind. / [At this point seeds are put in the fire.] May the eye of the envious and of envy burst." [The burned seeds and ashes are then moistened with spit and rubbed on the palm of the right hand of the child for whom the verses have been recited. Additional ashes are rubbed on the sole of his left foot and from the eyebrows down to the point of his nose.]
(2) From Fīrūzī, near Abāde: *esfand-e dūne dūne / ye dūne sad dūne / češm-e hasud betareke.* "*Esfand*, seed by seed, / One seed, a hundred seeds, / May the eye of envy be burst."
(3) From Najafābād-e Tāt: *espand o espand-dūne / espand sī o se dūne / be haqq-ī xodā-ī yegūne / Mohammad kāštes, Alī čīdes / Fāteme barā Hasan o Hoseyn-eš dūd kardes / nām-ī xodā, nām-ī rasūl / betereked češm-ī hasūd o hasad.* "*Espand* and *espand* seed, / Thirty and three *espand* seeds, / By the grace of the One God, / Muḥammad planted it, ʿAlī collected it. / Fāṭima made it smoke for the sake of Ḥasan and Ḥusayn. / In the name of God, in the name of the Prophet / May the eye of the envious and of envy burst!"
(4) From the area of Bushehr: *esband o esband dūne / esband sī o se dūne / čašme xīš o bīgūne / harke esmet bedūne / harke esmet nadūne / betarake čašme hasud o hasad.* "*Esband* and *esband* seed, / Thirty and three seeds, / The eye of a relative or of a stranger. Whoever knows your name, / Whoever doesn't know your name. / May the eye of the envious and of envy burst."
(5) From the area of Isfahan: *esband o namak / šas o šīš dūneye band / Mostafā sūxte kard bahr-ī Yaman / betereked češm-ī hasud o hasad.* '*Esband* and salt / Sixty and six seeds bound [together on a string] / Muḥammad burned (them) for the sake of Yemen. / May the eye of the envious and of envy burst.' [With the recital of the last verse, one seed, together with salt, is put in the fire for each person suspected of casting the evil eye.] (M. Schwartz reconstructs the beginning of this verse to have originally been *esband o namak / namak o esband /*, with rhyme */ šaš o šīš dūneye band/*.)

Thou art *Üzerlik*, thou art the air [scented with *üzerlik*].[8]
Thou art the remedy for a thousand diseases.
Wherever thou art found the evil eye and illness will disappear.
Üzerlik, seed by seed, may it be poured to save the body,
Whether a relative or a stranger, may his eye be burnt in the fire.
Golden-colored *Üzerlik*, thy clothing is white, *Üzerlik*.

§70 How is the unique importance of *Peganum harmala* in Iranian folk religion to be explained? On the basis of the argument that *Peganum harmala* was sauma, its folk uses may be seen as the direct and unbroken continuation of ancient sauma practices. The place of sauma in popular beliefs and customs in pre-Islamic Iran, as against its role in the established religion, has hitherto been little investigated. To show the parallelism with the present-day role of *Peganum harmala* we must briefly consider the place of sauma in ancient Iranian society as evidenced by Zoroastrian literature.

§71 In Zoroastrian literature sauma is presented as if it existed in Iranian culture only as an adjunct to Zoroastrianism, but such a view is actually contradicted by the texts themselves. The very presence of *haoma* in these texts testifies to the enduring importance of sauma in Iranian beliefs since long before the time of Zarathushtra. The purpose of including these texts in the Zoroastrian canon has not been to promote *haoma*, which is irrelevant to any essential Zoroastrian doctrine, but to promote these doctrines—or rather the authority of the Zoroastrian institutions to decide them—by invoking already recognized sources of legitimacy. The traditional reverence for sauma was appropriated by Zoroastrianism, for example, in the connection with *haoma* of Zarathushtra's birth (see §93). Since this reverence for *haoma* was prevalent in Iran earlier and the hegemony of Zoroastrianism would not have diminished it, it may be expected to have continued independently during and after the ascendence of that religion.[9]

§72 It is an accepted fact that popular beliefs and attitudes towards sauma were a strong and persistent element in the Iranian tradition, strong enough, indeed, for some scholars to suppose that *haoma* achieved its important place in Zoroastrian ritual despite the Prophet Zarathushtra himself having condemned and prohibited the use of sauma, as these scholars believe he did (against this view, see below, §§158–160).

§73 The Avesta itself indicates in one place that sauma had folk uses which differed markedly from the ritual drinking of its extract with which the scriptures are chiefly concerned. This is *Yasht* 14.57, a verse apparently referring to its protective value as an amulet:

vərəθraɣnəm ahuraδātəm	We worship the Ahura-created Vṛthraghna
yazamaide	(Victory).
haoməm baire	I carry on me *haoma*.
+sairi.baoɣəm haoməm	I carry on me the head-saving,
vərəθrājanəm baire	victorious *haoma*.
nipātārəm vohu baire	I carry on me the protector (as) the good thing.
pātārəm tanuye baire	I carry on me the protector for the body.
haoməm yim nivizaiti[10]	When one attaches *haoma*,
nivandāṯ apayeiti	he escapes from the grasp
dušmainyaoṯ pəšana hača	of the enemy in battle.

§74 Such a use of sauma would not have required the approbation of priests and would have persisted whether or not sauma was recognized in the prevailing religion. Although nonritual uses of sauma itself, unextracted and not drunk as an intoxicant, were presumably widespread, we can hardly expect the ceremonially oriented Zoroastrian literature to give extensive recognition to such practices.

§75 Just as sauma was important before and during the establishment of Zoroastrianism, the harmel plant continued to be important in Iranian folk religion during and after the Islamization of Iran in the seventh century. It may therefore be of interest to consider what parallels may exist between the relationship of *Peganum harmala* to Islam and that of sauma in the pre-Islamic period to Zoroastrianism.

§76 In the folk verses quoted above, the apotropaic use of *Peganum harmala* is said to have originated with the primary figures of Shīʿa Islam, namely, with the Prophet, ʿAlī, Fāṭima, Ḥusayn, and Ḥasan. The association of the plant with these personages appears to represent an accommodation of ancient folk beliefs to the official religion, in this case not as a result of concessions by the formulators of Muslim doctrine, but as a spontaneous development within folk religion itself. The ascription of prevailing folk attitudes toward harmel to the founders of Islam is also manifest in more official literature of Shīʿa Islam, for example in the following *ḥadīṯẖ* series, which is found in the *Ḥulyat al-muttaqīn* of Muḥammad Bāqir Majlisī (d. 1699),[11] probably the most eminent theologian of Iranian Shīʿism. On his authority we must conclude, against Henning, that the place of *isfand* in the Iranian tradition is not to be assigned to mere witchcraft.

> It is related from the Prophet that over each leaf and seed of the *isfand* plant an angel is appointed so that through its bark and roots and branches grief and sorcery are set aside.[12] In its seeds is the cure of seventy-two diseases. Therefore, make medical treatment with *isfand* and frankincense [*kundur*].
>
> From the [Shīʿa] saint Jaʿfar al-Ṣādiq it is related that the Devil is made distant seventy houses from a house where there is *isfand*. It is a remedy for seventy illnesses, of which the easiest is *xūra* [black leprosy?].
>
> And in another account it is related that the Prophet complained to Allah that his people were cowardly. A revelation came down to him to command his people to ingest *isfand* so that by means of it they might become brave.[13] He ordained that it be the incense [*kundur*] chosen by the Prophet. No smoke rises more quickly to heaven than does its smoke, which expels devils and averts misfortunes.

§77 The evidence for *Peganum harmala* in its Islamic contexts, furnished by the three texts we have examined above—the Iranian folk verses, the Azari invocation of *Üzerlik*, and the *ḥadīṯẖ*s collected by Muḥammad Bāqir Majlisī—may now be compared with *haoma* in the Avesta:

8 Hüseyin Kāzim Kadri 1927: 383-384, where it is stated that the verses first appeared in the journal *Mullā Naṣruddīn* (published in Baku from 1906 to 1911). Professor Hasan Javadi has kindly provided the translation.

9 An analogous situation exists regarding the Iranian celebration of the New Year, which one might conclude from Zoroastrian texts alone to have been a purely Zoroastrian observance but which in reality both preceded Zoroastrianism and has continued in Islamic Iran, albeit redefined as a secular event (see Moghadam 1938).

10 For *nivizaiti* see below, §250 n.8.

11 Chapter 9, part 12 (Tehran, edition of 1371*q*., pp. 220-221; edition of 1341*š*, p. 191), cited by I. Shokurzade (1967: 220 n.4).

12 Sunni sources appear also to record this *ḥadīṯẖ*: see L. Leclerc (1874: 137n.), M. Vonderheyden (1937: 460), and L. Trabut (1935: 186).

13 This *ḥadīṯẖ* is transparently Persian rather than Arabic in origin. It seems to be a "Magian" explanation for the success of Arab armies in the seventh century conquest of Sasanian Iran to claim that "Muḥammad's people" were cowards until provided with sauma. A sense of bravery is often associated with harmine intoxication resulting from the consumption of *yagé*.

***Peganum Harmala* in Texts of Islamic Iran**	***Haoma* in the Avesta**[14]
1. Use is instituted by four persons of the lineage of the founder of the religion:	
The institution of *isfand* (including planting, collecting and burning) is attributed to Muḥammad (and/or ʿAlī), and Fāṭima, Muḥammad's daughter, for the sake of her sons Ḥusayn and Ḥasan.	Four persons, Yima, Athwya, Thrita and Zarathushtra's father Pourushāspa, are listed as Zarathushtra's predecessors in instituting the use of *Haoma (Yasna* 9.3–14; see below, §§91–92).
2. Is directly endorsed by God:	
Allah commands Muḥammad to use *isfand.*	Ahura Mazdah created *Haoma (Yasna* 10.17; 11.8).
	Ahura Mazdah invested *Haoma* with the Zoroastrian religion (*Yasna* 9.26).
3. Brings apotropaic benefits to the house where it is kept:	
The Devil is made seventy houses distant from a house where there is *isfand.*	*Haoma* should be present in an Ahurian house so that demons flee from it (*Yasna* 10.1).
	"Let contamination, as soon as it is manifested, vanish from that house, as soon as one brings forth... *Haoma*" (*Yasna* 10.7).
4. Instills courage:	
Muḥammad's people are made courageous by *isfand.*	*"Haoma* gives courage" (*Yasna* 9.22).
	"(*Haoma*) I invoke thee for courage and for victory for my body and for strength that brings salvation to many" (*Yasna* 9.27)
5. Expels a thousand demons/diseases:	
"*Üzerlik,* thou art the remedy for a thousand diseases."	The least extraction, praise, or ingestion of *Haoma* smites a thousand demons (*Y.* 10.6).
6. Bears the epithet 'golden/yellow':	
"Golden-colored [*altun*] *Üzerlik.*"	"Yellowish [*zāiri-*] *Haoma*" (*Yasna* 9.16, etc.).[15]

CORRESPONDENCE IN ATTRIBUTES AND INVOCATIONS

§78 *Haoma* is mentioned frequently throughout the Avestan books in connection with the worship of the ancient Iranian deities. Usually this consists of nothing more than naming *haoma* as something consecrated to the gods. *Haoma* is also associated with the roles of deities in contexts which do not contribute to our understanding of sauma (see Gray 1929; Boyce 1970), but with few exceptions the only material in the Avesta which refers to *haoma* as a plant is found in the *Hōm Yasht*, the part of the Avesta devoted to the worship or invocation of *Haoma.* This text, consisting of about 1,700 words, is today included in the liturgy of the *Yasna* ceremony (as chapters 9-11.15) and is recited immediately before and during the consumption of *haoma* in that ritual.

§79 Perhaps the closest parallel to the *Hōm Yasht* outside of Zoroastrian literature is a text of the Mandaeans, who dwell in southern Iran and Iraq, and whose ancient gnostic baptist religion was strongly influenced by Iranian ritual and lore. This Mandean text is entitled *Šafta ḏ Šambra* ("The Scroll of [Wild] Rue"), and was intended for recitation when *Peganum harmala* (Mandean *šambra*), pounded in a mortar and "mixed with water, wine, *šakir*,[16] or the urine of a red bull"[17] was administered as a drug. A noteworthy difference between the two texts is the insertion of the name of the person for whom the invocation is recited at various points in the Mandean text; this practice is alien to the recitation of the *Hōm Yasht.* Furthermore, while the *Hōm Yasht* is recited by the priest who is about to drink *haoma*, the *Šafta ḏ Šambra* is recited by the person who administers the extract (who, however, must often have been a Mandaean priest).

§80 Although Mandaic is a language used only by those adhering to the Mandaean religion, and almost all literature written in it consists of religious works, the *Šafta ḏ Šambra* is not a part of Mandaean canonical literature. The text is of a decidedly magical character, and the gods are called forth wholly for the purpose of furthering the effectiveness of the spirit of harmel in a specific situation, that of purging someone of sickness, that is to say, of demons. Wisdom or knowledge is not among the benefits sought, nor is intoxication mentioned in the Mandaean text, even though this effect may well have been experienced as an outcome of drinking preparations of that plant.

[14] In order to preserve the textual ambiguity of *haoma* in Avestan texts, the word may be capitalized whether or not it obviously refers to a personification.

[15] Golden/yellow is the color of harmel during most of the dry season in the Middle East, as noted by Viktorov (1973): "Growths of *Peganum harmala* L. are especially well marked from the air: dark green in summer, having a characteristically golden orange color in autumn". For the meaning of Avestan *zāiri-* see §260 below.

[16] *škr* was translated 'syrup' by E. S. Drower (1934), but later as 'liquor (or syrup)' in the *Dictionary* of E. S. Drower and R. Macuch (1963: 441). Aramaic *škr*, indicating an indeterminate alcoholic drink other than wine, may correspond to Avestan *hurā*, Middle Persian *hur*, for which *ŠKL* (i.e.**škr*) is the Pahlavi logogram. Because *hurā-* and wine were drunk at the recital of the Gathas (according to *Nērangistān* 29-30), which presumably means in the *Yasna* ceremony, it may be inferred that both of these alcoholic drinks sometimes accompanied the taking of sauma. The drinking of alcohol together with harmala alkaloids is frequently reported for *yagé* ceremonies.

[17] These ingredients recall more the Zoroastrian preparation called *nērang*, than the *haoma* of the *Yasna*. It is indeed possible that the Mandaeans would have been most familiar with sauma as an ingredient of *nērang*, since the *Yasna* could not be witnessed by non-Zoroastrians and the drinking of *haoma* is one of the less conspicuous Zoroastrian practices (e.g. it seems *never* to have been recorded in any Islamic source on the "Magian religion"; the *hawm al-majūs* known to Muslims was not a plant consumed but only held by Zoroastrian priests). *Nērang* is not only drunk in the initiation rites of *nō-šwā* and *nōzādī* (formerly undergone by all Zoroastrians in Iran) but is also consumed in the daily ritual of *kustī bastan* 'tying the sacred cord' (Soroushian 1956: 166), which must have been often witnessed by the Mandaeans during the centuries when they were under Persian administration. One form of *nērang* is prepared from *hōm*, bovine urine, fruit juice, and wine (*ibid.* 166). A. Houtum-Schindler (1885: 83) describes *nērang* as made from "*hōm*" mixed with cow urine. He claims the mixture was given to the new-born and the dead, taken daily during [the nine days of] *barešnum*, and was also used as a remedy against sickness. I am informed by Mary Boyce (letter of October 7, 1978), however, that *hōm* is not an ingredient of *nērang* in any orthodox usage.

The drinking of bull urine is not originally a Mandaean but an ancient Iranian practice. The Iranian inspiration for the Mandaean text and associated harmel practices is especially marked by the mention of bull urine as an additive to the extract of the plant, for the Mandaic term used for bull urine, *gumiza*, is clearly borrowed from Iranian ritual (cf. Middle Persian *gōmēz*).

§81 An unusual feature shared by both texts is the use of the names *haoma* and *šambra* respectively, at once for the plant, the drink prepared from it, and the personification of the plant. The association of the plant with other divine and semi-divine beings is parallel in both texts and, since the personification of *Šambra* as a deity is unknown elsewhere in Mandaean writings, its appearance in the *Šafta ḏ Šambra* may represent a borrowing from a non-Mandaean source and possibly the influence, if not directly of the Avestan *Hōm Yasht*, then of a similar early Iranian invocation of sauma. The highly formulaic character of the *Šafta ḏ Šambra* indicates that it was composed orally and transmitted perhaps for many centuries before it was written down, although existing manuscripts are no older than the early nineteenth century (Drower 1934). Considering the antiquity of most Mandaean texts, the work could easily date from before the Islamic period; that is, from the millennium when the areas inhabited by the Mandaeans were under Iranian political domination. The Mandaeans during that time adopted many religious and magical practices from their Iranian neighbors, and it would seem natural for them then to have given attention also to the most important single element in Iranian ritual, *haoma,* and therefore to the traditional Iranian attribution of supernatural power to sauma. There may be a reflection of the Iranian *haoma* in Mandaean ritual practice,[18] but reference to *haoma* by name is absent from Mandaean literature. The textual correspondences we shall now examine suggest that the *šambra* in the *Šafta ḏ Šambra* may be a Mandaean adaptation of the sauma of Iranian tradition.

§82 Comparison of habitats of Mandaean *Šambra* and Avestan *Haoma*

Mandaean *Šafta ḏ Šambra* (Translated by E.S. Drower, 1934)[19]	**Avestan *Hōm Yasht*** (Translated by M. Schwartz)
(O) good plant (son of) the god of the mountains, son of the lord of mountains, son of the lord of the high mountains, son of deep ravines and son of peaceful valleys (337.1).	Good is *Haoma,* created by Mazdah. I praise all the *Haomas*,[20] be they those on the heights of the mountains, be they those in the depths of the valleys, cut for the bundles bound by women[21] (*Yasna* 10.17).
Further I abjure thee, glorious medicine, by the male gods and female astartes by Shamish (the sun) that shineth on thee: by Sin (the moon) that traveleth over thee; by wind, fire and water: by the mountains which bore thee: by the gorges and craggy heights that reared thee: and by the waterways in them (343.6).	Thou (*Haoma*) hast been upon the mountain heights throughout all ages (*Yasna* 9.26). I praise the cloud and the rain which make thy body grow on the heights of the mountains. I praise the high mountains where, *Haoma,* thou growest. I praise the wide, broad, energetic, blessed earth, thy bearer. I praise the field of thine earth by which thou growest fragrant and swift, and the good growth of Mazdah. *Haoma,* mayst thou grow on the mountains and mayst thou prosper; truly thou art the Fountain of Rightness (*Yasna* 10.3–5).
I abjure thee by the mountains that bore thee, by the uplands that reared thee, by the north wind that breathed over thee (344.16).	
[O] *Šambra,* go below like water which gusheth from the peak of a high mountain (344.15).	
The Lady of Gods and Men took thee and carried thee off to the male gods and the female astartes and she gave favorable testimony concerning thee. And they sent (it) to everyone that was ill, working a cure, and healing was found in it (344.30).	The beneficent god has placed thee upon High Haraiti. From there the learned *spənta-* [!] birds carried thee in all directions, to the peak above the eagles, to the Hindu Kush, to the star-topped peaks . . . to the white-colored mountains. There on those mountains thou growest, *Haoma,* who art of many sorts, rich in sap, verdant. Thy healings are connected with the joys of Good Thinking (*Yasna* 10.10–12).
Thou didst spring forth of thine own strength, and didst come forth and camest into being (342.8).	*Haoma,* who through thine own power art thine own master (*Yasna* 9.25).

§83 Much mention is made in the Mandaean text of the mountains as the home of *Peganum harmala.* Throughout the Middle East, harmel is generally regarded as a mountain plant; this is seen not only from names identifying harmel as "mountain rue" (e.g. Arabic *saδāb al-jabal;* Persian *sudāb-i kūhī*), but from Persian folk verses, for example, the following from Lorimer (1977: 65; pointed out to me by Dr. Mahmoud Omidsalar):

esfand-i sar-i-kuh	O *Esfand* of the mountain top.
esfand-i kamar-i-kuh	O *Esfand* of the mountain waist.
esfand-i bun-i-kuh	O *Esfand* of the mountain base.
esfand tu ke mīdūnī	O *Esfand,* you who know,
behaqq-i suleymūn-i peyγambar	By the grace of Solomon the Prophet
čišmzaxm-rā bigardūnī	Turn away the evil eye.

Although harmel is abundant in the mountains of Iran, it is hardly less so in the lowlands north of the Persian Gulf where the Mandaeans live (see A. Patzak 1964: 401). The emphasis given in the text to the lofty and remote origins of a plant that is in fact a common weed available from the nearest rubbish heap would seem then to have been intended not to describe its habitat, but, rather, to counter its banal provenance. This same consideration may be applied to the Avestan descriptions of *haoma* as growing in the mountains. There are thus no grounds for concluding from the Avesta that sauma grew exclusively on mountains.[22]

18 According to E. S. Drower (1956:210 n.1), the preparation of the Mandaean *miša* ("oil of unction"), consisting of date-pulp pounded in a mortar with sesame oil and strained through a white cloth, possibly reflects the preparation of Iranian *haoma.* For the use of sesame oil in preparing *Peganum harmala* as a drug see §44C and cf. also §137.

19 Occasional words in Drower's translation have been replaced by the original Mandaean, e.g. 'rue' by *šambra*, etc.

20 This plurality of *haomas* may be compared with Reichel-Dolmatoff's (1972:97-98) account of the various *yagés* distinguished by Tukano shamans in Colombia:

"From each *yagé* plant the Indians choose branches or pieces of different colors . . . . These colors do not refer solely to the external appearance of the vine but above all to the predominant color of the hallucinations experienced through its use. A *yagé* taken by the Desana produces visions of 'jumping feather crowns', or snakes shaped like necklaces that coil themselves around the houseposts. Another kind of *yagé* is said to produce hallucinations of 'snakes that jump' . . . . it is possible that at the base of this classificatory system there lies traditional knowledge that certain parts of the vine . . . contain different concentrations of the hallucinogenic component and therefore cause different visions. As a matter of fact, one of the chief concerns in the preparation of the drink is precisely the knowledge of how to combine portions of different vines.

"The effect is therefore highly unpredictable, and the consumer of *yagé* runs the risk of having some extremely unsettling experiences. This fact worries the Indians, who, apart from the combination of components used, attempt to influence the effects magically to eliminate the more unpleasant aspects. To this end there is a long series of spells and songs to be recited while the drink is being prepared".

The problem of determining the exact strength and constitution of sauma extracts may have similarly influenced the development of Indo-Iranian rituals.

21 *Peganum harmala* is frequently collected in bundles by women. A. Gabriel (1970: 141) compares the bundles of Zoroastrian *barsom* with bundles of harmel: "Das Bündel geweihter Zweige erinnert an die noch jetzt bisweilen auch bei Muslimen übliche Verwendung der syrischen Raute (*Peganum harmala*) zur Segnung von Gästen" (see below, §124 n.10).

22 On the other hand, if the Mandaean text is modeled on an Iranian original, the mountainous

§84 Comparison of gracious attributes of *Šambra* and *Haoma.*

Mandaean *Šafta ḏ Šambra*	**Avestan *Hōm Yasht***
And there will be healing, victory, sealing, armed-readiness, gladness, and medicine, and joy to him that drinketh it (335.8).	I ask of thee, O golden (one), intoxication, power, victory, health, healing, success, increase, strength of the whole body (*Yasna* 9.17).
. . . that drinketh thee, either in wine, or in *šakir*, or in water, or in the urine of a red bull (337.17).	Thou (*Haoma*) makest rich in men, more *spənta-*, and more insightful whomever aportions thee combined with *gav-* ['flesh/cattle-product'] (*Yasna* 10.13).
And the medicine (bringeth?) joy and healing to the drinker and riches to him who administereth it. Thou (O) sprig, givest salvation and not perdition, for thou make them strong (and art) a healer, thou workest healing and yieldest not (344.1).	Thee I invoke for courage and for victory for my body and for strength that brings salvation to many (*Yasna* 9.27).
Cure, my cure! Victorious Medicine, my victorious healer! (344.8).	(O) *Haoma*, give me of thy healing by which thou art a healer, (O) *Haoma*, give me of thy victoriousness, by which thou art a victor (*Yasna* 10.9).
Protection, son of Protection art thou, lofty is thy throne. "Protection son of Protection" they call me (335.15).	**From other Zoroastrian texts** I carry on me the... victorious *Haoma*. I carry on me the Protector (as) the good thing. I carry on me the Protector of the body (*Yasht* 14.57).
I am *Šambra*, the good neighbour, king of all drugs (335.17).	(*Haoma*) is the chief of medicinal herbs (*Bundahišn* 17.20]).

§85 Comparison of punitive attributes of *Šambra* and *Haoma.*

Mandaean *Šafta ḏ Šambra*	**Avestan *Hōm Yasht***
Thou hold back...those evil spirits... like lightning that is sent and loosed against that evil serpent, driving it out and turning it aside by its force from that house (334.22).	O golden *Haoma*, loose thy weapon for protecting the body of the righteous against the yellow loathsome poison-emitting serpent, against the evil-doing, bloody, injurious murderous one, against the lying mortal *sāstars*...against the Truth-mocker... against the sorcerous witch (*Yasna* 9.30-33).
Turn away that evil serpent that makes for him: scare it off, thou Medicine, frighten it away by thy potency. And receive from me these spells and conjurarations... harass, drive away and make impotent those who hate him and all his enemies, and *šids*, demons (*daiwia*), incubi, hobgoblins, malign spirits, amulet spirits, evil apparations, spectres and fearsome shades of darkness, evil enchantments, wicked machinations (343.15).	I ask this, that I may overcome all the enmity of the enemies, demons (*daēva)* and men, of *yātu* spirits, of *pairika* spirits, of *sāthras*, of *kavis* and *karapans*, of two-legged scoundrels, of two legged Truth-mockers, of four-legged wolves, and of hosts having a broad front, roaring, scampering (*Yasna* 9.18).
Healing Medicine that cureth spirits and souls, before whōm *šids* tremble and evil spirits quaking are driven (337.5).	(O *Haoma*) throw aside the plot of that one who curses me, throw aside the various plots of him who stands as my curser (*Yasna* 10.12).
In the name of him who is a Healer that healeth...thou shatterest, drivest away and renderest impotentkgods and male idols and all evil beings male and female that slay embryos in the womb of their mothers and... vows, curses and provocations (imprecations?) of gods and men (324.9).	Even the smallest *Haoma*-preparation, the smallest *Haoma*-laudation, the smallest *Haoma*-potation, serves to smite a thousand demons. Let the contamination vanish from that house as soon as it is created, as soon as, indeed, one brings it forth...and praises the excellent healing of him who confers healing, *Haoma* (*Yasna* 10.6-7).

§86 The effects actually experienced from a preparation of harmel were well known in Middle Eastern lore: as reported in early Islamic materia medica, they are chiefly vomiting, sleep, intoxication, and an inclination toward coitus (see §44). There is no reason to think the Mandaeans were unfamiliar with these characteristics of the drug, or that they would not have been anticipated by those for whom this invocation was recited. It is doubtless the very predictability of these effects that made useful the invocation of the plant in the hope of ameliorating them. If this were not the situation, it is hardly likely that persons suffering illness would have been subjected to a 2,500-word conjuration of the medicine before consuming it, nor is it probable that the *Šafta ḏ Šambra*, which is not a text of religious value to the Mandaeans, would have been preserved at all.

§87 The Mandaean *Šafta ḏ Šambra* has implications not only for determining the plant referred to in the Avestan *Hōm Yasht* but also for understanding the content of that text and the purposes underlying its recital in sauma rites. The very recitation of the *šambra* invocation appears to be intended to compel a preparation of *Peganum harmala* to yield certain results. The *Šafta ḏ Šambra* explicitly declares that the text itself contains spells and conjurations and that the recited words "will be a cure that will free" the subject (336.9). Similar statements appear in the *Hōm Yasht*, the words of which "bring health and victory against enemies" (*Yasna* 10.18). Whether or not the words were believed to compel *haoma* after the manner of magical conjurations or to exert more gentle influence upon *haoma* to do what was asked, the motivation for reciting the *Hōm Yasht* should not be overlooked: "(*Haoma*) understands the many truly spoken sayings. . . . *Haoma* . . . does not question . . . the truly spoken word" (*Yasna* 9.25). The practical purpose of the *Hōm Yasht* does not seem to be to communicate observations about the properties of sauma, but to influence the outcome of drinking it. In general, it may be assumed that the effects attributed to sauma in the *Hōm Yasht* are only the desirable ones the recital of the text was believed to further.

§88 The aspect of sauma most extolled in the *Hōm Yasht* is the quality of its intoxication, but one cannot assume that the characteristics sought were those actually expected. The focus upon the benign effects may be taken as reflecting an actual concern that the effects may be unpleasant.

Attribution of generative powers

§89 We may next turn to another property shared by harmel and sauma. The very end of the *Šafta ḏ Šambra* recommends the preparation of *Peganum harmala* for a purpose quite different from the apotropaic healing with which the invocation is otherwise concerned:

> Read it over them and administer the potion to a woman that desires to bring forth (a child) and for one that desires to have children (346.20).

The same virtue is claimed in the *Hōm Yasht:*

> *Haoma* gives pregnant women the birth of an excellent son and righteous progeny (*Yasna* 9.22).

§90 The *Hōm Yasht* also alludes to the power of *Haoma* punitively not to assist certain women to have desirable offspring.

avaŋhərəzāmi janyaoš ūnam	I renounce the vulva/burrow
mairyayå əvītō.xarəδayå	of the filthy roguish wench[23]

provenance ascribed to the plant may simply repeat the Indo-Iranian conception of sauma as originating in mountains. In Anatolia, it should be noted, harmel seems to be exclusively confined to the interior highlands (K. O. Müller 1932).

[23] For this reading see below, §180.

yā mainyeinti davayeinti	who plots to deceive
āθravānəmča haoməmča	the priest and *Haoma.*
hā yā dapta apanasyeiti	She herself, deceived, fails,
yā tat̰ yat̰ haomahe draonō	sitting down to consume
nigåŋhənti nišhaδaiti	the *draonah*[24] of *Haoma*:
nōit̰ tam āθravōpuθrīm	He does not make her the mother of priests
naēδa dasti hupuθrīm	He does not make her the mother of fine sons.[25]
(*Yasna* 10.15)	

§91 By contrast, the birth of illustrious sons is the only benefit which the beginning of the *Hōm Yasht* claims to have been realized by the first four mortals who extracted *haoma.*

> (*Yasna* 9.1) At the mortar time [the first period of the day], *Haoma* came upon Zarathushtra, purifying the fire and intoning the Gathas. Zarathushtra asked him: (2) "Who, man, art thou, whom I see as the most beautiful in all the material world, luminous with thine own life?"[26] Then the righteous *dūraoša Haoma* answered: "I am, O Zarathushtra, the righteous *dūraoša Haoma.* Take me, Spitāma, extract me that I may be drunk, praise me with might, as the other *saošyants* [saviors] have praised me." (3) Thus spake Zarathushtra: "Praise be to *Haoma!* Which mortal in the material world first extracted thee? What reward was granted him? What benefit came to him?"

§92 *Haoma* responds to Zarathushtra's questions about the first four mortals who extracted him, saying that the benefit they received was the birth of sons, whose merits he then briefly describes. For example, *Haoma* says (*Yasna* 9. 13–15) the fourth to have extracted him was Pourushāspa, with this result:

> To him were you born, you, righteous Zarathushtra, in the house of Pourushāspa, opposed to the *daēvas*, following the law of the *ahuras.* (14) Famed in Aryana Vaējah, you were the first to sing out the *Ahuna Vairya* prayer; four times, each (time) sung out louder. (15) You who made all the demons disappear beneath the earth, those who had earlier rushed against this earth in the form of men. You who are the strongest, who are the bravest, who are the most active, who are the swiftest, who are the most victorious of the creatures of the Two Spirits.

§93 How *Haoma* was able to cause the birth of sons to these men is not stated, but one explanation, perhaps the only one for how a drug could have such results in the material world, is that it was thought to act as a sexual stimulant. This, indeed, is a property clearly indicated for sauma in the account of the birth of Zoroaster, epitomized from lost Avestan texts in *Dēnkird* VII (2.26–35): Zoroaster's father, Porushāsp, had his wife prepare a decoction of the *hōm* plant mixed with milk, which they both then drank (apparently without reciting the *Yasna* liturgy ordinarily accompanying the drinking of *haoma*). In consequence they lay together for the first time and, despite repeated interruptions by the demons, in the fourth attempt accomplished the conception of Zoroaster.[27] In this account, the only effect of sauma upon Porushāsp or his wife seems to have been sexual stimulation. As has already been noted, this is one of the effects of drinking a preparation of harmel reported in traditional Near Eastern pharmacopoeias.

SIMULTANEOUSLY BOTH INCENSE AND INTOXICANT

§94 So far the correspondence of the role of *Peganum harmala* in Iranian folk religion with that of *haoma* in the Avesta has been supported by evidence that *Peganum harmala* is: (1) invoked or described by terms similar to, or identical with, those used of *haoma*; (2) characterized by the same epithets; (3) assigned similar properties; (4) associated in a similar manner with sources of religious authority; and (5) used for apotropaic purposes, for healing, and to promote procreation. However, there

24 Where the *draonah* ('portion', especially 'portion allotted as payment to a priest') of *haoma* is mentioned again in the *Hōm Yasht* (*Yasna* 11. 4-7), it refers to the organs of sight and of speech of the *haoma*-drinking priest (who surrenders his body [=*gāuš* of *Yasna* 11.7] to *haoma;* see below §150 n.3). *Haoma,* being a drug, would most likely work its effects on someone who drinks *haoma,* i.e. in the context of the *Hōm Yasht,* on the *Yasna* priest; yet here the "he" who could make a "filthy roguish wench" the mother of priests must be the priest and not *haoma* directly. The verse apparently alludes to sexual/reproductive aspects of the drug, although to whom or what the wench or her empty place may refer is completely obscure.

25 A preparation which probably contained sauma is described by Pliny from the *Chirocmeta* (*Naturalis historia* XXIV:166; see below, §151): "Democritus [Bolus of Mendes] gives the name *hermesias* to a means of procreating children who shall be handsome and good. It is not a plant, but a compound of ground kernels of pine nuts with honey, myrrh, saffron, and palm wine, with the later addition of *theombrotion* and milk. He prescribes a draught of it to those who are about to become parents, after conception, and to nursing mothers. This, he says, results in children exceeding fair in mind and body, as well as good. Of all these plants he adds also the magical [or Magian?] names". *Theombrotion* ('food for the gods, divine food') which the *Chirocmeta* describes as a finely scented plant growing thirty *schoeni* (i.e. about 200 km.!) from the Choaspes (Karkha) River and like a peacock in its colorings, may be identified with sauma. For "peacock" see below, §§172–177. Pseudo-Democritus also says of *theombrotion*: "The kings of Persia take it in drink for all bodily disorders and for instability of intellect and of the sense of justice [meaning perhaps as a test for these instabilities, since a king would hardly have confessed himself to be in need of treatment for them] and that it is also called *semnion* from the majesty of its power". Greek-Latin *semnion* is from Greek ςεμν́Ÿ 'awesome, sacred', and may be a translation of Avestan *spənta*- as the name of the plant.

26 Because plants do not speak, the human appearance of *Haoma* more probably reflects a characteristic of the subjective experience of the drug than the morphology of a plant species. Hence we cannot conclude from these words of Zarathushtra that a given specimen of the *haoma* plant, or of the roots of the plant, actually had the appearance of a luminous and beautiful man. Gernot Windfuhr (1986), however, makes this passage the basis for arguing that *haoma* was the (geographically remote and psychopharmacologically irrelevant) ginseng plant because (the most highly valued) ginseng roots have a homunculus shape (with one eye). To Windfuhr's discussion may suitably be added reference to the identical ideas for identifying ginseng with *soma* of P. Andreas Eckard (1928: 226–230).

Klopin's (1980) proposal that *haoma* was *Mandragora turkomania* seems inspired by associating with the reputed man-like shape of mandrake roots a similarly concrete interpretation of Zarathushtra's salutation of *Haoma.* Encounters with human incarnations of plants are often reported by *yagé* users; indeed, the skills of the *yagé* healers studied by Luna (1986 and 1987) are *only* learned by means of encounters after drinking *yagé* with a human incarnation of the *Banisteriopsis* plant.

27 According to Abū al-Mutarrif ʿAbd al-Raḥmān ibn Wāfid (*c.* 1050) in Ibn Bayṭār (see above §44C): "By means of causing intoxication and sleep, it is useful to persons given up to passionate love." An anonymous authority is also quoted by Ibn Bayṭār as saying: "it clears the complexion and stimulates coition." For the sexual aspects of harmaline intoxication, see C. Naranjo (1975:140-144). The report of clinical studies by C. Caller Ibérico (1941) in which small doses of harmaline were found to have pronounced effects directly on sexual organs, cited by R. S. De Ropp (1951:267), should be mentioned, though such results are not usual. C. Naranjo recorded an aphrodisiac effect of harmaline upon subjects only at dosages less than those required for hallucinations.

A curious account that the Turkish Sultan Süleyman administered the seeds of *Peganum harmala* to excite women in his harem is given by O. R. Alander in his dissertation "Inebriantia" (1763: apparently the earliest published attempt to inventory the world's intoxicating plants); it seems, however, to have had as its basis only Alander's fantastic misunderstanding of a remark published by Pierre Belon (1555:207) speculating that the notorious drunkard Sultan Selim may have made use of harmel seeds to intoxicate himself! Nevertheless, the reputation of harmel as an aphrodisiac was well known to the Turks and, as Schwartz (§278) suggests, could explain its Turkish name *(y)üzerlik.*

remains one important aspect of the use of harmel which does not at first seem to accord with the use of sauma, namely the burning of the seeds of *Peganum harmala* in folk religion, in contrast with the Avestan extraction and drinking of *haoma*. How can this disparity be resolved?

§95 While burning is the usual use reported for harmel in modern Iran, there is evidence in folk religion that an extract was also drunk; Mandaean materials recommend the drinking of a preparation of harmel for healing and procreation, as we have seen. However, the Mandaean texts also recommend ingestion of the plant for wholly apotropaic ends, as in the following passage where the plant is called by its Persian name, *isfand/ispand*:

> Solomon then asks, "O demon, what is the charm that exorcises thee?" . . . The demon replies giving a recipe and a magical formula, the latter usually being Arabic in Mandaic script. The recipes are various, for instance: "black *ispand* in the milk of a red cow: boil it over the fire and eat it" (Drower 1943: 156).

§96 According to the Shiʿa *ḥadīth* quoted earlier (§59), Muḥammad was commanded by God to have his people ingest *isfand* for bravery. This *ḥadīth* is interesting in the present connection because it is followed by the recommendation not that *isfand* be ingested, but that it be burned. The *ḥadīth* concludes: "He ordained that it [*isfand*] be the incense chosen by the Prophet. No smoke rises more quickly to heaven than its smoke, which expels devils and averts misfortunes." Since the *ḥadīth* is prescriptive, the consumption of *isfand* by Muḥammad's followers seems to be mentioned in order to encourage the burning of the plant. Another of the *ḥadīth*s quoted states that "an angel is appointed over every leaf and seed of *isfand*," but in this case also, the moral drawn is that one should burn *isfand*. How the relationship of the simultaneously recommended ingesting and burning *isfand* was meant to be understood by those who heard these *ḥadīth*s is not immediately obvious. What is important for us is that they reflect Iranian traditions in which ingestion and burning were held to have the same effect.

§97 While there is evidence connecting the burning of *Peganum harmala* with its ingestion, it is insufficient to explain the fact that burning has been the chief mode of using *Peganum harmala* throughout the Islamic period in Iran, as presumably it was in Iran earlier. The question which must then be asked is whether sauma was indeed burned in pre-Islamic Iran. Although the fact has gone largely unnoticed, there is evidence for the burning of sauma both in Zoroastrian rituals and in the Avesta, indeed in the very earliest Iranian sources, the Gathas.

§98 In *Yasna* 32.14, Zarathushtra speaks of certain miscreants who "set their thoughts on helping the wicked one, whereby the bovine is ordered to be slain, (the wicked one) who burns the *dūraoša-* for help." Here sauma is referred to as *dūraoša-*, which is known in the Avesta only as a fixed epithet of *haoma*.[28] This passage, which has much importance for the identification of sauma and for its history in Iran, is further discussed below (§§136 and 159-160); here we need note only that it clearly shows that sauma was something in the Avesta which was burned.

§99 It is important to point out now that sauma is represented as being burned in the *Yasna* rite itself. During the recital of the hymn to Fire in *Yasna* 62, the residue of the plants from which the *haoma* extract has been obtained is placed in the fire.[29] The burning of haoma is also represented where the plant used as the chief ingredient of the *haoma* drunk in the *Yasna* and commonly called *hōm* in Iran today, *Ephedra*, is burned as fuel incense which Boyce (1970: 64-65) reports takes place on almost all occasions when an animal is slaughtered for food among the Iranian Zoroastrians (see §§115 and 131).[30]

28 For discussion of the meaning of Avestan *dūraoša-* see §§226-227 below. Bailey has reported (1964) that Khotanese "seems to have preserved the most ancient and famous word for the intoxicant, the *dūraoša-* of the Avesta." The passage (in P2925, Bailey 1969: II, 101.34) is translated by Bailey (1979: 161-162): "he here draws to me as one draws an exhilarant draught (*durauśa' ttraha*)." If Bailey is correct, this would be the only Iranian attestation of the word *dūraoša-* outside of the Avesta and this passage would be the most explicit reference to sauma drinking in Iranian literature that is not part of the Zoroastrian tradition. Bailey's reading of the passage is, however, questioned in the following note on Khotanese *durauśa'*, graciously contributed (October 6, 1983) by Professor Ronald Emmerick: "*durauśa'* occurs only in P 2925.33 KT 3.101. According to Bailey (1979:161 *s.v.*), it means 'elatant, exaltant, exhilarant' and is an 'epithet of a beverage'. See also Bailey 1982: 51. Bailey appears first to have compared Khotanese *durauśa'* with Avestan *dūraoša* in 1964: 4. He did not mention the Khotanese word in his discussions of *dūraoša-* in 1936: 95-97; 1953: 22; 1957a: 30-32; or 1957b: 53-58. There is a formal difficulty involved in Bailey's comparison. He tries to deal with it by deriving Khotanese *durauśa'-* from a hypothetical **duraušya-* but does not account for the *-ya-* suffix. He offers no proof that **šy* could result in Late Khotanese *ś*, since his only parallel, Khotanese *khaṇauśa'*, which he derives from **kanaušya-*, is equally uncertain: the related forms have neither **šya* nor **ya*.

"Bailey's explanation of *durauśa'* involves a still more serious difficulty of a semantic nature. He describes *durauśa'* as an 'epithet of a beverage' but the only evidence he offers in support of the idea that a beverage is involved is an etymology. According to Bailey *durauśa' ttraha* means 'an exhilarant draught', but *ttraha* is nowhere attested in the meaning 'draught'. The etymology he offers for *ttraha* is not without its own difficulties. It is based on a root *tar-* attested only in the modern Iranian languages Ormuṛī and Parāčī and poses the question why **tr-* did not become *dr-* as in *drrai* 'three', cf. Avestan *θrāiiō*, Old Indic *tráyaḥ*.

"There is a well-attested Khotanese word *ttraha* meaning 'radish': see Bailey 1979: 143, *s.v. ttrahā-*. Its meaning is guaranteed by several bilingual passages in which it corresponds to Sanskrit *mūlaka* and Tibetan *la-phug*. The soundest method of procedure would seem to be to see whether *ttraha* in the passage in question could not bear its normal meaning. In fact the use of the verb *thaṃj-* with *ttraha* would suggest that it may well do so. Here *ttraha thaja* may mean 'one pulls out a radish' rather than 'one draws an exhilarant draught'. For this use of *thaṃj-* one may compare in Old Khotanese *kho ju ye viysu thaṃjāte khārja* 'as one pulls a lotus out of the mud' (Emmerick 1968: 5.90). This parallel is particularly apt. In Emmerick 1968: 5.90 the comparison is between pulling a lotus out of the mud and rescuing someone from the ocean of birth. Now Bailey describes the context of *ttraha thaja* as 'an amorous context' but the immediately preceding lines 31-2 refer to *vauma vi ī parauysadā* 'of those drowning in the ocean' and to *satsaira* 'the cycle of existence'. The context is thus clearly similar to that of Emmerick 1968: 5.90.

"On this analysis *durauśa'* may be expected to be the locative of the source of motion like *khārja* in Emmerick 1968: 5.90. Formally it has the appearance of the locative from a noun **durauysa-*. In view of the use of Khotanese *dūra-* 'hard' in connection with *uysmā-* 'soil' as in *uysmīnai pṛḍai dūrä* 'a hard clod of soil' Ch 00268.170 Bailey 1951: 67 [Deśanā 22]), one is tempted to regard *durauśa'* as miswritten for **durauśma'* 'in hard soil'. The locative form would be like *rraśma* from *rraysmā-* 'battle-rank' (Emmerick 1968a p. 277). The omission of the lower portion of a complex akṣara is a not uncommon kind of scribal error. However, one cannot be absolutely certain that *durauśa'* is not an adjective qualifying *ttraha* 'radish'.

"As a tentative rendering of *ṣa' ma 'v thajai khū *durauśma' ttraha thaja* I would suggest 'he pulls me out as one pulls a radish out of hard soil'. For confirmation it will be necessary to scan Buddhist literature for such a comparison."

29 "When [the solid remains of the twigs out of which the liquid has been well squeezed by the fingers in the strainer are] thoroughly dry, they are put into the fire at the time of *Atash Nyayish*" (Haug 1884: 402 n.1). This must refer to *Yasna* 62.9, after which ritual instructions are for the *raspī* to place *hōm* and *urwarām* upon the fire ("*hōm ud urwarām kustag ō ātaxš dahišn*", Darmesteter 1892-1893: I, 389 n.28). The burning of the residue of *haoma* is also reported by A. Khodadadian (1975: 228-229), F. M. Kotwal (in Boyce 1975b:167 n.134 and 323) and F. M. Kotwal and J. W. Boyd (1977:31).

30 The *hōm* is burned together with frankincense during the recital of *Yasna* 7 and 8 in a *drōn* ceremony (Boyce 1970: 64-65). The older practice still survives at the festival of *Mihragān*,

§100 Where we find reference to the burning of sauma in the Avesta, the plant is called *dūraoša-*, not *haoma*. This is probably best explained by the fact that the literal meaning of *haoma*, 'extract', refers to an aqueous state which will not burn. To speak of burning an extract would seem especially inappropriate in view of the Avestan prohibition of mixing fire and water, which excluded even the use of moist wood as fuel for ordinary household fires.

§101 The placing of incense on fires is a dominant motif in ancient Iranian iconography and was of great importance in Iranian rites, focused as these rites were on fire, for which fragrant fuel (Avestan *aēsma- baoiδī*) was required. The above noted ritual uses guarantee that sauma was a suitable offering to the fire. Since sauma was the most sacred of plants, it should have been a preferred offering. Frankincense and sandalwood, the incense favored by Zoroastrians (and other Iranians) today, are foreign products that were not readily available in ancient Iran and were probably unknown to the early Iranian pastoralists. Because there are few plants indigenous to the Iranian area useful for incense, sauma must have met this need whenever it was available.[31] Of the few native substances used as incense, the seeds of *Peganum harmala* seem consistently preferred in Iran during Islamic times,[32] and there is every reason to believe that they were also preferred in Avestan times, in full accord with the identity of harmel as sauma.

5

THE EVIDENCE OF ZOROASTRIAN RITUALS

§102 This chapter will examine the use of plants to represent sauma not only among the Zoroastrians in India, the Parsees, but in greater detail among the small groups of Zoroastrians in and around the cities of Kerman and Yazd in central Iran, who have maintained a tradition of rituals and religious customs apparently unbroken since pre-Islamic times. We shall consider how under varying circumstances both of the two plants extracted for Zoroastrian *Yasna* rituals, *Ephedra* and pomegranate, and a third plant, rue (*Ruta graveolens*), are ritually used to represent sauma and how the role of each of them provides evidence that sauma was harmel.

§103 The most explicit Iranian representation of the consumption of sauma is found in the *Yasna* ritual, which lasts about two hours and is performed several times each morning by priests in Zoroastrian fire temples. During the *Yasna* a priest in the role of *zōt* (Avestan *zaotar*) executes the following three major ritual actions: (1) after reciting *Yasna* 8.4 he consumes some of the *drōn* bread (which appears to be a vestige of sauma, as is discussed separately §133); (2) during the recital of *Yasna* 11.10 he consumes a *haoma* extract; and finally, (3) while he recites *Yasna* 22–27 he prepares a second *haoma* extract, differing from the *haoma* he has drunk only in that it contains milk. This second *haoma* extract (the *āb-zōhr*, see §131) is poured down a well after the ceremony has concluded.

§104 The *haoma* extract consumed by the *zaotar* is not prepared during the *Yasna*, but before it, by the other priest participating in the ritual, the *raspī*. To prepare it the *raspī* sits alone within the consecrated area and pounds in a mortar, with water, three twigs of a species of *Ephedra*, referred to as *hōm*, and a piece sliced lengthwise from a twig of the pomegranate tree (Kotwal and Boyd 1977). From these crushed plant materials he squeezes out the liquid and passes it through a plate with nine holes, and then through a metal ring wound with three hairs from a bull, and into the *haoma* cup from which the *zaotar* will later drink. The residue from this extraction is thrown on the floor and is eventually burned (see §99 n.28). Only after the *raspī*'s preparation of the extract is complete does the *zaotar* join the *raspī* in the ceremonial area and begin recital of the seventy-two chapters of the *Yasna* liturgy. Thus, when, about a quarter of an hour after the rite begins, the *zaotar* is handed the "*haoma*" to drink, it consists of an extract which has been pressed out from two plants. One of these plants presumably represents sauma while the other represents a secondary constituent, or additive, to the primary drug.

§105 The Indian *soma* rites do not attest a parallel to this use of two plants, but, as will be seen (§114), this situation cannot be the basis of an argument against two plants being part of the original ceremony. The extraction of two plants is indicated in the text of the Avestan *Yasna* liturgy as well as being represented in the ritual actions accompanying its recital and, since Iranian ceremonies have been consistently simplified (see Pavry 1918), not embellished, it is *a priori* unlikely that the second plant would be an innovation. We shall now consider the relationship to sauma of each of these two constituent plants, *Ephedra* and pomegranate.

EPHEDRA

(a) The relationship of *Ephedra* to sauma

§106 For centuries the Zoroastrians of central Iran have collected the leafless, much branched, jointed twigs of small shrubs of the genus *Ephedra* (locally known as *hōm*) in the mountains and have used them as *haoma*.[1] In areas of eastern Iran where these *Ephedras* are particularly abundant (and where Zoroastrian influence has long been absent) they have such vernacular names as *hōm, hum-i bandak, xuma, um, uma, ōmə, oman, yūmana, amojak, uroman, humb, narōmb, nārom*, and so forth (see Table 3), all of which names derive from Old Iranian **hauma-*. This

however, when under otherwise identical circumstances, it is not the plant called *hōm* but *Peganum harmala* which is burned, see §115.

[31] While the names of other incense plants (such as *vohu.gaona-* or *vohu.kərəti-*, see §238) are obscure in the Avesta, the burning of juniper (Avestan *hapərəsi-*) is linked there with the otherwise unknown "Vyāmbura" *daēva*-worshippers. Burning juniper could not have been a practice limited to *daēva*-worshippers, however, because juniper is abundant and valued as a fragrant fuel over much of eastern Iran and the Indo-Iranian borderlands. Juniper is burned apotropaically together with harmel in the Shina and Hunza areas (Jettmar 1975: 217 n.134, 258, 270, 421), and in Wakhan (Grjunberg and Steblin-Kamenskij 1976:249-250). The burning of juniper together with a fragment of "*hōm*" (*Ephedra*) in modern Khorasan (Aitchison 1889:434) is presumably a reflection of the same practice but, again, with the replacement of harmel by *Ephedra*.

[32] The seeds of *Peganum harmala* are regularly burned in offerings to open fires by the Zoroastrians of Iran today (see J. S. Soroushian 1956, *s.v. būtī sven*, and *čaryū*). W. Eilers and M. Mayrhofer (1962:68n.) report that in Yazd the Zoroastrians burned as incense *kundur* (apparently locally designating pine resin), sandalwood, *senjed* (oleaster), and *isfand* (*Peganum harmala*). In the nineteenth century, the seeds of *Peganum harmala* were exported by the Zoroastrians of Iran to those in India for use as incense; see J. E. Polak (1874: 703). The fact that the modern burning of *Peganum harmala* is not for aesthetic but for apotropaic ends is consistent with what Zoroastrian tradition indicates must have been the case with sauma: "The burning by the Parsees of sandalwood incense on the holy fire during the performance of all religious ceremonies and prayers . . . is intended not so much to propitiate the good spirit of the holy fire, as to scare off the evil spirits by the fumes of the materials burnt" (Ruttonshaw Kershaspji Dadachanji [1911: 341]).

[1] The *Ephedra* plants used ritually are one to two-foot high shrubs having many thin, yellow-green branches emerging from a somewhat woody base. They are characterized by leafless, jointed stems, the ends of which (in female plants) sometimes bear globular 1/4-inch fruits. They therefore have a gross similarity in appearance to harmel plants in winter, although confusion between *Ephedra* and harmel is hardly likely. Botanical differentiation of species of the genus *Ephedra* is often difficult. Presumably several of the ten species occurring in Iran (Riedl 1963) could serve as *haoma* in ritual. Boyce's (1970: 62) samples were *E. pachyclada* Boiss. (see Figure 4) or *E. intermedia* Schrenk & Mey., var. *Persica* Stapf. Bornmüller (1893: 43) reported "*E. distachya*" to be the plant used as *hōm* in Yazd, but no species of this name is included in the *Flora Iranica*. Pictures of *Ephedra* plants used as *haoma* appear in J. Darmesteter, (1892-1893: I, lix); A. V. W. Jackson (1906: 387), and J. R. Hinnells (1973: 127; photograph by Mary Boyce).

establishes that *Ephedras* were well known by the name *haoma* in Avestan times and even earlier. What is more, still farther east in areas where Dardic and Indic languages are spoken, these species of *Ephedra* bear such names as *soma, som, sumanai, asmania, amsania, asmina-butī* and *soma-latā*, indicating that in Old Indic they were called *soma*. A point which is of obvious importance to determining the botanical identity of sauma but which seems not noted previously, is that the naming of *Ephedra* from *hauma* in Iran, and from *soma* in Indic, indicates that *Ephedra* was called *sauma already in the common ancestral Indo-Iranian language.

§107 Moreover, the use of *Ephedras* in present day Iranian *haoma* rituals was probably paralleled by the use of *Ephedras* in the *soma* rites of the north Indian Vedic schools, which endured until the tenth century Islamic invasions of north India. Today *soma* rites are rare and are found only in south India, where schools of Vedic priests were to some extent reestablished by refugees from these invasions. The plant which reports uniformly indicate to be used as *soma* in these south Indian rites is an asclepiadacious, leafless climber, *Sarcostemma brevistigma* Wight & Arn.[2] The twigs of this plant contain a milky sap, but when dry they may be difficult to distinguish from *Ephedra* stems.[3]

§108 *Sarcostemmas* are tropical species and could not have been available for use as *soma* in Vedic times because they are absent from the flora of north India, and must therefore have been adopted only when, long after the Vedic period, Brahman priests emigrated to south India. These priests must have then selected *Sarcostemma* to substitute for the plant traditionally used as *soma* in north India. *Ephedra* species do not seem to occur in south India, nor in fact near the ritual centers on the northern plains themselves, so, to have been used there during the many centuries of Vedic practices, they would have to have been imported from adjacent uplands to the north and northwest.[4] The greater distance and political barriers would, however, have precluded importation of *Ephedra* to the *soma* rituals once the sites of these rituals had shifted to south India.

§109 That it was *Ephedra* which *Sarcostemma* replaced as *soma* is evidenced by the fact that in Nepal today *Ephedra* is called by the Sanskrit name *somalatā* '*soma* creeper' (Singh 1979; Shrestha 1979; Manandhur 1980). The Islamic invasions resulted in the flight of Hindu refugees both to south India and to Nepal. Although these refugees do not appear to have established Vedic rites in Nepal, they introduced the Sanskrit language there. Sanskrit names for plants in Nepal date from the arrival of these refugees (J. F. Staal). The designation of *Ephedra* in Nepal by the Sanskrit term *somalatā* can only mean that when the Brahmans reached Nepal they found *Ephedra* growing there and they recognized it as the same plant they had known in north India as *somalatā* when it was being imported for *soma* rituals.

§110 This ceremonial use of *Ephedra* for millennia in both Iran and India must reflect some unique intrinsic property of the plant. The only characteristic of *Ephedra* markedly distinguishing it from the numerous xerophytes of similar appearance among which it grows is a pharmacological one, and this certainly must underlie its ceremonial role, that is, consumption as a drug. Some of the *Ephedra* species known by names reflecting *haoma/soma* contain, in quantities conditioned by rainfall and season, ephedrine, a sympathomimetic alkaloid somewhat similar in physiological action to adrenaline. The claims of several modern authors (e.g. Qazilbash 1960; Mahdihassan 1963, 1974, 1985; Falk 1987) notwithstanding, the pharmacological action of ephedrine as a stimulant is of insufficient intensity and too inconsistent in character with what is indicated for sauma by the Iranian evidence to allow identification of *Ephedra* itself as sauma, but it must nevertheless be its pharmacological action which underlies the specificity of *Ephedra* use in sauma ceremonies and consequently the common names of these plants. The cultural history of *Ephedra* also shows that it was not sauma. It is unknown in traditional Indic or Iranian folk medicine,[5] while in China, where it has been recognized for many centuries as a medicine, it is not regarded as intoxicating and its consumption lacks ceremonial or religious associations.[6]

§111 The clearest demonstration that *Ephedra* cannot have been sauma exists in the very fact that *Ephedra* extracts are today drunk as *haoma* by Zoroastrian priests who do not become intoxicated from them and whose predecessors, moreover, apparently consumed *Ephedra* extracts for centuries without so much as knowing that *haoma* is said in the Avesta to be intoxicating (see §22). It is also clear that, whatever pharmacological effects Zoroastrian priests may experience from drinking *Ephedra* extracts, it is not for the purpose of experiencing those effects that the extracts are drunk, whereas the object of drinking sauma preparations was precisely for their effects. What then will explain the identification of *Ephedras* as *soma* and *haoma*, both by priests and throughout numerous Iranian and Indic dialects since near the time when sauma ceremonies first began?

[2] Synonyms for *Sarcostemma brevistigma* Wight & Arn include *Asclepias acida* Roxb., *Sarcostemma acidum* Voigt., and *Sarcostemma viminale* Wall. ex Decne. A. C. Burnell (1878: viii n.), states that, while *Sarcostemma* was used for *soma* on the east coast of India, on the west coast two species of *Ceropegia*, "*C. Decaisneana*" and "*C. Elegans*" were used, but he does not say how he knew of the ritual use of these species. The two *Ceropegias* are also asclepiadacious vines and probably merely substitute for *Sarcostemma brevistigma* in local rites.

[3] The twigs of *Sarcostemma brevistigma* which J. F. Staal (1979: 156) observed in ritual use were, in fact, mistaken for *Ephedra* stems by the first botanist he consulted.

[4] The importation of *soma* plants is reflected in the ritualized enactment of the purchase of a cart of *soma* plants described in *Śatapatha Brāhmaṇa* 3.3.1.1*f* (see Hillebrandt 1980: 160-167; Dandekar 1973: II, 112-144; Kashikar 1964: 270-277; and Staal 1979).

[5] Ephedrine is contained only in the stem bark of *Ephedra* plants with none in the roots or stem wood, and can easily be extracted by preparing an infusion of the stems in a mortar. Ephedrine may constitute up to 2.5% of fresh stems of some *Ephedra* species (Hegnauer 1962-1973:I, 450-457) so that perceptible pharmacological effects may be expected from less than a gram of such twigs. The ephedrine content of *Ephedras* is much influenced by the amount of moisture available to the growing plant and the season of its collection, and not all *Ephedra* species produce the drug (see Chopra *et al.* 1965: 146 *seq.*; Nadkarni 1954: 486 *seq.*). If, as is argued below, *Ephedra* was valued only as an additive to sauma, with the omission of sauma from the ceremonies, the pharmacological potency of *Ephedra* plants would have ceased to be significant, and the precautions necessary to preserve the effectiveness of ephedrine, which is easily destroyed by heat or moisture (Blakelock and Gillett 1966: 83), seem indeed not to be observed in the handling of the *Ephedra* plants employed in modern Zoroastrian rituals. The procedure prescribed in the *Vidēvdād* (5.42-43) of burying polluted *haomas* under the floor of one's house for one year could nullify the potency of any drug plant. While *Ephedras* are easily recognizable as a distinct class of plants, the various species look much alike and it is unclear to what extent the early Indo-Iranians distinguished between the species recognized in modern botany. It seems that names reflecting Indo-Iranian **sauma-* are now applied to all the species of *Ephedra* commonly encountered in the east Iranian-northwest Indian uplands. Application of such names to the only local species growing at lower elevations, *E. ciliata*, which contains no ephedrine, although also attested, is apparently less pervasive. The *Ephedra* species most probably imported and purchased for ancient north Indian *soma* rites was *E. Gerardiana*. The creeping habit of this species probably explains the conception of *soma* as a creeper (Sanskrit *-latā*) and thus ultimately accounts for the selection of the climbing plant *Sarcostemma brevistigma* to serve as *soma* in south India. There is no evidence that *haoma* was ever supposed in Iran to be a climbing plant.

[6] Alison Bailey Kennedy has determined that the supposed references to *Ephedra* in early Chinese sources may actually pertain to species of *Equisetum*. She reports that at Kew Gardens in 1984 she examined the plant specimens recovered by Sir Auriel Stein from graves near Turfan and described by him (1931) as *Ephedra* twigs, and discovered them to be in fact *Equisetum* also. She has promised to present arguments that a similar confusion of *Ephedra* with *Equisetum* may underly the association of *Ephedra* with **sauma*.

TABLE 3: MODERN INDO-IRANIAN NAMES FOR *EPHEDRA* SPECIES

Names underlined derive from PIIr. **sauma*—.(see §106).

EPHEDRA GERARDIANA Wall.	
amsania	Punjab (5)
asmani-booti	Punjab (1)
asmānia	Jhelam (31), Punjab (1, 10)
būdsūr/būtsūr	Punjab (10)
budagur	Punjab (12)
čewa	Punjab (1, 10)
ehewa	Punjab (22)
khanda	Kunawar (10)
khanda-phog	Bushahr (12)
khanna	Sutlej (31) Kunawar (10)
oman	Pashto (14)
phok	Sutlej, Janusar (19)
raci	Bushahr (12)
sang-kaba	Sherpa (Nepal) (16)
soma	Sanskrit (1)
somalata	Nepal (27)
somlata	Nepal (16, 28), Sanskrit (16)
thayon	Ladakh (29)
tootagantha	Hindi (1)
trano	Ladakh (10)
tsapatt(-tsems)	Ladakh (10, 31)
tse	Piti or Spiti (31) Ladakh (10)
tutgantha	Jaunsar (11,13) Hindi (15)
uman /uroman	Pashto (14)

EPHEDRA INTERMEDIA *Schr. & Mey.*	
hōm	Central Persia (9)
hum/huma	Baluchistan (23)
imom/imik	Wakhan (30)
khanna	Kunawar (11)
maha/mawa	Khyber/Hindu Kush (24)
marizad	Baluchistan (8)
oman	Pushto (12)
porgaz	Brahui (8)
rogangaz	Baluchistan (8)
sumani	Chitral (11)
um/uma	Baluchistan (23)

EPHEDRA NEBRODENSIS *Tineo.*	
gwatham	Baluchistan (8)
omah/umah	Baluchistan (11)

EPHEDRA PACHYCLADA *Boiss.*	
asmina-buti	Gilgit (14)
hōm	Afghanistan (9)
hum/huma	Afghanistan (2)
kōreš	Qayen (Khorasan) (2)
maha/mawa	Khyber/Hindu Kush (24)
mao	Khyber (2)
som	Gilget (14)
oman	Pashto (3)
soma	Kafiristan/Nuristan (24)
um	Afghanistan (2)
uma	Afghanistan (2), Baluchi(24)
uman	Afghanistan (24)
xōreš	Afghanistan (2)
xušk-targ	Qayen (2) Baluchi (20)
yehma	Afghanistan (4)

EPHEDRA CILIATA *F. & M.*	
andho-khimp	Indian desert (6)
bandak-māu	Pashto (26)
bandukai	West of Indus (31)
brata/bratta	Punjab (10, 31)
drāksa	Sanskrit (3)
hīb	Jaz Murian (Baluchi) (15)
hum-i-bandak	Afghanistan (3)
kucan	Punjab (10, 11, 31)
kūrkan	Punjab (10)
lana	Indian desert (6)
lastūk	Salt Range (Punjab) (31)
nangarwal	Bari Doab (Punjab) (31)
nikki	Punjab (10)
phog/phōk	Punjab (21) Rajputana (10)
sou-phogaro	Indian desert (6)
tandala	Salt Range (Punjab) (31)
um/umbar	Kashmir and India (3)

EPHEDRA *(species not specified)*	
acilig	Azerbaijan (12a)
amojak	Khufi (30)
asmania	Kagan Valley (14)
bandak-e-kōhī	Afghanistan (26)
budsur	Punjab (22)
buzak	Afghanistan (26)
dundula	Punjab (22)
ehewa	Punjab (22)
hōm	Brahui (7), Pashto (22)
hum/humb	Baluchi (4)
jarkana	Pashto (26)
kučan	Punjab (22)
medrāx	Khowar (30)
modrag	Tajik-Wakhan (30)
nārom	Brahui (7)
nar-ōmb	Baluchi (4)
nawa	Pashto-Waziristan (14)
rīš-e-buz	Afghanistan (26)
oman	Pashto-Waziristan (14)
ōmə	Pashto (17)
usmania	Kagan Valley (14)
(w)umān	Tajik-Afghanistan (30)
xumḍ	Tajik-Zerafshan (30)
(y)imik	Wakhan (30)
yūmana	Munjani (30)
yūmenä	Yidga (30)

1. Ahluwalia 1967. 2. Aitchinson 1891. 3. Aitchinson in Watt 1889-1896. 4. Bailey 1972. 5. Bamber 1916. 6. Bhandari 1916. 7. Bellew 1874. 8. Blatter in Parsa 1941-1956. 9. Boyce 1970a. 10. Brandis 1879. 11. Brandis 1921. 12. Chopra *et al.* 1965. 12a. *Flora Azerbaidzan* 1950. 13. Gupta 1928. 14. Hocking 1958. 15. Leonard 1984. 16. Manandhar 1980. 17. Morgenstierne 1973. 18. Morgenstierne 1974. 19. Nadkarni 1954. 20. Nāşerī 1971. 21. Nair 1978. Pakistan Forest Reseach Service 1956. 23. Parsa 1943-1952. 24. Qazilbash 1960. 25. Sabeti 1966. 26. Schapka & Volk 1979. 27. Singh *et al.* 1979. 28. Srestha 1979. 29. Srivastava & Gupta 1982. 29a. Stapf 1889. 30. Steblin-Kamenskij 1983. 31. Stewart 1869.

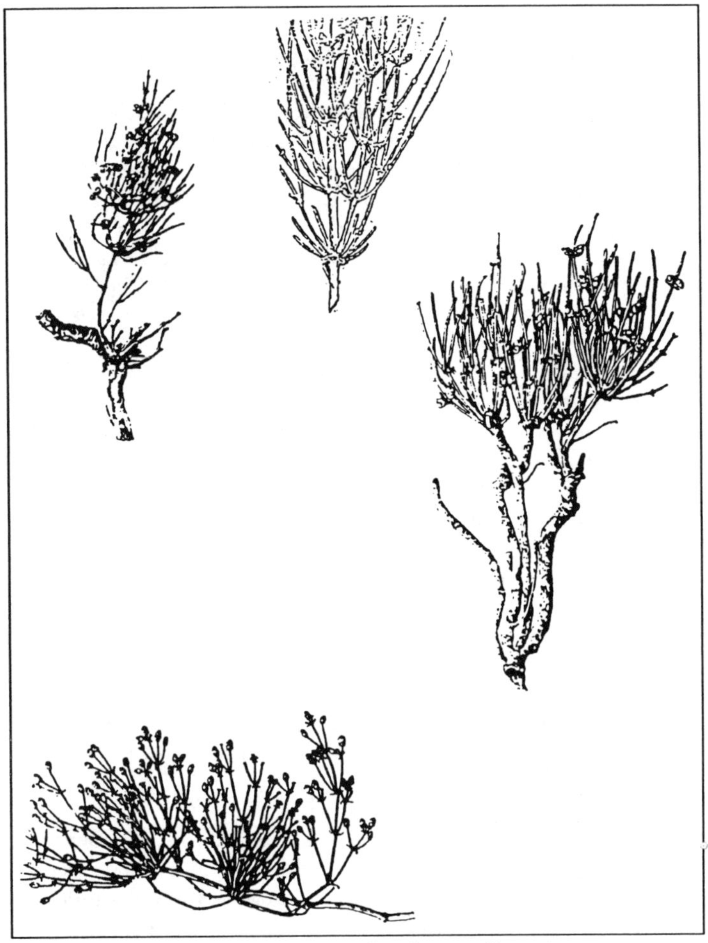

FIGURE 4. EPHEDRA SPECIES OF THE EAST IRANIAN—NORTH INDIA AREA.

§112 It has sometimes been supposed that *Ephedra* was symbolically substituted for the original intoxicant, but there are many reasons to doubt this. First, it would be strange that a merely symbolic substitute should itself have unique pharmacological properties. Furthermore, sauma must have been commonly known in ancient Iranian society as an intoxicating plant in order for the credibility of the sauma ceremonies, and the authority Iranian priests claimed from them, to have been maintained. Despite being commonly designated *haoma* (and the like), *Ephedra* is without suitable psychoactive potential in fact (and is not regarded in traditional ethnobotany as having any psychoactive properties at all) and, therefore, it cannot have been believed to be the means to an experience from which priests could claim religious authority or widely believed to be the essential ingredient of an *intoxicating* extract. Nor is it likely that *Ephedra* would be uniquely designated by vernacular names like *haoma* if it had been introduced into the ceremonies as a symbolic substitute for sauma, for this purpose could have been served equally well by many other plants without prejudice to the outcome of the ceremony. Moreover, for a single, arbitrarily chosen substitute for sauma to be so universally adopted would have required an implausibly uniform Indo-Iranian society (and priesthood); once such a choice were made, there would have been no means to communicate or enforce it. Even if that had been possible with respect to the conduct of ceremonies, it would remain to explain how the adoption of such a convention among priests could result in the popular designation as *soma/haoma* of *Ephedra* species.[7]

§113 It is therefore neither likely that *Ephedra* was a substitute for sauma nor that it was sauma itself, yet, according to both Iranian and Indian traditions, *Ephedra* was essentially linked with the extract drunk during the ceremonies. The only way of reconciling this fact with the considerations of the preceding paragraphs is to view *Ephedra* as an archaic additive to the extract. Thus, *Ephedra* too would have been a *soma-/haoma-* 'pressed out (plant)', though not the only (or fundamental) one. The Avesta clearly indicates there was more than a single *haoma. Haoma* is *pouru.sarəδa-* 'of many kinds' (*Yasna* 10.12) and the word *haoma-* frequently appears in the Avesta as a plural, particularly in that part of the *Yasna* and its supplement, the *Vīsperad*, recited while preparing the *haoma* drink. Also both *haoma-* and *para.haoma-* 'subsidiary *haoma*' are named at those points in the *Yasna* liturgy where there occur a list of the items to be consumed by the *zaotar* (i.e. at *Yasna* 3.2; 4.1; 7.26; and 8.1).[8]

§114 The pre-Islamic use of *Ephedra* as *soma* in Indian rituals casts light on its function as a constituent of the ritual extract. In the Indic tradition, after sauma came to be omitted from the ceremonies (which appears to have been a necessary precondition for their continuation; see §155), *Ephedra* continued to be pressed out as *soma*. No additional plant was introduced as a replacement for sauma. On the other hand, *Ephedra* itself could not have been a substitute for sauma because of the rationale of the *soma* rituals: *soma* was an offering to the gods, and it was in order to receive *soma* that gods made themselves present. It is hardly possible that rituals would be undertaken to summon the gods to partake of specious *soma*. Presumably the gods might be expected to supply a missing ingredient in the *soma* offered them, but would not have been expected to be taken in by a false offering. The fact that *Ephedra* is used alone in the later Indic rituals is a further argument that it was an original constituent and not a substitute plant and thus confirms the Iranian evidence that at least two plants were originally present in the ritual extract.

The ritual use of *Ephedra* as evidence that sauma was harmel

§115 *Ephedra* seems to have been used in Iranian rituals almost exclusively as an additive to the *haoma* mixture of the *Yasna*. Since *Ephedra* was identified with *haoma* in rituals, however, it would be remarkable if it were not also occasionally used to symbolically represent sauma. This is undoubtedly the case when *Ephedra* is burned, for *Ephedra* is not an incense plant. The burning of *hōm* (i.e. *Ephedra*) together with frankincense occurs in the ordinary Iranian rites sanctifying the slaughter of meat animals (see §101). This ritual burning of *Ephedra* must be a reflection of the earlier practice of burning *Peganum harmala* (together with frankincense [i.e. Persian *kundur*; cf. §§76 and 99]) which is still car-

[7] The cognate Indic and Iranian names for *Ephedra* may aid in locating where the Indo-Iranians came from, for there are almost no other plants bearing cognate names in Indian and Iranian languages. The vernacular survival of the Indo-Iranian name for *Ephedra* implies continuous association with the plant by both Indo-Aryan and Iranian groups. While ephedrine containing species of *Ephedra* occur in alpine areas of Europe and China as well as in the Hindu Kush-Pamir-Himalaya highlands they are discontinuously distributed in Eurasia. In areas where they are not abundant, as in western Iran, *Ephedras* have ceased to be known by *haoma*phoric names. An alternative to the widely held view that the differentiation of Iranian and Indic languages occurred in the course of two waves of eastward migration from southeastern Europe, is the hypothesis that this differentiation took place in the Helmand valley in eastern Iran. This would be consistent with the distribution of these *Ephedra* species as well as with the fact that Indo-Iranian culture developed around the herding of cattle. G. Gnoli (1980) has argued attractively that this area was the site of the ancient Iranian society reflected in the Avesta. Its unique regional suitability for a cattle rearing economy is also relevant to locating Proto-Indo-Iranian origins.

[8] In Pahlavi *parāhōm* denotes the liquid extract as against the plant, nevertheless, the earlier Avestan term *para.haoma-* did not specify the liquid extract as against the plant and may never have been used for the extract at all. The term *haoma-* must primarily have referred to the drink and in the Avesta it is not *para.haoma-* but *haoma-* which occurs as the object of the verb 'to swallow' (*x*ᵛ*ar-*, *Yasna* 9.16).

ried out (with precisely identical ritual procedures) in connection with the most important annual sacrifice, that of the *Mihragān* festival, by the Zoroastrian priests of the city of Yazd.[9] Thus, where *Ephedra* is used alone, it is manifestly as substitute for *Peganum harmala*, another indication that harmel was sauma.

§116 If *Ephedra* was an original constituent of the ritual extract, its pharmacological properties must have been consonant with or complementary to those of sauma. It has been noted (§110) that ephedrine is a sympathomimetic drug, stimulating the sympathetic nervous system and thus interfering with sleep. The physiological effects of harmaline are in some respects the very opposite of those of ephedrine, for harmaline lowers blood pressure and may induce sleep (as was recognized as an effect of harmel in Islamic materia medica [§44]). It is not possible to precisely predict the pharmacological action of a combination of ephedrine and harmaline, but it is reasonable to expect that the action of ephedrine would diminish the tendency of harmaline to induce sleep and could thus facilitate the experience of visions. Indeed, no plant available in the Iranian environment seems better suited to be consumed as a means of averting sleep than *Ephedra*. In general, there is reason to believe that harmel used for the purpose of visions would probably have regularly been in the form of mixtures with other plant drugs, since, as has been noted (§38), the harmaline containing preparations of *Banisteriopsis* consumed in South America for visions typically involve the admixture of other plants. Likewise, when clinically administering harmaline orally in order to induce visions, Claudio Naranjo found that harmaline most effectively induced visions when it was combined other psychoactive substances. Apparently over many generations the shamans of South America have discovered how to induce a wide range of experiences by varying the additives to the *Banisteriopsis* drug and a parallel body of empirical lore may have developed around the preparation of harmel as a drug. Not only do the properties of *Ephedra* seem specifically suited for use with harmaline, but the mere datum that sauma was prepared in mixtures is particularly consistent with its identification as harmel, for the effects of most plant drugs are not to such a degree modified by other drugs consumed with them.

Pomegranate

(a) Pomegranate and the identification of sauma with *haδānaēpātā*

§117 If it is allowed that *Ephedra* may have originally been an additive to sauma, then, of the two plants compounded for the modern *Yasna* ritual, it should be pomegranate rather than *Ephedra* whose original purpose was to symbolize sauma. The prevailing view, however, has been just the reverse: that pomegranate was an additive plant. The Avestan term *haδānaēpātā,* which is named in the *Yasna* liturgy as a plant consumed together with *haoma* and to which the ritual use of pomegranate corresponds, is widely supposed to *mean* 'pomegranate'. This is first because in places where the Avestan *Yasna* liturgy calls for the presence of *haδānaēpātā*, the modern Zoroastrian ritual employs pomegranate twig, root, or leaf. Secondly, the identification of *haδānaēpātā* as 'pomegranate' is due to etymological assumptions. These etymological issues are discussed in §§231-251; here it need merely be said that the fact that the element *haδāna-* 'having seeds, seedy' is the basis of words for 'pomegranate' in some later Iranian languages does not prove that the entire compound *haδānaēpātā* also means 'pomegranate'. Moreover, the data, when examined closely, actually preclude the meaning 'pomegranate' for *haδānaēpātā* in the Avesta.

§118 In the Avesta *haδānaēpātā* is specified for two uses: as an ingredient of the intoxicating extract and as incense; yet for neither of these uses is pomegranate in any way suitable, nor should any feature of the pomegranate earn it the prominence of the *haδānaēpātā* plant. The pomegranate's fecundity symbolism, which accounts for its role in certain other religious contexts, is irrelevant here. It is the fruit which lends itself to this symbolism, but the fruit is not used in preparing the *Yasna* drink, nor could the *haδānaēpātā* collected as loads of fuel incense (*Vidēvdād* 14.5; 18.71) refer to the fruit. The Avestan *haδānaēpātā* is in fact never interpreted as pomegranate in the Pahlavi textual tradition, where the Avestan word is simply transcribed and left undefined. What is even more decisive, however, is that Avestan *haδānaēpātā,* in addition to being described as a fragrant plant substance, is clearly classified as a soft (*varədva-*) as against a hard (*xraoždva-*) wood (*Vidēvdād* 14.2-3), whereas pomegranate wood is exceptionally close grained and slow burning, and is burnt in Zoroastrian sacred fires for these very qualities (Boyce 1977: 75).

§119 The term *haδānaēpātā*, no cognates of which survive in any later language, was probably not common (if used at all) in ordinary speech, but belonged rather to priestly usage (like other Avestan terms for ritual substances, see further §237), and may have been one of the terms which designated sauma. The ambiguity of *haoma* as a term for sauma existed already in Avestan (and indeed far earlier as proven by the Indian use of names connected with *soma* for *Ephedra*); in the context of the ceremony, "*haoma*" implied the intoxicant but was commonly used to name the nonintoxicating *Ephedra* which was also, and more regularly, present. Whereas ordinary "*haoma*-containing" *Yasnas* might or might not actually include sauma, Avestan may be expected (especially in light of the ordeal functions of the *Yasna* discussed in Chapter 6) to have had a means of more emphatically asserting the presence of sauma in the extracts prepared for the *Yasna*. The characterization of *zaoθras* (see §129) as containing both *haoma* and *haδānaēpātā* (in *Yasna* 22, 24, 66, etc.) may indeed have been intended to assert that they really did contain sauma, although in the course of time a nonintoxicating plant was substituted in most and eventually in all yasna performances. The identity of *haδānaēpātā* and sauma is further indicated by the coincidence that the two uses which the Avesta assigns to *haδānaēpātā*, namely, as incense and intoxicant, are precisely the uses of sauma. It is unlikely that this unusual combination of functions would characterize both sauma and yet another Avestan plant. Pomegranate, by reason of representing *haδānaēpātā* in the modern *Yasna*, may therefore be regarded as the substitute for the sauma plant.

§120 This appears also to be the function of pomegranate elsewhere in Zoroastrian rituals. For example, Modi, in his account of *The Religious Ceremonies and Customs of the Parsees* (1937: 52), reports that "instead of the juice of the *haoma* plant, if [it is] not available at hand, the juice of a few grains of pomegranate . . . is dropped into the mouth of the dying person." In the older initiations described in texts, and in the modern initiations of priests, drinking *haoma* is required. Although according to *Pahlavi Yasna* 9.26 "one has not accepted the Religion until he drinks *hōm*", it is by no means sure that all persons espousing Zoroastrianism were required to consume sauma. However, as all members of this faith must today pass through an initiation modeled in part on the initiation of priests, it seems likely that sauma is reflected by the infusion of crushed pomegranate leaves and twigs which is administered to the novice at the beginning of these rites. Moreover, pomegranate seeds (Modi 1937: 338; Drower 1944: 87) or twigs (Haug 1884: 407) appear to represent sauma when—as is the usual practice among Zoroastrian priests in India—they are placed on the *drōn* bread to replace the *sadāb* called for by the Pahlavi scholia to the *Nērangistān* (see below, §132 with n. 24).

§121 The choice of pomegranate to represent sauma may result in large part from the availability of the pomegranate, its being evergreen, and the importance of its fruit in other Zoroastrian observances, as well as its

[9] Compare Boyce's detailed description of the burning of *hōm* and frankincense in the village of Sharifabad, cited in §99 n.28, with her (1975a: 112) account of burning *Peganum harmala* and frankincense by the more conservative priests of Yazd in the identical ritual procedure.

partial association by name with *haδānaēpātā*. But pomegranate is also characterized by a resemblance to *Peganum harmala*; in particular, by the likeness of its wild fruits to harmel seed capsules. This similarity is reflected in Arabic by the use of **ḥuraymla* (or **ḥurmayla*), a derivative of *ḥarmal*, and *ʾumm ḥarmal* 'mother of harmel' as names for pomegranate.[10]

§122 The present-day substitution of pomegranate for harmel in Zoroastrian ritual has a long history, as is shown by accounts (written in Islamic times) of practices observed at the ancient festival of *Isfandagān*. This festival occurs on the day *Isfandarmuδ* (< Middle Persian *Spandarmat* <Avestan *Spənta- Armaiti-*) (the fifth day) of the month *Isfandarmuδ* (the twelveth month), 30 days before the New Year. Accounts of a parallel Iranian festival occurring one month earlier, that of *Bahmanjana*, observed on the day *Bahman* (the second day) of the month *Bahman* (the eleventh month), say that that festival featured the consumption of the plant *bahman*.[11] If any plant was analogously consumed at *Isfandagān*, it should be *isfand*, as indeed, according to an informant of Anjavī Shīrāzī (1973:1, 53), *isfand* (presumably in quite small quantities), mixed with milk, was still consumed in Kerman at *Isfandagān* during the early years of the present century. A sixteenth-century account of *Isfandagān*, written in central Iran by Zoroastrian priests (see below §131 n.17), states that the festival was marked by preparing and burning a mixture containing (among five ingredients) raisins and *isfand*. This account also provides the detail that at the same time an exorcism against the poison of noxious creatures was written on saffron paper or deer skin and fastened outside the house. Al-Bīrūnī, in his tenth-century *Chronology* (ed. Sachau 1878:220), reports that the festival of *Isfandagān* was famous as the occasion for writing (between dawn and sunrise) an exorcism (essentially identical to the one described by the Zoroastrian priests) accompanied, rather than by the burning of *isfand*, by pulverizing together raisins and pomegranate seeds and eating these to nullify the poison of scorpions. Pomegranate seeds were not traditionally regarded as an antidote, but the seeds of harmel were (see, e.g. al-Bīrūnī quoted by Togan 1941:117). Originally the festival must have featured the consumption of *Peganum harmala* (i.e. *isfand*) in order for the sauma effects to be experienced. In popular survivals of the festival later on, when most participants were no longer prepared for such effects as visions that drinking sauma might bring, the *isfand* was merely burnt, or else it was replaced by a non-intoxicating plant. Al-Bīrūnī's report shows that the substitute plant was pomegranate.

(b) Pomegranate and the identification of sauma with *barsom*

§123 Pomegranate appears to have a further substitute function in Zoroastrian ritual when it is used as the Zoroastrian *barsom* (Avestan *barəsman-*). The Middle and New Persian term *barsom* designates certain twigs which, during various rituals and, with special importance, while preparing *haoma* before and again during the *Yasna*, are held in the left hand of the *haoma*-preparing priest, whose his right hand grips the *haoma* pestle. In the Avesta, *barəsman-* is more often characterized as strewn than as held in the hand. Existing Avestan and Pahlavi texts say nothing about the source of *barəsman-/barsom* except that it is a plant substance, nor about the connection of holding it in the hand with strewing it. Zoroastrian works in New Persian state that *barsom* should be cut from either the pomegranate or the tamarisk (*Rivāyat of Kaus Kamdin* and *Rivāyat of Kamdin Shapur:* M. R. Unvala 1922:I, 484; II, 32–33; Dhabhar 1932:418), or else that *barsom* should consist of *hōm* (presumably *Ephedra*) or tamarisk, or, if neither of these is available, pomegranate (Shea and Troyer 1901:158; Dehkhudā 1947–1973: B 893). Since, except for tamarisk (whose presence is probably an intrusion of non-Iranian origin, see §126), the plants named (i.e. *Ephedra* and pomegranate) are the very two plants which are pressed out and drunk ritually as *haoma*, their use as *barsom* suggests that *barsom/barəsman-* may originally have been the s a m e plant as sauma. The mutual identity of *barsom* and *haoma* may also be indicated by the accounts of the plant called in Arabic *hawm al-majūs* 'the *haoma/hōm* of the Magi'. Islamic pharmacological texts (from as early as the 10th century C.E.) furnish only vague and conflicting botanical information about *hawm al-majūs* (see above, §54

[10] "*Imḥarmal*: small black fruits of a variety of pomegranate which are not edible but are used to make a local medicine" (Guest 1933: 48, 79). "*Immḥarmal*" is a pomegranate according to Henry Field (in D. Hooper 1937:160, 226). According to Abū Ḥanifa al-Dīnawarī (d. 895) (Lewin 1953:104.8): "the *ḥrymlh* (vocalized *ḥurraymila* [«ἰ] by Ibn Manẓur [*c.* 1300], *Lisān al-ʿArab* [1966: 13, 195] is like the small pomegranate." M. Vonderheyden (1937: 456 n.1) says "Le diminutif "ἰdesigne une plant toute différente, une sorte de petit grenadier."

[11] The analogy is particularly evident in a Zoroastrian text written in Yazd in 1719 in which *sapand* (=isfand=*Peganum harmala*) is stated to be the plant consumed at the festival of *Bahmanjana*: "In the matter of the *Behemanjeh* [*sic*] *Jashan*. This *Jashan* is solemnized on the day *Behman* of the month *Behman*. Some say that the Parsis on that day used to partake of vinegar mixed with *sapand* [i.e. *Peganum harmala*], while others say that they used to swallow *sapand* mixed with fresh milk, so that Behman Amashasfand might sharpen the memory and perfect wisdom and intelligence" (translated by M. R. Unvala, from an unpublished text [1908: 208; cf. MS. no. 100[283] in Dhabhar 1923: 63]).

This account was apparently derived from descriptions of this festival by Islamic writers of the tenth century (e.g. al-Bīrūnī [*al-Qānūn al-Masʿūdī*, see Sachau 1879: 424; *Kitāb al-Tafhīm li-awāʾil ṣināʿat al-tanjīm*, ed. Wright 1934: 181-182], Asadī Ṭūsī [ed. Dabīr Siyāqī 1957: 158]; Minūčihrī [ed. Dabīr Siyāqī 1959: 86]; cf. also the thirteenth-century account by al-Qazwīnī [ed. Wüstenfeld 1849: 2, 83]). The plant consumed at *Bahmanjana* in these Islamic accounts is not referred to as *isfand* or the like, but as the roots and petals of the (white/yellow and/or red) *bahman* plant. Although substances continue to be sold in bazaars as *bahman*, there is perplexity about its identity throughout Islamic pharmacognostic literature (see Meyerhof and Sobhy 1932-1940: 294-298; Renaud and Colin 1934:71; Stewart 1869:161). The plants usually identified by modern writers as red and white *bahman*, namely *Statice limonium* (Plumbaginaceae) and *Centaurea behen* (Compositaceae), respectively, are Mediterranean species unknown in the Iranian area, while the variety of straw for which the name *bahman* is used locally in southwestern Iran (Eqtedārī 1955: 50–51; Soroushian 1956: 23) seems wholly incongruous with accounts of the *bahman* plants in the materia medica. Incongruous also is the mention of "white *bahman*" as a superior compote in the late Sasanian text *Xusrau ud Rēdag* 45 (J. M. Unvala 1921: 23).

The term *bahman*, rather than referring to yet another plant, may have been, like *haoma*, *dūraoša-*, and *haδānaēpātā-*, etc., a name for sauma in a particular context of its use. The form *bahman* goes back, via Middle Persian *Wahman*, to Old Iranian **Vahu- Manah-*, Avestan *Vohu- Manah-* 'Good Thinking', the *Aməša Spənta* (hypostatic aspect of the divinity) most associated with sauma (see Boyce 1970: n.85). In the *Dēnkird* VII 3.52 (Madan 1911: 624.6) account of Zoroaster's initial revelation, it is said that he saw Good Thinking (i.e. Vohu Manah = Bahman) as a giant man carrying a white twig (*arus tāg*, regarding which see §260). This white "plant of Bahman" seems to be the precedent for the white *bahman* plant of the *Bahmanjana* festival. It may be conjectured that the reports of the consumption of *bahman* at *Bahmanjana* were based on the precedent of the consumption of *isfand* at *Isfandagān*.

While the Yazdi account of *isfand* at *Bahmanjana* is probably taken ultimately from the tenth century Islamic sources, it is relevant for what it reveals of the attitude of Zoroastrian priests in the eighteenth century toward harmel. The fact that the *bahman* of the earlier accounts has been emended to *sapand* in the Zoroastrian version shows that harmel was believed by Iranian priests to have at one time been consumed to achieve psychoactive results (such as perfecting wisdom and intelligence), results which are otherwise attributed in the literature of Zoroastrianism only to *haoma*. It also discloses that there was an enduring awareness of *Peganum harmala* in the role of sauma among priests. The preparation of *Peganum harmala* with milk in both the account of *sapand* at this *jashan* and in the account of the more recent consumption of *isfand* at the *Isfandagān* festival in Kerman should be compared with the mixing of *haoma* with milk (discussed below, §138). Regarding the alternative preparation of *isfand* with vinegar above, cf. §43 n.1 and the preparation of *sīr-o-sedōw* (§137).

n.11), but it is significant that they do not report that the Magi extracted and consumed *hawm al-majūs* in their rituals (i.e. as *haoma*), but rather they say that the Magi, while reciting prayers, held *hawm al-majūs* (and thus that the plant corresponded with *barsom*). We then have attestation of the very same plants which are ritually prepared and drunk as *haoma/hōm* (i.e. *Ephedra* and pomegranate) being used as *barsom*, and complementarily, *haoma/hōm* described as if it were *barsom*.

§124 In addition to the use of pomegranate twigs both to represent sauma in *haoma* extracts and to serve as *barsom*, a further fact should be noted. At the very time a piece of pomegranate twig, apparently symbolically representing sauma, is being pounded in the mortar with the right hand, *barsom* is held in the priest's other hand (Kotwal and Boyd 1977). This suggests not only that *barsom* and sauma were identical, but also that sauma stems, rather than being cut into short lengths to fit into the mortar (as are the *Ephedra* and pomegra-nate pieces now used), were originally grasped together as *barsom* while their ends were being crushed in the mortar (*see* Figure 5, p. 179).[12] The active drugs of harmel are concentrated not along the stems but, depending on the season, in either the roots or the seed capsules at either end of the stems (see above, §47). From the beginning of the year until the ripening of the seeds, the roots are the part of the plant richest in the harmala alkaloids. Because harmel typically grows in hard ground, only by grasping together the stems at their base and pulling off the upper few inches of root can roots of the plant be easily harvested. To extract a drug from roots thus obtained, the uprooted end of the stems could be held firmly over a mortar with one hand while operating a pestle with the other. Similarly, during the later part of the year when harmaline and harmine are concentrated in the seeds, these drugs might be most efficiently obtained by holding with one hand bundles of stems cut off at the base while pulling away and crushing numerous seed capsules into a mortar with the other hand. The *Yasna* ceremonies of ancient Iran took place out of doors in areas defined by furrows, and in most parts of Iran these furrows could have been drawn to enclose an area containing live harmel plants.[13] From the plants within the ritual area itself the drug could then be freshly prepared by holding together successive handfuls of stems and crushing in a mortar whichever end was appropriate for the season of the year, then discarding the stems. Wherever this process had been carried out, the numerous stems remaining from it would constitute a very visible (and perhaps also highly pungent) indicator of the site of sauma ceremonies. Thereby the act of preparing sauma might become associated with the strew of these stems. If it is to these strewn stems that Avestan *barəsman-* referred, then the act of strewing *barəsman-* would betoken the performance of the *Yasna;* which is to say, the act of consuming sauma, hence "strew *barəsman-*" would in effect amount to an idiom for "consume sauma". The chief means of serving the gods in the Avesta is the performance of *Yasnas*, and in the Avesta there is no indication of any way in which gods would be served by the strewing of plants except in connection with the performance of the *Yasna*. This would account for the frequent mentions in the *Yasna* liturgy of serving the gods with strewn *barəsman-*.

§125 This explanation of barsom contrasts with the widely accepted view (see Paul Thieme 1957) that in origin Avestan *barəsman-* is essentially identical with Indic *barhis-*, which in the Vedas is also frequently said to be strewn (*stṛ*), and in Indian ritual consists of grass spread as a cushion for the gods (*devas*), upon which they would sit and receive offerings of *soma*. While the Avesta preserves an exact cognate of Indic *barhis*, Avestan *barəziš-* (> Persian *bāliš*) meaning simply 'cushion', it is not mentioned in connection with ceremonies and need never have had anything to do with a ritual cushion for gods. In Iran the deities of Zoroastrianism seem to have been regarded as incapable of making use of a tangible cushion, so that if the spreading of grass as a seat for the gods was ever a custom inherited by the Iranians, it would early on have been discontinued. Whereas etymologically Avestan *barəsman-* has a common origin with the words for 'cushion', Avestan *barəziš-*, Indic *barhis-* (see below, §§252-258), there is no justification for concluding that *barəsman-* meant 'cushion', still less that it referred to a cushion of grass to be sat upon by the gods. It is possible that the tender foliage upon which the sacrificial victim was laid in Magian rites, as described by Herodotus (I. 152), is a reflection of the ancient ritual usage, and a cushion was still known in connection with animal sacrifice by the Sasanian commentators on the *Nērangistān*,[14] but this cushion is nowhere associated with the terms *barəsman-/barsom* in Iranian texts.[15] There is in fact no trace of a strew of grass for use by the gods, for sacrifices, or for any other purpose in the *Yasna* or in any existing Iranian ceremony,[16] yet during the performance of the *Yasna* the Avestan liturgy frequently proclaims the strewing of *barəsman-* as a part of the ceremony. Rather than suppose that ritual representation of this apparently important act of strewing *barəsman-* has simply disappeared without a trace from the ceremonies, one could more convincingly maintain that the strewing of *barəsman-* never referred to the preparation of a sacrificial cushion but referred instead to the act of extracting and consuming sauma (or later, the symbolic enactment thereof). In this figurative sense the gods have continued to be worshipped by "strewing *barsom*", although in concrete terms, in the *Yasna* today the *barsom* is held rather than being strewn during the pounding of "*haoma*"

12 An important part of some Zoroastrian rituals is the tying of the *barsom* twigs into a bundle. This procedure may be a reflection of binding together the stems of mature *Peganum harmala* plants in order to efficiently crush the terminal seed capsules in a mortar (cf. §82 n.21). The shape of the harmel plant (see Figure 5) is particularly consistent with the uniquely descriptive reference (*Nērangistān* 98 [*f.*179.10-15]) to the source of *barəsman-* as *+hamō.varəšajim paouru.fravāxšəm* 'having many [glossed in Pahlavi "30"] stems from the same root'.

13 Sauma ceremonies developed among a nomadic population and must have taken place in open country. The Iranians had no temples at all until Achaemenian times (Boyce 1975c) and seem to have performed *Yasnas* out of doors, perhaps until the Islamic conquest. Since *Yasnas* may not be witnessed by outsiders, they are now conducted in fire temples, but in earlier times security must have been achieved by locating them at relatively remote sites. "All that was needed for solemnizing the high rituals was a clear, flat piece of ground which could be marked off by a ritually drawn furrow" (*ibid.* 455). Living plants are preferred in Zoroastrian ceremonies, and since harmel plants are found in proximity to virtually all human activities in Iran, the extract would have been prepared from plants obtained within the ceremonial area itself.

14 *Nērangistān f.*128*v* (concerning killing a sheep): "[Placing] the rump toward the *zōt*, breast to the fire, dig a hole, put down a cushion without recitation (*nērang*). If no hole is dug the cushion will be damaged" (*bē ka maɣ nē kand bāliš rēš bawēd*).

15 Boyce (1970:69 n.1) renders a passage at *Nērangistān f.*85*v*.11 as a reference to killing an animal "on" *barsom*, but such a translation is precluded by the context: *ka Srōš drōn xward barsom ne pad nigērišn a-pādyāb be bawēd a-š be šōyišn u-š be rāyēnišn u-š gūmānīg wizard bawēd ka gōspand pad yast a-š ō kušišn ka yast pad zōhr a-š zōhr ō dahišn Afarg guft had pad barsom ī a-pādyāb gospand nē kunišn u-š zōhr ō nē *dahēd.* 'When the *Srōš drōn* is consumed (and) *barsom* inadvertently becomes impure it should be washed and put right; the recitation becomes doubtful. When an animal is in the worship it should be killed. If the worship includes *zōhr*, the *zōhr* should be offered. (However,) Afarg spoke thus: "With impure *barsom* no animal should be killed nor should *zōhr* be *offered."' The *barsom* to which Afarg refers here is that present in the *Srōš Drōn* ceremony, which consists of *hand-held* twigs of *barsom*. This passage makes it clear that it was necessary also to *hold* these twigs when animals were sacrificed, and says nothing about *where* the animal was to die.

16 The *Nērangistān* commentary *Griftan ī Drōn* (see below §132 n.24) mentions cutting (or not cutting) grass to prepare a cushion "not for the comfort of the priest but for the ritual power (*nērang*) of the *drōn* (ceremony)," but, possibly because the *drōn* ceremony is now only performed inside fire temples, this is no longer done.

(and at other prescribed moments) and then laid aside in an orderly fashion on a special stand.

§126 Stems of *Peganum harmala* are insubstantial and, like grasses, wilt rapidly (cf. Avestan *ną̄my-ąsu-* '[*haoma*] having a soft stem', *Yasna* 9.12, see §182). Whether one believes *barsom* to have originally been grass or sauma stems, he must explain why it is that *barsom* has historically consisted of woody twigs. The practice of holding twigs as the Iranian priestly insignia was undoubtably adopted from earlier Near Eastern traditions of holding tamarisk branches, as Peter Calmeyer (1975) has shown. In order for the Iranian priests to have adapted *barəsman-/barsom* to serve the ritual and emblematic functions of the hand-held twigs, it would have been necessary for them to have replaced the original *barsom* plants by stouter ones, such as twigs of the pomegranate or of *Ephedra*, or else by the anciently used tamarisk branches. The identification of these emblematic twigs with *barsom* indicates that *barsom* was in some essential way connected with the distinctive office of the Iranian priesthood. Since the priesthood was ultimately defined by the performance of sauma rites, it seems again highly probable that it was to these rites that *barsom* referred and, indeed, that the plant represented by the *barsom* twigs would have been sauma, the plant whose use must have *actually* been emblematic of the priesthood.

RUTA GRAVEOLENS

(a) *Ruta graveolens* in rituals represents harmel

§127 *Ruta graveolens* L., the garden rue, called in Persian *sudāb* or *sadāb*, is essential to the rituals of the Iranian Zoroastrians, who grow it in the precincts of each of their fire temples (Boyce 1966b: 54). Although the word *sudāb/sadāb* is likely Iranian (and seems itself to link *Peganum harmala* with sauma, see below, §§274-286), the plant it now names, *Ruta graveolens*, is not Iranian at all. Except in the coastal districts of Anatolia, Syria and Palestine and parts of central and southern Arabia, species of the genus *Ruta* (i.e. *Ruta graveolens, Ruta chalepensis* or *Ruta montana*) have not been reported as wild plants in Asia.[17] Rue seems to have first been cultivated in (or near) Greece, where wild species of *Ruta* occur.[18] The plant cannot have been known to the early Iranians and, therefore, *Ruta graveolens* itself cannot have been the plant originally used, unless the rituals wherein it figures (which we shall presently consider) are late innovations (and given the antiquity and pronounced conservatism of the Zoroastrian tradition, this hardly seems likely). In other words, there can be no doubt that in Iranian ritual *Ruta graveolens* is a substitute; the only question is, what is the plant for which it substitutes? The unique, intimate relationship of *Ruta* to *Peganum harmala* (see §53), the fact that in the Middle East, names for *Ruta graveolens* are frequently derived from names for *Peganum harmala*, and the direct evidence from the Zoroastrian rituals themselves, show that *Ruta graveolens* must be the ritual replacement of *Peganum harmala*. I shall next present evidence to establish that in these rituals *Ruta graveolens* has the role of sauma, indicating further that sauma was *Peganum harmala*.

§128 Among the Zoroastrians in Iran *Ruta graveolens* is reportedly tasted on all religious occasions (see Sheriyar 1914: 311–312). This constant presence of *Ruta graveolens* is best explained by the precedent of sauma. This is confirmed by the representation of sauma by *Ruta graveolens* in three concrete situations: (a) as the chief plant used in the preparation of offerings (*zaoθras*) to Water and to Fire; (b) as the plant to be consumed in the *drōn* rite; and (c) as the plant corresponding to Avestan *dūraoša*, a designation for sauma, at *Gāhāmbār* festivals.

(b) The use of *Ruta graveolens* in *zaoθras* represents sauma

§129 In Avestan, *zaoθra* means 'that which is poured', hence, 'liquid offering'. The term usually seems to refer to the extracted sauma, drunk by a priest in the worship of a divinity. In two cases, however, *zaoθras* are prepared which are not drunk: when offered to Fire and Water they are poured into the material manifestations of these elements.

§130 The *zaoθra* to the Waters, called *āb-zōhr* in Middle Persian, survives in two forms. When the *āb-zōhr* is offered after a *Yasna* it consists of the mixture of the extract of pomegranate and *Ephedra*, together with milk, which the *zaotar* prepares during the *Yasna* (see §104). This shows that the *āb-zōhr* originally contained sauma. At other times, when the pomegranate-*Ephedra*-milk mixture made during a *Yasna* is not freshly available, Zoroastrian priests in Iran make the *āb-zōhr* offering with a mixture consisting of grains, fruits, garlic, milk and *Ruta graveolens*;[19] this mixture then seems to serve in the place of the pomegranate-*Ephedra* mixture in representing sauma.

§131 Analogous to the Water offering is the Fire offering, the *ātaš-zōhr*. The essential part of the *ātaš-zōhr* is the fat of a sacrificial animal (Boyce 1966a), although a paring of its horn or even some hair may also be used, together with a plant constituent which, in parallel with all other *zaoθras*, should be sauma. Two occasions when the *ātaš-zōhr* was still made were observed in 1964 by Mary Boyce among Zoroastrian communities in Iran: one at the *jašn-i Mihrīzed* (ancient *Mihragān*), when an animal was sacrificed and its fat offered to the fire accompanied by the burning of *Peganum harmala* (see §115); the other at *čahārom*, the ceremony of the fourth day after death. Boyce (*ibid.* 107) reports that the

[17] The species classed as *Ruta* in some Asiatic floras (e.g. *R. tuburculata, R. abiflora*, etc.) are apparently all species of the related genus *Haplophyllum* A. Juss. (see Townsend 1966a and 1966b).

[18] Further confirmation that the cultivation of *Ruta* spread from a single location is the consistency of magical and supernatural powers assigned to *Ruta graveolens* and particularly the universal attribution to it of the ability to ward off and counteract the poison of noxious creatures. These powers are not ones which can be rediscovered by simple observation and represent beliefs which must have been borrowed along with the cultivation of the plant. (For a survey of the powers attributed to rue in European folklore see H. Marzell in Bächtold-Stäubli [1927-1942:7, 542-548], Branky [1901], and Gunther [1905]). The ascription of these powers to *Ruta graveolens* is probably not historically independent of their assignment to *Peganum harmala*. Since *Peganum harmala* has borne names meaning 'sacred' since Proto-Iranian times, it is likely its ethnobotanic importance as a source of supernatural powers is far older, and that Greeks exposed to Iranian beliefs about harmel (in Anatolia) transferred them to *Ruta graveolens* in Greece, providing an impetus for its cultivation, which eventually had a role in the spread of the plant to other Mediterranean lands and, in Roman times, throughout Europe. A major claim for the value of "rue" (Greek π῾ηανον) in the Classical World was its being a chief ingredient of the antidote of Mithridates Eupator (d. 64 B.C.E.), the last Iranian ruler of Pontus, but is is likely that the "rue" traditionally used by an Iranian prince as an antidote would have been *Peganum harmala* (Greek π῾ηανον ἤριον, "wild rue"). The success of *Ruta* as the successor to harmel even where harmel is a native plant must be largely due to the ease with which *Ruta graveolens* can be propagated from cuttings (as against the difficulty of cultivating harmel, despite its proliferation as a weed), and also to the fact that *Ruta graveolens* is evergreen, a factor of particular symbolic importance in its replacement of harmel in Zoroastrian rituals. For the history of rue as a spice in Rome (but not so used in Greece), see A. Andrews (1948).

[19] This information, like most of the details on Iranian ritual, comes from Mary Boyce, who made a unique study of the practices in Zoroastrian villages in 1964. The modern libation (*ōwzūr*), which she identifies with a form of the ancient *āb-zōhr*, as prepared by a priest, was from "five things, namely, milk, garlic, rue, rice, oleaster- [misprinted oleander-] fruits, and bread" (1966a:112 n.1). The essential place of sauma as an ingredient in the offering to Water is substantiated by Boyce (*ibid.* 113), citing *Nērangistān* f.140.16 to the effect that *parāhōm* (meaning here the pomegranate-*Ephedra*-milk mixture, see above, §113 n.6) and *āb-zōhr* are identical. She further observes: "In the Pahlavi texts the *āb-zōhr* is sometimes referred to as the pouring of *hōm* into the waters. This is readily understandable, since *haoma* regularly stands first among the ingredients of the libation and gives its name to it as the *para.haoma, parāhōm*" (1966a:117). This provides so much more reason to believe that the modern *āb-zōhr/ōwzūr* she describes contains a representation of sauma.

ātaš-zōhr at *čahārom* consists of some fat, a paring from the horn of, and a scrap of wool from, the sheep sacrificed at the last *Mihragān*, pounded up with the root of an aromatic plant (*būd-i nākōš*), garlic, and *Ruta graveolens*. The five ingredients of this *ātaš-zōhr* parallel the composition burned on the festival day of *Isfandagān* (§122), which also included a paring of the horn of a sheep sacrificed at *Mihragān* and garlic, but contained raisins and *Peganum harmala* instead of *Ruta graveolens*.[20]

(c) Use of *Ruta graveolens* in the *drōn* ceremony represents sauma

§132 Apart from the classification of *sadāb* (i.e. *Ruta graveolens*) as a herb (i.e. as a *tarrag: Bundahišn* 117.28: B. T. Anklesaria 1956:149), the earliest Iranian mention of *sadāb* is in the *Nērangistān*, or 'ritual code'.[21] This text consists of brief passages in Avestan with interlinear Pahlavi translation interspersed with Pahlavi commentaries. The longest of these commentaries gives views of various Sasanian authorities (much in the style of the Mishnah) on the conduct of the abbreviated form of the *Yasna* ritual known as the *drōn* rite.[22] In this commentary (*Nērangistān* 28) *drōn* refers to small cakes of ritual bread, together with which alcoholic drinks or drugs may also have once been consumed (though this is no longer the case),[23] and in this text *sadāb* is specified as the plant to be placed on the bread cake consumed as *drōn* by priests.[24]

§133 The Avestan liturgy of the *Yasna* ceremony is a compilation of texts of differing origins. It does not seem to have been recognized previously that, by reason of its relationship to the liturgy, the consumption of the *drōn* bread must represent the act of consuming sauma as practiced before the insertion of the three chapters which comprise the *Hōm Yasht* (*Yasna* 9–11.15) into the text of the *Yasna* liturgy. The *Hōm Yasht* differs in content and form of expression from most of the text now surrounding it in the *Yasna* (see Schlerath 1968: xi) and must itself have originated as the liturgy of a separate and independent sauma ceremony (Boyce 1975b:266). The proposition that the consumption of the *drōn* bread represents consumption of sauma follows from these four considerations: (1) The parallel consumption of *soma* in the Indic *Yajña* shows that the *Yasna* originally included the act of drinking sauma. (2) If the three chapters which comprise the *Hōm Yasht* were deleted from the present *Yasna* liturgy, the *drōn* bread would be consumed at precisely that point in the recital of the liturgy where the drinking of *haoma* now occurs. (3) For the *Hōm Yasht* to have been inserted in its present position in the *Yasna*, sauma must have been drunk at that very point of insertion. (4) The only substance whose consumption is presupposed by the *Yasna* rite is sauma; there is no other Avestan substance to which the *drōn* bread can be likened. Thus the consumption of the *drōn* bread in *Yasna* 8 is historically equivalent to the consumption of the *haoma* in *Yasna* 11 as a representation of drinking sauma, and the specification of *sadāb* as the unique plant eaten with the *drōn* bread assigns it to the place of sauma.

(d) The Use of *Ruta graveolens* to represent Avestan *dūraoša*

§134 The use of *Ruta graveolens* in place of sauma is again manifest in the legend of the origin of the obligatory holy days of the Zoroastrians, the *Gāhāmbārs*. These are six feast days, distributed over the seasons, on which is performed an extended form of the *Yasna*, the *Vīsperad* ('all the judges', see §150), the nature of which makes it especially likely that these festivals were characterized by the use of sauma. The *Gāhāmbārs* are quite ancient. They were reportedly celebrated before the time of Zoroaster, who appears from one account (see *Zātsparam* 21) to have had his initial vision in connection with one of them. The legendary origin of these six holy days is recounted in a letter sent from the priests of central Iran to Zoroastrians in India in 1628 in response to the discovery that *Ruta graveolens* was not being used in the rituals of the Indian congregations. Some *Ruta graveolens* plants were apparently sent with the letter, and the recipients were especially advised to use them at *Gāhāmbārs* and in the ceremonies performed to assure the safe passage of the soul on the third day after death.

§135 According to the legend related in that letter, the *Gāhāmbārs* originated under King Jamshid (the Avestan Yima), who during his reign of universal weal and prosperity was visited by a demon of greed disguised as a needy stranger. As hospitality required, the visitor was offered his fill of whatever the king could provide, whereupon he proceeded to devour the vast herds and everything edible that this richest of all monarchs possessed. King Jamshid prayed earnestly for help from Ohrmazd, who in response sent Bahman (Avestan Vohu Manah 'Good Thinking') to King Jamshid with the following message:[25]

> "Go and capture a yellow bovine and in the name of Ohrmazd kill it and command that it be cooked in old vinegar, and put garlic and *sudāb* into the caldron and place it before the demon so that he eats it."
>
> This was done, and when the demon ate the first mouthful, he withdrew and became non-existent.

[20] According to the description provided by H. Anquetil du Perron (1771: 2, 577) from the *"vieux Ravaef" f.*252, a fifth ingredient of the mixture burned at *Isfandagān* was cotton seed. Variations of the constiuents (always five in number and always including *isfand*) are given (from the *Rivāyat of Kamdin Shapur*) in M. R. Unvala (1922:I, 526–527; Dhabhar 1932: 341-342) and in S. D. Bharucha (1906: I, xiv).

[21] Still earlier, in the latter part of the Syriac *Book of Medicines* of the sixth century C.E. (ed. W. Budge 1913: 675), *sdb* occurs (without definition as either *Ruta* or harmel) in recipes apparently copied from some non-Greek (Iranian?) source.

[22] This commentary precedes the part of the Avestan text dealing with the failure to sing the Gathas due to intoxication during ceremonies. In particular, the Avestan (*Nērangistān* 29–30) discusses intoxication from consuming a *draonah-* 'portion payed to priests' consisting of wine or kumiss.

[23] "When one desires to take a drug, when a drug is among the edibles assembled and set out with the *drōn*, he should taste the drug before (tasting the *drōn*)" *ka dārūg ē ō kāmēd xwardan ud ka dārūg az ān ī pad xwarišn mehmānīh pad drōn frāz nihišn u-š čāšnīg pēš ēn az dārūg kunišn* (*Nērangistān f.*46.5; equivalent to *Pahlavi Rivāyat* 182.4). The Middle Persian word *dārūg* seems to have been of similar meaning to, and may be the etymological antecedent of, English *drug*, French *drogue*, etc. (but for alternative views see E. Sluszkiewicz 1977). Because of the relative position of this passage within the text, Middle Persian *dārūg* cannot here refer to wine or an alcoholic drink. Wine and *hur* (or perhaps the mysterious beer *"wašag"* [see Henning 1953]; *Nērangistān* has *wš'k'*) are subjects of a separate discussion in *Nērangistān f.*40.16 (corresponding to *Pahlavi Rivāyat* 175.7).

[24] *Nērangistān f.* 40.11; *Pahlavi Rivāyat* 175.4. The whole of the commentary of which this is a part comprises a distinct Pahlavi treatise having the title *Griftan ī Drōn*, "The Conduct of the *Drōn* Ceremony." I shall present elsewhere a collocation of the two versions of this text and also an examination of the *Čim ī Drōn* which accompanies it in the *Pahlavi Rivāyat* (pp. 166-169). It accords with the hypothesis that pomegranate and rue both represent sauma, that on the one hand the *Nērangistān* specifies *sadāb* as placed upon the *drōn* bread, and that, on the other hand, it is pomegranate which is placed upon the *drōn* bread in actual practice. Although *Ruta graveolens* resembles harmel more distinctly than does pomegranate, ingestion of an extract of *Ruta graveolens* causes gastroenteritis. Hence for the *Yasna*, where the drinking of an entire cup of *haoma* extract is required, pomegranate has been particularly preferred. The same consideration may have lead to abandoning the consumption of *Ruta graveolens* in the *drōn* rite, although in general the representation of sauma by pomegranate is the more ancient practice, since pomegranate is a native plant.

[25] Translation based on the text in M. R. Unvala (1922: II, 162–163, with parts also in I, 159.11 and 428.9) and (from another MS. of the same *rivāyat*) in J. J. Modi (1921). The same tale also occurs as the latter part of Chapter 94 of the metrical version of the *Sad Dar*, a Latin translation of which is given by Thomas Hyde (1700: 485–486) and a paraphrase from this by A. Christensen (1934: 645). The metrical *Sad Dar* was composed in Kerman in 1495 C.E., 132 years earlier than the letter quoted above, but its account differs only in the detail that a red, rather than a yellow, bovine was to be killed. For the later use of *sadāb* at the *Gāhāmbārs* of Zoroastrians in India, see J. K. Katrak (1941: 215–216).

> Then, from that day on, they instituted the *Gāhāmbār*, and whenever famine and want arise a bovine should be slain and garlic and *sudāb* should be cooked and eaten so that famine and want disappear. For *Gāhāmbār* it is absolutely necessary that *sudāb* compounded with garlic be burned in the *Gāhāmbār* fire and (also necessary) that it be tasted.

§136 This legend must have had its origin in an interpretation of the section of the Gathas which includes the passage referring to the burning of sauma by its distinctive epithet *dūraoša* (see §98). The Pahlavi translation of the relevant Gathic verses, which occur in the thirty-second chapter of the *Yasna* liturgy, states that a demon, who overhears Yima/Jamshid announce his intention to provide the people with meat, greedily sets about to slaughter the cattle himself. The Pahlavi recommends burning *dūrōš* (i.e. *dūraoša*) for assistance in counteracting this demon.[26] Equating, as we must, the burning of *dūraoša* (i.e. of sauma) with the burning of *Ruta graveolens,* we see that the latter is a substitute for sauma.

§137 The form in which *Ruta graveolens* is now present at *Gāhāmbārs* and at other religious occasions is in a mixture known as *sīr-u-sedōw* 'garlic and rue.' The following is a first-hand description by Mary Boyce (letter of February 19, 1970; cf. Boyce 1977:42) of its preparation among the Yazdi Zoroastrians:

> The *sedōw* (rue) is used either fresh or dried. It is crushed in a mortar with the *sīr* (garlic), and there is added chopped coriander leaves and turmeric, cumin seed, pepper, and salt. Fat (which must be the rendered fat of a sacrificial animal) is melted or oil (necessarily sesame seed oil) is heated in an iron pan. When this is very hot, the mixture is poured in from the mortar; and when it is heated right through, vinegar is added and then pure water. Occasionally a beaten egg is also added at this point. The hot mixture is then poured into a ritually pure utensil, usually a silver-plated bowl, containing chopped dried mint. A few bits of bread are added, and the bowl is carried at once to where the priest is officiating.

In *sīr-u-sedōw* the yellow bovine of the legend is represented only by fat from a sacrificial animal, and to the rue and garlic[27] are added spices (perhaps to rationalize the concoction as merely culinary),[28] but this mixture clearly has a common origin with that called for in the *Gāhāmbār* legend.

§138 The yellow *Gāhāmbār* cow and the fat representing it in *sīr-u-sedōw* have a correspondent in Zoroastrian eschatology that further establishes sauma as the plant to be consumed with them. At the end of the world a final *Yasna* will be performed in which the bull Haδāyuš will be slaughtered and its fat mixed with the "white *haoma*" to provide the draught of immortality for the resurrected dead.[29] Although the "white *haoma*" differs from ordinary *haoma*, just as the Haδāyuš bull differs from ordinary cattle, this mythological *Yasna* seems to be a paradigm for (or reflection of) the *Yasna* ceremony as it was ordinarily performed. Throughout the Avesta, *gav-* 'flesh/bovine' is mentioned as a constituent of *haoma* preparations. The individual deities of the *Yashts* are regularly worshiped with *haomayō gavā* (or **haoma yō gava* [cf. Hoffmann 1967]) 'flesh/bovine with *haoma*', and the *zaoθras* which the Avesta proclaims to contain *haoma* and *haδānaēpātā* are also said to contain *gav-*. In ritual usage *gav-* is often represented by milk (which is mixed with *soma* in India), and it was milk which was mixed with *hōm* to engender Zoroaster (§95),[30] but in some other rituals *gav-* may be represented not by milk, but by urine,[31] or horn, or in the account of *Gāhāmbār* beginnings above, by meat, whereas in the drink consumed at the final *Yasna,* it is in the form of the fat of the bull Haδāyuš.[32] The only modern ritual preparation involving the fat of sacrificial animals with which this "white *haoma*" mixture could be said to correspond is *sīr-u-sedōw*, in which *Ruta graveolens* has unmistakably the role of sauma.

§139 That the use of *Ruta graveolens* in Zoroastrian ritual must be in place of *Peganum harmala* was first recognized by W. B. Henning, who thought the replacement resulted from a superstitious regard for *Peganum harmala* as a plant (only) of sorcerers: "In late times *sudāb* was admitted to Zoroastrian ceremonies, probably as a substitute for *isfand,* in a concession to popular superstition" (1965: 39 n.2). The need to mollify Muslim suspicions of sorcery may indeed have been a factor encouraging the replacement of *isfand* in ritual by other plants.

(e) *Ruta graveolens* and the history of *soma* in India

§140 The Sanskrit term *somalatā*, used for *Sarcostemma brevistigma* and *Ephedra Gerardiana* in different places in the Indian area, also reportedly identifies *Ruta graveolens* (Fleming 1812, Piddington 1836, Monier-Williams 1899), as do also the synonyms *saumyā, somavallarī,* and other relevant Sanskrit terms (see Table 2). There does not seem to be any attestation of the use of *Ruta graveolens* as *soma* in Indian rituals, which is not surprising since an extract pressed out from *Ruta graveolens* is toxic. There is, moreover, no property of *Ruta graveolens* which could readily explain these names. However, since *Ruta graveolens* necessarily reached India via Iran, where it appears to serve analogously to *soma* in certain rituals, it may be that the Sanskrit names are modeled upon Iranian terminology of ritual substitutes for *Peganum harmala.* Although Achaemenian, Parthian, Saka and Kushan incursions into India may have exposed some Brahmans

26 Translations of the relevant parts of *Pahlavi Yasna 32* may be found in M. Molé (1963: 230), and E. W. West (1904: 189). Both of these scholars (as also H. Humbach [1974]) observed that the legend quoted above must have originated as an interpretation of *Pahlavi Yasna* 32.8-14.

27 Garlic is an ingredient of the *Peganum harmala* mixture prepared on *Isfandagān* (§§119 and 133), with which the *sīr-u-sedōw* mixture probably shares a common origin. Garlic may owe its presence here to its having been esteemed in its own right as an apotropaic in ancient Iran. There appears to have once been a *Sīr-sūr* 'Garlic-feast' on the fourteenth day of the tenth month, with the object of gaining protection against demons (al-Bīrūnī, *Chronology,* tr. Sachau 1879: 212). The third Old Persian month, *θāiγṛčī-*, may have been named for garlic (Eilers 1953: 43n., but doubted by Boyce 1982: 25). In the Indian tradition, by contrast, garlic was regarded as impure (see Bedi 1960).

28 A secular form of this preparation seems to have survived elsewhere in Iran as *āb-kāma,* an infusion of spices eaten with meat. Historically, *āb-kāma* could be prepared with either *Ruta graveolens* (Dehkhudā 1947-1973: *s.v.*) or *Peganum harmala* (Minorsky 1953: 255), showing once again the equivalence of the two plants in Iran. Since *Peganum harmala,* which has no role as a spice in Iran, was probably the older ingredient, its presence in *āb-kāma* suggests that the origin of this bitter sauce may have been in the ritual connection of sauma with the sacrifice of meat animals for food (see §153).

29 *Bundahišn* 226.3: *yazišn pad rist-wirāyišn Sōšyans kird abāg ayārān kunēd ud gāw ī Haδāyuš pad ān yazišn kušēnd, az pih ī ān gāw ud hōm ī spēd anōš wirāyēnd ud ō harwisp mardōm dahēnd ud harwisp mardōm a(h)ōš bawēnd* 'Sōshyans with helpers will perform the *Yasna* at the Resurrection of the Dead and they will kill the Haδāyuš bull at that *Yasna,* and from the fat of that bull and white *haoma* they will prepare immortality and will give it to all men and all men will become deathless' (similarly *Dādistān-ī Dēnīg* 48.16 and *Zātsparam* 3.15).

30 Milk is present in the putative sauma mixtures mentioned in §90 n.25 and §130 n.16. Harmel extract is drunk with milk according to the passage quoted in §95 and at the observance of *Isfandagān* in Kerman (see §122).

31 For the combination of *hōm* (*Ephedra*) with bovine urine in a form of *nērang,* see §79 n.17.

32 Because of the variation in the form in which *gav-* is ritually present, it seems unlikely that the bovine constituent served a pharmacological function. "Bovine" may have been consumed with sauma to facilitate for the drinker contact with the soul of the slaughtered beast and a means thereby of negotiating immunity from the ordinary consequences of killing sentient beings. The need to forestal retaliation by the slain animal's spirit in this way could have been a factor in the persistence of the centrality of sauma in priestly traditions (see Chapter 6). In the liturgy, at the conclusion of the *Hōm Yasht* (*Yasna* 11.1 and 7) recited just before the *zaotar* drinks *haoma, gav-* is a metaphor for the flesh of the *zaotar* (see §150 n3).

to Iranian rituals, there is nevertheless little reason to think that late Iranian ritual use of *Ruta graveolens* could have prompted adoption of the plant under the name *soma* in Sanskrit.

§141 If the Sanskrit names for *Ruta* do not then reflect Iranian use of the plant, the alternative is that the names were given to *Ruta* in the course of its propagation in India. It has generally been supposed that the dispersion of *Peganum harmala* across northern India resulted from Muslim transportation of the seeds for medical or apotropaic uses. However, peoples entering India from Iran probably used and esteemed harmel much more before the advent of Islam, and the conditions for its distribution have remained the same from the period antedating the immigration to India of the Indo-Aryans themselves. Although harmel may be locally abundant in its characteristic ruderial environment, it is not a common plant in India. It seems unlikely that *Ruta graveolens*, on the other hand, reached India much earlier than the Hellenistic period, since there is no evidence for its cultivation anywhere outside of Greece before that time, and since *Ruta* is not a part of the traditional Indian Ayurvedic herbal. As happened in Iran, when *Ruta* was introduced into India, it must have acquired the names of the wild species it most resembles, that is, *Peganum harmala.* If this is so, then harmel must have been recognized as sauma and designated *soma* in some quarters of India long after Vedic times.

§142 The problem of the availability of sauma in Vedic India has frequently been misunderstood. There is no reason to think that the absence of sauma has ever impeded the performance of Vedic rituals. The fact that sauma intoxication has been absent from the *Yajña* throughout historical times shows that sauma is unnecessary for the viability of that rite as an institution. Apparently, even before the completion of the ṚgVeda, a major use of the priests' knowledge of Vedic hymns and ritual was for magical purposes, for which the intoxicating effects of sauma would not necessarily have been required. Historically, sauma seems not to have been essential to the magic of Indian priests. Sauma itself was doubtless potentially useful for such purposes, but the power attributed to sauma would presumably have been regarded as inherent rather than due to special priestly knowledge, and access to the plant by nonpriests, and particularly by non-Aryans and the intended victims of Vedic magic, would only have lessened the relative advantage of the Aryan priests in the conduct of magic. Whether or not sauma grew in India or only at a great distance from it, access to the plant by Indians would have been the same for the priests and their enemies alike. The problem for the Vedic priests would have been less how they were to obtain the plant themselves than how to prevent others from doing so.

§143 Just as knowledge of Vedic hymns and ritual techniques was jealously restricted by Indian priests, in the context of the Indian caste system it would have been useful for them to have controlled access to sauma. Since the actual growth and distribution of the plant could not be controlled, the only means of curtailing access to it would have been to obscure its identity. This was accomplished by the combination of elaborate obscurantism in the composition of hymns to the plant drug (an extension of a characteristic already found in certain Indo-Iranian genres [see Boyce 1975b:9]), with a corresponding proliferation of irrelevant ritual details. The *Brāhmaṇas* (*c* 600 B.C.E.) list a variety of plants, few of them clearly identifiable and many patently fantastic, for use as *soma* substitutes (e.g. *Śatapatha Brāhmaṇa* 4.5.10; 5.3.3; 6.6.3; see R. E. G. Müller 1954). These hypothetical substitutes do not seem to share features that could be related to a common original plant and do not at all show similarities with *Ephedra/Sarcostemma.* Because of the similar appearance of the *soma* of present-day Indian rituals (i.e. *Sarcostemma brevistigma*) and the *Ephedras* used in Iran, it can be supposed that there has in fact been a continuous tradition of the ritual plants used as *soma* and that the substitutes proposed in the *Brāhmaṇas* had no reality in actual practice.

§144 Although such tactics would have succeeded in obscuring the identity of the plant among the laity, outside of Aryan society knowledge of the identity of the intoxicant plant as a sacred object would persist among the servants of the priesthood and be adopted by them. This would have been regarded as a defilement of the plant which could not be prevented. The priests, who by this time may anyway have had no need for the intoxicant plant, would have tended to stop using it. At this point the sanctity of the plant would have become manifest as a taboo.

§145 Now may be appreciated the significance of the otherwise unexplained reports by E. Balfour that *Peganum harmala* was "the plant sacred to the Pariah caste" (1885: II, 18), and "the [*Peganum harmala*] plant is . . . not to be touched by Sikhs or Hindus" (*ibid.* III, 172).

§146 This explains why *Peganum harmala* disappeared from all Hindu rituals and folk traditions and is no longer associated with its ritual substitutes. Thus, the Indian situation, so closely linked to its unique social history, is markedly different from the Iranian, where the ancient ethnobotanic tradition is unbroken. It is this Iranian ethnobotanical tradition that yields the ultimate identity of the plant which stands behind Iranian *haoma* and Indian *soma*, *Peganum harmala* L.

6

THE HISTORICAL PERSISTENCE OF THE SAUMA RITES

§147 To this point we have been exclusively concerned with examining evidence for the botanical/pharmacological identity of sauma. Before summarizing the arguments identifying sauma with harmel, some of the historical aspects of this identification need to be considered. The purpose of this chapter is to clarify how harmel was used in order to account for how the ceremonies symbolically representing harmel consumption continued to be at the core of the Zoroastrian tradition after the actual consumption of the plant in those ceremonies had ceased and had even been forgotten.

§148 It will be recalled that in the *Ardā Wīrāz Nāmag* quoted in §24, Wīrāz was sent forth to the spirit world to resolve the question of whether souls were helped in avoiding hell by the ceremonies (which were historically based directly or indirectly on drinking sauma) practiced by Zoroastrian priests (or more precisely, in view of the probable pre-Sasanian origin of the *Ardā Wīrāz Nāmag*, by the Parthian Magi). The administration of the drug to Wīrāz could not have been merely intended to convince Wīrāz, who anyway had no doubts about the truth of Magian teachings, but was meant to persuade those summoned to observe him. Since it was the people's doubt about priestly claims that led to the project of sending Wīrāz, the Magi could not have supposed that the people would accept the report of Wīrāz, who was experienced in the intoxicant use of sauma and hence surely a priest himself, without being shown some evidence of his reliability. The drug which was meant to bring Wīrāz visions was at the same time the means of exposing him to an ordeal (as shown by Göbrecht 1969) that would publicly attest his personal trustworthiness. He passed this test by remaining tranquil.

§149 A contemporary (mid-second century B.C.E.) account of the use of drug plants by the Parthian Magi survives from the *Chirocmeta* by Bolus of Mendes (in Egypt), a book quoted in Pliny's *Naturalis historia* 24, 160–67 (translated by W.H.S. Jones 1956: 7, 113–17) where it is wrongly attributed to Democritus (see Bidez and Cumont 1938: I, 117–19, and above, §90 n24). Since sauma is the only plant known from Iranian religious sources with attributes similar to the magical plants described by Bolus under various Greek names, it is probable that some, or perhaps all of those plants refer to sauma (which as we have seen was already also diversely named in Iranian texts, e.g. by Avestan *dūraoša-, haδānaēpātā-, barəsman-, haoma-*). Bolus' account attests that the potential of plants as ordeal drugs was exploited by the Parthian Magi. The capacity of sauma to produce visions of a credible spirit world would certainly have qualified it for the uses that Bolus reports the Magi made of the following plants:[1]

> *Thalassaegle:* "To drink *thalassaegle* ['sea radiance'] causes men to rave, while weird visions beset their minds."
> *Achaemenis:* [A name which has obvious reference to the Persian world.]: "Criminals, if they drink it in wine, confess all their misdeeds because they suffer diverse phantoms of spirits that haunt them. Mares have an intense aversion to it . . . for which reason it is known as *hippophobas*" (see above, §55, n.14).
> *Nyctegreton:* ['That which keeps one up all night'.]: "The Magi and the kings of Parthia use the plant to make their vows."
> *Ophiusa:* "To take *ophiusa* ['that which is characterized by snakes'] in drink causes such terrible visions of threatening serpents that fear of them causes suicide; wherefore those guilty of sacrilege are forced to drink it." (Cf. the prominent role of snakes in *yagé* visions, §82, n.20.)

§150 This ordeal aspect of the use of sauma also appears in the liturgy on both occasions where sauma consumption is represented in the *Yasna*, that is, accompanying both the consumption of the *drōn* bread after *Yasna* 8.4 and the drinking of *haoma* extract during *Yasna* 11.10. In the first case, when the *zaotar* is about to partake of the surrogate sauma represented by the *drōn* bread (see §133), he invokes the drug to expose him in the following words (*Yasna* 8.3) if he is falsely representing himself:

8.3 *aməša spənta daēne māzdayasnē*	O Aməša Spəntas, Vision of Mazdaworship,
vaŋhavašca vaŋuhīšca	Good Males, Good Females,
zaoθråsca yō aēšva	*Zaoθras*! Whoever among these
mazdayasnaēšva	Mazda-worshippers here, calling himself a
mazdayasnō aojanō ašahe rāθma	Mazda-worshipper, an adherent of the Truth,
jīštayamnō yāθwa gāθå ašahe	ruins the world with witchcraft,
mərəγənte avi tū dim disyata	O you waters, plants and *zaoθras*,
yå apasca urvaråsca zaoθråsca	make him known!

8.4 *yasca aētaēšąm mazdayasnanąm*	Whoever of these Mazda-worshippers,
pərənāyunąm aiwi.zūzuyanąm	of full age, invoking diligently,
imå vacō nōiṯ vīsaite framrūite	is not ready to recite *these* words
aētąm ā yātumanahe jasaiti	will get the punishment for sorcery.

[At this point the *zaotar* consumes the *drōn* and then recites *Yasna* 8.5-8, which propound curses upon deceivers and which are identical to the words that are recited following the drinking of *haoma* (i.e. *Yasna* 11.11-15)].

Whereas originally in the *Yasna* these "plants, waters, and *zaoθras*" must have referred to the sauma drink, in the shorter *drōn* ceremony they must refer to the *drōn* bread and whatever is consumed with it. The announced function of the plants, waters and *zaoθras* to expose duplicitous participants indicates that the ceremony must have once been an ordeal for the priests who performed it.[2] The function of testing the drinker is again asserted in *Yasna* 11, (the last of the three chapters of the *Hōm Yasht*) which the *zaotar* recites just before he consumes the *haoma* extract. *Yasna* 11 consists of an elaborate warning that woeful consequences will befall anyone who attempts to resist the effects of the drug, and that the *zaotar*, following Zarathushtra, surrenders his body to *haoma* and thus shows himself to be a follower of Truth.[3] In the more elaborate *Yasna* performed at *Gāhāmbārs* and at the initiation of priests, the *Vīsperad* ('all the judges'), the *zaotar*, before drinking the *haoma*, interrupts his recital of the *Hōm Yasht* to make a roll-call of six additional priests who, as well as the usual *raspī*, were apparently at one time regularly assembled on such occasions to witness (and judge) his response to the drug. What most decisively shows that administering sauma functioned as an ordeal is the construction of the *Yasna* itself: at near the beginning of the ceremony the *zaotar* is handed a cup containing as *haoma* an extract whose composition is unknown to him, since it is prepared in his absence before the *Yasna* starts [see §104], but which is supposed to be a powerful drug, and he must drink it under scrutiny of other priests and all the spirits summonsed as witnesses.

§151 The use of sauma ceremonies as tests must have been effective in maintaining fidelity among Iranian priests, all of whom must periodically assume the role of *zaotar*, while at other times they must prepare the extract to be consumed by their fellows. The willing participation of persons in the role of *zaotar* in the *Yasna* would have insured that they were accepted as qualified by the other priests. By being willing to take the role of *zaotar*, one would demonstrate his preparedness to expose his soul to judgment by the spirits and show his confidence that other priests would recognize his spiritual acceptability. If one had already gained acceptance in this manner, it would have been largely unnecessary for the extract administered to him in the *Yasna* to have as much pharmacological potency as that administered to someone whose suitability was in doubt. The *Ardā Wīrāz Nāmag* shows that the drug was not taken casually to induce visions, but was reserved for occasions when there was genuine need to obtain information about the spiritual world.[4] In the usual con-

[1] Although in other contexts Pliny uses *Magi* for charlatans active in the Roman world of the second century C.E., in the *Chirocmeta* the term has the older meaning 'Iranian priests'.

[2] The ordeal character of the text of *Yasna* 8 has been demonstrated by Darmesteter (1892-1983: I, 75), J. C. Tavadia (1948) and M. F. Kanga (1950).

[3] *Yasna* 11 requires that, just as a sacrificial animal submits to the *zaotar* priest (*Yasna* 11.1), the *zaotar* priest must in turn surrender himself to *haoma*, who is "the swiftly-sacrificing *zaotar* of Ahura Mazdah" (*Yasht* 10.89 [Boyce 1970:69]). Because the Pahlavi translators of the Avesta were unaware that *haoma* had originally been an intoxicating drug, they could not have understood the thematic coherence of *Yasna* 11 nor its relevance to the act of drinking *haoma*. In consequence, the command at *Yasna* 11.7-8 for the drinker to cut free his organs of sight and speech and allow them to be acted upon by the drug has been misinterpreted, apparently since Sasanian times, as an injunction to mutilate the heads of sacrificially slain animals to propitiate the abstract deity *Haoma*. This interpretation has prevailed despite the fact that there is no animal sacrificed in connection with the *Yasna* ceremony today nor any other passage in the *Yasna* liturgy to suggest that an animal ever was sacrificed or dismembered during that ceremony.. I shall discuss elsewhere the unitary structure of *Yasna* 11 and its constant relevance to the ritual actions actually accompanying its recital.

The traditional interpretation of *Yasna* 11 exhibits a wholly symbolic conception of *haoma*, as a result of which the substitute plants were seen as equivalent representations of a spiritual entity and not as standing for a particular species. This explains why no priority seems to be accorded to harmel among ritual plants and why the question of botanically distinguishing the primary species from its substitutes did not arise among the Zoroastrian priests. In Iran the botanical identity of sauma became obscure because the issue was not meaningful, and not as the result of any compact among priests to conceal it or willfully to compromise the authenticity of rituals.

[4] Among the situations where sauma seems most likely to have been used was at the inauguration of pre-Islamic Iranian rulers. This is indicated by King Wishtāsp's consumption of "*hōm* and *mang*" at his "initiation" (as Molé [1963: 383–84] has justifiably interpreted the passage quoted in §28), which is still commemorated by Zoroastrians at the New Year. The New Year was the occasion when the inauguration of Iranian rulers traditionally occurred and when the use of sauma for divination (in this case of the qualifications for authority) may be expected to have been most exploited. A reflection of the initiation of kings with sauma may

duct of ceremonies there may have been little or no need to induce visions. Thus, virtually from the inception of the ceremony as an institution, the extract administered in it would frequently not have been sauma at its full potency and need not have been sauma at all.

§152 The story of Wīrāz suggests that although the vision-inducing drug was available, it was only rarely used, chiefly because people did not desire it. Even Wīrāz, who apparently had no reason to be apprehensive about its effects, did not want the drug. If the practitioners of the ceremony determined through visions that it was not necessary in each case actually to travel to the other world but that they could accomplish their purposes through ritual procedures alone, then the extract would not have to contain the vision-inducing ingredient. The ceremony without sauma would demonstrate equally well the acceptability of the *zaotar* to the spirits and exclude unqualified persons from attempting to act as priests.

§153 The value of the ceremony as a test by which to exclude imposters would have been important in connection with the payment of priests and may explain why sauma ceremonies came to be associated with animal sacrifices. The exclusive ability of Indo-Iranian priests legally to oversee the sacrifice of animals was doubtless at one time basic to their livelihood. In the early situation the payment of priests must have been in kind and must have consisted of a portion of the animal sacrificed. Long after the establishment of a priestly hierarchy, priests apparently continued to be itinerant and in each new situation would have required a means quickly to demonstrate their authority to superintend sacrifices. Sauma may have once been necessary to the priests' authority to conduct sacrifices because by means of it they could reliably convey the animal's spirit to the other world. But regardless of whether this was the original relationship of sauma to animal sacrifices, the value of sauma as a means of protecting the prerogative of priests to receive a share of every feast must have been the major factor linking sauma drinking and animal sacrifice. Their conjunction must have developed also out of the necessity of sacrifices to pay priests for conducting sauma ceremonies for other purposes, such as to benefit souls after death. The minimum price claimed by priests for such services can be supposed to have been a good meal, and, as late as Avestan times, a good meal could only have been a meal of meat, which was synonymous with food (Avestan *pitu-*; Boyce 1975b).

§154 Under such conditions the employment of priests for any purpose would necessarily include sacrificing an animal. Since priests were thought to be able to bring benefits to human souls through sauma ceremonies, one might as well have commissioned the priests to conduct a sauma ceremony on behalf of his soul even if the primary objective of employing priests was to have an animal killed and eaten in a feast, since the charges would be no more. Consequently, although it is certain that it was sometimes essential to have animals killed for food, and this must have involved hiring priests to do it, there is no direct attestation of the employment of priests solely for this purpose. Rather, whenever a feast was called for or it was desirable to obtain meat for any reason, priests would be employed to perform sauma ceremonies for the benefit of whatever human souls the donors of the animals would designate.

§155 The sauma ceremonies have continued throughout their history to be the chief activity by which priests obtain their livelihood and maintain their exclusive claim to their livelihood, and not as a means of obtaining visions. Thus, for the ceremonies to have so effectively served these secondary functions, it was necessary that the extract routinely administered in them, year by year, be without the uncertainties inherent in potentially hallucinogenic plant materials. Since the ranks of the priesthood in both Iran and India came to be decided by social processes (chiefly kinship) rather than by the tests for which harmel could be used, once this change had occurred it would be essential that priests carefully avoid putting their colleagues to the test; to hand a colleague an extract that so much as tasted of harmel and could imply doubts concerning his fitness would have risked insulting him. Courtesy has thus disallowed even a vestigial presence of harmel in the extract drunk in rituals. Safe, nonintoxicating alternatives to sauma/harmel have therefore been essential for the survival of the sauma ceremonies. Thus the ceremonies, originally structured for controlling the intoxication of sauma, developed into independent rituals excluding intoxication—so that no amount of the original plant is consumed in their modern enactments.[5]

be preserved in Plutarch's *Life of Artaxerxes* III.1–3 (as translated by B. Perrin 1914–1926: Bk. XI, 130-31):

"A little while after the death of Darius [II], the new king made an expedition to Pasargadae that he might receive the royal initiation at the hands of the Persian priests. Here there is a sanctuary of a warlike goddess whom one might conjecture to be Athena. Into this sanctuary the candidate for initiation must pass, and after laying aside his own proper robe must put on that which Cyrus the Elder used to wear before he became king; then he he must eat a cake of figs, chew some turpentine-wood, and drink a cup of sour milk. Whatever else is done besides this is unknown to outsiders."

Zoroaster also put on a garment when he came up from the *hōm* liquid (*Zātsparam* 21.4 and *Dēnkird* VII 3.53, 4.57 [Madan 1911: 625.1, 636.1; Nyberg 1964: 56.17, 57.16]) as, it seems, did his father Porushāsp when he approached the *hōm* (*Dēnkird* VII 2.32 [Madan 1911: 606.14; Nyberg 1964: 41.7]) and as also did Ardā Wīrāz (see §24). This suggests that a change of clothes may have been a regular feature of sauma rites and therefore gives further reason to believe that the above account reflects sauma-drinking in the initiation of Iranian rulers.

[5] For Iran, the evidence we have seen from the *Ardā Wīrāz Nāmag* and Bolus' *Chirocmeta* indicates that intoxication by the drug still had an important role within the religious establishment at least into Parthian times. Apart from its importance as a means to Truth, however, informal use of harmel for intoxication for other religious purposes among Iranian priests may well have simultaneously continued outside of the ceremonies.

Among the Indo-Aryans, after they settled in India, the reliance upon livestock for food greatly declined, and with the diminished importance of animal sacrifice so did the value of the ceremonies as a means of demonstrating the qualification of priests. By the time of the ṚgVeda the ceremonies had ceased to have any place for sauma. Nevertheless, there is reason to suppose that completely apart from the *soma* ceremonies a role for sauma intoxication would have survived in India also. The effectiveness of harmel as a drug is particularly susceptible to modification by admixture with other plants, and these seem always to have had a place in sauma preparations. The opportunities for controlling the effects of sauma through additives must have caused the Indo-Aryans to examine thoroughly the resources of the flora they encountered in India. If the pre-Aryan Indian cultures were familiar with psychoactive plants, the Aryans would surely have investigated those plants. In any event, for centuries after the Aryans entered India, the value of *soma* intoxication asserted in the Vedic hymns and rituals kept alive belief in the value of psychotropic plants as adjuncts to religious experience and sustained interest in local ethnopsychopharmacological resources. It is therefore relevant to note that (as was pointed out to me by Leonard Enos) several indigenous Indian *Desmodium* (Leguminosae) species are rich in N,N-dimethyltryptamine, the same substance found in plants added to *Banisteriopsis* extracts in South America (Banerje and Ghosal 1969; Ghosal *et al.* 1972; Ghosal 1972). This substance is pharmacologically inert orally unless it is combined with harmala alkaloids (which modify its metabolism through the inhibition of MAO or other enzymes). It appears the only way *Desmodium* species could have been effectively consumed as psychoactive drugs in India would have been by ingesting them with extracts of *Peganum harmala*, the one local source of these alkaloids. It may, then, be significant that one Indian *Desmodium* species, *Desmodium gangeticum* DC. (=*Hedysarum gangeticum* L.) is reportedly designated by Sanskrit names associating it with *soma* ceremonies, namely (according to Kirtikar and Basu 1935) *saumyā-* (also given as a name for *Ficus glomerata*, *Abrus precatorius* (=rosary pea), *Glycine debilis* (=soybean) and *Ruta graveolens* [see §140]) and (according to Monier-Williams 1899) *aṃśúmat-* 'rich in *soma* juice'.

7

SUMMARY OF ARGUMENTS SHOWING IDENTITY OF SAUMA AND HARMEL

§156 No detail concerning either sauma or *Peganum harmala* appears to disagree with their equation. If one would still claim that the botanical identity of sauma is unproven, he would need to supply a different explanation both for how harmel came to have every one of the nonintoxicating uses known for sauma (e.g. as apotropaic, incense, aphrodisiac, etc.), and for how it came in some cases to occupy the place of sauma in Zoroastrian rituals, and, on the other hand, account for what became of sauma in popular religion and priestly ceremonies after the time of the Avesta. However, even if one could explain away each of the correspondences we have examined, to claim that harmel was not sauma would in fact require assuming that there were simultaneously two sacred apotropaic intoxicant plants, both used both as incense and drunk in nearly identical ceremonies in ancient Iran. Vestiges of the distinction of harmel as a sacred plant exist among all Iranian peoples. That distinction can only have come about in response to some unique property of this plant and only if that property was exploited and valued. But *Peganum harmala* is a commonplace weed without significant economic value, as compared with other Iranian plants, and in general unremarkable, except in the one respect that it alone among Iranian plants contains the visionary drugs harmaline and harmine. This property is not exploited today, but because it is the sole significant distinctive feature of harmel, the only way the plant could have acquired sanctity among all Iranian peoples was for these drugs to have been used and for their effects to have been widely experienced and esteemed. It is clear that the effects of this drug in ancient Iran could only have been interpreted in religious terms, and since it must have been used, it is therefore to be expected that some trace of that use should exist in the data of ancient Iranian religion. In other words, if the use of a sacred intoxicant, that is, of sauma, had not already been deduced from the Indo-Iranian texts and rituals themselves, it would be necessary to propose it on the basis of the properties and cultural history of harmel in Iran. However, the correspondences we have seen between the two independent sets of evidence for harmel on the one hand and sauma on the other, point to a single intoxicant plant, and in addition, verify the historical reality of the use of its drugs as a major feature of ancient Iranian culture.

§157 Major arguments for the identity of sauma and harmel

1. GEOGRAPHICAL CORRESPONDENCE

Sauma must have been widely available to many Indo-Iranian groups over large parts of the Iranian area, and was not a localized or rare species. No known psychotropic plant is so abundant and conspicuous as a source of psychoactive drugs over the Iranian area as is harmel, and harmel has been long known in Iran to have psychoactive properties.

2. PHARMACOLOGICAL CORRESPONDENCE

The pharmacological suitability of the drugs of harmel for use as sauma is objectively demonstrated by the parallel roles played in ancient Iran by sauma and in certain South American cultures by *Banisteriopsis* extracts containing the same drugs. In both cases (1) the plant extract is the basis of mixtures with other psychoactive plants; (2) the intoxicant use of the plant is chiefly in ceremonies supervised by trained specialists; (3) the effects of the drugs are valued for visually revealing a simultaneous, intangible spirit world interpreted as being a higher reality; and (4) the experience of these visions is central to beliefs and religious institutions.

3. EVIDENCE FROM IRANIAN FOLK RELIGION

The chief evidence for *haoma* comes from the record of ancient Iranian folk religion which is preserved in the Avesta. The survival of this ancient text among the Iranian Zoroastrians (chiefly as oral literature) manifests a conservatism which may be expected also in Iranian folklore and ethnootany.

Sauma in ancient Iran	*Harmel in later Iran*
Name:	
The name "*haoma*" was apparently restricted to ritual contexts, and was not the common name of sauma.While intoxicant use was limited to specialists, the property of chief popular interest was the sacred power sauma's psychoactive use proved it to possess. Sauma was the sacred (i.e. Avestan *spənta-*) plant.	Modern Iranian names for harmel show that it was named 'sacred' in ancient Iran. Only the identification as sauma provides a plausible explanation of the Iranian names for harmel.
Ethnobotanic attributes:	
In pre-Islamic Avestan and Pahlavi texts *haoma* is invoked in verses which: (A) Attribute the origin of the use of *haoma* to the founding figures of Zoroastrianism. (B) Assert that •*Haoma* brings healing, victory, salvation & protection. •*Haoma* originates in mountains. •*Haoma* promotes childbirth [as aphrodisiac(?)]. •*Haoma* is chief of drugs, etc.	In post-Islamic Persian, Mandaic, and Turkish texts harmel is invoked in verses which: (A) Attribute the origin of the use of harmel to the founding figures of Shiʿa Islam. (B) Assert that •Harmel brings healing, victory, salvation & protection. •Harmel originates in mountains. •Harmel promotes childbirth (as aphrodisiac). •Harmel is king of drugs, etc.
Use as apotropaic incense:	
The chief nonpriestly use for sauma was as an apotropaic, a use which is inherently independent of formal religion. Sauma was burned as incense apotropaically. Sauma was apparently the chief incense plant of Avestan times (e.g. *dūraoša, haδānaēpātā* = sauma).	Harmel is the chief apotropaic plant of Iran today and this role is demonstrably pre-Islamic. Harmel is the most widely used native incense plant in Iran and the only one containing known psychoactive drugs.

4. EVIDENCE FROM ZOROASTRIAN RITUALS

The purpose of sauma intoxication was to gain knowledge from visions which could be obtained from the plant. Belief in the validity of such visions (and skill in using the drug to obtain visions) disappeared from Iran. Visions are no longer sought from the rituals representing the use of sauma and the original plant is therefore not consumed in them. In various ritual contexts where the *consumption* of sauma is represented, the selection of the three other plants which are used, i.e. ***Ephedra***, pomegranate and ***Ruta graveolens***, is explained by the relationship of these plants to harmel. The ancient addition of *Ephedra* to sauma mixtures is explained by the pharmacology of harmel. Pomegranate is a native Iranian plant which has had demonstrable use in Iranian ethnobotany as a replacement for harmel. The presence of ***Ruta graveolens*** in Zoroastrian rituals is explicable only as a harmel substitute. In Zoroastrian rituals where sauma is *burned* instead of being consumed, the plant used has always been harmel.

Part 2
By Martin Schwartz

AVESTAN PASSAGES RELEVANT TO *HAOMA*

ALLEGED GATHIC REFERENCES TO *HAOMA* (see §7, §72 and §98)

§158 The alleged opposition of Zoroaster to the use of the intoxicant *haoma* is based chiefly on the interpretation of one passage, *Yasna* 48.10, concerning which I showed the following in a recent detailed study (Schwartz 1985a): Instead of *madahyā,* genitive of *mada-* 'intoxication', one must read *magahyā* (cf. Pahlavi translation *mayīh*). The form *maga-* means 'gift of reciprocity', especially that given to poet-priests (cf. Old Indic *maghá-*), but also 'ditch, pit' (=Younger Avestan *maga-*). The homophony is exploited by Zoroaster in a complex pun. I translate *kadā ajə̄n / mūθrəm ahyā magahyā // yā . . . karapanō urūpayeintī //* as 'when will they ban(ish) the filth of that ditch/reciprocity-gift whereby . . . the *karapans* commit plunder' (*aj-ə̄n* 'ban, remove, set aside as accursed or sacred', cf. Arabic *ḤRM;* to Old Indic *ā́gas-* 'sin, vice'; Greek *ήθΫ* 'stain, pollution; holiness, sacred precinct; i.e. *sacratum*'. *Karapan-* /karpan-/ *'singer, poet', cf. Old Indic *kr̥panyú-* 'singer, poet' from *kr̥panyá-;* also *kr̥pámāna-* with *kaví-;* and *urūpaya-* < **rupāya-*, cf. Middle Persian *rubāy-* 'swipe, snatch', *rōb* 'robbery, plunder'). The phrase *mūθrəm ahyā magahyā* is contrasted (with phraseological and phonic parallelism in the respective surrounding verses) by *mīždəm . . . ahyā magahyā* (*Yasna* 53.7) 'the prize of that gift', referring to the reward for the commitment to Zoroaster, which entails prosperity for the righteous, while the *karapans* and their supporters disappear into the ground. Thus *Yasna* 48.10 contains no reference to intoxication, let alone condemnation of *haoma.*

§159 I recognize another play on words in the other Gathic passage cited in discussions of *haoma, Yasna* 32.14, which reads, *ahyā grə̄hmō *ā hōiθōi / nī kāvayascīt̰ xratūš (nī.)dadat̰ // *varəcåhīcā fraidivā / hyat̰ vīsəntā drəgvantəm avō // hyat̰cā gāuš jaidyāi mraoī / yə̄ dūraošəm saocayat̰ avō //.* The occurrence of the same word, *avō,* twice in the same position at the end of consecutive lines, is unusual, as is also the syntax of *avō* in c, where the dative **avaŋ́hē* 'for help' is expected. I assume two Avestan words *avō,* 1) = Vedic *ávas(-)* 'help, sustenance' and 2) = Old Indic *avás, ávas* 'down(ward)'. The latter *avō* may now also be recognized in *Yasht* 8.40, where the context demands 'downward', rather than a pleonastic hapax 'water'; cf. also *avō* as preverb, *Yasht* 13.44. The implication of *avō* is that the *kavis,* by patronizing the wicked *karapan* in connection with sacrificing the bovine (cf. *Yasna* 32.12) and burning the *haoma*-plant (*dūraošəm*), in the long run lead him downward, i.e. to hell. I translate, 'For the loot [*grə̄hmah-,* cf. Old Indic *gras* 'to devour', Sogdian *γrāmē* 'wealth', etc.] of which (world) some *kavis* have constantly put their thoughts and energies down into the trap, whereby they set about to help the wicked one, whereby the bovine is ordered to be slain, (the wicked one) who burns the *dūraoša*-plant, for help/hell'. The form *avō* 'downward' concretizes the directionality suggested by *nī.* The phrase 'in the snare' is paralleled in the preceding stanza by 'in the House of Worst Mind' (*acištahyā dəmānē manaŋhō*) in which the destroyers of the world have sought loot (*grə̄hmō *īšasat̰*). That both phrases refer to hell is shown by *Yasna* 46.6a, *drujō . . . dąmąn haēθahyā* 'the bonds of Lie' alongside *Yasna* 46.11a *drūjō *dəmānē* 'the House of Lie' (note that *dāman-* = Old Indic *dāman-* 'bond', cf. Persian *dām* 'trap', etc., but probably with play on **dāman-* 'establishment, dwelling', cf. Vedic *r̥tásya dhāman-* 'foundations of Truth'). My interpretation of 32.14 is supported by the stanza immediately following it, 'Because of these things, the *kavi*hood and *karapan*hood is going to perdition, along with those they ensnare (**daintī;* Insler 1975), who will not be brought to those who rule at will over life in the House of Good Mind'.

§160 Thus *Yasna* 32.14 does not provide evidence for Zoroaster's rejection of the commonplace sacrifice of cattle, nor does it prove that Zoroaster condemned the burning of *dūraoša* (the *haoma*-plant), much less that he repudiated the pressing and drinking of *haoma.* It does provide evidence for the ritual burning of the plant, of greatest importance for Dr. Flattery's identification of the plant as *Peganum harmala.*

§161 The use of word play, together with syntactic ambiguity, reflect a general stylistic obscurantism characteristic of Indo-Iranian priestly poetry (for which cf. Boyce 1975b:9; Gonda, cited §244; on Zoroaster see Schwartz 1985a and 1986). An extension of play on sound is found in *Yasna* 11.9, where there occurs a series of forms based on Gathic words which resemble, in some instances only vaguely, the names of the numbers from one to ten. This bizarre paronomastic use of the Gathas provides a "count-down" (Schwartz 1986: 331-332) preceding the drinking of *haoma,* as Flattery has observed. This important connection of the text of the Gathas with the ritual use of *haoma* is of relevance for Flattery's observations of parallelisms with the *yagé* cult, where sacred chants accompany the taking of the drug; cf. especially §§120 and 124 above.

ANNOTATIONS TO THE *HŌM YASHT*

Yasna 10.8: *urvāsman-* (see §21)

§162 The association of *urvāsman-* (Old Avestan *urvāzəman-*) 'bliss' and *aša-* 'Rightness, Truth' probably has visionary connotations; cf. Kuiper (1964: 105). Kuiper's general views are not vitiated by taking the key passage, *Yasna* 30.1c *ašā yecā yā raocə̄bīš darəsatā urvāzā,* as '. . . and [via hymns] for *Aša* (**ašāyecā* for **/ašayācā/*), the things which are to be seen in bliss (*urvāzā*) amidst the lights'. The paradisiacal aspect of the visionary experience is seen from *Yasna* 11.10, *vahištəm ahūm ašaonąm raocaŋhəm vispō.xᵛāθrəm* 'the Best Existence of the righteous, full of light, having every comfort', which echoes *Yasna* 31.7c: *raocə̄bīš . . . xᵛāθrā* 'the spaces/comforts amidst the lights', where the context is literally visionary, as shown by *Yasna* 31.8 (see further Schwartz 1986:367-369).[1]

§163 *Yasna Haptaŋhāiti* 36.2, where 'the Fire of Ahura Mazdah' is addressed as 'most blissful' and bade to come to the worshippers 'with the most blissful of bliss' (*urvāzištahyā urvāzyā*), is also relevant for the visionary aspect of *urvāsman-*, for as is made explicit in the final stanza, *Yasna* 36.6, Fire is the 'corporeal manifestation' (*kəhrpə̄m*) of Ahura Mazdah, these lights here (*imā raocā*), i.e. on earth, whose 'highest (manifestation)k is called the sun'. Since *Yasna* 36.1 begins with the theme of the 'communion of Fire' *(vərəzə̄nā āθrō),* keeping in mind the connection of Fire and *Aša* (*Yasna* 34.4; 46.7, etc.), one may compare *Yasna* 49.8: *urvāzištąm ašahyā karə̄m* 'the most blissful union of *Aša'* (cf. *Yasna* 49.9, where *sarə̄m* is connected with *daēnā* 'visions'), and with *Yasna* 32.1–2, which relates *urvāzəmā* 'bliss', *sarə̄mnō* 'united', and *ašā huš.haxā xᵛə̄nvātā* 'the Good Associate of sunny *Aša'*.[2]

[1] *Gāhāmbār* 3.6 (whence *Visperad* 18.2 and in turn *Pursišnīhā* 37, mentioned by Kuiper 1964:105) further collocates bliss (*urvāsma-*), Best Existence (*vahištəmca ahūm*), Endless Lights (*raocā*) and boundless comforts (*xᵛāθrā*) as shown to the soul eschatologically (in contrast to the sufferings for the deceitful, *sādrā drəgvatō*); the background here probably involves *inter alia* (see e.g. *Yasna* 12.1 and *Yasht* 12.36) a conflation of *Yasna* 31.7-8 with *Yasna* 45.7-8, which are united by *cašmainī* 'in a vision' and other parallel features (Schwartz 1986: 368).

[2] For the relation of *Yasna* 32.1–2 and *Yasna* 49.8–9, and the connection of *vərəzə̄na-* and *urvāzəman-,* see Schwartz (1986:342-347). The centrality of the term *urvāzəman-* (**vrāzman-*) in Iranian visionary experience explains the unique and elaborate oral acrostic suggestion of the word at *Yasna* 33.2c (cf. *ibid.* 342-345).

§164 The contrast in *Yasna* 10.8 of *aēšma-* 'violence, fury' and *urvāsman-* 'bliss' may ultimately also go back to the visionary contexts of the Gathas; *Yasna* 49.4 collocates *aēšma-* and the vision of the deceitful one (*drəgvatō daēnā*), contrasting with *Yasna* 49.5, 'he who has united (*sar-*) his vision with Vohu Manah', and 'the most blissful (*urvāzištąm*) union of Truth'; cf., in the parallel and concentrically related *Yasna* 49.8–9, the motif of "yoking" the vision with Truth. There is also an implied opposition of *urvāzā* and *aēšməm, Yasna* 30.1 and 6. The visionary associations of *urvāsman-* in *Yasna* 10.8 are amplified throughout the rest of the text by the request for lightness, brightness, and clarity of intoxication.

§165 The reading *rənjaite,* with expected middle voice (cf. Old Indic *ráṅjate*), has support from manuscript variants. The form *rənjaiti* is not impossible in intransitive sense (cf. *rənjat̰.aspa-*, if 'having horses which move lightly'. The factitive/causative form would be not *rənjaiti* but **rənjayeiti.* Intransitive meaning for *rənjaiti/e* would parallel *Yasna* 10.19 *rənjyō vazāinte* 'waft (quite) lightly', where *rənjyō* is adverbial accusative neuter of the *comparative stem *rənjyah-*.

Yasna 10.14: Avestan *drafša-* (see §21)

§166 Apart from the unsuitability of *āsitō* to be the subject of the sentence, it is obvious that the translation of Bartholomae (Wolff 1910), with *drafša-* as 'flag, banner', is rather forced, and not very apt for the larger context. Particularly obscure here would be the relationship it introduces between the supposedly fluttering consumers of *haoma* and the "speaker" ('me') whose experiences of intoxication is the topic of the text.

§167 The translation I have suggested for *Yasna* 10.14 differs considerably from the interpretation of Bartholomae-Wolff, which reads: "Nicht sollen sie mir beliebig wie das Stierbanner sich einherbewegen, (wenn) sie (dich) geniessen; stracks vorwärts sollen sie gehen, (die) sich an dir begeistern; mit energischem Schaffensdrang sollen sie sich einstellen". The translation of the rest of the passage (which I do not contest) reads: "Ich weihe dir, o ašaheiliger ašafördernder Haoma, diesen Leib hier, der mir schön gewachsen scheint". My own interpretation for the disputed text is as follows: '*May they (your intoxications), besetting me at their own impulse, not move me about as the trembling of a cow. May your intoxications come forth clear(ly); may they arrive bringing straightness of mind.' My rendering is based on the following considerations:

(1) The construction *mā mē . . . caire* is parallel to *mā tē nīre* 'may nothing of yours flow away' at *Yasna* 10.17; the unusual construction of the prohibitive particle with an infinitive in *-e* based on the present stem is characteristic of *Yasna* 10. The question thus is, what is the subject of *caire*?

(2) For Bartholomae and others the subject is *āsitō,* taken as nominative plural of a stem *āsit-* 'consuming', but the latter is highly suspect. A verb *as-* 'to eat' is unknown in Iranian outside of *kahrkāsa-*, originally *'chicken-eater', Avestan *kahrkāsa-*, Sogdian *čarkas* 'buzzard, vulture', Ossetic *cærgæs* 'eagle', which may be regarded as a formation antedating Proto-Iranian. The attested verb for 'consume' (used with *haoma-*) is *xᵛar-*. Furthermore, *āsit-*, with formant *-it-*, would also be isolated. By contrast, *huzāmit-* and *(daēvō.)γnit-* are formed from attested stems in *-i-*, respectively *huzāmi-* and *-γni-* (cf. *vārəθraγni-*); similarly Bartholomae s.v. *huzāmit-*. Rather than assign *āsita-* to **as-*, one may take it with the attested stem *āsita-* 'lying upon' (in *āsitō.gātu-* 'lying upon a place'), past passive participle of *ā-say-* 'to lie upon'. In the present context *āsitō* may be either nominative plural of a root-stem *āsit-* or nominative singular of the participle *āsita-*, agreeing with *drafšō.*

(3) The interpretation of *gaoš drafšō* as 'bull-banner' ('banner bearing the image of a bull') is problematic in many ways. Contextually it is unlikely that this specific flag, allegedly a symbol of Iranian victory, would be introduced in a negative context. Formally, for 'bull-banner' one would expect a compound **gao.drafša-* rather than *gaoš drafša-* 'the bull's (or, more usually without masculine specification, cow's) banner'. Bartholomae elaborated Darmesteter's acceptance of the Pahlavi translation *gāw drafš* 'bull banner' and his equation with the flag which, according to sources of the Islamic period, was established as the Iranian national standard, the *dirafš-i Kāviyān,* by the blacksmith Kāva, who made a banner out of his leather apron (or leather bag, or turban), which he attached to a pole or lance. According to Bartholomae's theory, the *drafšō* 'banner of the bull', Pahlavi *gāw drafš,* originally referred to a flag representing a bull, but was later reinterpreted as 'flag made of the skin of a bull'. While A. Christensen (1925: 37), in his fine study on Kāva's banner, accepted Bartholomae's views (and the translation upon which it is based), the numerous early descriptions he assembled of the *dirafš-i Kāviyān* (*ibid.*, 35-36) in no way support the thesis that the banner had a bovine device, or was made of bull hide. Thus there is no ground for taking *drafšō* as 'banner' in a phrase with genitive *gaoš.*

4) An abundance of evidence points to the meaning 'flag, banner' as only one specific application of a broad original signification of *drafša-*. Old Indic *drapsá-* is 'banner' at *RV* 4.13.2, but it is more commonly attested in the meaning 'drop, droplet', and in fact refers to the drops of *soma-*. It is even possible (I shall not press the point) that at *Yasna* 10.14 *drafša-* echoes an old word-play on 'droplet' (of sauma) and 'fluttering, trembling'; cf. R̥gVeda 1.64.2, where *drapsínaḥ,* describing the atmospheric and martial Maruts, means both 'bearing banners' and 'pouring out drops', while in hymns to Agni, the god of fire, *drapsá-* 'droplet of soma' may also mean 'spark' (Gonda 1975: 242-243). Middle Iranian attests not only the noun *drafša-* 'banner' (Middle Persian *drafš,* Sogdian *'rδ'šp, 'rδ'yšp,* cf. Armenian *drauš*), but also a verbal stem *drafša-* 'to tremble' (Middle Persian *drafš-*) as well as 'to shine' (Middle Persian *drafš-*), 'to blaze' (Parthian *drfš-*, Manichean Sogdian *wyδrfš-*). The association of meanings 'tremble' and 'shine', etc. is found for other words, e.g. Old Indic *tviṣ-* 'violent agitation'; 'brilliance, glitter, splendor'; Greek *ςεέφ* 'shake, quake', *ΣεέριοΫ* 'burning, Dog Star'; or Old Indic *sphuráti* 'darts, rebounds, springs, trembles'; 'flashes, glitters, gleams', and *sphuraṇa-* 'glittering, sparkling'; 'trembling, throbbing, vibrating', etc. The latter has more distant cognates with similar semantic range, e.g. Old Norse *sparkr* 'lively, brisk', English *spark, sparkle,* Latvian *spirgsti* 'glowing coals', Swedish dialects *spräker* 'lively'; 'shining, radiant'; *spräkkle* 'spot, speckle'; Norse *spronge* 'ride quickly, sprinkle', English *spring,* etc. Clearly the image of agitating motion gave rise to words for flashing and flickering light, as well as sprinkled droplets, etc.

§168 Thus the entire range of forms in Indic *draps-*, Iranian *drafš-*, may be relegated to a single etymon with meaning 'to be in agitated motion'. The old etymology of *drapsa-*, *drafša-* 'flag' from PIE *drep-* 'to cut (cloth, etc.)', whence Old Indic *drāpi-* 'mantle, garment', Lithuanian *drāpanas* 'clothing', Middle Persian *drab-* (Pahlavi *dlp-* [*Nērangistān* 170.10 and 25; Waag 1941: 92, 94]) 'to wear', must be abandoned. Old Indic *drapsá-*, Avestan *drafša-* 'flag'; *drafšaka-* > Armenian *draušak* 'streamer on a crown', are semantically parallel to Old Indic *dhvaja-* 'banner', Avestan *dwō.ža-* (*dwaža-*) 'to flutter'. Parallel to the developments of *drafša-* *'be in agitation, shine' on one hand, and *'flutter' on the other, would be Sogdian *ərδēf-* (Manichean *'rδyf-*, S. *'rδyp-*) 'to shine' and Khotanese Saka *drāh-* (ppp. *drautta-*) 'to fly' (< *'flutter the wings' and/or 'dart about'), both of which go back to a single stem, Old Iranian **drāfaya-*. The *-f-* of the latter is probably due to the influence of *drafša-* < *drapsa.* This *drapsa-* should be from earlier **drab-sa-* (and *drāfaya-* from **drābaya-*, with Old Iranian *-f-* from *drafša-*), Iranian root **drab-*, from PIE **dreb-*. The latter is also reflected by Lithuanian *drebėti,* 'to tremble' (and Old English *treppan* 'to tread', Dutch *trappen* 'to stomp', Middle High German *trampfen* 'to run'; cf. the relationship of Old Indic *sphur-*

'tremble, dart', etc. to Iranian *spar-* 'to tread, kick', etc.).

§169 It has been seen that Old Iranian *drafša-* meant not only 'banner', but also 'trembling, convulsion(s)'. The latter meanings suit *Yasna* 10.14, and would refer, in accordance with Flattery's analysis of the realia, to the undesirable spasms of harmel intoxication. The trembling is compared to that of a terrified cow, and its uncontrolled nature is expressed by *vārəma* (**vārəm-ā*) 'at impulse', literally 'at its own will'. While one can construe 'let not trembling, besetting (*āsitō*, literally 'lying upon') me like that of a cow, move me about', where *āsitō* (singular) agrees with *drafšō*, this would be syntactically contorted. I therefore take the subject of *caire* to be not the first item of comparison, *gaoš drafšō* 'the trembling of a cow', but *āsitō* (*tē . . . maδō* 'your intoxications . . .) besetting . . .', with *āsitō* plural of root-stem *āsit-* 'lying upon, settling upon, besetting'.

§170 The correct translation of *tē maδō* follows from the newly established context. Contrasted with the unnerving spasms are the characteristics described by the plurals *frašа* (note the phonic relationship *drafša-: fraša-*) 'clear, splendid' (see below) with predicate *frayantu* 'may they go forth', and *vərəzyaŋuhåŋhō* 'bringing straightness of mind' (cf. Gershevitch 1974:49) with predicate *jasəntu* *'may they come'. According with the subject to which these refer, the phrase *tē maδō* should not mean those 'who are intoxicated (or inspired) by you', but 'your intoxications', which the priestly hymnist prays will bring not the tremors indicated by *drafšō*, but straightness of mind (*vərəzyaŋuhåŋhō*), clarity, and lightness. Thus we would have accord between verses 19 and 8, *rənjyō vazåinte (*tē) maδō* 'may (*thy) intoxications move lightly' and *rənjaiti haomahe maδō* 'the intoxication of *haoma* is light'. See §178.

§171 The form *maδō* would ordinarily be the nominative plural of a root-stem *(-)mad-*, which could, in theory, mean 'becoming intoxicated' (cf. Vedic *soma-mad-*), but, as is actually shown by **aγryō.madu.mad-* (see below, §184), means 'intoxicating (someone)', from which an independent noun *mad-* 'that which intoxicates, intoxication' could easily arise. The gender of *mad-* is feminine, as is shown by *imåsə, Yasna* 10.19; see below, *ad loc.*

Yasna 10.14 and 19: Avestan *fraša-* (see §21)

§172 The word *fraša-* here is not the adverb 'forward' (as in the alliterative cliché *fraša fra-ay-*, limited to passages in the *Vidēvdād*, 6.27, 7.52, 18.29, which is probably a reinterpretation of *fraša fra-ay-* of the passage under discussion). Instead, *fraša* is nominative plural of the adjective *fraša-* discussed by Bailey (1971a: vii-xvi). Bailey has demonstrated beyond doubt that *fraša-* means 'conspicuous, spectacular, splendid, wondrous'. Important among the evidence he martials are (1) the translation of Old Persian *fraša-* as Akkadian *bunū*, verbal noun from *bānu* 'be bright, lively; make beautiful, be magnificent'; (2) the Avestan collocations, *Yasna* 19.10, *srīra-* 'beautiful', *abda-* 'wondrous', and *Vidēvdād* 1. 20, *bāmya-* 'radiant'; (3) the Pahlavi collocation *abd fraškard;* (4) Armenian *hrašk'* 'marvel', *hrašakert* 'extraordinary'; (5) Middle Persian *frašagar* translated by Persian *ẓāhir* 'manifest'; and (6) Middle Persian *frašemurw*, Georgian *p'aršamangi* 'peacock', literally 'marvelous bird, bird with spectacular colorations'.

§173 The identification of *fraša-* in *Yasna* 10.14 and 19 with *fraša-* 'conspicuous', etc. now becomes clear from the parallelism of *fraša frayantu tē maδō* and *raoxšna frayantu tē maδō*, where *raoxšna* is 'brilliant, bright, splendid'; both adjectives *fraša-* and *raoxšna-* are appropriate descriptions of intoxications (referring to the vivid quality of the visions), but could hardly be used of those intoxicated. It may be noted in passing that the use of *fraša-* as an epithet of *haoma* is probably connected with *frāšmi-*, occurring exclusively as an epithet of ***haoma***, *Yasna* 10.21 (where it is parallel to the color term *zairi-*), and further *Yasna* 57.19, *Yasht* 8.33. The meaning of *frāšmi-* should be something like 'glowing', but the relationship with *fraša-* may have been associative, rather than etymological; compare Gershevitch (1959:233).[3]

§174 The identification of *fraša-* as an epithet of ***haoma-*** now also helps explain the characterization, transmitted by Bolos of Mendes *apud* Pliny, of the Persian plant *"theombrotion"* (whose description otherwise suits *Peganum harmala* used as ***haoma***, see §93 n.25), 'like a peacock in its colorings'. The Old Iranian phrase **fraša- mrga-* 'spectacular bird' yielded the word for 'peacock' not only in Middle Persian *frašemurw*, but also in Parthian **frašamarg*, reflected in the Georgian form. The adjective *fraša-* appears to have disappeared from everyday Iranian speech, for it is not attested beyond Old Iranian, except in Armenian *hrašk'*, which may go back to an older stratum of the Parthian vocabulary; its absence not only from our large corpus of Middle Persian texts, but also from the fairly abundant Sogdian texts, points to the relatively early general desuetude of *fraša-*. Thus, by the time of Bolos of Mendes, the Persians called the peacock by a term no longer comprehensible, 'the *fraša-* bird', or 'the bird *Fraša*'. The word *fraša-*, constantly heard alongside *raoxšna-* 'bright' in the liturgy to *Haoma*, could then be associated with 'peacock'. This could give rise to a popular belief in a particular variety of ***haoma*** plant with the colors of a peacock.

§175 The disappearance of the word *fraša-* in Persia eventually affected the word for peacock as well. Middle Persian *frašemurw*, *frašamurw* was replaced by New Persian *firišta-murγ* 'angel-bird', where *firišta* 'angel' (Middle Persian *frēštag*) replaced the no longer meaningful *fraša-*. From Arabic, Persian has the better known word for peacock, *ṭāvūs*.

§176 I would explain the early obsolescence of *fraša-* as due to its being subsumed by its development as a technical term of theology. The starting point is the Gathic phrase *fərašə̄m (ahūm) kar-/dā-* 'make (the world) *distinguished, excellent'. In the Gathas this referred to a situation regarded as imminently possible; note especially *aṯcā tōi vaēm hyāmā yōi īm fərašə̄m kərənaon ahūm* 'Thus may we be those who will make this world excellent' (*Yasna* 30.9). It is probably significant that the three other Gathic attestations of *fəraša-* are connected with *haiθya-* '(something) actual, real, true' and *vasnā* 'according to wish': *xšmākā xšaθrā ahurā fərašə̄m vasnā haiθyə̄m dā ahūm* 'By your power, Lord, Thou shalt make this world in actuality excellent', *Yasna* 34.15; *yō mōi ašāṯ haiθīm hacā varəšaitī zaraθuštrāi hyaṯ vasnā fərašō.təməm* 'He who, in accordance with righteousness, shall accomplish as actual for me, Zarathushtra, that which is most excellent, in accordance with (my?) wish', *Yasna* 46.19; *dātā aŋhəuš arəδaṯ vohū manaŋhā haiθyā.varəštąm hyaṯ vasnā fərašō.təməm* 'The Creator of the world shall promote, through Good Thinking, as an actual accomplishment, that which is most excellent, in accordance with (His) wish', *Yasna* 50.11. The *fraša-* is here something brought into reality, *haiθya-*, from the plane of wish, *vasnā* (the concept of *vasnā* may involve more than 'will'; see Schwartz [1986:387 n.15]). While ***haiθya-*** may correctly be translated 'true' (like its cognates Old Indic *satya-*, Ossetic *æcæg*) the Pahlavi inevitably translates it throughout the Avesta not by the usual words for 'true', *rāst, wābārīgān, wizurd*, but by *āškārag*

[3] To Benveniste's (1936:230-231) etymology of *frāšmi-*, to which Gershevitch refers, add now the evidence from Sogdian for **šam-* given by N. Sims-Williams (1985:180). The meaning 'blush' for the Sogdian goes well with Av. *frāšma-* *'sunshine', and the semantic parallelism with *zāiri-* as 'golden-colored, yellowish' suggested by Gershevitch.

For the meaning of *fraša-*, see now J. Narten (1986:197-203).

'patent, overt, manifest'. This glossation must be based on an early exegetic tradition where *haiθya-* 'true' was understood as that which is patent, verifiable, ascertainable, in contrast to truth as a matter of ethics or religious faith. This accords precisely with the prehistory of *haiθya-* < PIE **Esn̥tyo-*, from **Es(e/o)nt-*, participle of **Ees-* 'to be'; hence **Esn̥tyo-* is basically 'as something is', cf. Old Indic *sa(n)t-* 'real (English cognate *sooth*), virtuous', but German *Sünde,* English *sin.*

§177 With regard to the statement in Pseudo-Democritus that *theombrotion* is drunk by Persian kings against bodily disorders and instability of intellect, cf. the attributes of *haoma* (healing, increasing insight, etc.) in the *Hōm Yasht* (§84). For Pseudo-Democritus' statement that the Persian kings drank *theombrotion* to increase the sense of justice, cf. the *Hōm Yasht*'s characterization of *haoma* as 'truly the source of Truth/Rightness' (*haiθimca ašahe xå*), *Yasna* 10.4, and the epithet 'furthering Truth' (*aša-vāzah-, aša-vazah-*) uniquely applied to *haoma* (*Yasna* 10.1 and 14, etc.). The institutional application of the justice-manifesting consumption of *haoma* was the ordeal; see §§150-159. For Pseudo-Democritus' term *hermesias,* see §90 n.25.

§178 In *Yasna* 10.19, the separation of *imåsə* from from *tē maδō,* which has previously impeded translation, parallels that of *āsitō . . . tē maδō* at *Yasna* 10.8, again with *fraša frayantu.* Note the alliteration *fraša frayantu,* the assonance *fraša . . . raoxšna* and the alliteration *raoxšna . . . rənjyō.* For reasons of meter/rhythm and parallelism, **tē maδō* must be posited after *vazåinte,* whose *-te* caused haplological disappearance of **tē.* The form *vazåinte* 'waft, fly, move forth' may echo *Yasna* 10.14 *ašavāzō* 'making Rightness/Truth move forth', cf. *Yasna* 10.1 *ašavazåŋhō,* both epithets of *Haoma.*

§179 In *Yasna* 11.10, while *pairi.tē haoma . . . daδāmi* is repeated from *Yasna* 10.8, it is expanded by the request of reciprocity, *pairi.mē . . . dayå . . . haoma*; this parallelism may extend to *ašava . . ašaonąm.* Cf. also the parallel of *havaŋuhāi* 'for well-being' (from *hu-* 'good' and *ahu-* 'existence') plus *ašavastāi* vis-à-vis *vahištəm ahūm* 'Best Existence' plus *ašaonąm.* I emend *(θwaxšāi) *haomahe (maδāi)* for *haomāi* in consideration of both form and meaning; cf. *haomahe maδō* (*Yasna* 10.8). The erroneous *haomāi* is a simple instance of "attraction" to the surrounding datives.

Yasna 10.15: Avestan *ūnå-* (see §90)

§180 The interpretation of this passage rests on the meaning of two words, *ūnąm* and *ǝ̄vitō.xarəδayå.* I take the first simply as accusative of *ūnā-* = *unā-,* literally 'empty place, hole (cf. H.-P. Schmidt 1969: 124 *seq.*; 1983), here probably = *'cunnus'.* For the second hapax, *ǝ̄vitō.xarəδayå,* I follow the reading preferred in Geldner's edition. I see the form as parallel to *mairyayå,* i.e. the gen. of an *-ā-* stem fem. adj., *ǝ̄vitō.xarəδā-,* obviously a compound. The first member, **ǝ̄vita-,* I take as 'endowed with, characterized by', and identify it with the second element of *satǝ̄vita-* and *utǝ̄vita-,* where **-ǝ̄vita-* is equivalent to the possessive suffix of the parallel forms *satavant-* and *ūtavant-* in *Yasht* 2.14. **ǝ̄vita-* would be the past passive participle of *avi-ay-* 'herzugehen zu, ankommen'. The second member, **xarəδa-,* has been recognized as the cognate of Khwarezmian *pcxrδ,* New Persian *payxāl* 'excrement (of animals and birds), refuse', New Persian *āxāl* 'peel, trash, discards', New Persian (loan word) *xard* 'mud', Shughni *šarδ-,* Yidgha *xawd-,* Yaghnobi *xərd-,* Pashto *xaṛ-el* 'to defecate', Khotanese *saṃkhal-* 'to stain', etc. Thus, *ǝ̄vitō.xarəδå* would mean 'filthy, dirty'. The Sanskrit translation *paribhraṣṭabuddhi-* 'with impaired intellect', which misled Bartholomae into making his improbable analysis **ǝ̄vitō.xarəδāy- < *a-vitaxra-dāy-,* is probably based on an erroneous interpretation involving *xarəδ-* as equivalent to Middle Persian *xrad (xraδ)* or New Persian *xirad* 'wisdom, intellect' (Avestan *xratu-*); this also motivated the misreading *ǝ̄vitō.xraδayå.*[4]

[4] This interpretation of *ǝ̄vito.xarəδayå* was made in the unpublished 1975/1976 revision of my dissertation "Studies in the Texts of the Sogdian Christians", pp. 62-63; cf. also Bailey (1979:417). For *xard-* see also Schwartz (1969:447; 1970:290) with literature.

Yasna 11.2: Avestan *bāšar-*

§181 Hoffmann's (1986:166 and 179, fn.4) translation of *bāšar* as "Pfleger" instead of 'rider' is hard to accept, in view of the clear context for 'rider' ('may thou not be a yoker of steeds, a mounter of steeds, a harnesser of steeds, who do not entreat me for [showing] strength in the crowded district assembly of many men'), and the symmetry horse : rider (*bāšar-*) :: *haoma* : drinker (*x^{v}āšar-*). There may have been a general expansion of the agent suffix to include middle voice verbs, or a special creation of *bāšar-* in the specific context of *Yasna* 11.2 by analogy with *zaotar-* and *x^{v}āšar* (where there is also rhyme).

Yasna 10.5: Avestan *nąmy-(ąsu-)* (see §87)

§182 Against Gershevitch's (1974:48) translation of *nąmy-(ąsu-)* as '(having) sweet (stalks)' stands the Pahlavi translation *narm-tāg,* 'soft stalked'. The meanings 'soft' and 'sweet' are also found for Sogdian *namr-* in C 2 (spelled *nmr-*) and glossed 'sweet' in *Psalm* 19.11 (*nmry-str*). Furthermore note Avestan *nąmišta-,* superlative of the quality expressed by *nəmah-* 'homage' < 'bending', both words being collocated at *Yasna Haptaŋhāiti* 36.2 in a series of *figuræ etymologicæ.* Clearly **nāmi-* is a Caland's Law variant of Old Iranian **namra-* 'pliant, soft'. The semantic development of the vr̥ddhi **nāmra-* to 'sweet' is an inner-Sogdian phenomenon, cf. French *doux,* etc.

Pahlavi translations of Avestan *mad-* (see §22 n.2)

§183 It is a curious fact that the Pahlavi translators did not understand straightforward forms of the Avestan root *mad-* 'to intoxicate' (except for where the context permits equation of the noun *maδa-* 'intoxication' with *maδu-* = 'wine'). The relevant Pahlavi glosses are based on *mʾd-* (which Iranologists have tacitly rationalized to **md-,* for example Bartholomae's *madišn* for *mʾdšn',* *madēnitan* for *mʾdynytn'*; etc. In the translations of *Vīsperad* 8.1 and apparently *Nērangistān* 30, the Pahlavi glosses in *mʾd-* are interpreted as forms from *meh* 'greater' (*mehēnīdan* 'to increase', etc.). In the translation of the *Hōm Yasht* (*Yasna* 9-11), this *mʾd-* is elaborated by glosses which show it was taken as referring to knowledge. Thus *maδō* (*Yasna* 10.14; 10.19) is glossed *vidyā* by Neriosengh, and *maδəm mruye* (*Yasna* 9.17) is glossed *mʾdšn' gōw tis-ē-m pad frahang gōw ku-m dānāgīh bawād* 'speak **māyišn,* i.e. say something to me in instruction: that I may have knowledge'. (For the latter passage Bartholomae's emendation of the straightforward ... *tis-ē-m* 'something to me' as ... *az ēn may* 'from this wine' must be rejected as unjustified). For *Nērangistān* 29, which pardons priests who do not recite the Gathas 'after (their) drinking intoxicating (alcoholic) beverages' (*maiδyanąm parō x^{v}arətōit),* there occurs the gloss *az may xwarišn* 'after drinking wine', further explained as *may xwarēnd mast be-bawēnd* 'they drink wine, they become drunk'. Avestan *maδa-* is translated as Pahlavi *may* in *Nērangistān* 30, where *hurąm x^{v}araiti maδō aspaya.payaŋhō* 'drinks kumiss, (i.e.) the intoxicant beverage (not 'Wein'!) of mare's milk' is glossed by Pahlavi *hur xwarad may ān-iz asp pēm* 'drinks kumiss, the "wine" which is mare's milk'; the mistranslation was no doubt furthered by the genuine collocation of *hurā* and the proper word for wine, *maδu-,* in *Vidēvdād* 14.17 *(hurayå vā maδǝ̄uš vā).* Here the phonically similar (but originally unrelated) words for 'wine' and 'intoxication, intoxicant' merged in translation as an *ad hoc* broadened concept of wine (*may*) for any alcoholic beverage. This is of interest for the solution of the general glossation in Pahlavi of the Avestan words pertaining to intoxication.

§184 The Indo-Iranian verbal stem for 'bring about intoxication' would have been a causative stem *mādaya-,* well attested in Old Indic. One may assume for Old Persian a cognate **māδaya-,* which lies behind the relevant Pahlavi forms in *mʾd-.* Thus the earliest stratum of Pahlavi glossation correctly rendered the Avestan forms in *mă̄δ-* for 'intoxicate, intoxication.' However, **mā̆δ(aya)-* underwent the regular change to Middle Persian *māy-*, homophonous with forms for 'copulate' (from the old root *māy-;* thus *m'dšn'* is both 'intoxication' and 'copulation'!), bringing about the Middle Persian exploitation of the old past participle *masta-* for the concept of intoxication, and making *m'd-*, i.e. *māy-* *'intoxicate', no longer correctly comprehensible. Hence *m'd-* was treated differently in various contexts. It was also taken from *meh* 'greater', or left unexplained, e.g. for *Yasna* 10.8, where *m'dšn'* merely elicits a statement of helplessness, *m'dšn' abāyēd guftan* 'one must say *m'dšn'*.' The Avestan refer-ence is to the violent intoxications, *maδå̄ŋhō,* against those of *haoma.* However, the word *mad(a)-* in reference to *haoma* was foregrounded by the importance of the sacred beverage; some interpretation was necessary. Two factors determined the interpretation: (1) the belief that *haoma* conferred spiritual benefits; and (2) the apparent sense of *maδa-* (and *maiδya-*) elsewhere for an intoxicating beverage used ceremonially, i.e. 'wine'. Taken together, the two factors would give the impression that the *maδa-* of *haoma* was in some way a spiritual analogue of the intoxication of alcohol. As noted earlier, the Middle Persian word for 'intoxicated' is *mast,* whence *mastīh* 'intoxication'. The Avestan cognate was observed to occur in *aγryō.maδu.mastəma-* 'highly intoxicated by the first treading of wine' (*Pursišnīhā* 31), which, as analyzed by K. M. Jamaspasa and H. Humbach (1971:I, 49), is superlative of **aγryō.maδu.-mad-*, for which the Pahlavi has *kē-š ān ī mast ud aγrāy mastīh* 'whose intoxication is that of one who is intoxicated, which is of high value'. A form almost identical to Pahlavi *mastīh* is Avestan *masti-* 'knowledge' (from the root *mand-*), correctly translated by *frazānagīh* for the two attestations in the *Hōm Yasht, Yasna* 9.17 and 9.20. In the second Avestan passage it is stated that *haoma* grants, to those who avidly study the sacred text, holiness (*spānah-*) and *masti-*. In the first passage *masti-* concludes a series of nine things for which *haoma* is invoked; the series begins with *maδa-*, so that *maδa-* and *masti-* both frame the list. This associative parallelism of *maδa-* and *masti-* allowed the following analogy: Pahlavi *mastīh* (Avestan **masti-*) 'intoxication' : Avestan *maδa-* 'intoxication, intoxicant, alcoholic beverage' :: Avestan *masti-* 'knowledge' : *maδa-* 'x', whereby 'x' = 'knowledge'. The latter development could not have taken place if, during the later period of Pahlavi glossation, it was believed that *haoma* was intoxicating, which would exclude "spiritualization" of *maδa-* via *masti-* 'wisdom'.

2
AVESTAN TERMS FOR THE SAUMA PLANT

Etymology of *soma-/haoma-* (see §45)

§186 This is the proper place to take account of an unusual explanation of *soma/haoma* offered by a distinguished Iranist, Sir Harold Bailey (1971; 1972:105; 1975:19; 1979:491; 1984; 1985). As against a universal consensus that *soma-/haoma-* has its origin in the Indo-Iranian root **sau-* 'to crush or grind by pressing with a pestle in a mortar' with suffix *-ma-* (see §262 below), Professor Bailey, in a favorable response to Mr. Wasson's theory that the sauma plant is a mushroom, proposed that **sauma-* have its origin in a word meaning 'mushroom'. It would be a remarkable phenomenon for there to have arisen a central ritual of pounding a mushroom (and, eventually, a twiggy substitute of wholly different appearance) because of similarity in sound between 'mushroom' (unattested for **sauma-*) and 'pound in a mortar'; it would be as if English-speaking ritualists, having instituted a cult of a psychotropic mushroom, would have the word *mushroom* prompt them to innovate a ritual of constructing sacred rooms (and piously fill them with oatmeal mush).

§187 Before proceeding to the etymology itself, it is worth observing the attestation ṚgVeda 1.84.8 (as translated by Bailey 1984:17) has 'when will (Indra) spurn [*sphurát*] the giftless mortal, like the *kṣúmpa*-plant with foot?' This is the only clear mention of mushrooms in the ṚgVeda, and it is interesting that here the mushroom is the exemplum of something despised. This is not definitive evidence against the *soma*-mushroom theory, but is nevertheless relevant. Bailey attempts to bridge the forms *kṣúmpa-* and Indo-Iranian **sauma-* by taking *k-* as prothetic. While he does not note the fact, all the other instances of Indo-Iranian *k-* prothesis involve Proto-Indo-European (PIE) **sw-*. Thus Old Iranian **xšv(a)ib/p-* 'to move quickly from side to side, to whip' (the respective meanings of Old Norse *svífa* and Latvian *svaipīt*), cf. Avestan *xšvaēpā-* 'rear, *tail', Old Indic *kṣip-* 'throw, swing' (probably dissimilated from **kṣvip-*); Avestan *xšvīd-* 'milk', Old Indic (lexicographical) *kṣvidyati* 'becomes moist' (Latvian *svaidīt* 'to smear', *sviēst* 'butter'); and Old Indic *kṣvedati* 'hums', Pashto *špel-* 'to whistle' (Old Slavic *svistati* 'to whistle'). Some of these forms were indeed alluded to by Bailey, who also cites the words for 'six'. However, the initial velar is lacking for 'six' in Old Indic, and the *ch* of the Prakrit forms, rather than reflect **kṣ-* and unmotivated palatalization, may go back merely to *s-*, cf. Pischel (1900:§211). Possibly one should proceed from PIE **sweks,* becoming Proto-Indo-Iranian **svakš;* the Indic form may reflect lost *-v-* by analogy with *sapta* 'seven', and subsequent assimilation of **saṣ* to *ṣaṣ;* an independent assimilation of **svaš* to **švaš* may lie behind the Iranian *xšvaš,* with *x-*, as regularly, preceding an older initial cluster **šC-*. Thus 'six' should not be ranged with the other forms in Proto-Indo-Iranian that have **kšv-* alongside cognate forms, in other languages, reflecting **sw-*.

§188 If *kṣúmpa-* belongs with German *Schwamm,* etc., it would be a replacement of **kṣvámpa-* or the like. This situation could be explained by a PIE ablaut alternation **swómPo-: *sumPó-* (perhaps originally nominative **swómb(h)s* > **swómps:* genitive **sumb(h)ós*, etc., cf. English *swamp: sump*), giving, via analogical levelings, **kṣvámp: *kṣumpás,* and finally a single compromise thematic *kṣúmpa-*. Thus the *k-* of *kṣúmpa-* would ultimately have the same origin as the *k-* of *kṣvidyati,* etc.

§189 While the *(*)kṣv-* of *kṣúmpa-* thus has parallels in such forms as *kṣvidyati,* the *k-* is nevertheless remarkable, for one would regularly expect **sv-*, and not Proto-Indo-Iranian **kšv-*, Old Indic **kṣv-*, for the entire series of words, 'mushroom' included. It is notable that an irregularity is also found in Greek ςομζŸ 'spongy, fungous', against the expected *ήμζŸ (<*μ̂ζŸ <*ʽϝομζŸ < **swombho-*). It therefore becomes conceivable that the irregularities of both the Indic and Greek forms for 'fung(o)us' represent a single PIE variant of **swombh-*, i.e. **kswombh-*. PIE **ksw-* would have been simplified via **sw* to Greek ς-. A PIE variation **(k)sw-* would also explain the hitherto puzzling series of Greek words with cognates pointing to PIE **sw-*, words which, apart from the initial sigma, appear, like ςομζŸ, to be Hellenic in phonology, and have meanings which make it unlikely that they were borrowed from a non-Hellenic language. These include ςαρδᾶωφ 'deride' (Welsh *chwarddu* 'to laugh', Sogdian *sxwarδ-* [Old Iranian **us-hvard-*], 'to shout', Avestan *kaxᵛarəδa-* 'sorcerer, ήθŸ', ςλαŸ 'gleam', ςελ῀νθ 'moon' (Old Indic *svarati* 'shines', Greek λθ 'sunlight', λᾶνθ 'torch'); ς̀η῀ 'silence' (German *Schweigen*) and ςιφπ῀ 'silence' (Old High German *giswiftōn* 'conticescere', etc.); and ςυρζετŸ 'sweepings, draggings', (Gothic *afswaírban, biswaírban* 'to wipe off', Old Frisian *swerva* 'to crawl'); semantically Greek ςαἔρφ 'sweep, clean', ς̆ρφ 'sweep, drag, crawl' from PIE *twer-* 'to turn' may have been influenced by PIE **swerbh-*.

§190 Particularly interesting is Greek ς̀μύŸ 'bending upwards, convex, snub', with cognates not only in Germanic (Norwegian *svīma* 'to reel', Old English *svīma* 'vertigo', Middle Low German *swāien, sweimen* 'to swing, sway', and Celtic (Welsh *chwid* 'agile turn', *chwin* 'movement'), but also in Slavic (Ukrainian *xvíjaty* [*-s'a*] 'to tilt [reel]', Russian *xvéjat'sja* 'to move'). These words are from the same ultimate root as Avestan *xšvaēpā-*, Old Norse *swífa*. Here Slavic *xv-* (against regular *sv-* from PIE **sw-*) would parallel Indo-Iranian **kšv-* (Old Indic *kṣv-*, Old Iranian *xšv-*) and Greek *s-* as the reflexes of PIE **ksw-*, variant of **sw-*. The same Slavic cluster is found in Russian *xvóryj* 'ill' (Middle High German *swër* 'pain, illness, swelling', Avestan *x^vara-* 'wound'), where again PIE **(k)sw-* should be reconstructed. Note that the regular Slavic reflex of PIE **ks-* is *x-*, e.g. Polish *chybać*, Czech *chybati* 'to swing, sway, be in agitation': Old Indic *kṣubh-*, Avestan *xšaob-* 'be in agitation'; Old Slavic *xudŭ* 'small', *xuždii* 'smaller': Old Indic *kṣudra-/kṣodīyas-* *small/smaller'.

§191 The language groups concerned, i.e. Indo-Iranian, Greek, and Slavic, are precisely those where a difference in the reflexes of **ksw-* and **sw-* is expectable. In phonetic terms, the **k-* prothesis of **ksw-* may be explained phonetically as originating in a tense onset accompanying a fortis pronunciation of the cluster *sw-*, and is due to the close relationship of *w* and velarity (cf., among many examples, **sw-* and **tw* becoming *k'* in Armenian). This phonetic intensification would correspond to the "expressive" nature of words in question, which refer to raucousness and high-pitched noise, glowing and glimmering, agitated motion, etc. In some instances the original "expressive" factor can no longer be precisely identified. In these cases the relevant feature may have developed secondary sound-symbolism. Thus, in Greek ς̂η̂ and ςιφπ̂ the sigma may express sudden cessation of sound; cf. English *shh, hush*. In Avestan *xšvid-* 'milk' the *xšv-* is hard to separate from that of Avestan *xšvipta-* (**xšvifta-*) 'milk (obtained from a milch animal)', Sogdian *xšift-*, Sarikoli *xevd*, etc. 'milk', explainable as 'that which is obtained by rapid or agitated motions' or 'sped forth', root **xšv(a)ip/b-*, but the relative chronology of the semantic developments is unknown, as is the connection of Old Indic *kṣīra-*, Persian *šīr* 'milk'. The meaning 'milk' for **xšvifta-* may be based upon *xšvīd-*, where the prevelarization could be related to a basic word for dripping, trickling, soaking through, etc. For Sogdian *xšift-*, see further §203 n.1.

§192 The latter possibility would be supported by Old Indic *kṣúmpa-*, Greek ςομζŸ < PIE **(k)swomP-*. For **swomP-* I assume a basic meaning 'swamp(y)', whence 'fung(o)us', *a priori* more likely than the reverse order of semantic development. For the further connections I would compare PIE **seup/b-*, whence Old Indic *sūpa-* 'soup', Germanic names for 'soup' (and the like), 'sop, soppiness', and verbs for 'slurp' and 'sip'; **seup/b-* is itself one of several PIE roots **seu-* 'to exude liquid, be moist', whence various words for soakage, sogginess, etc. Thus, with nasal infix, **sumP-* and (with reverse ablaut) *swomP-* 'soppiness, swamp(iness)'.

§193 There is in fact a considerable difference between **sauma-* and the Germanic words for 'mushroom', etc., which would have given in Indic not **svama-* (**suama-*) or **suma-*, let alone **sauma-*, but **svamb(h)a-* or **sumb(h)a-*. The PIE etymon 'mushroom' ('swampy, boggy, moist') is reconstructed **swomb(h)*. The **-mb(h)-* is clearly reflected in Germanic, e.g. Old Norse *svǫppr*, Danish *svamp* 'mushroom' and 'sponge'; cf. English *swamp* and, with zero grade, *sump; *-mbh-* is reflected by *-mm-* in Gothic *swamms* (*sic*), Old English *(mete-)swamm* 'mushroom', etc., Old High German retains, alongside *swam(m)*, German *Schwamm*, the cluster *-mb-* in *swamb;* Greek ςομίŸ stands to *swamb, Schwamm*, as Greek ήμïοŸ 'lateral tooth' stands to Old High German *kamb*, German *Kamm* 'comb'. As in Germanic, the disappearance of *b* after *m* is inconsistently realized in Iranian: Khotanese *huma-* would be like Khotanese *dumaa-*, Avestan *duma-*, against Sogdian *δumb*, Middle Persian *dumb* (alongside *dum*) 'tail'; PIE **dumb-*, cf. Old High German *zumpfo* 'penis'. Since there is no way to bridge the Proto-Indo-Iranian forms **svamb(h)a, *sumb(h)a-* 'spongy object, mushroom' and **sauma-*, the connection must be abandoned.

§194 Bailey (1979) himself has recently seemed to abandon the sauma-mushroom identification while apparently still advocating the possibility that **sauma-* is *'the spongy plant' (note that he now adds Khotanese *hąba-* 'balsam' from **humba-* to the etymon). Bailey (1979: 162) writes:

> In *ṚV* 10.94.3 reference to the stalks of *soma* cites the *vṛkṣásya śâkhām aruṇásya* 'the branch of the red *vṛkṣa*-plant'. Avestan *varəša-*, Old Indic *vṛkṣá-* seem to have survived in Yazghulami *warš* 'a herb which blinds cattle', and Shughni 'a hill grass', if these are from **varša-*; it could then give a meaning 'plant with root, shoot, or stalk', whence later 'tree'. The phrase *vṛkṣá- . . . aruṇá-* with 'branch' hardly suits a mushroom.

§195 Again on a relationship of Khotanese *huma-*, etc. to *soma-*, Bailey notes (1979: 491): "The use of the 'branch of the red tree', *vṛkṣásya śâkham aruṇásya*, causes difficulty"; here he also refers to *ṚV* 10.94.3 together with the Middle Persian description of *hōm ī spēd* 'the white *haoma*' as a tree (*draxt*) or plant (*urwar*) (see also Bailey 1974: 374 and 371). It may be added that this Vedic and Middle Persian evidence for the unmushroomlike nature of the sauma plant is completed by the Avestan mention of trunks (*varšajīš*), shoots *(fraspar*ə*yō)* and outgrowths (*fravāxšō*), as well as stalks (*-ąsu-* = Vedic *aṃśu-*), *Yasna* 10.5; *Yasna* 9.16. The picture of a chlorophyll-producing plant is further borne out by Avestan *zairi.gaona-*, to which correspond Aramaic *zargōn* 'vine', Middle Persian and Parthian *zargōn*, Sogdian *zarγōn* 'greenish, vegetable'. All of this goes against the identification of sauma as the mushroom *Amanita muscaria*, but is suited by the identification as *Peganum harmala*.

§196 Bailey (1985), following Benveniste (1929), connects **haoma** via Plutarch's ήμφμι (on which see §52 n.10) to Greek ώμφμĕŸ, and thence to Greek μφμιον, Syriac *humāmā* and Arabic *humāma*. For the series of forms he claims an original Iranian **humāma*, consisting of **huma** 'soft' plus suffix *-ama-*. The connection of *haoma* with ώμφμĕŸ, is, however, untenable (see §269) and derivation from Iranian **huma-* 'soft', and thereby connection at the linguistic root level with *haoma-*, provides no botanical specificity. Bailey's citation of Old Indic *saumya-* 'soft' alongside *soma-* does not make it clear that *saumya-* really means 'like *soma-*' and hence, *inter alia*, 'gentle' (rather than 'physically soft'). Against Bailey's etymological manipulations, whereby *haoma-* would be 'something soft', the traditional explanation of *soma-/haoma-* remains unshakable, supported as it is by proper morphological analysis, by its textually associated cognate forms for 'mortar', 'ritual pressing', etc., and by the actual method of preparation.

More on mushrooms, and the alleged PIE **bhongo-* 'psychotrope'

§197 There exists a series of phonologically similar words in Indo-European, Uralic, and northeastern Siberian languages which seems to bring together mushrooms and other plants under a shared characteristic, a narcotic effect. This linguistic material has had a significant role in the history of the identification of *soma/haoma* and other issues pertaining to the use of psychotropic plants by the Indo-Iranian peoples. The forms consist of (1) words for 'mushroom, squamous substance' and likely cognates. These include: in Indo-European, Latin *fungus* and Greek ςΐηηοŸ; in the Finno-Ugric branch of Uralic, Mordvin *paŋgo* 'mushroom, fungus, lichen', Ostyak *paŋk*, etc., Vogul *paŋx, poŋk*, etc. *'Amanita muscaria'*; Ostyak *paŋkəl-, paŋkət-* 'after eating *Amanita muscaria*, become intoxicated and/or sing; prophesy, heal shamanistically'; Vogul *pōŏŋkl-*, etc. 'become intoxicated (by any means)'; in the Samo-yed group of Uralic, Ket *haŋgo 'Amanita muscaria'* and Tavgi *faŋka-* 'be intoxicated'; and in Chukotkan languages, Chukchi, Koryak, and Kamchadal *poŋ-* 'mushroom'; (2) Words for drug plants in Indo-Iranian: Old Indic *bhaṅgá-*, *bhaṅgā-* (already AtharvaVeda) 'hemp', also (ṚgVeda) epithet of *soma;*

Avestan *baŋha-* 'an abortive plant'; Middle Persian *bang* 'henbane'; Persian *bang* 'henbane, hemp'.

§198 Before discussing the views on the history of drug plants to which these linguistic data have given rise, it will be of help to discuss the forms of the first ("mycological") group. The etymology of Greek ςίηηοΫ (and its variant ςπηηοΫ), Latin *fungus*, have been usually discussed by Indo-Europeanists together with Armenian *sunk* (*sounk*), with the conclusion that all derive from an unknown "Mediterranean" source. This position allows an escape from accounting for the difficult phonological details. Another solution, proposed by H. Pedersen (1900; I have not been able to obtain the original article and am dependent on the summary of Roman Jakobson *apud* Wasson 1968: 319-320), also operates with the Greek, Latin, and Armenian forms, to which it adds also Old Slavic *gǒba* 'sponge' and kindred Slavic forms also meaning 'mushroom'. Pedersen suggested that *gǒba* and Old High German *swamb* could go back to PIE **sgwhombho-*, but, in order to account for the Greek, Latin and Armenian forms, he alternately proposed an original **sphwongo-*, becoming through metathesis **sgwompho-*, with variant **sgwombho-*.

§199 An original **sphwongo-* is *a priori* unlikely, since PIE initial clusters of two labials, PIE **p(h)w-* and **bhw-*, cannot otherwise be reconstructed. Furthermore, PIE **sp(h)-* would give Armenian **p'*, not **s-*, while the proposed variant of the metathesis, **sgwombho-*, would yield Old Slavic **gvǒmba* and ProtoGermanic **skwambaz*, not **swambaz* (cf. Old Norse *svǒppr*).

§200 Old High German *swamb*, etc. should be (against Pedersen) related to Greek ςομζοΫ (see above, §181), and separate from Greek *sp(h)óngos* and Latin *fungus*. Armenian *sunk* does not belong here either. It is of Caucasic origin, most likely South Caucasian (Kartvelian), cf. Georgian *sok'o* 'mushroom'; (see Klimov [1964: 165] where Armenian *sunk* (and *sokon*) are given, with Ossetic and Nakh-Daghestanian forms, which are probably also from the Kartvelian). The *-n-* of *sunk* may be due to the influence of Armenian *spung* 'sponge' (from Greek), cf. *sung*, variant of *sunk*, which therefore need not be of "West Armenian" origin.

§201 This leaves Greek *sp(h)óngos*, Latin *fungus*, and Old Slavic *gyba* to account for. If we start with PIE **bhongo-*, we get *fungus* as regular reflex, *sp(h)óngos* via *s*-prothesis, perhaps with additional influence of ς(ϝ)ομίΫ, and *gǒba* via metathesis of **bǒga*. This metathesis would be motivated by the semantic similarity of Balto-Slavic **gumba-*, Lithuanian *gum̃bas* 'convexity, round excrescence', *gum̃bras* 'boil', cf. Pashto *γumba* 'boil', and also by Old Slavic **gǒba* 'lip, snout'; for the relevant forms see Vasmer (1950-: 316).

§202 It is noteworthy that the meanings and geographical distribution of the forms Greek *sp(h)óngos* 'sponge', Latin *fungus* 'mushroom, fungus, lichen, mildew' and Slavic **gǒba* 'mushroom, sponge' points to the meaning of **bhongo-* not as 'sponge' (originally a specific Mediterranean development of the Greek), nor even as 'mushroom', but 'spongy, soppy, swampy substance', of which fungi are the most common exemplars. The meaning would come close to that of German *Schwamm* 'sponge/mushroom', whose cognates include words for swamp and sump. As I have proposed (§191), **swombho-* ultimately means 'soupy moisture', to root **seup-*; thus **bhongo-* could have doublet **bhogno-*, whence Russian *bagnó*, 'low swampy place', Ukrainian *bahnó* 'swamp', etc., and perhaps also German *Bach* 'stream', Irish *búal* 'water' (see Vasmer 1950-:36). For the phonological relationship of **bhongo-* to **bhogno-*, cf. Latin *fundus:* Old Indic *budhna-* 'bottom', but the inserted nasal of **bhongo-* could also be sound-symbolic. Cf. also **swomp/bho-*, root **seup-*.[1]

§203 It is quite possible that **bhongo-* was borrowed as **p8ŋk8-* in Uralic in some very remote period of contact with the Indo-Europeans; cf. the later borrowings of 'mushroom' in Uralic from Indo-European, Hungarian *gomba* from Slavic, probably Finnish *sampa* from Germanic **swamb/pa(z)*, and also Turkish *mantar* 'mushroom, fungus, cork' from Greek μανιτάρι (ancient ὠμανἔτα). It is noteworthy that **p8ŋk-* is reflected with the general meaning 'mushroom, fungus, lichen/mildew' in Cheremis and Mordvin, but is specifically 'fly agaric' in Vogul and Ostyak. There is no evidence to suggest that **bhongo-* in Indo-European meant specifically 'fly agaric'; this sense could have developed in Uralic (more precisely, Ob-Ugrian) territory, where this was the mushroom *par excellence*.

§204 This brings us to the second series of words, i.e. the Indo-Iranian words formally reminiscent of **bhongo-* but referring to non-mycological drug plants. B. Munkácsi (1907: 343-344) first connected the Ob-Ugrian words for '(fly agaric) mushroom' with the phonically similar Indo-Iranian words referring to various drug plants, and concluded that the Ob-Ugrian originally meant 'intoxicating, narcotic', and comes from Indo-Iranian. See further the extracts of subsequent relevant literature most usefully gathered and discussed by Wasson (1968: 226 *seq.*); note particularly Wasson's judicious criticisms of M. Eliade's (1964) thesis that "the magico-religious value of intoxication for achieving ecstasy is of Iranian origin", which is the most extreme extension of Munkácsi's view. Most recently the issue has been discussed again by F. Crevatin (1983: 109-15), who seems to believe that PIE **bhongo-* (and **spongo-*), whence he derives the Uralic forms, originally referred to the fly agaric mushroom, and that the same etymon gave rise to Uralic and Indo-Iranian terms with application of 'intoxicant potion' to plants other than mushrooms. Crevatin also seems cautiously favorable to the thesis that the Indo-Iranians originally used a psychotropic mushroom, but is reluctant to identify *soma/haoma* thus.

§205 As against the evidence for PIE **bhongo-* 'mushroom', there is in fact no real evidence for such a form meaning 'narcotic or intoxicant plant'. The apparent Indo-Iranian **bhanga-* with such a meaning is based on illusory data, as I shall now try to show.

§206 With regard to 'hemp', called *bhaṅga-* (and *śaṇa-*) in Sanskrit, there is no evidence for its use as an intoxicant in either India or Persia before well within the Islamic era. It is true the Scythians were exceptional in this regard, for their inhalation (!) of hemp is noted by Herodotus and confirmed by the Scythian tomb artifacts from Pazyryk. But it is clear also from Herodotus and other sources that the Scythian religion was different from that of other (Indo-) Iranians, and that the nomadism of the Scythians involved them in a different cultural complex, including particular shamanistic practices. It is perhaps relevant that in Ossetic, the surviving Scytho-Alanic language, 'hemp' is *gæn(æ)* (cf. **kæn-* 'flax' in *kættāg* 'linen'), whose prototype was early disseminated not only in the Caucasus (Svanetic *kan*, Abkhaz *a-k°no*), but independently among the Turks (*kendir*), and also yielded, in Uralic, Cheremis *keŋe*. This form (like Sanskrit *śaṇa-* 'hemp', with *ś* from palatal *k̂*?!) lacks the labial which follows the *n* in the *cannabis* word in Assyrian, Middle Persian, Greek, Slavic and Germanic on one hand, and the East (Central Asiatic) Middle Iranian on the other: Khotanese *kaṃhā-* 'hemp', Sogdian **kinbā* or **kenbā (kynp')*, Khwarezmian *knbynk* (adj.), Khotanese *kuṃbā-* 'flax', from earlier disyllabic **kanbā-* (and **kanfā-*, from **kanphā-* for Khotanese *kaṃhā-* ?).

§207 The latter forms are of further interest. Words for 'hemp' and 'flax' often merge. If the source of Sanskrit *bhaṅga-* 'hemp' also referred to flax, and (as Mayrhofer 1956-1976, *s.v. bhaṅgā-* suggests) had the original form **kaṃbhă-*, **gaṃbhă-*, or the like, a metathesis to *bhaṅga-* could have been motivated by the association of flax (and hemp) with the beating (Old Indic *bhaṅg-*) necessary for the plant fiber to be used. W. Eilers (1985: 25) has suggested more simply a theoretical Proto-Indo-Iranian

[1] [For these forms cf. also Toporov (1985:301–305)].

**bhang-* 'to beat' as the source not only for Old Indic *bhangā-, bhanga-* 'hemp', but also Avestan *baŋha-* and Middle Persian, New Persian *bang/mang* 'henbane', which he wrongly also takes as 'hemp'.

§208 Against the opinion of Crevatin (1983: 112–113), the data of the Atharva-Veda do not show that hemp was used as a psychotrope. In *AV* 11.6.15 we are dealing with a series of holy plants. *Soma* was obviously the most sacred ritual plant, whether or not it was used psychotropically at the time the AtharvaVeda was composed. The presence of barley in the text is due not to a use in beer, as Crevatin suggests, but due to its long venerability as the Indo-European food grain *par excellence.* The numinous force ascribed to barley (Avestan *yava- ašavan-* 'the barley endowed with *Ṛta',* Persian *jordā*) is not only evident in the Avesta, where the mere cultivation of this grain is said to counter demons, but in a variety of Hittite, Vedic, and Greek data; see in detail Watkins (1978). *Darbha*-grass provided the seat of the god Agni on the fire-altar, and was used to sweep the sacrificial area, whence the numinous power of this grass (cf. *AV* 19.32). Crevatin's confidence that *darbha* was psychoactive is based on *AV* 6.43, where *darbha* figures in a charm to appease the anger of stranger and kin, but here we are not dealing with a tranquilizing drug, a "*sedativo*": the AtharvaVeda is not medical, but magical.

§209 Finally, the inclusion of hemp (*bhaṅgā-*) in the list is due to its use as the traditional means of binding, which, as is well known, is an operation which has a profound and multifaceted role in archaic magic and its symbolism, being the medium of control, alliance, incapacitation, and delimitation; it is also the means of fastening amulets. Cf. *AV* 2.4.3-4. As a name for hemp, out of which snares were ritually prepared, *bhaṅgá-* 'smashing' would be a propitious indication of the desired effect. Cf. *AV* 8.8.6, where the bonds of death, specified as hempen by *Kauśikā-sūtra* 16.15-16, 14.28, are associated with fatal hammers.

§210 It may be added that *bhaṅgá-* 'smashing, breaking through', as epithet of *soma* in *ṚV* 9.16.13, amplifies the immediately preceding *aptúr-* 'overcoming the waters'. This numinous epithet, with its victorious resonances, could have been another factor in the naming of hemp *bhaṅgá-, bhaṅgā́-,* although the fact that *bhaṅgá* occurs with regard to *soma* only in a single, contextually conditioned passage makes a connection questionable. In any event, it can be concluded that *bhaṅgá-*, either as a name of hemp or an epithet of *soma,* is independent of psychotropic reference.

§211 Passing now to the Iranian material, Avestan *bangha, baŋha-*, and Middle and New Persian *bang* and *mang* (Arabic *banj*), I shall now try to show that these names too do not go back to an Old Iranian **banga-* 'psychotropic or narcotic plant'.

§212 W. B. Henning (1951: 33 *seq.*) noted that Avestan *baŋha-/bangha-* is better derived phonologically from Proto-Iranian **dvaŋha-* (=Old Indic *dhvaṃsa-* 'destroying') than from a Proto-Iranian form with **-anga-*. Obviously this would suit the name of a plant at issue in *Vidēvdād* 15.14, where *baŋhəm* is listed as an abortive plant (I shall return to this passage). This also neatly fits *Vidēvdād* 19.20, the divine epithets of Ahura Mazdah *axᵛafnō, abaŋhō* 'sleepless, indestructible', and *Vidēvdād* 19.41, *daēvəm kundəm baŋhəm vī.baŋhəm* 'the demon Kunda, destructive, full of destruction'. However, this meaning also seems to occur for the name of a righteous person whose memory is revered, *Pouru.baŋhəm* (*Yasht* 13.124); 'full of destruction, having much destruction' (or 'destroying many'), a warrior's name, seems more likely than 'he who has many narcotics', which would suit a drug merchant or (given the context of *Vidēvdād* 15.17) an abortionist. But if a *nom de guerre* is not involved here, I suggest *'having a large abdomen', cf. Old Indic *bhā́ṃsas-, ṚV* 10.163.4.

§213 That in *Vidēvdād* 15.14 *baŋha-* should mean merely 'destructive, destroying' is shown by the larger context: *baŋhəm vā šaētəm vā γnānəm vā fraspātəm vā kąmcit̰ vā vitācinąm urvaranąm 'baŋha-* or *šaēta-* or *γnāna-* or *fraspāt-*, or any of (the) (foetus-)dissolving plants'. The last two terms are clearest etymologically. First, *γnāna-* 'beating, killing', is from the root *gan-* 'strike, kill', cf. *Vidēvdād* 13.51 *ava.γnāna-* masculine 'killer', *γənąna-* neuter *Yasht* 10.27 'a blow' (delivered by Mithra against evil beings)'. Next, *fraspāt-* means literally 'throwing forth' (=Pahlavi *frāz abgandan*). This may now be understood as a term for 'abortive', cf. Persian *bačča andāxtan* 'throw a child' = 'have an abortion', and also Modern Greek *ἀποβολή* 'abortion, miscarriage' (originally 'throwing off/out'). The same semantic development occurs in Sogdian: Manichean *pš'q* 'abortion' (in Manichean texts referring to the 'Abortion-demons'), from *pšāy-* 'to throw, abort', S. *nš'y-* *'to be aborted',[2] which points to *šaēta-* also meaning 'abortive'.[3]

§214 Thus we see that all three words following *baŋha-* in *Vidēvdād* 15.14 are adjectives which are in effect synonymous with *vitācinąm* 'liquidating (a foetus)', modifying 'plants' at the end of the sentence. It is now obvious that *baŋha-* at the head of the list is semantically like the rest of the series. The series may be translated 'destroying or aborting or killing or inducing miscarriage, or any of the plants which liquidate'. The series is therefore ordered: [A] a general word for 'destructive' alternating with [B] a term for 'abortive': ABA'B'(A''). It is doubtful that this is anything more than a pleonastic way of saying 'any abortive plant at all', and that any specific plant is named.

§215 One must account for the fact that the Pahlavi translation of *baŋha-* in the latter passage is not *bang,* but the less similar variant *mang,* with the specific gloss *mang ī Wištāsp* 'the *mang* of Wiṣhtāsp'. The situation may be explained thus: the scholiasts were confronted with two terms, which they thought to form a pair of botanical designations (whereas the next two words they recognized as common nouns for abortifacients). They of course assumed *baŋhəm* to be *bang/mang,* while for *šaētəm* they thought of Middle Persian *šēd* 'bright(ness)' (Persian *šēd,* cf. Armenian *ašxēt;* Avestan *(-)xšaēta-*). Taking *baŋha-* as *bang/mang,* they identified this with the *mang ī Wištāsp,* seeing *šaēta-* as a more splendid *mang,* and invented a symmetrical counterpart, *mang ī Zarduxšt,* 'the *mang* of Zoroaster'. If my explanation is correct, there is no ground for Belardi's (1979: 115-116) speculation that the realia involve two plant juices, one abortive, the other intoxicant.

§216 While it was almost inevitable that the Pahlavi scholiasts would have rendered Avestan *baŋha-*, in the context of harmful plants, as the virtually homophonous *bang* (or its variant *mang*) 'henbane', it is most unlikely that *bang/mang* derives from Avestan *baŋha-*, which is not a botanical designation. Nor is a derivation from 'destructive' appropriate

[2] S. *nš'y-* occurs in the Paris Text 22.18, untranslated by Benveniste (1940: 156). The passage means (starting from the end of Line 22): '(Her) deficient milk (restore *γš'β[t]y,* cf. Yagnobi *xšift*) will dry up, and the pregnant woman's foetus will be aborted *(nš'yt)* in her womb'. One should reconstruct an active form **nišāy-* from **ni-šāya-,* related to Khotanese *biṣṣāta-* 'dislocated', Old Indic *sā́yaka-* 'missile', from PIE **seE- (*sē-), *sē(y)-* 'to throw, cast'. Cf. already Schwartz (1969: 446).

[3] It is clear that *š,* the regular reflex of PIE **s* after *i,* was generalized from the *-šāy-* of *nišāy-* *'throw down, abort' to the parallel form *pšāy-,* where *p-* reflects the preverb *apa-,* after which one would expect Old Iranian *-hāy-* for PIE **(-)sēy-*. This resulted in a new "root" **šāy-* 'to abort'. See the parallel examples in Gershevitch (1974:72); in support of Gershevitch's **šaiča-* 'pouring, forming pools, sprinkling', note the medieval place name *Šēz* in Azarbaijan, at the site of a spring-fed lake. From this **šāy-* was formed an early East Iranian form *šaēta- [šaita-]* 'abortive', parallel to that of the cognate Old Indic form *setā-* 'furrow' from PIE *sēy-* 'to throw (seed), sow' (cf. also Old Indic *senā* 'missile'). For **seE->*sēy-, *sey-,* see Schwartz (1980b). It may be added that B. T. Anklesaria (1950) and H. Jamasp (1907) have taken *šaēta-* as 'abortive' by comparing Sanskrit *śāyayati* 'cause to lie down', regarded as possible by W. Belardi (1979: 115). One must object that the cognate of Sanskrit *śī* 'lie' is Avestan *sī (say-),* with expected *s-,* not *š.* Belardi's preferred connection with the other Avestan *šaēta-,* 'acquisition, possession, wealth' (not 'power'!), is unconvincing.

for *bang/mang,* as shall presently be seen. Phonologically it is very improbable that *bang/mang* is from Proto-Iranian **dvanha-,* which would give Middle Persian **dax.* The change *dv-* to *b* does occur in Parthian, e.g. *bar* = Middle Persian *dar* 'door' from **dvara-,* but **-anh-* to **-ang-* is unknown in Parthian or elsewhere in Middle Iranian. Obviously Zoroastrian Middle Persian *-ang-* in scholia as approximation of Avestan *-aŋh-* in proper nouns is irrelevant for our present instance.[4]

§217 It now becomes necessary to explain Middle Persian, New Persian *bang/mang* 'henbane', Arabic *banj* 'henbane, datura' (which, as most scholars have agreed since Henning's [1951: 33 *seq.*] discussion, must not be confused with the later Persian *bang* 'hemp' from New Indic *bhang,* Sanskrit *bhaṅga-*). An ingeniously novel explanation was offered by W. Belardi (1979:119): Assuming *banha-* and *bang/mang* are 'henbane', Belardi reconstructs Proto-Iranian **dvanga-,* Proto-Indo-Iranian **dhvanga-* '*Solanacea;* plant containing solanine'. From this **dhvanga-* Belardi also derives Sanskrit *dhvāṅkṣi-* (lex.) 'a particular medicinal plant', *dhvāṅkṣatuṇḍa-, dhvāṅkṣanāsā-, dhvāṅkṣavallī- 'Ardisia solanacea', dhvāṅkṣamācī- 'Solanum indicum',* all forms which would arise by popular etymological modification via *dhvāṅkṣa-* 'crow' (all these forms are misprinted *dhvaṅkṣa-,* as Crevatin [1982], who is sceptical of the etymology, has noticed).[5]

§218 Belardi's etymology, for all its erudite combinations, is very problematic. It is difficult to think that the word in question would embrace so broad a botanical spectrum. In detail, the genus *Ardisia* does not belong to the order *Solanaceae* (which includes e.g. the potato and eggplant), and neither *Ardisia solanacea* nor *Solanum indicum* contain the same alkaloids as *Hyoscamus* (hen-bane), as Belardi thinks (D.S.F.). While the Sanskrit forms are self-explanatory at face value, i.e. named for their resemblance to a crow's beak, etc., an etymon **dhvanga-* remains unexplained (Belardi wisely refrains from any temptation to mention *dhvaj-* 'to flutter'). Furthermore, it is a fact that the Sanskrit and Iranian names of shrubs, herbs, and fruits, are rarely (if ever) cognate.

§219 The assumption that *bang/mang* means 'henbane' has been countered by Flattery, who instead argues for it being a more general word for 'psychoactive drug'. In favor of this one could note Arabic *banj* as both 'henbane' and 'datura'. More importantly, as Flattery argues (§26 n.3), there is nothing to show that *bang/mang* necessarily referred to a potentially lethal drug, not even in the Ardā Wīrāz legend. Wīrāz drinks the *mang ī Wištāspān,* apparently the same *mang* Wishtāsp took for the trance in which the truth of Zoroaster's mission was revealed. In the *Iranian Bundahišn* 4.20 (Anklesaria 1908: 43.12), the drug which mercifully palliates the death throes of the Primordial Bovine is called *mang ī bēšāz kē hast ī *bang-(i)z (banj?) xwānīhed* 'the medicinal/healing *mang,* which is (also) that which is called *bang*'.

§220 The key to the etymology of *bang* is the variant form *mang,* again referring to a psychoactive substance. This form occurs in the Pahlavi accounts of the Primordial Bovine, divinely given *mang* for soothing the pangs of death; of Wishtāsp, who enters the long trance which precedes his acceptance of Zoroaster's religion; and of Wīrāz, who has his vision after drinking *mang ī Wištāspān.* The first two myths are based on lost Avestan texts. In the two versions of the first myth, *Iranian Bundahišn* 4.20 (quoted above) and *Zātsparam* 2.7, the word *mang* is glossed as 'that which is called *bang*'. These data indicate that *mang* is the more antique form, possibly an adaptation of an Avestan form, and that *bang* is of later origin. While in Iranian *b-* could be dissimilated to *m-* before *n-* (Eilers 1953: 73 *seq.*), *m-* becoming *b-* is not unusual, particularly when a nasal follows.[6]

§221 Thus we arrive at **mangă-* 'psychotropic substance', which could give specific senses 'henbane, datura', and, with Flattery (§§26-27), '*Peganum har-mala*'. The etymology would be PIE **meng-* 'to create attractive illusions, to charm, appear charming, deceive' (cf. Pokorny 1959: 731 'schöner machen, schwindelhaft verschönern') whence Old Indic *mañjú-, mañjulá-* 'attractive', and probably also *maṅgalá-* 'good omen, fortune'; Greek *μάηηανον* 'means of charming, bewitching, or tricking; philtre; device'; *μαηηάνευμα* 'quack remedy' (occurring with *ἴάρμακα* 'drugs'); Middle Irish *meng;* Ossetic *mæng,* Sogdian, and Persian *mang,* all 'deceit, trickery'. It may be assumed that Iranian inherited two homophonous words, **manga-* 'deceit, trickery' and **manga-* (or **mangā-*) *'magic potion, hallucinogen'.[7]

§222 It may be concluded Indo-European **bhongo-* did not mean 'psychotrope' but merely meant *fungus* and the like; it is a coincidence that Ostyak *paŋk* 'intoxicating mushroom', Old Indic *bhaṅga-* 'hemp', Avestan *baŋha-,* characterization of abortive plant ('destructive'), and Middle Persian *bang* 'henbane' are similar in form. A parallel of sorts to this situation is the accidental similarity of English *hemp* and *henbane.* If I may close this unavoidably ponderous section with levity, the alleged **bhongo-, *banga-* 'hallucinogen' turns out to be merely an attractive illusion.

Haoma and hops

§223 Abaev (1975) has proposed to derive Ossetic *xumællæg* 'hops' from **hauma- aryaka-* "Aryan *haoma*". This would be conceivable if it were known that the Scytho-Alanic (West Saka) ancestors of the Ossetes regarded *haoma* as paradigmatic of intoxicant in general (which would probably involve a desacralization of the beverage). Unfortunately nothing is known about the Saka usage of *haoma* (the background of the epithet *H-u-m-v-r-g* applied to certain Sakas by the Achaemenids unfortunately remains wholly conjectural; against Khotanese *durauśa'* reflecting

[4] I am not convinced that Elamite *-nk-,* Greek *-ηη-* [-ng-] represents an actual *[ng] as against *[nh] in the examples discussed by Gershevitch (1969: 212-214). The instance of Middle Persian *frasang* (and *frasax*), Greek *παραçάηηθ* '*parasang*' is complicated by possible influence of Persian *sang* etc. 'stone', cf. English *milestone.*

[5] And even if, against all likelihood, the Iranian name of 'henbane' were related to the Sanskrit names in *dhvāṅkṣ-* for such different plants, even granting *dhvāṅkṣ-* represents **dhvaṅga-,* the correspondence of the Iranian would be irregular. As noted above, **dhvanga-* would give (Late) Avestan **banga-,* not *baŋha-,* and (if my arguments that *baŋha-* is not a phytonym are correct), the only reason to have thought that *baŋha-* is a misspelling of **banga-* (i.e. *baṇga-* in Hoffmann's [1971] system), the equation with Middle Persian *bang,* etc., is no longer tenable. I shall not quibble that **dvanga-* should have given Persic **dang;* interdialectal exchange is theoretically possible. The vast formal and semantic gulf between *dhvāṇkṣatuṇḍa-,* etc., and *bang/mang* suffices to make one seek another explanation.

[6] Thus *maizman-* 'urine' gives Khotanese *bīysman-,* cf. Sogdian *βizm-δānē* 'bladder', and, with *-n-,* Avestan *maiδyāna-* 'middle', Persian *miyān* 'middle, waist': Yagnobi *bidon* 'middle' and Ormuri *biyān* 'waist', and Avestan *maγna-:* Sogdian *βaγnē,* Khwarezmian *βaγnək,* Ossetic *bæγnæg,* Middle Persian *brahnag.* The examples can be multiplied.

[7] As a semantic parallel to the etymology of *mang/bang* 'hallucinogen, henbane' (Arabic *banj* 'datura'), I would compare the etymology of Sanskrit *dhattura-* 'datura (*Datura alba*)', where *dhūrta-, dhūrtakāra-* 'deceptive, tricking' is clearly involved; see the material in Turner (1966; 1973:384 and 393 under *dhattūra-, dhūrta-,* and **dhūrtakāra-*). There is now all the less reason to involve dubious etymologies in **dhwes-, *dhus-,* or an unknown substratic etymon without further derivatives, and the role of "popular etymology", cf. Mayrhofer (1959:88-89). Old Indic *dhūrta-* gives Prakrit *dhutta-* 'rogue' and 'datura'; from **dhūrtakāra-* would come Marathi *dhutāra-* 'cheat', etc. and by metathesis Marathi *dhaturā* 'trickery', with compromise forms Buddhist Hybrid Sanskrit *dhutturaka-,* Hindi *dhutūrā,* Bengali *dhutura,* Assamese *dhūturā,* etc. The *-tt-* forms could be due to forms like *dhutta-* with *tt* from *rt,* and also have expressive value; and Sanskrit *dhustūra-* could have *st* as "learned" overcompensation replacing Middle Indic *th* (found e.g. in Maithili *dhuthur*), in reality the product of assimilatory aspiration by *dh-;* similarly the forms with *dhvas-* in the first syllable. Thus *dhūrta(kṛt-),* literally 'deceptive, causing deception', glossed as 'datura', is not a baseless lexicographical fabrication.

Avestan *dūraoša-*, see Emmerick's note §98 n.27). Earlier attempts to connect the hops word with *haoma-* have been justly rejected by most scholars. The fermentation of beer is quite different from the pressing of *haoma;* note that extraction by mortar and pestle cannot be applied to hops. There is no evidence for the cultivation of hops originating among the Scyths; this would in fact be contradicted by the application of **hauma-* as a name for 'hops', which have no intoxicating property in themselves, but are used to facilitate the production of beer, enhance and preserve it (Burgess 1964). The situation with, for example, Russian *xmel'* 'hops, intoxication' is different, for here hops would be associated with the production of an intoxicant beverage introduced by another people. Henning (1946: 720) connects Greek *ω ĎŸ* 'beer' with Sogdian *zwt'k* 'some intoxicant beverage', but this is too uncertain as evidence for Scythian brewing of beer. The former word, if of Greek origin, may be connected with *ωυμŸ* 'leaven, ferment', and the latter may be from an ancient **zūta-* 'poured (as a libation)'. The modern Ossetic word for 'beer', *bægæni* (whose **g* [as in the case of Khwarezmian *bkny*] cannot be from Old Iranian **g* [which gives ɣ], seems to be of Turkish origin, suggesting external influence in development of brewing techniques. Sogdian *βɣ 'ny* has nothing to do with *bægæni* and beverages; see Henning (1968: 244-245).

§224 It is likely that the 'hops' word originated among the Germanic peoples, for whom beer has a long tradition of importance. Indeed Germanic uniquely provides a convincing etymology (German *hummeln* 'to grope, grasp around' has been compared, in reference to the distinctive growth of the clinging vines). From Germanic the word for 'hops' (Old Norse *humli, humla, humall,* whence eighth century Latin *humulus* and Finnish *humala,* traveled eastward and southward (note Slavic **xŭmel^*, thirteenth century Greek *γοέμελι*, and cf. especially Old Norse *humli*, Old English *humele*) to the region north of the Black Sea, where it likely was borrowed into Scythic as **xumall-ag* (with the productive suffix *-ag, -ak*), whence, likely via a Turkic intermediary **qumlaq/ *xumlaq*, the word was further disseminated in Chuvash, Vogul, Hungarian, etc. From Scythian **xumallag* comes, as the expected development, Ossetic *xumællæg.*

§225 This trajectory seems confirmed by the history of the 'ale' word: Germanic **alud-* (Old English *ealud*, etc.), representing a West Indo-European word for *'bitterness' (cf. Latin *alumen*), gave Finnish *olut*, etc. and ultimately Scythic **alud/t-*, whence Ossetic *æluton, ilæton* (whose fabulous nature suggests an exotic origin), Georgian *ludi*, for which cf. further Abaev (1955: I, 130). It may be concluded that Ossetic *xumællæg* has no relevance for the history of *haoma.*

Avestan *dūraoša-* (see §98)

§226 Since no noun or adjective **dura-* is found in either Indic or Iranian, and *dūra-* 'far' occurs in both, and **-auša(s)-* is reflected in Iranian and Indic only in the sense of 'destroying, destruction' (rather than its etymological meaning 'burning'), the simplest explanation would be that Avestan *dūraoša-* 'keeping destruction far away' reflects the original form and meaning, whereas the Old Indic *duróṣa-* has shortened the first syllable by popular etymology (*dur-* 'bad, difficult'). The Vedic hapax *oṣám* 'quickly' may be from older 'burning', but it is unclear if the latter meaning was still extant when the compound **dūrauša-* was created; the difficulty of the Vedic attestations are probably due to poetic plays on the meanings 'hard to destroy' and/or 'hard to burn', which await another occasion for discussion.

§227 The usual interpretation of *dūraoša-* as 'keeping death afar, averting death' associates *haoma* with a drink of immortality. Except in an eschatological context, however, immortality is not a prominent objective of haoma-drinking. Considering that *dūraoša-* in the Gathas refers to sauma in the context of burning it and that burning is the chief way of using an apotropaic plant in Iran, together with the fact that *haoma*'s apotropaic function is quite marked elsewhere in the Avesta, it seems more likely that *dūraoša-* had the sense 'keeping destruction far away' as referring to the apotropaic powers of the plant. For the etymology of *dūraoša-/duróṣa-*, see, in addition to the references to Bailey in §98 n.28, Gershevitch (1975:49) and Bailey (1985a).

Avestan *haδānaēpātā- 'Peganum harmala'* (see §§117-121)

§231 From considerations of realia Flattery (§§117-122) has rejected the equation of *haδānaēpātā-* with pomegranate (for which see Morgenstierne 1973: II, 190; Klingenschmitt 1965: 32 n.8, with reference to Bailey 1957b: 53), and has indicated instead that *haδānaēpătā-* should be a designation for harmel.

§232 It is true that *haδānaēpātā-* seems to be a compound whose first member is comparable with an Old Iranian etymon for 'pomegranate', **haδānā-*. From a purely linguistic viewpoint however, the two items cannot be directly and unqualifiedly equated, since *haδānaēpātā-* has the additional element *pātā-* apparently added to the first member, *haδānaē-*, terminating in a diphthong *-aē-* which itself requires explanation. The presence of the additional material in fact suggests that *haδānaēpătā-*'is not pomegranate but some other plant thought to bear some relationship to it.

§233 Both details have been addressed recently by Bailey (1985: 871), who still takes *haδānaēpătā-* as 'pomegranate'. For *-pătā-* Bailey compares West Iranian words for 'poplar', Persian *pad, pada,* Baluchi *paθk, patk,* etc. I fail to see the relevance of 'poplar' here. That it is listed in Pahlavi together with willow as a tree, which like *haδānaēpătā-*, is a soft wood, in no way concerns pomegranate, which has hard wood. Furthermore, Bailey's citation of the second part of the Avestan word as *pātā-* is fallacious; the basic form is *haδānaēpătā-*, with *pāt-* retained in the nominative (and normalized in the Pahlavi transcription), and *-pat-* in other cases showing the common Avestan secondary shortening of unstressed *ā*. Earlier Bailey (1979: 197) had compared Baluchi *paθk,* Kirmani *patk,* and Mazandarani *palak* with Ossetic *fætk'u.* The latter, apart from its semantic difference from 'poplar', is probably of Caucasic origin, as indicated by the termination *-tk'u* (see Abaev 1973: 203), with replacement of the inherited **(ha-)marnā-*. If the analysis is *fæ-tk'u* < **pa-*, cf. perhaps Latin *pom-um?* Alternatively *fætk'u* could be from the ultimate etymon of Hebrew *tappūaḥ*, etc., cf. Ossetic *færæt* 'axe', etc.: Middle Persian *tapar*, etc. I believe that such a metathetic relationship may be found in the Slavic word for 'poplar', on whose problematic PIE antecedent the unobserved Iranian correspondence sheds new light: Old Slavic **topol^* < **potol-*, as also Proto-Iranian **patar-* feminine, nominative **patā* (whence the New Iranian forms cited above), **potol-* was itself dissimilated, like Latin *pōpulus* (and Old Slavic **topol^*, if not directly from **potol-*), from PIE **poptol- or *ptoptol-* (perhaps *'the fluttering', from reduplicative stem of **pet-* 'to fly' and noun formant **-e/ol-*).

§234 For the *-aē-* of *haδānaēpătā-* Bailey reconstructs **-as/-az,* comparing Khotanese *biśśvāraa-* 'high-born, princely', which he reconstructs to Proto-Iranian **visas-puθra-* (*sic*, similarly Bailey 1979: 292). This analysis rests on several assumptions, each unsupportable: (1) That Indo-Iranian **-as* would remain in Proto-Iranian as **-as* before *p-*, rather than become *-ah*, as is ordinarily assumed. This is refuted by the Elamite transcription of the word for 'prince', *misapušas* (literally 'son of the [royal] house'), cf. Bailey (1972: 292). This renders Old Persian **visah pusa-*, where *visah* is genitive of *vis- (viθ-)*. (2) That the Khotanese outcome of Proto-Indo-Iranian **-as* became **-ai*, then **-ē*, then *-ī*. Rather, Proto-Indo-Iranian **-as* became Proto-Iranian **-ah,* which in East Iranian became a fronted simple vowel, cf. already Gathic *-ə̄* in *kə̄* 'who', etc.;

Armenian *sepouh* (with short *e*, rather than *ē*, Middle Iranian *ē*, Old Iranian *ai*), which is hardly from Alan (with Bailey 1979:293), but from Parthian **wisepuhr*, shows Parthian *e* < **-ah*. Khotanese (and Sogdian) have *-i* as the regular outcome of **-ah*, as in the nominative singular of thematic stems; in Khotanese *biśīväraa-* the *-ī* is lengthened under stress at morpheme juncture. It is Younger Avestan, where **-ah* became *-ō* (as apparently in part also Gathic), that is erratic, cf. Avestan **-āh* > *å*. (3) That Avestan *-ō(.)-* at the end of thematic first members of compounds reflects a Proto-Iranian substitution of the thematic vowel *-a-* by the ending of the thematic nominative singular. Rather, as shown by East Middle Iranian compounds, this development occurred within Avestan; it may even be a matter of scholastic orthography. The Digorun Ossetic alternation *dzæbēdur, dzæbōdur* 'mountain goat' probably has nothing to do with **-as/h C-* (cf. Abaev 1958:390-391), let alone with the Avestan developments. Nothing, in fact, supports the alleged alternation of *-aē-* and *-ō(.)-* .

§235 The second element of *haδānaēpātā-* is identical to the past passive participle of the root *pā-* 'to protect, preserve, contain, keep, hold in, hold back', well attested in Avestan and throughout Iranian. The past passive particle was taken over in Armenian with the meaning 'covered', etc.; cf. *oskiapat* 'covered with gold, gold plated', further *patak* 'cover', reflecting an early Parthian form **pātak*, and Armenian has as denominal verb *patem* 'I cover, surround, enclose'. (Bailey [1979: 197] invents for the Armenian words an Iranian root **pat* 'to cover', whence he also derives Shugni *pūθč* 'eyelash', Persian *palk* 'eyelid', etc., which are more likely to be partially sound-symbolic reflexes of **pet-* expressing fluttering and flapping.) As for the *-aē-*, it is simply what it appears to be, the locative of a thematic stem at morpheme juncture, cf. e.g. *raθaēštar-* 'one who stands in a chariot'.

§236 Thus *haδānaēpātā-* would mean 'the (plant) contained in the pomegranate fruit (*haδāna-*)'. Applying this to Flattery's independent equation of the *haδānaēpātā-* plant with *Peganum harmala*, we may compare the colloquial Arabic designation *'umm-ḥarmal* (*imḥarmal*, etc.), literally 'mother of harmel', for 'pomegranate' (§121). It is quite possible that this curious appellation for the pomegranate ultimately derives from Iran, the source of other Arabic lore concerning *Peganum harmala* (e.g. §66, n.5); note especially the likelihood of Arabic *ḥarmal* based on a calque of Iranian *svanta-* (§265). A folkloric view of pomegranate as the matrix/origin/prototype of *Peganum harmala* would have as a corollary *Peganum harmala* as 'contained', i.e. latent, in the pomegranate fruit. Possibly too the term *haδānaēpātā-* may refer not only to the harmel as 'contained', but also to the capsules containing (cf. Armenian *pat, patak*) the harmel seeds, with a complex word play '(having) containers at the thing which is accompanied by seeds' (*haδāna-*, neuter?). It is precisely the many capsules of *Peganum*, with their abundant seeds (30 to 40 per pod), which is strikingly similar to a small pomegranate (reflected also in the Arabic *ḥurraymila, ḥurrmayla*, etc. [§121 n.10]).

§237 The term *haδānaēpātā-* emerges as a kind of priestly kenning, a special ritual designation. One may compare, in the *Vidēvdād*, priestly inventions replacing the ordinary secular designations (which are overtly disdained as belonging to 'people of bad/evil speech/words' (*duž.vacah-*). In *Vidēvdād* 13, against profane *dužaka-* for 'hedgehog', there stands *vaŋhāpara-*, which I take as 'stickleback', from *vaŋhā-* (*F.*3g), glossed by Pahlavi *pušt* 'back', and *-para-* probably related to Greek *περνθ* 'point, needle, quill', Russian *perjat'* 'to pierce', but with *para-* as preposition, perhaps paronomasically 'having a superextensive back'? In *Vidēvdād* 13.2, as against profane *kahrkatāt-* for 'rooster', there stands *parō.darəs-* 'that which sees first'. In these instances the secular terms may have been interpreted as pejorative. Thus *dužaka-* (whence Persian *žūža*, etc.) would have been associated with *duž-* 'bad' (perhaps as *duž-aka-* 'having nasty barbs': *-aka-*) and/or as 'little-bad-thing' and 'bad evil' (*aka-*). While the *kahrka-* of *kahrkatāt-* is represented by Pashto *čirg* 'rooster' (and Persian *kark* 'chicken', etc.), the *-tāt-*, which is the productive suffix forming (feminine) abstract nouns, requires explanation. I suggest that *kahrkatāt-* amounts to 'cluckdom', where *-tāt-* enhances the onomatopoeic quality of *kahrka-*. Thus, via focused magnification of merely potentially pejorative aspects of these ordinary words, they become characterized as words of malice. The "elevated" terms for 'hedgehog' and 'rooster' reflect their position in the priestly world view, i.e. creatures who belong to the world of Good, who combat the forces of Evil (the rooster combats the demon of sloth, and the hedgehog destroys the ant). The opposition of the approved (priestly) words to words of "bad-speaking men" (=ordinary words!) is a dualistic partial recasting of the Indo-European opposition of words of divine language to words of human language. Both oppositions are compatible with a more basic opposition, poetic vs. ordinary language (cf. Toporov 1980: 208 *seq.* with literature).

§238 The poetic traits of metaphor and ambiguity characterize not only *haδānaēpātā-* but also terms for parallel ritual objects. At *Vidēvdād* 8.2 and 18.71, *haδānaēpātā-* is accompanied by the names of two other (fragrant) fuel plants, *vohu.gaona-* and *vohu.kərəti-*. The meaning of the latter is obscure; a possibility is 'having/conferring good praise/glory' (*kərəti-*), but a meaning 'having a good make', apparently equal to 'well made, having a fine shape', would be paralleled by the transparent interpretation of *vohu.gaona-* as 'having good color'; thus Pahlavi *hugōn* preceded by *hukard*. Yet these meanings would be oddly vague as designations of fuel plants. In fact Avestan has a different, more descriptive meaning, 'blackish' (*'blood-colored') for *vohu.-gaona-*, as at *Yasht* 8.58 (Pahlavi *siyā-gōn* 'of black color'), the reference is to sheep. Possibly then *vohu.kərəti-* is 'having a blood-like aspect'? Cf. Schwartz (1982: 195). As with *haδānaēpātā-*, a complex word play seems involved.

§239 The oldest attestations of *haδānaēpātā-*, *Yasna* 3.3 and *Yasna* 22.1, occur with yet another roundabout designation for a ritual object, *gav- jīvyā-* 'living flesh/cow' traditionally understood to designate ordinary *xšvid-* 'milk' (but see §138 n.32 above). The form *jīvyā-* is remarkable for the preservation of *jīv-* as against *jv-*, which is found everywhere else in Avestan (including the orthography of the Gathas), and shows the great antiquity of the ritual phrase. Perhaps the term *haδānaēpātā-* is equally old.

On *pāṭā́-*, *AtharvaVeda* 2.27

§240 Could *haδānaēpātā-* be of Indo-Iranian origin? The question arises from its new identification as another name for *Peganum harmala*, and in consideration of the proposal of W. W. Malandra (1979: 220-224) and M. Stutley (1980:130) that *pāṭā́-* in *AtharvaVeda* 2.27 is *soma*. The meaning of this hapax is unknown. The plant with which it is later identified, *pāṭhā- 'Stephania* (or *Clypea*) *hernandifolia'* is phonemically different, and Malandra (1979:220) rightly looks for a different explanation. Malandra notes a number of parallels between *pāṭā́-* and *soma:* The eagle discovered them both, Indra consumed both, Indra's use of the *pāṭā́-* amulet in overcoming the Asuras, as prototype of human use of it to overcome opponents in disputes, is parallel to Vasiṣṭha's invocation of Indra(-)and(-)Soma to overcome and countercurse his false accusers, *ṚV* 7.104. From *ṚV* 7.104.12, where it is said that *soma* favors the honest and smashes the untrue, Malandra deduces that *soma* was thought to be instrumental, like Varuna, in discriminating truth from falsehood and destroying the liar or perjurer.

§241 One may now bring in some data from the Iranian side. For *soma* as showing forth truth, cf. Flattery's discussion of *haoma* as an ordeal medium (§§147-155), and compare further the invocation of *Haoma* at *Yasna* 10.4 *haiθīmca ašahe xå ahi* 'really thou art the well/source of Truth' with the parallel invocation of Varuṇa, *ṚV* 2.28.5 *ṛdhyā̃ma te varuṇa khā̃m ṛtásya,* cf. Kuiper (1960: 248). Furthermore, *haoma* also was used as an amulet against one's foes in battle (see §73), which matches the statement at *AV* 2.27.4 that Indra wore the *pāṭā́-* on his arm.

§242 The association of the *pāṭā́*-charm with defeat of the enemy in battle also follows from *AV* 2.27.5 'By means of it (the *pāṭā́-*) I shall conquer the enemies, as Indra (conquered) the Sālāvṛkas'. This passage was cited by Kuiper (1960: 251) in supporting his hypothesis that the verbal contest as a reiteration of Indra's primordial battles. Kuiper here has in fact anticipated Malandra's observation of the similarity between the *pāṭā́*-text and the *soma* myth (includ-ing the parallel role of the eagle). But it is Malandra who takes the bold further step and explicitly suggests the identification of *pāṭā́-* with *soma.*

§243 Malandra, focusing on the text's statement that the *pāṭā́-* was dug up by the *sūkará-* (hog or boar) with his snout, ventures to identify the plant as a tuber, since lexicographers attest many names of tubers which begin with *sūkara-* or *varāha-* 'boar'. In view of the boar's fondness for truffles, Malandra suggests that the *pāṭā́-* was a truffle. However, Malandra also holds open an identification of *pāṭā́-* as a mushroom, in view of Buddhist traditions identifying *sūkaramaddava-*, the food (pork?) whose ingestion was held responsible for the Buddha's death. Malandra makes very clear that he is "not among those who are convinced that the ṚgVeda offers evidence that *soma* was a mushroom" (1979:222, cf. 223, lack "strong evidence to support the *soma* = mushroom equation"). Nevertheless, he concludes that if *pāṭā́-* were a truffle, it could then have been a substitute for an earlier mushroom, and thus be admissible as "circumstantial evidence" for Wasson's *soma*-mushroom theory.

§244 The assumption underlying Malandra's approach to the identification of the plant in question is, in itself, a reasonable one: Salient statements of a text have a close relationship with the object which is the focus of that text, and in the instance of an object whose identification is obscure, such statements may be identificatory. This is expectable with regard to descriptive prose but is hardly axiomatic for the poetry of magical charms. As J. Gonda (1949:3) remarks concerning his earlier work on the language of *AtharvaVeda Saṁhitā* 1-7 (cf. also Gonda 1940 and 1975):

> A good number of stylistic peculiarities in Vedic literature, such as alliteration, anaphoric repetition, paronomastic juxtaposition, rhyme and homoioteleuton and other 'figures' must not be considered as ornaments, as stylistic 'embellishments' (at least not primarily), . . . on the contrary, they had another function: in the sacral or ritual *'Sondersprache'* a certain stereotypy in the construction of the sentence (parallelism, etc.), . . . [and] repetition of various kinds, etc. possess a very real and essential expressive value, they intensify the magic power or religious value of the text, have a hallowing effect, render the text solemn.

It is precisely such devices that are the *raison d'ētre* of various "statements" of our Vedic texts, of which the AtharvaVeda is the most explicitly incantatory.

§245 The use of phonic repetition may be illustrated for *AV* 2.27 from the first stanza: (a) *(néc chátruḥ) prā́śam jayā̃ti* '(May not the enemy) win the argument': the last words are echoed by (c) *prā́śam prátiprāśo jahy* 'smash the argument of the arguing opponent', which is repeated as the refrain of the following stanzas, (c) doubly echoes the *prā́ś-*, with the further strong alliteration by *pra-* of *prati-* 'opposed, counter-', and at the end of the line *-prā́śo jahy* echoes *prā́śam jāy-*. The role of phonic factors in producing an entire topic may be illustrated by another AtharvaVedic datum. *AV* 4.85.1, addressed to the apotropaic plant *varaṇā-*, features a play on the name of the plant and the verbal root *v(a)r-* 'to ward off'; more at *AV* 10.3.1-6. But what is more interesting is *AV* 4.7.1, proclaiming the effects of the water, *vār*, of *varaṇāvatī-* 'that which is associated with *varaṇā-'* (probably a river near which the plant grew), as able to 'ward off', *vārayātāi.* The verb is repeated in the recitation, *vāraye* 'I ward off'. Here focus on the water, with *vār-* chosen instead of the alternative common forms *udaka-*, *jala-*, etc.), and on *varaṇāvatī,* instead of address to the plant itself, is phonically motivated. From a viewpoint of magical use of language, extra dimensions of calling forth apotropaic powers are thereby gained.

§246 We may now consider the detail of the *sūkará-* digging up the *pāṭā́.* The phonic aspects after the relevant passage can be best appreciated after an analysis of other aspects of its background as a poetic text. These factors, while essentially heterogeneous, underwent a complex interaction with the phonic factors through the associability of their similar elements. The text in question is thus a result of an interhierarchical convergence of diverse data, formal, structural, and conceptual (I call this convergence "syntropy"):

(1a) A myth of the origin of the use of the plant. The myth specific to *soma* is its being brought by an eagle (*śyená-*, *suparṇá-*) to Indra. This connection of the eagle and the plant *par excellence* explains why, e.g. in *AV* 1.24, addressing the 'dark plant of even color', the first statement is 'the *suparṇá-* that was born in the beginning, you were his gall'. The text goes on to say how the Asurī gave it to the trees for color, and made it a cure for leprosy. (1b) A statement of how the plant was first dug up by a mythological being is a topos in the AtharvaVeda; for example, 4.37.1: 'That which Jamadagni dug up to make his daughter's hair grow, Vitavya has brought here from the dwelling of Asita'; *AV* 4.4.1, 'You, the plant which the Gandharva dug up for Varuṇa when his virility declined, you, who produce erections, do we dig up'. Cf. also 6.109.3. This topos combines the format of origin myth and a statement of digging up the plant for purposive use; note e.g. *AV* 6.136.1 'As a goddess you were born upon the goddess Earth, Plant! We dig you up, O Nitatnī, that you may strengthen the hair'. Cf. *AV* 6.21.1; further 4.7.5-6 and 6.6.8.

(2a) The pig/boar is the rooter, i.e. digger, *par excellence.* (2b) The Boar (sometimes called Emuṣá) is, like the *suparṇá-* (who brings the *soma* that energizes Indra's cosmogonical act), a protological beast. Cf. Kuiper (1960: 251): ". . . this plant . . . is said to have been dug put by a boar with his snout—just as a boar has dug out the earth from the bottom of the cosmic waters before Indra could expand it". The Boar, in fact, was regarded as an avatar of Viṣṇu, but also identified with the cosmogonic god Prajāpati (*Taittirīya Saṁhitā* 7.1.5.1, *Taittirīya Brāhmaṇa* 1.1.3.5, cf. *Śatapatha Brāhmaṇa* 14.1.2.11).

(3a) The pairing of the eagle and the boar as discoverers of the plant makes for a parallelism (3b) which achieves a contrast of items, (3c) themselves complementary, their respective domains of operation, heaven and earth, together indicating a cosmic totality. Cf. the statement in the *Hōm Yasht* that *haoma* grows on the highest mountains and deepest valleys, etc. (§83).

Now the phonic aspect: (4) Of the words for the mythic animals, which included *śyená-*, the primary name of the eagle in the *soma*-myth, and *varāhá-*, the usual word for 'boar' (as against the tame hog), or *Emuṣá-*, as it is called in some texts, the forms *suparṇá-* (which is found instead of *śyená-* in some ṚgVeda texts), and *sūkará-* ('hog, boar', also used of Emuṣa) have detailed phonic similarity, suitable to their being chosen for contrastive/complementary celestial and terrestrial mythical discoverers of the plant:

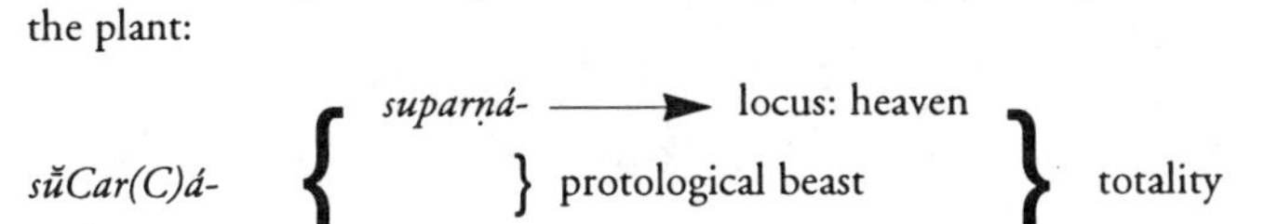

§247 The phonic relationship is foregrounded by the shared initial positions of the animal names, and by the structural parallelism of the rest of their respective lines, *AV* 2.27.2ab:

suparṇás tvā̊nvavindat
sūkarás tvā̊khanan nasā̊

The mantric power of the two lines explains why they recur as the opening of *AV* 5.14, a charm devoted to a nameless plant, which may or may not be the *pāṭā́-*.

§248 If the above analysis is correct, it is likely that the connection of the plant with the eagle was primary in the poet's mind, so there is a good chance that *pāṭā́-* was regarded by the poet as another name for the *soma*-plant (i.e. whichever plant he identified as *soma*); the possibility is increased somewhat by the parallels drawn from Indra's career. Both data may, however, be merely a matter of poetic adoption of material from the *soma*-hymns.

§249 The *pāṭā́*-plant was also treated by M. Stutley (1980:130). Stutley's discussion parallels that of Malandra in several respects, but is more confused. In the midst of the summary of *AV* 2.27, she remarks: "The *pāṭā́ (Clypea hernandifolia)* has a bitter root and is much used in India as a medicament." Despite this identification (where *pāṭā́* is written instead of *pāṭhā*), she returns to *AV* 2.27: "It was said to have been discovered (or seen) by an eagle and then [*sic*] dug up by a pig, which suggests that it may have been a truffle." Stutley even goes on to note that according to *Kauśikā-sūtra* 38.18-21, 'He ties on his arm an amulet of *pāṭā́* root and wears a wreath of seven of its leaves'. Clearly this seven-leaved wreath (*mālam saptapalāśim, Kauśikā-sūtra* 38.21) contradicts the identification of *pāṭā́* as a truffle (or any tuber or mushroom). The impression that *pāṭā́* was conceived of as sappy (i.e. containing chlorophyll) is conveyed by *AV* 2.271: *arasā́n kṛṇv oṣadhe* 'make them [the opponents] sapless, O plant!'. Note also that *Kauśikā-sūtra* 38.18 with Dārila's commentary (for which see M. Bloomfield 1886: 481) indicates that the *pāṭā́* has a root which the plant's user chews (*pāṭāmālāṁkhadann*) when he speaks.

§250 This further shows that the *pāṭā́* may not actually have been expected to be consumed. The oral application of the plant was here probably connected with efficacy of speech, just as binding the plant onto the arm (as attributed to Indra) was thought to confer victorious strength. For the latter detail may be compared the binding on of the *haoma* amulet (§73).[8]

§251 If, as must remain uncertain, *pāṭā́-* was a (magic?) name for some plant regarded as the *soma*-plant (used in a manner other than pressed), then a relationship with Avestan *haδānaēpātā-* is conceivable, but rather improbable. Unless, as is very dubious, the term started as Indo-Iranian **pātā-*, of unclear meaning ('protection' is formally unlikely), one would have to posit a truncation of the original compound. Such a truncation would also be a difficulty for regarding *pāṭā́-* as inspired by an Iranian priestly term, a notion which intrinsically has nothing to recommend it. Finally there is the *ṭ* for expected *t;* a spontaneous palatalization is possible but not ideal. Etymologically *pāṭā́-* could be partially inspired by *pāṭhā-*, and partially by the root *paṭ* 'to split, to sunder', cf. *paṭu-* 'acute, keen, trenchant', *vākpaṭu-* 'eloquent, successful in speech'. In any event, *pāṭā́-* has no real relevance for the identification of the *soma*-plant.[9]

Avestan *barəsman-*, Indic *barhís-* (see §§123-126)

§252 Avestan *barəsman-* (Pahlavi and Persian *barsom*) has been constantly compared with Vedic *barhís-*. Both words refer to pieces of vegetation which are used ritually in connection with offerings; both are said to be strewn (*stṛ-/star-*) and, since *barəsman-* goes back to Proto-Iranian **barzman-*, both are reconciled by an Indo-Iranian root **bharźh*. The same root also furnishes in Iranian a formally identical cognate of *barhís-*, Old Iranian **barziš-* (Avestan *barəziš-*), Persian *bāliš* 'cushion, pillow', which accords with the fact that *barhís-* grass was used as a cushion upon which the gods were thought to accept the offerings.

§253 These facts have given rise to an assumption that has prevailed among most commentators on the subject, that *barəsman-* originally had the same meaning as *barhís-*, both referring to a cushion of foliage; see most recently P. Thieme (1957: 71-75). The conclusion that the meaning 'cushion' is basic has also lead to a preference for deriving *barhís-/barəziš-* and *barəsman-* from PIE **bhelǵh-* 'to blow up, swell' whence Old Prussian *balsinis,* Serbo-Croatian *blàzina* 'cushion, pillow' as against derivation from the Indo-Iranian root **bh(a)rźh-* 'to make high'. For these views see Mayrhofer (1956-1976: II, 415-416). It will now be shown that these conclusions are fallacious.

§254 The provision of foliage as a seat for the gods is a custom of Indo-European origin. This institution reflects a period when grasses were ordinarily heaped up to form cushions. The strewing of grasses for this purpose was probably originally designated by the PIE verb **ster(H)-*, whose close association with long, twiggy grasses may be seen from Latin *strāmen,* English *straw* (although the same verb could be used of the spreading of cloth upon which to lie). In *barhís-*, precisely because of its ritual context, there is a preservation of the early material realia, grasses employed as a cushion; in *barəziš-, bāliš* there is generalization of the function served by the grasses, 'cushion', whence the development 'pillow', just as 'cushion' is designated in Old Indic by another derivative of the root, *upabárhaṇa-* (cf. Khwarezmian *βžnyk* 'pillow' < **barzanaka-*, Parachi *bāna-pāī* 'pillow' reflecting **barz-n-*, etc.).

§255 These data are ideally suited by derivation from a root meaning 'to heap up'. This definition suits the meaning not only of Indo-Iranian **bh(a)rźh-*, but also its Indo-European etymon **bherǵh-;* from 'heap up' one not only gets the very numerous Indo-Iranian forms for 'high, elevated object', matched in Germanic by Old English *beorg* 'tumulus, hill', German *Berg* 'mountain', etc., but also words referring to solidity, e.g. Old Indic *bṛṁhati, (pari)bṛḍha-,* Latin *forctis, forctus,* as well as the sense of 'cover over' found in the Saka Iranian Ossetic *æmbærzun*, Khotanese *vūḍa-* 'covered', and matched by German *bergen,* etc. By contrast Old Prussian *balsinis* and Serbo-Croatian *blàzina* refer originally to a stuffed or inflated bag (i.e. the modern type of pillow), cf. especially Slovenian *blazína* 'pillow, handball, football'. Against the derivation of

8 Regarding the 'binding' of *haoma* in *Yasht* 14.57 it may be noted that since *nivizaiti* is a hapax for which Bartholomae could furnish no cognates, his translation 'attaches (*ansteckt*)' seems based solely on the context, which involves the *haoma* being borne on one's person during battle. However, further evidence from Iranian is now available. Bailey (1979:387) brings *ni-viz-* together with Avestan *a-vaēza-* *'unbound (by sin)', comparing Khotanese *vīysāna-* 'a binding', and also Baltic and Slavic forms meaning 'to plait, to bind' from PIE **wei-ǵ(h)-*. I have furnished similar comparisons from Baltic, etc., venturing also to explain Av. **Višta-aspa-* 'having bound/tied horses', parallel to *Yuxtāspa-* and *Hitāspa-* (Schwartz 1980a:126). I hope there to have met the objection to my earlier, similar explanation for *Vištāspa-* (Schwartz 1985b:659), recently voiced by Mayrhofer (1985:327), who asks whether one can still conceive any alternative to the equation with ṚgVedic *víṣita- áśva-* forwarded by O. Szemerényi and refined by J. Narten. Note especially pp. 581-582 in the article of Insler to which I last refer, where the derivation of *víṣita-* from **sHto-* is refuted in favor of PIE **-sito-*. The latter form would also necessarily be continued in Av. *Hitāspa-*. In Schwartz (1985b:659) I merely meant to range *Jāmāspa- (Dājāmāspa-)* with *Hitāspa-*, *Yuxtāspa-*, and *Vištāspa-* semantically, not formally; *Jāmāspa-* (on which see now Schwartz 1980a:125; 1986:345, 347, and 389) is of course not a past participle.

9 For *pāṭā́*, see now Das (1987), who has treated the matter in detail. From the additional AtharvaVedic material Das has brought to bear upon its identification, the *pāṭā́* is a leafy plant with "hooks" (Das 1987:36).

the Indo-Iranian words in question from the same etymon as the Balto-Slavic words for 'pillow' is the fact that forms like Old Indic *upabárhaṇa-* show an inner-Indo-Iranian formation from a still productive verbal root. There is no evidence for an Indo-Iranian verbal root **bharźh-* 'to swell up'. In fact there is no evidence for the latter as a verbal root even in PIE. The various forms from Celtic, Germanic, Baltic, and Slavic given by Pokorny (1959-1969:125-126) under **bhelǵh-* 'schwellen' point only to an old noun for 'inflatable animal skin, leather bag'. The exception, Old Irish *bolgaim* 'I swell' alongside *bolg* 'bag', should therefore be a denominative, parallel to English *bulge,* etc., ultimately from Gallic *bulga* 'leather bag'. In place of the alleged verb **bhelǵh-* I suggest a nominal formation in *-ǵh-* from **bhel-* 'to blow up'.

§256 A vestige of the institution of "strewing" a heap of grass as a seat for the gods may have been preserved in Western Iran; Herodotus I. 152 reports that the Magi deposited the sacrificial victim upon tender grasses, but this may be due to a projection of Greek ritual ideas upon the Iranians. There is no support for the theorization that *barəsman-* originally referred to vegetation used as a cushion. Since the root means 'to heap up' without necessarily referring to a cushion, *barəsman-* need merely refer to some heap of vegetation whose laying out would be indicated by the verb *star-;* see above on English *straw* and Latin *strāmen.* The formation of *barəsman-* (**bherǵh-men-*) would in fact be parallel to that of *strāmen.*

§257 As it happens, there exists possible evidence for a Middle Persian scholastic retention of the original sense of *barəsman-* as 'heap (of vegetation)', in *Pahlavi Vidēvdād* 18.3. In a list of tokens of the priestly office, Avestan *urvarā* 'vegetation' is glossed as *barsom,* which is further glossed *hast kē gōwe(n)d* 'there are those who say'. The unclear word cannot, from its context, be *kwtyn'* (i.e. *kūdīn* 'mallet, sledgehammer' [also Persian]) as at *Nērangistān* 129.5, 17, 18 (*bis*), 22, 23, 29, nor its homograph at *Nērangistān* 172.25, *kntgr* (elsewhere *kntgl*), i.e. *kantigr, kantīr* 'quiver'. The second letter, between the unambiguous *k* and *t,* may in theory be *w, r, n,* or *O* (ideographic *'ayin*). In practice only *w* is likely, since [r] is spelled *l* in less common words, and, since *[kVnVt-] is dubious, Old Iranian *[nt] would appear as Pahlavi **nd,* not *nt,* and *O* is excluded, as the word is obviously not an ideogram. The sequence *kwt-* suggests **kōt (*kōd),* whence Armenian *koit* 'heap', Persian *kōd* 'heap of grain, collection'. The last three letters are ambiguous; if *-gwn,* read *kōdgōn* (or, less likely, if *-yn',* read *kōdēn*) *'like a heap'? A more satisfying possibility is a scribal error for simple **kwt,* with a false start for **gwb-* of the *gōwēnd* which follows; then we would simply read *kōd.* We would thus emerge from this analysis with a scholium for *barəsman-,* 'heap (of plant matter)'.

§258 In any event, the pressing of *haoma* would require a preparatory accumulation of stems. The identification of these heaps with the *barəsman-* would explain the frequent mention of strewing the *barəsman-* as a specific act of worship in the *Yasna* ceremony, and accords with the other Avestan references to this act. The "strewing" of the *barəsman- (*barzman-)* would be comparable, in name and action, to the "strewing" of the **barziš-,* the grasses serving as a cushion for the offerings. This circumstance may have had a role in the disappearance of the latter institution in Avestic religion, what with the greater importance of the *haoma* ritual.

3
NAMES FOR HARMEL

Iranian **svanta 'Peganum harmala'* (see §§57-64)

§259 The Proto-Iranian form **svanta- (=*su̯anta-)* 'sacred' must be reconstructed as the foremost name for harmel. This is especially significant in view of the fact that the representatives of this form in modern Iranian languages are the sole reflexes of the ancient word for 'sacred', apart from compound fossils of ancient fixed phrases (i.e. the month name, Persian *Isfandarmuδ* [of which *isfand* is a modern abbreviation] = the Avestan goddess Spəntā Armaiti, and the word for 'sheep', Persian *gusfand,* etc., Avestan *gav- spənta-*). Thus harmel was 'the sacred (plant)' *par excellence,* as Flattery notes. This phytonymic evidence in itself points *a priori* to the conclusion that the *haoma*-plant is *Peganum harmala.* In fact *spənta-* actually is adjective of *haoma-* at *Vīsperad* 9.3. The etymon is reflected by a variety of forms whose phonological characteristics show independent evolution, rather than borrowing from Persian *isfand, sipand* or the like. Here may be cited the vocalism of Pashto *spānd,* and cf. the interesting *spalanai* 'harmel-seed', which must be explained as the expected Pashto outcome of earlier **spadān-,* itself dissimilated (via **spand(δ)ān-*
) from an ancient compound **spanta-δāna-(ka) < *svanta-dāna-*); the vocalism of Oroshori *səpān,* as well as its development **-nt- > *-nd- > -n-*
; and contrastively the lack of voicing of *-nt-* in Baluchi *sipantān* (old plural, or, like Pashto *spalanai,* Ishkashmi *səpandona < *svanta-dāna-* *'harmel-seed', with expected East Iranian *sp*) reflecting Proto-Iranian *svanta-; isfand* itself has the characteristically Persic *sf* (as against *sp*), reflecting Proto-Iranian **svanta-,* cf. Persian *gusfand* alongside *guspand,* Avestan *gao.spənta-* 'sheep' (*sacral, i.e. ritual, bovine), etc. An alternative Persic reflex of **sv (*su̯)* is *s* (cf. Old Persian *asa-,* Avestan *aspa-,* Sanskrit *asva-*) with **svanta-* giving Old Persian **santa-,* reflected in Kuhgiluya *gusend* (Lum'a 1960:180), Kumzari *"gosan"* (Thomas 1930) 'sheep', and Armenian *sandaramet* representing the name of the earth divinity (=Avestan *Spəntā Armaiti;* Persian *Isfandarmuδ;* Cappadocian Σονδαρα may have Σο- from **sva-*). Thus one may expect Persic forms for *'Peganum harmala'* from **santa-.*

§260 The latter may well be the source of Lari *sandolos* 'the *esfand* which is placed on fires' (Eqtedārī 1955: 136) and *sondoros "esfand"* (Bastakī 1980); Syriac *sndryg* 'harmel seed'; and Persian *ṣandaldāna* (Persian-Arabic *ṣandal-dānaj*) 'harmel-seed'. The termination of the Lari form is curious. It is tempting to reconstruct **alus/arus* = Middle Persian *arus* 'white' (Ossetic *urs* 'white', Avestan *auruša-,* Proto-Indo-European **Elu-so-*); one could compare Pahlavi *arus tāg* 'the white twig' of Wahman (above §87 n.24), the 'white *isfand'* (*sipand-i siped*) of the Islamic pharmacopoeias, and even the Pahlavi *hōm ī spēd* 'white *haoma'.* But this combination is unlikely. It is not white *esfand* which is indicated for the Lari form; rather "the *esfand* placed on fires" should refer without color distinction to harmel seeds, the meaning found for Syriac *sndryg* and Persian *ṣandaldāna.* Moreover all three words are formally connected: Syriac *sndryg* (for **sndrg* = Middle Persian **sandarag*?) is inseparable from Greek ςανδαρᾶκθ 'sandarac' (the tree *Callitris quadrivalvus* or *Tetraclinis articulata,* whose resin is used for varnish and incense), just as Lari *sandolos, sondoros* calls for comparison with Perso-Arabic *sandarūs* 'sandarac', *sandalus* 'the resin of *Trachylobium Hernemannianum'* (sold in Indian bazaars). The *-l-* of *sandolos* (and *sandalus*) also necessitates comparison with Perso-Arabic *ṣandal* (< Sanskrit *candana-*), properly 'sandalwood', found again, oddly, with *-dāna* 'seed', in reference to harmel. Note also Mandaic *sandlus, sandrus* compared by Drower and Macuch (1963) with Perso-Arabic and Syriac *sandarūs* 'sandarac' but glossed as 'sandalwood' (the form occurs with *riha* 'incense'). One may assume an ancient Persic **santa-* giving **sand* 'harmel' with special reference to the seeds, burned as an apotropaic incense, and used for preparing a dye. This **sand* would recall *sandarus* 'sandarac', also an incense and dye-stuff, and further the fumigant sandalwood, *ṣandal,* with confusion of **sand* with each, and further interaction between *sandarus* and *ṣandal,* as independently probably also Mandaic *sandlus* (*sandrus*). The form *sandalūs* for 'resin of *Trachylobium Hernemannianum'* would derive its name similarly. The presence of such a form in Lari is probably connected with commerce via Bandar ʿAbbās.

§261 Forms in modern Iranian languages which preserve gender, such as Pashto *spānda* and Oroshori *səpān* in the east and Vafsi-Ashtiyani *esbanda* in the west, would regularly reflect for 'harmel' an old feminine **svantā-* (see Morgenstierne 1952: 206). This would disagree with the masculine gender of *haoma-*. In theory, the feminine gender could be a secondary development; for example, for 'finger', **angušta*, feminine, is reflected by forms in various modern Iranian languages (*ibid.* 205), but Old Iranian actually had masculine *angušta-*, attested in Avestan, in agreement with Sanskrit *aṅguṣṭha-*; note Morgenstierne's account of the transformation of masculine collective plurals to feminine singular (*ibid.* 204). But in view of the wide distribution of the **-ā-* feminine in the word for 'harmel', it is likely the Proto-Iranian form was feminine as well. The feminine gender predominates for plant names in later Iranian (see the examples in Morgenstierne 1952) and seems to reflect an Old Iranian tendency; cf. such clear Avestan feminines as *hapərəsī-* 'juniper' and *haδānaēpātā-*. As an adjective **svantā-* agreed with *urvarā-* 'plant', and as a noun may have been an abbreviation of the phrase **svantā urvarā.* Agreement with *urvarā-* may have had a role in the general tendency for plant names to be feminine.

§262 Perhaps the gender difference between **svantā-* and *haoma-* arose because **svantā-* exclusively designated a plant, while *haoma-* referred to a plant, a god, and the juice pressed from the plant. In *haoma-* (=Proto-Iranian **hauma-*, Old Indic *soma-*) we have an action noun in **-ma-*, a suffix which in both Old Indic and Old Iranian is typically masculine and frequently refers to ritual objects and institutions. Other examples are Old Indic *stoma-*, Avestan *staoma-* 'hymn' from *stau-* 'to praise'; Old Indic *homa-* 'oblation' from Old Indic *h(a)u-* 'to pour'; Avestan *aēsma-* (Old Indic *idhma-*) 'fuel' from **aidh(-s-)* 'to burn'; Avestan *maēsma-* 'urine (used for ritual purification)' from Old Iranian **maiz-* 'to urinate'. Thus properly Old Indic *soma-*, Old Iranian **hauma-* from Indo-Iranian **sau-*, Iranian **hau-* 'to press (in a mortar)' = 'that which is pressed', and **hauma-* is the product of the sacred plant, or the plant itself, or the god embodying both—all three used inseparably from the ritual pressing of the plant. Hence **hauma-* was not a general name for the plant, but for one ritual manifestation of it, whose institutional naming has a different basis from the more general term, *svanta-*. Since our texts refer to the plant in the context of the pressing, it is Avestan *haoma-* (and Vedic *soma-*) which they employ.[1]

§263 Some derivatives of **svanta-* require explanation. Tajik has conservative *sipand, sipandən* (= Persian *sipand, sipandān;* the second form, combining **sipand-ān* plural/collective of *sipand,* and *sipand-dān* 'harmel seed'), but also has the colloquial *sipandar* (Andreev 1953: 50, 53, 237), cf. also Wakhi *spandr* (alongside *spand*), Shughni *ispandur,* Shina *spandur,* Burushaski *supándur* (differently Berger 1956:14). Possibly *sipand* interacted with *kundur* '(frank-)incense', giving *sipandur,* then *sipandar.* In some forms of *ispand/sipand, p* became *m* under the influence of *n,* note in Persic Lenjān-i Tāt *esmand* (§68 n.7); and, if borrowed from Eastern Persian, *isman* in Balti, and compare Kirghiz *adraspan, adrašman.*

§264 I would explain the form *sepaxt 'Peganum harmala'* occurring in one of the dialects of Bashkardi (according to a private communication to me by I. Gershevitch, who did field research in this Persic language) as a blend of *sepand* (represented elsewhere in Bashkardia according to Dr. Gershevitch) and **sepext* < Middle Persian *spixt* 'sprouting/blooming'; cf. Khotanese *spāta-* 'flower' < *spixta-;* further Pahlavi *spēg* translating Avestan *fraspara γa-* 'bloom (of *haoma*)'.

Arabic *ḥarmal* and its Old Berber equivalent (see §53)

§265 In the form γουρμᾶ attributed by Dioscurides to the "Africans" (Ἄφροι), under which Dioscuridean designation early Berber forms are uniquely attested, I recognize **ḥurma* as the Old Berber prototype of modern *(i)urmi, awerma,* etc. *'Ruta chalepensis, Ruta graveolens'* (for which see above, Table 2). The Dioscuridean form is therefore of interest for the chronology of the general disappearance of **ḥ* in Berber. But it is not likely that the relationship of the Berber and Arabic words is due to a common origin in Afro-Asiatic; the absence of comparable words for harmel in the indigenous languages of Africa, and the lack of clear cognates in Semitic for Arabic *ḥarmal* (Dioscurides, who attributes ὑρμαλᾶ to the "Syrians", may well have confused Arabs and Syrians), the Iranian area as the likely center for the diffusion of harmel, and considerations of linguistic geography, make it probable that **ḥurma* represents a borrowing from Arabic. Since Arabic *ḥarmal* does not seem to continue an old Semitic plant name, one would seek an Arabic etymology. The root *ḤRM 'sacer esse, sacratum esse'* yields *ḥaram* and *ḥurma* 'sacred, sacred thing' (which would be a calque of Iranian *svanta-* 'harmel' = 'sacred', see §§259-264). *Ḥaram* and/or *ḥurma* would then be influenced by the names of the botanically kindred *Zygophyllum simplex* L., *jarmal, qarmal* (Migahid 1978). These are formed like *xardal* 'mustard', *ḥanẓal* 'colocynth', with the formant *-l* common in Arabic plant names. In fact names for *Zygophyllum* species occur without the formant: *qurma* (with vocalism like that of Arab *ḥurma* 'sacred thing'), and, more significantly, *ḥarm 'Z. simplex'* and *'Z. decumbens'.* In the latter we may recognize a confusion of *'Zygophyllum'* with *'Peganum harmala',* for *ḥ* does not ordinarily alternate with *j* or *q* (whereas a *j/q* alternation is possible, since both *j* and *q* are pronounced dialectally as *g*), and there is nothing 'sacred' about *Zygophyllum* species, weeds much resembling harmel used marginally for camel fodder. In *ḥarm* one may therefore recognize an old form for *ḥarmal* lacking the *-l.* This makes it possible that the Old Berber **ḥurma* is borrowed from an Arabic form without *-l* (Arabic **ḥurma,* like *qurma,* or with Berber *u* < *a* because of the labial *m*), rather than with early dissimilatory loss of *-l.* The Arabic triconsonantal form would also confirm the derivation from 'sacred'. A loan translation would have arisen under early Persian-Arabic bilingualism. The calque would be paralleled by the later Turkish calque *yüzerlik = sadāb,* see §280. Eilers (1974:126) compares the formation of Arabic *ḥarmal : ḥaram* ("Tabu") to that of Hebrew *karmel : kerem* 'vineyard', with the remark that *ḥarmal : ḥaram* shows parallel semantic development (semantisch gleichentwickelt) to Persian *isfand* "Raute") from Old Iranian *spənta-* 'holy'.

Egyptian πνουβοε̈ (see §52)

§266 In MSS of Dioscurides the name of an Egyptian plant, πνουβοε̈ appears after Latin **ruta hortensis* (or *montana*) and is followed by "Syrian" ὑρμαλᾶ and βθςαςᾶ the latter forms indicate that the reference is to wild rue (*Peganum harmala*), rather than to garden rue, and should therefore occur under the entry π῾ήγανον ἥριον rather than the preceding π῾ήγανον κῆπα ῾ν in the MSS edited by Wellmann. The form πνουβοε̈ is to be analysed as *(?)π-,* representing the Ancient Egyptian masculine article, and the word for 'gold', Ancient Egyptian *nb(w),* Coptic *noub.* This in turn furnishes the identity of the hitherto mysterious plant *nbw* occurring in the late Berlin Museum Papyrus 3027, K 7, 5-6. The text has most recently been treated in H. Grapow, H. von Deines, *et al.* (1958: 5, 504 [hieroglyphic text], 4:1, 1958, 293 [translation]): 'Ein anderes (Heilmittel): *ʿḫmw* (Blätterzweige) der *nbw*-Pflanze;

[1] Other harmel names with specialized religious significance may be reflected in modern vernaculars; e.g. Lurī *dēništ* 'harmel' may well be a form based on Avestan *daēnā,* Middle Persian *dēn* 'The Religion' (or 'Vision'? 'Consciousness'?). If the form is of Old Iranian provenience, one of many possible etymologies would be with second member of compound **-yašta-, *-yašti-* (or **-išti-*), hence 'pertaining to worship to/for/in accord with the *daēnā*'.

werde zerkleinert in einem Hin-Gefäss, werde veranlasst, das (das Kind) es trinkt'. The name *nbw/(π̃)νουβοε̃* 'golden' would be parallel to the Azari Turkish epithet *altun* for *Peganum harmala,* and Avestan *zāiri-* 'yellowish, gold-colored', a chief epithet of *haoma,* and the less common *zairi.gaona-* 'yellowish, yellow-green' (see §77). The sacral term *zāiri-,* it may be added, seems to be the etymon of Baluchi *zirаγ 'Ruta graveolens',* which should be added to the material on *Ruta* as ritual replacement of harmel (see §139).

§267 Twelfth century Coptic names for 'rue' (Arabic *saδāb*) are (Ibn Kalb *apud* Budge 1928) *bašouš* 'rue' (< Syrian *baššūšā* 'harmel'); **kanon* 'garden rue' (< **pikanon* = **π̃ηανον,* with metanalysis via the masculine article *pi-*); *emtotf* and *kefrios* (=*saδāb jabalī* 'mountain rue').

§268 The identification of Egyptian *nbw* as *Peganum harmala* on the basis of Dioscurides was independently made by Terence DuQuesne of the Psychopharmacology Research Committee, London, as he kindly informed Flattery and myself (letters of April 24, 1982 and May 8, 1984). DuQuesne further links *nbw* with *nbyt* to which the Papyrus Ebers 852 assigns an Eastern origin.

Greek *μ§λυ* (see §52 n.10)

§269 There is no support for Benveniste's (1929) view that Plutarch's *ἥμφμι* pounded in a mortar was something other than *haoma-*. The mixture with wolf's blood would suffice to characterize it as a *daēvic* offering, dualistically distinguished from *haoma* prepared in the usual manner for offerings to the "orthodox" divinities. Thus, rather than identifying *ἥμφμι* with the botanically obscure Greek *ὤμφμε̃Ÿ* and further Syriac *humāmā,* Arabo-Persian *humāma,* I suggest that *ἥμφμι* is a dittography of sorts, brought about by correcting the false start *ομ* to *φμι* (for**῞μι,* Middle Persian *hōm(-),* with the false start left unstruck, as frequently). The form *(ἥμ)φμι* would show the same pattern of integration as other Greek plant names of exotic origin (*κμμι, ςςελι, πἔπερι, ςε̃ναπι*).

§270 It is quite possible that *μ§λυ,* given by Dioscurides as the name of harmel in Cappadocia and Galatia, may have served as the origin of the mythical plant of the Odyssey. Harmel's reputation as a magical plant may have come to Asia Minor (and ultimately from the Iranian heartland); cf. above on its medico-magical use in Egypt. Possibly then the connection of *μλ̃υ* with Hermes may be due to the similarity of *ρ̃μς* with Semitic variants of Arabic *ḥarmal,* cf. Dioscurides' "Syrian" *ὑρμαλᾶ.* Note also in this connection the name *hermesias* given by Pliny for a Magian preparation which quite likely contained *Peganum harmala,* as Flattery indicates (§83 n.23). The connection with Hermes also suits the psychotropic (and psychopompic) "speediness" of the drug (cf. the various connections of *Peganum harmala* and words for 'swift' discussed in §64 n.3). Acquaintance with the narcotic potential of the plant would explain the later attested use of the name *μ§λυ* for the sleepy nightshade, *Withania somnifera,* but note Greek *μφλε̃Ÿ* 'weak, feeble, dull' (also used of the intellect). If the name *μ§λυ* originated in an indigenous Indo-European language of Asia Minor and already there referred to the psychotropic nature of *Peganum harmala,* then it would be related to Armenian *mol, molor, moli* 'raving, mad, insane' (cf. Tomaschek 1894: 27-28); the latter would be also paralleled by Egyptian Arabic *mogannana (mujannana)* 'that which drives mad' = 'harmel' (Ducros 1930). One may note here the likely relationship of Syriac *šabbārā,* Mandaic *šambra,* with the root *ŠBR* 'be childish, foolish, stupid', *šaβrā* 'childishness, folly, stupidity'; thus harmel would be named from inducing foolish behavior, cf. Brockelmann (1928: 754). Finally, from Anatolia again, cf. Turkish *mahmur çiçei* 'bloom of sleepy languidness (as from intoxication)'.

§271 Greek *μ§λυ* for a kind of garlic may have its meaning from *μφλε̃ωα* 'garlic', under the influence of *μ§λυ;* the association of garlic with *Peganum harmala* may have been effected by their shared apotropaic attribution. There is little to recommend the oft-claimed connection of *μλ̃υ* with Sanskrit *mūla-,* the usual word for 'root'.

Names for harmel in al-Bīrūnī's *Kitāb al-Ṣaydana* (see §54 n.13)

§272 The form *dwpw* could be an attempt to render in the Arabo-Persian script some Indic vernacular derivative of Sanskrit **dhūpa-* 'incense, fumigant'. In this event *hmlw* would be a misreading, although its resemblance to *hwm* = *hōm* (and to *ḥrml*!) is striking, and the general superiority of the Arabic version must also be taken into account. Possibly there was a conflation of two words. The texts of Bīrūnī's *Ṣaydana* also provide material for the word for harmel in the medieval language of Sanjar (in eastern Syria). The Persian text (Or. 5849) gives the Sanjari name as *ʾsbrw thlk* (in variant MSS: *ʾsbw nhlk, ʾspr thlk;* Sotoudeh and Afshar 1973:225), while the Arabic text has *ʾsbry thlk* (Said and Elakie 1973: 1545) and has (as do some Persian MSS) instead of · *Sanjarī* the erroneous *Sijzī* (as if = Persian *sagzī,* the language of Sijistān, Sīstān). The first part of the name should represent a vernacular equivalent of Syriac *šabbārā,* Mandaic *šambra;* hence **ʾšbr* = **əšbar* = Syriac **/šbar/* (construct state)?[2]

§273 The phrase *ʿrzʾd mγwšy* given in the unique Arabic MS of al-Bīrūnī's *Kitāb al-Ṣaydana* as the Syriac for *hawm al-majūs* must be corrupt. I propose Syriac **ʿrtnʾ *dmγwšy*= *ʿarṭānā da-m(ə)γūšē; ʿarṭānā* and allied forms are glossed in Arabic lexica of Syriac as *buxūr maryam* (see Payne-Smith 1879-1901:2, 2990). The latter gloss brings **ʿarṭānā da-m(ə)γūšē* 'cyclamen of the Magians' into line with Arabic *hawm al-majūs* '*haoma* of the Magians', itself sometimes identified with *buxūr maryam,* as Flattery notes. As for the latter identification, it may be explained from an association of "Magian" with "sun-worshipper" (i.e. *āftāb-parast*) as the Persian name of the marigold. It is thus probably in reference to this plant that *buxūr maryam* 'Mary's fragrance' originally glossed *hawm al-majūs.*

§274 Quite possibly *buxūr maryam* first meant *'Cyclamen europaeum',* while *'Calendula officinalis'* was originally designated *šajara(tu) maryam* 'Mary's plant', with subsequent confusion of names. Cf. Middle Low German *marienblome* and Middle Dutch *marienbloemkijn* 'Mary's flower' = English *marigold* (*'Mary's gold'), attesting an interesting correspondence of Eastern and Western botanical folklore. For *buxūr* 'fragrance' in the Arabic name of *Cyclamen europaeum,* cf. Syriac (from Middle Persian) *āδarbōy* 'fire-fragrance' = *ʿarṭānīθā 'Cyclamen europaeum'.*

Persian *sudāb/sadāb* (see §§53, 127, 132)

§276 The form *sudāb 'Ruta graveolens'* has hitherto lacked an etymology. As a preliminary to clarifying the origin of the word, it may be noted that the inscrutable initial syllable should have not had *u,* which was favored by Classical Persian lexicographers and continued in the predominant modern Tehrani pronunciation *sodāb,* but rather *a.* An older vocalism *sadāb* is indicated by (1) the Pahlavi spelling *stʾp* rather than **swtʾp;* (2) the Arabic form *saδāb,* which probably represents the Sasanian pronunciation (in confirmation of the Pahlavi spelling); (3) the vocalization *sadāb (saδāb)* in early New Persian, evidenced by the vocalization in Abū Manṣūr ibn al-Muwaffaq (c. 950 C.E.) (Bahmanyār and Maḥjūbī Ardakanī 1967), and etymologies and puns involving *ṣad āb* 'a hundred waters', in al-Bīrūnī (*Kitāb al-Ṣaydana: s.v. fijan,* and in Rūdakī (discussed

[2] Note the spellings and vocalizations of vernacular forms in Payne Smith (1879-1901:2, 4043): *šawrā, šəβārā, šaβrē, šəβarē(?), šaβrānē,* at least some of which probably mean 'wick' rather than 'harmel'. The spelling *šmrʾ* given there is relevant for the Mandaic form. The relationship tosuch Syriac names for harmel as *basbāsā, baššāšā, bišbaš, biššā,* etc., is not clear.

below); (4) twelfth or thirteenth century Armenian *satap/sadab,* from the Persian, and (5) Turkish *sedef,* a colloquial modification of the Persian form along usual patterns (cf. Persian *čirkāb* 'bilge' > Turkish *çirkef*); (6) *sedōw* in the Zardoshti speech of Yazd and Kerman, which may be regarded as an independent West Iranian form. Unlike *šabān,* Pahlavi *šp'n,* which expanded at the expense of the older vocalism **šubān* < Old Iranian **fšu-pāna-* (example provided in a letter [May 10, 1979] by Professor H. W. Bailey), *sudāb* appears to have expanded at the expense of *sadāb.* Motivations for the change *sadāb* > *sudāb* will be discussed below.

§277 While *Ruta graveolens* was introduced into the Near East from the Greek territory (where it was known as πήγανον, whence the Semitic "rue" words [see Table 2]), there is no non-Iranian word from which *sadāb* (etc.) can be derived. *Sadāb* should thus be of Iranian origin. In view of the common exchange of words for *'Ruta graveolens'* and *'Peganum harmala'* (for which see the data in Berber and Coptic, above, §265), it is plausible that *sadāb* originally was a name for harmel. This is borne out by a verse attributed by Classical Persian lexicographers to Rūdakī (tenth century C.E.). The lexicographers cite the verse in connection with a noun *sudāb* supposedly meaning 'strength' (i.e. = *quvvat, tavānī, qudrat),* as follows:

agar sudāb bi-kārand u az tu yād kunand
sudāb-i mardī dar tan fuzūn šavad zi sudāb.

The verse would then mean, 'If they plant *sudāb* and remember you (or, memorialize you), masculine *strength (*sudāb-i mardī*) will grow in the body from the *sudāb'.* Now, apart from this verse, there is no evidence for *sudāb* (or the like) 'strength', which would moreover be etymologically inexplicable. Nor is it apparent how *'Ruta'* could be named from 'strength,' or vice versa. Moreover, if one follows the traditional reading and interpretation of the verse, the word play on *sudāb* would be very heavy-handed.

§278 If however one replaces *sudāb* in the first hemistich and at the end of the second hemistich by the older form of that plant name, *sadāb,* and by two words, *ṣad āb,* at the beginning of the second hemistich, one gets:

agar sadāb bi-kārand u az tu yād kunand
ṣad āb-i mardī dar tan fuzūn šavad zi sadāb.

'If one plants *sadāb* and remembers you, a hundred fluids of masculinity (*ṣad āb-i mardī*) will grow in the body from the *sadāb.'* The specificity of *āb-i mardī* 'fluid(s) of masculinity,' i.e. 'semen', presupposes an association of the plant with the increase of masculine sexual fertility, a property commonly attributed in Iran to *Peganum harmala* (see §§89-93) but not to *Ruta graveolens,* which was in fact regarded as an anaphrodisiac (see Détienne 1977:63-64; Afshar 1967). Thus in this early attestation *sadāb* can hardly refer to *Ruta graveolens* but should designate *Peganum harmala.*

§279 It should be noted that New Persian *āb* 'water, liquid, fluid' may without further qualification mean 'seminal fluid, semen,' (e.g. Jamālzāda 1963: 1; reference supplied by Dr. Mahmoud Omidsalar). When specificity is desired, the more explicit *āb-i mardī* (as in our verse) or *āb-i mardān* 'fluid of males' is employed. Thus *sadāb* 'harmel' could have been understood as 'a hundred seminal fluids', i.e. 'furnishing a hundredfold virile potency'.

§280 It is likely that Rūdakī's verse plays upon an understanding of *sadāb* as 'supplying a hundredfold virility' common in the folklore concerning harmel among Iranians of Transoxiana. In accordance with the general pattern of cultural history, and specifically folklore concerning harmel (see the Azari verse quoted in §69), one may expect such a notion to have spread to the Turkish communities of the area. I would therefore venture to use my etymology of *sadāb* 'hundred(fold) fluids/virility' to clarify the widespread Turkic name for *Peganum harmala, (y)üzerlik,* which until now has lacked an etymology. Both *yüzerlik* and *üzerlik* (*yüzärlik, üzärlik*) are attested from the time of Kāshgharī (twelfth century C.E.), and are current in Turkey today (*yüzerlik* occurring in provincial speech). The loss of *y* before the front vowel *ü* is common and is already attested in Old Turkish. Taking *yüzerlik* as the earlier form allows us to analyze the word as a compound of *yüz* 'one hundred' and *erlik (ärlik)* 'masculine power'; thus one arrives at 'conferring a hundred virile potencies', which would be the calque of *sadāb.*

§281 The meaning *'Peganum harmala'* is not only attested for *sadāb* in the above material, but also for Armenian *sanam.* The form may have arisen via dissimilation from **sandab* (> **sandam* > **sanam*), the *-n-* being perhaps due to the influence of *sandal* (Persian *ṣandal*), cf. §260. However, the form *sandab* is attested for the Arabic of Cairo with the meaning *'Ruta chalepensis'* (Förskål 1775:146; Meyerhof 1918:196).

§282 It may be concluded that *sudāb* is from earlier *sadāb,* which originally meant 'harmel'. The alleged word *sudāb* 'strength' may now be rejected as a lexicographer's invention from the context of the misread verse of Rūdakī. It appears that, after a long period of co-existence of the meanings 'wild rue' (harmel) and 'garden rue' (named after the latter plant because of the similar appearance), the secondary meaning came to predominate, 'harmel' having a more common alternative form (Middle Persian *spand,* New Persian *sipand, isfand,* etc.) whose numinous associations (cf. Middle Persian *Spandarmad* and *Amahraspand,* referring to divinities) exclusively suited the plant's apotropaic virtues. It was probably while both meanings still co-existed for *sadāb,* the garden rue, which lacked all connection with virile potency (an association still borne by the form *sadāb* in the early Classical Persian period, as indicated by the evidence of *yüzerlik* and supported by Rūdakī), began being called by a distinctive form *sudāb.* This arose, perhaps dialectally, through anticipatory labialization of the vowel in the first syllable by the *b;* for long range labialization cf. Persian *urdēbihišt* (modern Tehrani *ordībehešt*) from Middle Persian *ard(ē)wahišt* '(month) *of Best Rightness' (Old Iranian **ṛtahya vahištahya*); and, with progressive labialization, Persian *Bahrām* < Middle Persian *Wahrān,* Middle Persian *awestām* < **awestān,* 'province', etc.

§283 It is unlikely that *sadāb* ('harmel') arose in Middle Persian, or referred originally to the plant with regard to male sexuality. Compounds in 'a hundred' are very common in Old Iranian (a feature of Indo-Iranian origin) but not in Middle Iranian. Persian *sadāb* etc. would continue an Old Iranian compound **satāp-* 'having (or giving) an hundred (*sata-*) waters (*āp-*).' As against later Iranian, Old Iranian *āp-* is not used for 'semen' (which is indicated by *xšuδra-* ('liquidity'), so that the sense of *āb* in *sadāb* must have undergone a reinterpretation based on the plant's independent reputation as an aphrodisiac and promoter of male fertility.

§284 An ancient epithet 'having a hundred waters' for sauma is justified by various data illustrating the conception of *haoma.* As the chief representative of plant life, *haoma* was inevitably connected with water; cf. *Yasna* 10.3 in §82. More importantly, *haoma* juice mixed with water (*haomyā- āp-*) was the liquid *par excellence,* so that *haoma* was regarded as beneficial to the waters and even having a role in the production of water. This is reflected in ritual by the practice of offering a preparation of the consecrated extract as a libation to the Waters, and in mythology by the statement in *Yasht* 8.33: After Tištrya brings on the cloud-forming mists, the wind flies "along those paths which *Haoma* traverses", and from there the wind drives down the rain, clouds and hail upon the earth. In the Pahlavi books it is even said that *Haoma* is a "collaborator" (*hamkār*) of Tištrya in the production of rain (*Bundahišn* VI b 3 [f. 33.5] *Dēnkird* III, 112; *Zātsparam* 3.8).

§285 The connection of the plant (and divinity) with water and the production of rain must be of Indo-Iranian origin, for it is also found in the ṚgVeda, where it has undergone a great deal of poetic elaboration. As A. A. Macdonnell (1917: 153) writes:

> *Soma*'s connection with the waters resulting from the admixture, is expressed in the most various ways. He is the drop that grows in the waters; he is the embryo of the waters or their child; they are his mothers or his sisters; he is lord and king of streams; he produces waters and causes heaven and earth to rain.

There is in fact a Vedic parallel to the Old Iranian epithet **satāpa-;* it is *śatádhāra-* 'having a hundred streams', which refers to *soma* (9.80.4; 9.86.11; 9.96.14) and the admixture of *soma* (9.86.27). It occurs (3.26.9) with regard to the hymnist as the source (*utsá-*) of inspiration in a figure modeled after *soma* imagery; this is clear from the reference to the three "sieves" of the hymnist, and the statement that he "intoxicates". Finally, in what is probably the most recent attestation, 10.107.4, *śatádhāra-* refers to the wind (cf. above on *Yasht* 8.33, with connection of wind, *Haoma,* and rain); this last Vedic passage is proceeded by an apostrophe to *soma.* It may be concluded that *śatádhāra-* is properly a *soma* epithet.

§286 In view of the correspondence **satāp-: śatádhāra,* it is likely that 'having/yielding a hundred waters/streams' was a Proto-Indo-Iranian epithet of sauma. If it is assumed that the more specific word, *śatádhāra-,* is the more original, its replacement in Iranian would be understandable: Indo-Iranian had *dhārā-* 'blade' and *dhārā-* 'stream', and homophony caused the elimination of the latter word in Iranian, leaving only *dārā-* 'blade' (Sogdian *δār* etc.). The old epithet may well have undergone reinterpretation as 'having a hundred blades'. Just this meaning is found in the Avestan description of Mithra's mace, the *vazra-* (*Yasht* 10.96): *satafštāna- satōdāra-* 'having a hundred mammaries (= protuberances, knobs), having a hundred blades'.

§287 It would seem that the characterization of the plant as 'having/yielding a hundred waters' did not have sufficient force, from a cultic viewpoint, for its canonization in what emerged as the authoritative religion; hence, *satāp-* is not found for *haoma* in the Avesta. As a nonsacral name for the plant it survived in folk traditions, where its meaning underwent reinterpretation.[3]

[3] The two meanings of **śatádhāra-,* 'yielding a hundred streams' and 'having a hundred blades', are connected in the conception of the mace as thunderbolt. This conception is of Indo-Iranian origin, and is attested not only in Indra's water-releasing *vajra-,* but is reflected by the Middle Persian *wēr* and *warz(ag)* 'lightning(-bolt)', from Old Persian **vaδra-,* Old Iranian *vazra-.* It is even not impossible that the collocation of *satafštāna-* with *satōdāra-* formulaically reflects the same word play, with *-fštāna-,* literally 'mammary, female breast', supporting the image of released streams; cf. Vedic *ūdhar-* 'udder' used of the cosmogonic source of the waters, produced by Indra's cleaving the primordial rock or mountain (*áśman-, parvatá-, girí-*) with the *vajrá-.* The connection of a paronomasic vazra- . . . satōdāra- with Mithra may go conceivably back to a myth where Mithra had Indraic traits; cf. the Western Mithraic representations of Mithras producing streams of waters by piercing a mountain or rock. The Western Mithras has another apparently archaic trait which parallels the Vedic Indra: Mithras is a cattle thief (*βουκλποŸ:* Commodianus; for details see Schwartz 1975:417-418) associated with a grotto; cf. Indra's removal of the cattle of the Paṇis or Vala (paralleled by the cattle-rustling exploits of Herakles and Cacus). The connection of Mithra(s) and Indra would be due to independent assimilation of traits of the Indo-Iranian *Vṛtraghna-, for which cf. G. Dumézil (1969, chapter 3, part 2).

REFERENCES

Abaev, Vasilij Ivanovich 1955. *Istoriko-ėtimologičeskij slovar' osetinskogo jazyka, I.* Leningrad.

______1973. *Istoriko-ėtimologičeskij slovar' osetinskogo jazyka, II.* Leningrad.

______1975. "Contribution à l'histoire des mots: 1. Vieil-iranien *hauma-* et le nom eurasien du houblon." In *Mélanges linguistiques offerts à Emile Benveniste.* Paris (*Collection linguistique publiées par la Société de Linguistique de Paris 70*), 1-3.

ʿĀfīfī, Raḥīm (Editor) 1972. *Farhang-e Jahāngīrī* [by Mīr Jamāl al-Dīn ibn Fakhr al-Dīn Injū Shīrāzī]. Mashhad, 1351.

Afshar, Iraj (Editor) 1967. *Faraḥ-nāma Jamālī* [by Abū Bakr Muṭahhar al Jamāl al-Yazdī (1184 C.E.)]. Tehran, 1346.

Ahluwalia, K. S. 1967. *British pharmaceutical codex: plants and their Indian substitutes.* Delhi.

Ahmad, B., et al. 1959. *Report on the medicinal plants and herbs of Azad Kashmir.* Karachi.

Ainslie, Whitelaw 1826. *Materia Indica.* 2 vols. London.

Aitchison, J. E. T. 1889. "A Survey of the botanical features of the country traversed by the Afghan Delimitation Commission during 1884-5." *Transactions of the Edinburgh Botanical Society* 17, 431-524.

______1891. "Notes to assist in a farther knowledge of the products of western Afghanistan and north-eastern Persia." *Transactions of the Edinburgh Botanical Society* 18, 1-228.

Alander, O. R. 1763. "Inebriantia." No. 111 in *Amoenitates Academicae,* edited by Linnaeus. Stockholm.

André, Jacques 1956. *Lexique des termes de botanique en Latin.* Paris *(Études et Commentaires 23).*

Andreev, M. S. 1953. *Tadzhiki doliny Khuf.* Vol. 2. Stalinabad.

Andrews, Alfred C. 1948. "Rue among Greeks and Romans." *Classical Journal* 48, 371-373.

Anjavī Shīrāzī, Abū al-Qāsim 1973. *Jašn-hā va ādāb va moʿtaqedāte-ye zemistān.* 2 vols. Tehran.

Anklesaria, Behramgore T. (Editor and translator) 1950. *Pahlavi Vendidad: transliteration and translation into English.* Bombay.

______1956. *Zand-ākāsīh, Iranian or greater Bundahišn: transliteration and translation into English.* Bombay.

______1957. *Zand-ī Vohūman Yasn and two Pahlavi fragments: Drayišn-ī Akaramanō Dīvān and Gāsān Awar Vitartakān Khānēd. With text, transliteration, and translation in English.* Bombay.

______1964. *Vichītakihā-ī Zātsparam, with text and introduction. Part I: Text and introduction.* Bombay *(Pahlavi Text Series* 9).

Anklesaria, Tehmuras Dinshaji (Editor) 1908. *The Bundahishn: being a facsimile of the TD manuscript no. 2 . . . with an introduction by Behramgore Tehmuras Anklesaria.* Bombay (*Pahlavi Text Series* 2).

Anquetil du Perron, Abraham Hyacinthe 1771. *Zend-Avesta, ouvrage de Zoroastre contenant les idées théologiques, physiques et morales de ce législateur, les cérémonies du culte religieux qu'il a établi, et plusieurs traités importants relatifs à histoire des Perses. Traduit en français sur l'original Zend, avec éclairir les matières qui en sont objet.* 3 vols. Paris.

Ascherson, P., and G. Schweinfurth 1887. *Illustration de la flore d'Égypte.* Cairo (*Mémoires présentés à l'Institut Égyptien* 2).

Bächtold-Stäubli, Hanns (Editor) 1927-1942). *Handwörterbuch des deutschen Aberglaubens.* 7 vols. Berlin and Leipzig.

Back, M. 1978. *Die sasanidischen Staatsinschriften.* Leiden (*Acta Iranica* 18).

Bahmanyār, A., and H. Maḥjūbī Ardekanī (Editors) 1967. *Kitāb al-abniya ʿan ḥaqāʾiq al-adwiya* [by Muwaffaq al-Dīn abū Manṣūr ʿAlī al-Harawī]. Tehran, 1346.

Bailey, Clinton, and Avinoam Danin 1981. "Bedouin plant utilization in Sinai and Negev." *Economic Botany* 35, 145-162.

Bailey, Harold W. 1934. "Iranian studies III." *Bulletin of the School of Oriental Studies* 7, 275-298.

______1936. "Indo-Iranica." *Transactions of the Philological Society,* 95-101.

______1951. *Khotanese Buddhist Texts.* London (*Cambridge Oriental Series* 3).

______1953. "Indo-Iranian Studies I." *Transactions of the Philological Society,* 21-42.

______1957a. "Veda and Avesta." *University of Ceylon Review* 15, 23-35.

______1957b. "*Dvārā matīnām.* " *Bulletin of the School of Oriental and African Studies* 20,

41-59.
______1959. *"Ambages indoiranicae." Annali dell' Istituto Universitario Orientale di Napoli. Sezione linguistica* I (2), 113-146.
______1964. "Lyrical poems of the Sakas." In *Dr. J. M. Unvala memorial volume.* Bombay, 1-5.
______1969. *Indo-Scythian studies: being Khotanese texts.* Vol. 2. 2nd edition. Cambridge.
______1969a. "Avesta and Saka." *Indo-Iranian Journal* 11, 289-292.
______1970. "Saka studies: the ancient kingdom of Khotan." *Iran* 8, 65-72.
______1971. "Trends in Iranian studies." *Memoirs of the research department of the Toyo Bunko* 29, 1-16.
______1971a. *Zoroastrian problems in the ninth-century books.* 2nd edition. Oxford.
______1972. "A Half-century of Indo-Iranian studies." *Journal of the Royal Asiatic Society,* 99-110.
______1974. "The Range of the colour *zar* in Khotan Saka texts." In *Memorial Jean de Menasce.* Edited by P. Gignoux and M. Tafazzoli. Louvain and Tehran, 369-374.
______1975. "The Second stratum of the Indo-Iranian gods." In *Mithraic Studies.* Edited by J. R. Hinnells. Manchester. I, 1-20.
______1979. *A Dictionary of Khotanese Saka.* London.
______1982. *The Culture of the Sakas in Ancient Iranian Khotan.* New York.
______1984. "Vedic *kṣúmpa-* and connected data." In *Amṛtadhāra: Prof. R.N. Dandikar felicitation volume.* Edited by S. D. Joshi. Delhi, 17-20.
______1985. "Plant names." In *Cambridge History of Iran. Vol.2: The Median and Achaemenian periods.* Edited by I. Gershevitch. Cambridge, 870-873.
______1985a *"Durauzha* the drink exhilarant." *South Asian Studies* 1, 157-161.
Balfour, Edward 1885. *Cyclopedia of India and of Eastern and Southern Asia: Commercial, industrial and scientific, products of the mineral, vegetable and animal kingdom, useful arts and manufacturing.* 3rd edition. 3 vols. London.
Bamber, Charles James 1916. *Plants of Punjab.* Lahore.
Banerje, P. K., and S. Ghosal 1969. "Simple Indol bases of *Desmodium gangeticum* (Legumenaceae)." *Australian Journal of Chemistry* 22, 275-257.
Baqā'ī, Naṣr 1959. *Fārsī-e Kermān.* Tehran, 1338.
Bartholomae, Christian 1883. "Avestisch *maδa-, mada.*" *Zeitschrift der Deutschen Morgenländischen Gesellschaft* 37, 459.
_________1904. *Altiranisches Wörterbuch.* Strassburg. Reprinted Berlin 1961.
Bastakī, Haj ʿAlī Akbar 1980. *Farhang-e Bastakī.* Tehran 1359.
Bedevian, Armenag K. 1936. *Illustrated polyglottic dictionary of plant names.* Cairo.
Bedi, Ramesh 1960. "Garlic." In *P. K. Gode commemorative volume.* Poona (*Poona Oriental Series* 93), 9-14.
Belardi, Walter 1979. *The Pahlavi book of the righteous Viraz I. Chapters I-II.* Rome (*Biblioteca di ricerche linguistiche e filologiche* 10).
Bellew, H. W. 1874. *From the Indus to the Tigris.* London.
______1901. *Dictionary of Pukkhto or Pukshto.* London.
Belon du Mons, Pierre 1555. *Les observations de plusieurs singularitéz et choses mémorables trouvées en Grèce, Asie, Judée, Egypte, Arabie, et autres pays estranges, rédigées en trois livres.* Paris.
Benveniste, Emile 1929. "Une rite zervanite chez Plutarch." *Journal Asiatique* 215, 287-96.
______1936. "Notes parthes et sogdiennes". *Journal Asiatique* 228, 193-239.
———1940. *Textes sogdiens: édités, traduits, et commentés.* Paris.
______1973. *Indo-European language and society.* Translated by E. Palmer. London.
Bergaigne, Able 1878. *La Religione védique d'après les hymnes du Rig-Veda.* Vol. 1. Paris.
Berger, H. 1956. "Mittelmeerische Kulturpflanzennamen aus der Burušaski." *Münchener Studien zur Sprachwissenschaft* 9, 4-33.
Bhandari, M.M. 1978. *Flora of the Indian desert.* Jodhpur.
Bharucha, S.D. 1906. *Collected Sanskrit writings of the Parsees.* 2 vols. Bombay.
Bidez, Joseph, and Franz Cumont 1938. *Les mages hellénisés: Zoroastre, Ostanès, et Hystaspe d'après la tradition grècque.* 2 vols. Paris.
Black, W. L., and K. W. Parker 1936. "Toxicity tests on African Rue [*Peganum harmala* L.]." *New Mexico Agricultural Experiment Station Bulletin* 240, 1-14.
Blakelock, R. A., and J. B. Gillett 1966. *"Ephedraceae."* In *Flora of Iraq.* Vol. 2. Edited by C. C. Townsend and Evan Guest. Baghdad, 82-89.
Blatter, Ethelbert 1919-1936. *Flora Arabica.* Delhi (*Indian Botanical Survey Records* 8).
Bloomfield, M. 1886. "Seventy hymns of the Atharva Veda." *American Journal of Philology* 7, 466-488.
Bommüller, J. 1893. "Reisebriefe aus Persien." *Mitteilungen Thüringischer Botanischer Verein n.f.* 3.
Borza, A. A. 1968. *Dictionar ethnobotanic.* Bucharest.
Boulos, Loutfy 1983. *Medicinal plants of North Africa.* Algonac, Michigan.
Boyce, Mary 1966a. "*Ātaš-zōhr* and *āb-zōhr.*" *Journal of the Royal Asiatic Society,* 100-118.
______1966b. "The Fire temples of Kerman." *Acta Orientalia* 30, 51-57.
______1970. "Haoma, priest of the sacrifice." In *W. B. Henning memorial volume.* Edited by Mary Boyce and Ilya Gershevitch. London, 62-80.
______1975a. "*Mihragān* among the Irani Zoroastrians." In *Mithraic Studies.* Edited by J. R. Hinnells. Manchester. Vol. I, 106-118.
______1975b. *A History of Zoroastrianism.* Vol. I. In *Handbuch der Orientalistik.* Edited by B. Spuler. Abt. 1, Bd. 8, Abschnitt 1, Lief. 2, Heft 2A.
______1975c. "On the Zoroastrian temple cult of fire." *Journal of the American Oriental Society* 95, 454-464.
______1977. *A Persian stronghold of Zoroastrianism.* Oxford.
______1982. *A History of Zoroastrianism.* Vol. II. In *Handbuch der Orientalistik.* Edited by B. Spuler. Abt. 1, Bd. 8, Abschnitt 1, Lief. 2, Heft 2B.
______1984. "On the antiquity of Zoroastrian apocalyptic." *Bulletin of the School of Oriental and African Studies* 47, 57-75.
Brandis, Dietrich 1879. *The Forest flora of north-west and central India.* London.
______1921. *Indian Trees.* London.
Branky, Franz 1901. "Die Rauten. Ein kleines Kapitel zur Sittenkunde des deutschen Volkes." *Archiv für Religionwissenschaft* 1, 104-110.
______1903. "Zur Volksmedizine." *Archiv für Religionwissenschaft* 3, 284-287.
Brauer, Erich 1934. *Ethnologie der jemenitischen Juden.* Heidelberg (1 *Reihe Technologische Bibliothek mit Einschluss der altorientalischen Kulturgeschichte* 7).
Brockelmann, C. 1908. "Ibn Quṭaiba's *ʿUjūn al-akbār.*" *Zeitschrift für Assyriologie und verwandte Gebiete.* Beiheft zum 21 Bd.
______1928. *Lexicon Syriacum.* 2nd edition. Göttingen.
Brough, John 1971a. "Soma and *Amanita Muscaria.*" *Bulletin of the School of Oriental and African Studies* 34, 331-362.
______1971b. "Problems of the 'soma-mushroom' theory." *Indologica Taurinensia* 1, 21-32.
Brunner, Charles J. 1974. "The Middle Persian inscription of the priest Kirdēr at Naqš-i Rustam." In *Studies in Honour of George C. Miles.* Beirut, 97-113.
Brunnhofer, Hermann 1910. *Arische Urzeit.* Bern.
Budge, E. W. 1913. *Syrian anatomy, pathology and therapeutics of "The Book of Medicines."* 2 vols. London.
_____1927. *Herb doctors and physicians in the ancient world: the divine origins of the craft of the herbalist.* Reprinted Chicago 1978.
Burgess, A. H. 1964. *Hops: botany, cultivation and utilization.* London.
Burkill, I. H. 1935. *A Dictionary of the economic products of the Malay Peninsula.* 2 vols. London.
Burnell, A. C. 1878. *Elements of South Indian palaeography.* Reprinted Delhi 1968.
Burtt, B. L., and P. T. Lewis 1954. "On the flora of Kuwait 3." *Kew Bulletin* 9, 377-410.
Caller Ibérico, C. 1941. *"Ayahuasco." Boletín del Museo de Historia Natural "Javier Prado", Universidad de San Marcos* 5, 313-321.
Calmeyer, Peter 1975. "Barsombündel im 8. und 7. Jahrhundert v. Chr." In *Wandlungen: Studien zur antiken und neueren Kunst: Ernst Homann-Wedeking gewidmet.* Waldsassen-Bayern, 11-16.
Cerquand, J.- F. 1873. *Ulysse et Circe.* Paris.
Chandrasena, J. P. C. 1935. *The Chemistry and pharmacology of Ceylon and Indian medicinal plants.* Colombo.
Chopra, R. N. B. L. Badhwar and S. Ghosh 1965. *Poisonous plants of India.* Delhi.
Christensen, Arthur 1925. "The Smith Kaveh and the ancient Persian banner." [Translated by J. M. Unvala]. *Journal of the K. R. Cama Oriental Institute* 5, 22-39.
_____1934. "Les types du première homme et du premier roi dans l'histoire légendaire des

iraniens." Stockholm (*Archives d'Études Orientales* 14).

Clauson, G. 1972. *An Etymological dictionary of pre-thirteenth century Turkish.* Oxford.

Clay, Jenny 1970. "The Planktai and *moly:* divine naming and knowing in Homer." *Hermes* 100:2, 127-130.

Correll, D. S., and M. C. Johnstone 1970. *Manual of the vascular plants of Texas.* Renner.

Cory, V. L. 1949. "African rue (*Peganum harmala* L.) in the United States." *Field and Lab* [Graduate Research Center, Dallas, Texas] 17, 20-23.

Crevatin, F. 1983. "Per incertam lunam sub luce maligna." In *Problemi di sostrato nelle lingue indoeuropee.* Edited by E. Campanile. Pisa, 109-115.

Crum, W. B. 1939. *Coptic dictionary.* London.

Dabīr Siyāqī (Editor). 1957. *Lughāt-i Furs* [by ʿAlī ibn Aḥmad Asadī-i Ṭūsī]. Tehran 1336.

_____1959. *Dīvān-i Mīnučihrī Dāmaghānī.* Tehran 1338.

Dadachanji, Ruttonshaw Kershaspji 1911. "Relics of the primitive spirit-scaring idea in the Avesta and in prevalent Parsee religious practices." *Journal of the Bombay Anthropological Society* 10, 322-344.

Dandekar, R. N. (Translator) 1973. *Śrautakośa, encyclopædia of Vedic sacrificial ritual. Vol. 2, English section. The Agnistoma, Part 1.* Poona.

Darmesteter, James (Translator) 1892-1893. *Le Zend-Avesta: traduction nouvelle avec commentaire historique et philologique.* 3 vols. Paris (*Annales du Musée Guimet* 21, 22, 24). Reprinted 1960.

Das, Rahul Peter 1987. "On the identification of a Vedic plant." In *Studies on Indian Medical History, Papers presented at the International Workshop on the Study of Indian Medicine held at the Wellcome Institute for the History of Medicine 2-4 September 1985.* Edited by G. Jan Meulenbeld and Dominik Wujastyk. Groningen, 19-42.

Dayton, W. A. 1937. "Notes on harmal or Syrian rue." *Journal of the Washington Academy of Sciences* 27, 349-352.

Dehkhudā, ʿAlī Akbar 1947-1973. *Lughat-nāma.* Continued by M. Muʿin. Tehran.

Delatte, A. (Editor) 1939. *Glossaires de botanique grecs.* In *Anecdota Atheniensia* ii. Liège (*Bibliotheque de la Faculté de Philosophie et Lettres de l'Université de Liège* 88), 279-454.

De Ropp, R. S. 1951. *Drugs and the mind.* New York. Reprinted 1960.

Détienne, Marcel 1977. *The Gardens of Adonis: spices and Greek mythology.* Translated by Janet Lloyd. New Jersey.

Dhabhar, Bahmanji N. (Editor) 1913. *The Pahlavi rivāyat accompanying the Dādistān-ī Dēnīk.* Bombay (*Pahlavi Text Series* 5).

_____1923. *Descriptive catalogue of some manuscripts bearing on Zoroastriansm and pertaining to the different collections of the Mulla Firuz Library.* Bombay.

_____1932. *The Persian rivāyats of Hormazyar Framarz.* English translation with notes. Bombay.

_____1949. *Pahlavi Yasna and Visperat. Edited with an introduction and a glossary of select terms.* Bombay (*Pahlavi Text Series* 8).

Dickson, Violet 1955. *The Wild flowers of Kuwait and Bahrain.* London.

al-Dimyāṭī, M. Muṣṭafā 1965. *Muʿjam asmāʾ al-nabātāt.* Cairo.

Dollfus, D., and H. Schlumberger 1842. "Matières colorantes du *Peganum harmala.*" *Bulletin de la Société Industrielle de Mulhouse* 16, 547-552.

Donaldson, Bess A. 1938. *The Wild rue: a study of Muhammedan magic and folk-lore in Iran.* London.

Dozy, Reinhart 1881-1927. *Supplément aux dictionnaires arabes.* 2 vols. Leyden.

Drower, Ethel Stephana 1944. "The Role of fire in Parsi ritual." *Journal of the Royal Anthropological Institute* 74, 75-89.

_____1956. *Water into wine.* London.

_____1965. "The Sacramental bread (*piḫtha*) of the Mandaeans." *Zeitschrift der Deutschen Morgenländischen Gesellschaft* 105, 115-128.

_____(Editor and translator) 1934. "A Phylactery for Rue (an invocation of the personified herb)." *Orientalia* 4, 324-346.

_____1943. "A Mandean book of black magic." *Journal of the Royal Asiatic Society,* 149-169.

Drower, Ethel Stephana, and R. Macuch 1963. *A Mandaic dictionary.* London.

Dubler, C. E., and Elias Teres (Editors and translators) 1952-1957. *La Materia medica de Dioscórides.* 6 vols. Barcelona.

Dübner, F. (Editor) 1868. *Plutarchi operum: Scripta Moralia.* Vol. 1. Paris.

Duchesne-Guillemin, Jacques 1982. "Apocalypse juive et apocalypse iranienne." In *La soteriologia dei culti orientali nell' Imperio Romano.* Edited by U. Bianchi and M. J. Vermaseren. Leiden, 753-761.

Ducros, M. A. H. 1930. *Essai sur la droguier populaire arabe au Caire.* Cairo (*Mémoires présentés à l'Institut d'Egypt* 15).

Dumézil, Georges 1969. *Heur et malheur du guerrier.* Paris. [English translation: *The Destiny of the Warrior.* Chicago 1970].

Dymock, William 1889. *Pharmacographia Indica.* Part 1. Simla.

Eckhardt, P. Andreas 1928. "Ginseng, die Wunderwurzel des Ostens." In *Festschrift publication d'hommage offerte au P. W. Schmidt.* Edited by W. Koppers. Vienna, 220-230.

Edel'man, D. L. 1966. *Jazguljamskij jazyk.* Moscow.

_____1971. *Jazguljamsko-Russkij slovar'.* Moscow.

Efron, E. H. (Editor) 1967. *The Ethnopharmacologic search for psychoactive drugs.* Washington, D.C.

Eilers, Wilhelm 1978. "Semitische Wurzeltheorie." In *Atti del Secondo Congresso Internazionale di Linguistica Camito-semitica, Firenze 16-19 aprile 1974.* Edited by Pelio Fronzaroli. Firenze.

_____1953. *Der Alte Name des persischen Neujahrsfestes.* Wiesbaden (*Abhandlungen der Geistes- und Sozialwissenschaftlichen Kl., Akademie der Wissenschaften und der Literatur in Mainz* 1).

_____1985. "Einige altiranische Etymologien." *Münchener Studien zur Sprachwissenschaft* 45 *(Festgabe für Karl Hoffmann),* 23-38.

Eilers, Wilhelm, and M. Mayrhofer 1962. "Kurdisch *būz* und die indogermanische 'Buchen-Sippe': Zugleich ein Beitrag zur Ulme und allgemeinen Pflanzennamenkunde." *Mitteilungen der Anthropologischen Gesellschaft in Wien* 92 (*Festschrift Franz Hančar*), 61-92.

Eliade, Mircea 1964. *Shamanism: archaic techniques of ecstasy.* [Translated by Willard R. Trask]. Princeton.

Emmerick, Ronald (Editor and translator) 1968). *The Book of Zambasta: a Khotanese poem on Buddhism.* Oxford (*London Oriental Series* 21).

_____1970. *The Khotanese Suraṅgamasamādhisūtra.* Oxford (*London Oriental Series* 23).

Engler, A. 1931. *"Zygophyllaceae."* In *Die Nāturlichen Pflanzenfamilien.* Edited by A. Engler and K. Prantl. 2nd edition. Leipzig. Vol. 19a, 154.

Eqtedārī, Aḥmad 1955. *Farhang-e Lāristanī.* Tehran, 1334.

Fahd, Toufy 1977. "Matériaux pour l'histoire de l'agriculture en Iran: *Al-Filāḥa n-Nabāṭiyya.*" In *Sources for the economic history of the Middle East.* In *Handbuch der Orientalistik.* Edited by B. Spuler. Abt. 1, Bd. 6, Abschnitt 6, Teile 1, 276-375.

Falk, Harry 1987. "Soma—the plant and its connotations." Paper presented at the VII World Sanskrit Conference, Leiden, August 27, 1987.

Flemming, John 1812. "A Catalogue of Indian medicinal plants and drugs with names in Hindustani and Sanskrit." *Asiatic Researches* 11, 153-196.

Fleurentin, J., G. Mazars and J.-M. Pelt 1983. "Cultural background of the medicinal plants of Yemen." *Journal of Ethnopharmacology* 7, 183-203.

Flora Armenij 1954-1966. Edited by A. L. Takhtadzhiana. 5 vols. Erevan.

Flora Azerbaidzhan SSR. 1950. Edited by V. L. Komarova. Vol. 1. Baku.

Flora Kirgizskoj SSR. 1957-1967.

Förskål, Patter 1775. *Flora Aegyptiaco-Arabica sive Descriptiones Plantarum.* Copenhagen.

Foucauld, C. de 1951. *Dictionnaire touareg-français, dialect de l'Ahaggar.* Paris.

Frass, C. 1845. *Synopsis plantarum florae classicae.* Munich.

Friedberg, Claudine 1965. "Des *Banisteriopses* utilisés comme drogue en Amérique du Sud." *Journal d'agriculture tropicale et de botanique appliquée* 12, 403-37, 350-94, 729-780.

Fritzsche, J. 1847. "Bestandtheile der Samen von *Peganum Harmala.*" *Justus Liebigs Annalen der Chemie* 64, 360-364.

Gabikean, Karapet 1968. *Hay busašxarh.* Jerusalem.

Gabriel, Alfons 1970. *Religionsgeographie von Persien.* Vienna.

Geldner, Karl (Editor) 1896. *Avesta: the sacred books of the Parsis. Text with introduction.* 3 vols. Stuttgart.

______(Translator) 1951. *Der Rig-Veda.* 3 vols. Cambridge, Mass. (*Harvard Oriental Series* 33-35).

Gennadiou, P. G. 1914. *Λεχικον Ζυτολοηικόν.* Athens.

Gershevitch, Ilya 1959. *The Avestan Hymn to Mithra.* Oxford.

______1969. "Amber at Persepolis." In *Studia classica et orientalia Antonino Pagliaro oblata.* Rome. Vol. 2, 167-251.

______1974. "An Iranianist's view of the soma controversy." In *Memorial Jean de Menasce.* Edited by P. Gignoux and M. Tafazzoli. Louvain and Tehran, 45-75.

Ghafoor, Abdul 1974. "*Zygophyllaceae.*" In *Flora of West Pakistan.* Karachi.

Ghālib, Idwār 1965-1966. *Al-Mawsūʿa fī ʿulūm al-ṭabīʿa.* 3 vols. Beirut.

Ghosal, S. 1972. "Occurrence of psychodelic [*sic*] substances in some Indian medicinal plants." *Planta Medica* 21, 200-209.

Ghosal, S., S. K. Banerjee, S. K. Bhattacharya and A. K. Sanyal 1972. "Chemical and pharmacological evaluation of *Desmodium Pulchellum.*" *Planta Medica* 21, 398-409.

Gignoux, Philippe 1979. "Corps osseux et āme osseuse: essai sur le chamanisme dans l'Iran ancien." *Journal Asiatique* 267, 41-79.

_____1981. "Les Voyages chamaniques dans le monde iranien" *Acta Iranica* 21, 244-265.

_____1984. "Der Grossmagier Kirdīr und seine Reise in das Jenseits." *Acta Iranica* 23, 191-206.

Gilliat-Smith, B., and W. B. Turrill 1930. "On the flora of the nearer East: a contribution to our knowledge of the flora of Azerbaijan, North Persia." *Kew Bulletin* 7, 237-312; 8, 375-398; 9, 427-463; 10, 480-493.

Gnoli, Gherardo 1980. *Zoroaster's time and homeland. A Study in the origins of Mazdeism and related problems.* Naples (*Istituto Universitario Orientale, Seminario di Studi Asiatici, Series Minor* 7).

Göbrecht, Gunter 1967. "Das *Artā Vīrāz Nāmak.*" *Zeitschrift der Deutschen Morgenländischen Gesellschaft* 117, 382-409.

Goebel, H. 1838. "Ueber die Gewinnung einer rothen Farbstoffes aus den Samen der Pflanze *Peganum Harmala.*" *Dinglers Polytechnisches Journal,* 373-376.

Gonda, Jan 1940. "Alliteration und Reim im Satzbau des *Atharvaveda* (I-VII)." *Acta Orientalia* 18, 50-79.

______1949a. "The Origin and meaning of Avestan *spəṇta-.*" *Oriens* 2, 195-203.

______1949b. *Remarks on similes in Sanskrit Literature.* Leiden (*Orientalia Rheno-Trajectina.* Edited by J. Gonda and H. U. Obbink).

______1975. *Vedic literature: Saṁhitās and Brāhmaṇas.* Wiesbaden (*A History of Indian Literature.* Edited by J. Gonda, Vol. 1, Fasc. 1).

Grapow, Hanns, H. von Deines, et al. 1954-. *Grundriss der Medizin der alten Ägypten.* Berlin.

Gray, Louis 1929. *The Foundations of the Iranian religions.* Bombay (*Journal of the K. R. Cama Oriental Society* 15).

Griffiths, J. Gwynn (Editor and translator) 1970. *Plutarch's De Iside et Osiride.* Mystic, Conn.

Grjunberg, A. L., and I. M. Steblin-Kamenskij 1976. *Vakhanskij jazyk.* Moscow.

Guest, Evan 1933. *Notes on plants and plant products with their colloquial names in Iraq.* Baghdad (*Bulletin of the Department of Agriculture, Iraq* 27).

Guest, Evan, and Ali al-Rawi (Editors) 1966. *Flora of Iraq. Vol 1. Introduction to the flora: an account of the geology, soils, climate and ecology of Iraq with gazetteer, glossary and bibliography.* Baghdad.

Guigues, Pierre 1905. "Les noms arabes dans Sérapion *Liber de Simplici medicina.*" *Journal Asiatique* [10] 5, 473-546; 6, 49-112.

Gunn, J. S. 1937. "The Harmine group of alkaloids." In *Handbuch der Expermentellen Pharmakologie. Edited by B. Hefter. Erg.-Werk.* 5, 185-196.

Gunther, R. T. 1905. "The Cimaruta: its structure and development." *Folklore* 16, 132-161.

______(Editor) 1934. *The Greek herbal of Dioscourides.* [Translated by J. Goodyer], New York.

Gupta, B. L. (Editor) 1928. *Forest Flora of the Chakrata, Dehra Dun and Shakarpur Forest Divisions, United Provinces.* 3rd edition. Calcutta. Reprinted 1979.

Habib, Kamal Muhammad 1979. "The '*Kitāb al-Ṣaydana*': structure and approach." In *Al-Bīrūnī commemorative volume.* Edited by H. M. Said. Karachi, 458-473.

Hādī Khān al-ʿAlawī al-Khurāsānī al-Shīrāzī, Ṣādiq M. 1824. *Maxzan al-adwiya wa-taδkirat ūlā ʾl-nuhā.* 2 vols. Hūgli.

Harlez, Charles de 1883. "L'Avestique *maδa* et le tradition persane." *Zeitschrift der Deutschen Morgenländischen Gesellschaft* 37, 133.

Harner, Michael 1968. "The Sound of rushing water." *Natural History* 77, 28-33, 60-61. (Reprinted in Harner 1973).

______(Editor) 1973. *Hallucinogens and shamanism.* Oxford.

Haug, M., and E. W. West (Editors and translators). 1892. *The Book of Arda Viraf: Pahlavi text prepared by Hoshangji Jamaspji Asa, revised and collated with further manuscripts, with an English translation.* Bombay and London. Reprinted Amsterdam 1971.

Haug, Martin 1884. *Essays on the sacred language, writings, and religion of the Paris.* 3rd edition. Edited and enlarged by E. W. West. London.

Hava, J. G. 1915. *Arab-English dictionary (al-Faraid al-durriya).* Beirut.

al-Ḥayla, M. al-Ḥabib (Editor) 1968. *Kitāb Siyāsat al-ṣibyān* [by Ibn al-Jazzār]. Tunis.

Hedāyat, Ṣādiq 1933. *Nayrangistān.* Tehran 1312.

Hegnauer, Robert 1962-1973. *Chemotaxonomie der Pflanzen.* 6 vols. Basal.

Henning, Walter B. 1940. *Sogdica.* London (*James G. Furlong Fund,* 21).

_____1946. "The Sogdian texts of Paris." *Bulletin of the School of Oriental and African Studies* 11, 713-740.

_____1951. *Zoroaster: politican or witch doctor?* Oxford.

_____1953. "The Middle Persian word for 'beer'." *Bulletin of the School of Oriental and African Studies* 17, 603-604.

_____1965. "A Grain of mustard." *Annali dell' Istituto Universitario Orientale de Napoli, Sezione linguistica* 6, 29-47.

_____1965a. "A Sogdian god." *Bulletin of the School of Oriental and African Studies* 28, 242-234.

Hillebrandt, Alfred 1980. *Vedic mythology.* Vol. 1. Translated by S. R. Sarma. Delhi.

Hinnells, John R. 1973. *Persian mythology.* New York.

Hocking, George M. 1958. "Pakistan Medicinal Plants I." *Qualitas plantorum et materiae vegetibilis* 5, 145-153.

Hoffmann, Karl 1967. *"Haomo yō gauua."* *Münchener Studien zur Sprachwissenschaft* 21, 11-20.

______1971. "Zum Zeicheninventar der Avesta-Schrift." In *Festgabe deutscher Iranisten zur 2500 Jahrfeier Irans.* Edited by W. Eilers. Stuttgart, 64-73.

Hooper, David 1937. *Useful plants and drugs of Iran and Iraq.* Chicago (*Field Museum of Natural History, Botanical Series* 9:3. Publ. 387).

Horn, Paul 1893. *Grundriss der neupersischen Etymologie.* Strassburg.

Hort, A. (Editor and translator) 1916. *Theophrastus. Enquiry into Plants.* 2 vols. London (*Loeb Classical Library*).

Houtum-Schindler, A. 1885. "The Soma plant." *The Academy,* Jan. 31, 1885, pg. 83.

Hübschmann, H. 1897. *Armenische Grammatik. Teil I. Armenische Etymologie.* Leipzig (*Bibliothek indogermanischen Grammatiken* 6, L. 1).

Humbach, Helmut (Editor and translator) 1959. *Die Gathas des Zarathustra.* 2 vols. Heidelberg.

______1974. "Methodologische Variationen zur arischen Religionsgeschichte." In *Antiquitates Indogermanicae. Studien zur indogermanischen Altertumskunde und zur Sprach- und Kulturgeschichte des indogermanischen Völker: Gedenkschrift für Hermann Güntert.* Edited by M. Mayrhofer, W. Meid, B. Schlerath, and R. Schmitt. Innsbruck, 193-200.

Ḥusaynī, M. Muʾmin b. Mīr M. Zamān Tanakābunī 1849. *Tuḥfat al-Muʾminīn* [written 1669]. Delhi.

Hyde, Thomas 1700. *Veterum Persarum et Parthorum et Medorum religionis historia.* Oxford.

Ibn Manẓūr, M. Ibn Mukarram 1966. *Lisān al-ʿArab* [written c. 1300]. Cairo.

Insler, Stanley (Editor and translator) 1975. *The Gathas of Zarathustra.* Leiden (*Acta Iranica* 8).

Ivanov, V., N. Nikolov and I. Tonev 1965. "Virxu polučavaneto na xarmin ot semenata na *Peganum harmala.*" *Farmacija* (Sofia) 15, 164-166.

Īzadpanāh, Ḥamīd 1964. *Farhang-e Lorī.* Tehran, 1343.

Jackson, A.V.W. 1906. *Persia past and present, a book of travel and research.* New York.

_____1911. *From Constantinople to the Persian Gulf.* New York

Jamālzāda, Muḥammad-ʿAlī 1963. *Farhang-e lughāt-e ʿāmmiyāna.* Edited by M. Jaʿfār Maḥjūb. Tehran, 1334.

Jamasp, Hoshang 1907. *Glossary to Pahlavi Vendidad.* Bombay.

Jamaspasa, Kaikhusrow and Helmut Humbach (Editors and translators) 1971. *Pursišnīhā: a Zoroastrian catechism.* Wiesbaden.

Jettmar, Karl 1975. *Die Religionen des Hindukusch.* Stuttgart.

Jones, Marcus Eugene 1933-1935. *Contributions to Western Botany.* No. 18. Robinson, Utah.

Jones, W. H. S. (Editor and translator) 1956. *Pliny, natural history.* 10 vols. Cambridge, Mass. (*Loeb Classical Library*).

Jones, William (Translator) 1794. *Institutes of Hindu law, or, the ordinances of Menu.* Calcutta. Reprinted London, 1796.

Kadri, Hüseyin Kâzim 1927. *Türk lügati.* Vol. 1. Istanbul.

Kaganoff, Benzion C. 1977. *A Dictionary of selected Jewish names.* New York.

Kamel, Shokry H., T. M. Ibrahim, A. A. Afifi and S. M. Mamza 1970. "Chemical studies on the Egyptian plant, *Peganum harmala." United Arab Republic Journal of Veterinary Science* 7, 61-68.

Kanga, Maneck F. 1950. "Pahlavi *Yasn Ha VIII:* a critical study." In *Siddha Bharati or the rosary of Indology being the Dr. Siddheshwar Varma presentation volume.* Hashiarpur. (*Vishveshvvaranand Indological Series* 1-2). Vol I, 143-149.

______1986. "Epistle I, ch. X of Manuščihr Yudānyimān, a critical study." In *Studia Grammatica Iranica, Festschrift für Helmut Humbach.* Edited by Rüdiger Schmitt and Prods Oktor Skjærvø. Munich, 283-295.

Karsten, Rafael 1964. *Studies in the religion of the South-American Indians east of the Andes.* Helsinki (*Societas Scientiarum Fennica. Commentationes Humanorum Litterarum* 29:1).

Kashikar, C. G. (Editor and translator) 1964. *The Śrauta, Paitṛmedhika and Pariśeṣa Sūtras of Bharadvāja. Part II. Translation.* Poona.

Kasumov, M. A. 1983. "Garmala obyknovennaja i ee ispolbzovanie dlja okrashivanija sherstjanoj prjazhi." *Izvestija Akademij Nauk Azerbaidzhanskoj SSR, Serija biologičeskikh Nauk,* 1938 (5), 19-25.

Katrak, Jamshid Kavasji 1941. *Oriental treasures.* Bombay.

Keith, A. B. 1925. *The Religion and philosophy of the Veda and Upanishads.* 2 vols. Cambridge, Mass. (*Harvard Oriental Studies* 31, 32). Reprinted Delhi 1970.

Khashimov, Kh., M. Telezhenetskaja, N. Sharakhimov, S. Junsov 1971. "O dynamyke nakopleni alkaloidov v *Peganum harmala." Khimija Prirodnykh Soedinenij* 7, 382.

Khattab, Ahmed, and M. Nabil el-Hadidi 1971. "Results of a botanical expedition to Arabia in 1944-1945." Cairo (*Publications of the Cairo University Herbarium* 4).

Khlopin, Igor 1980. *"Mandragora Turcomanica* in der Geschichte der Orientalvölker." *Orientalia Louvaniensia Periodica* 11, 223-231.

Khodadadian, Ardeshir 1975. "*Āb-zōhr* und *Ātaš-zōhr." In Wörterbuch der Mythologie.* Edited by H.W. Haussig, Abt. 1, Leif. 12,, 228-229.

Kirtikar, K. R., E. D. Basu and J. C. S. An 1935. *Indian Medical Plants.* 4 vols. Allahabad.

Kisljakov, N. A., and A. K. Pisarčik 1970. *Tadzhiki Karategina: Darvoza,* 2. Dushanbe.

Klimov, G. A. 1964. *Etimologičeski slovar' Kartvel'skikh jazykov.* Moscow.

Klingenschmitt, Gert 1965. "*ĕkṛd* 'Harzen' im Indoiranischen." *Münchener Studien zur Sprachwissenschaft* 18, 29-33.

Kotwal, F. M., and J. W. Boyd 1977. "The Zoroastrian *paragna* ritual." *Journal of Mithraic Studies* 2, 18-57.

Kramrisch, Stella 1975. "The Mahavira vessel and the plant *Putika." Journal of the American Oriental Society* 95, 222-235.

Kühn, Carolus Gottlob 1829. *Medicorum Graecorum opera. Vol. 25: Pedanium Dioscoridim Anazarbeum.* Lipsiae.

Kuiper, F. B. J. 1960. "The Ancient Indian verbal contest." *Indo-Iranian Journal* 4, 217-281.

______1964. "The Bliss of *Aša." Indo-Iranian Journal* 8, 96-129.

______1984. "Was the *pūtika* a mushroom?" In *Amṛtadhārā. Prof. R. N. Dandekar Felicitation Volume.* Edited by S. D. Joshi. Delhi, 219-227.

Kutlu, H., and H. Amal 1967. "Türkiyede yetişen *Peganum harmala* L. üzerinde kimyasal araştırmalar." *İstanbul Üniversitesi Eczacılık Fakültesi Mecmuasi* 3, 133-147.

Löffler, R., E. Friedl and A. Janata 1974. "Die Materielle Kultur von Boir Ahmad, Südiran. Zweite ethnographische Sammlung." *Archiv für Völkerkunde* 28, 61-142.

Lagarde, Paul Anton de 1866. *Gesammelte Abhandlungen.* Leipzig.

Lamb, F. Bruce 1975. *Wizard of the upper Amazon: the story of Manuel Córdova Rios.* 2nd edition. Boston.

Lane, Edward William 1863-1893. *An Arabic-English lexicon.* 8 vols. London.

Laoust, E. 1920. *Mots et choses berbères.* Paris.

Leclerc, Lucien (Translator) 1874. *Kachef er-roumouz (révélation des énigmes) d'Abd er Rezzaq ed-Djezairy.* Paris.

______1877-1888. *Traité des simples par ibn al-Beïthar.* 3 vols. Paris (*Notices et Extraits des Manuscrits de la Bibliothèque National* 23:1, 25:1, 26:1).

Legey, Françoise 1926. *Essai de folklore marocain.* Paris.

Leonard, J. 1984. *Contribution à l'étude de la flore et de la végétation des déserts d'Iran (Dasht-e-Kavir, Dasht-e-Lut, Jaz Murran).* Brussels (*Jardin botanique national de Belgique*).

Lewin, Bernhard (Editor) 1953. *Kitāb al-Nabāt of Abū Ḥanīfā Aḥmad b. Dāwūd al-Dīnawarī.* Uppsala (*Upsala Universitets ʿrsskrift* 1953:10).

Lincoln, Bruce 1981. *Priests, warriors and cattle, a study in the ecology of religions.* Berkeley and Los Angeles (*Hermeneutics, Studies in the History of Religions* 10).

Lindquist, Eda W. 1936. "Rue and the evil eye in Persia." *Muslim World* 26, 170-175.

Lokotsch, Karl 1927. *Etymologischer Wörterbuch der europäischen Wörter orientalischen Ursprungs.* Heidelberg.

Lorimer, David Lockhart Robertson 1975. *Farhang-e mardom-e Kermān.* Edited by Feridun Vahman. Tehran, 1354.

Löw, Immanuel 1881. *Aramäische Pflanzennamen.* Leipzig.

______1924. *Die Flora der Juden.* Vol. 3. Vienna and Leipzig.

Lumʿa, Manūčihr 1960. *Farhang-e ʿāmmiyāna-ye ašāyer-e Buyir Aḥmadī va Kūhgilūya.* Tehran, 1339.

Luna, Luis Eduardo 1984. "The Concept of plants as teachers among four Peruvian shamans of Iquitos, Northeast Peru." *Journal of Ethnopharmacology* 11, 135-36.

______1986. *Vegetalismo: shamanism among the mestizo population of the Peruvian Amazon.* Stockholm (*Acta Universitatis Stockholmiensis: Stockholm studies in comparative religion* 27).

Lushington, Alfred W. 1915. *Vernacular list of trees, shrubs and woody climbers in the Madras Presidency.* Madras.

Macdonnell, A. A. 1917. *A Vedic reader for students.* London.

McKenna, Dennis J., G. H. N. Towers and F. J. Abbott 1984a. "Monoamine oxidase inhibitors in South American hallucinogenic plants: part 1: tryptamine and β-carboline constituents of *ayahuasca." Journal of Ethnopharmacology* 10, 193-223.

_____1984b. "Monoamine oxidase inhibitors in South Americian hallucinogenic plants: part 2: Constituents of orally active myristicaceous hallucinogens." *Journal of Ethnopharmacology* 12, 179-211.

McKenna, Dennis J., L. E. Luna and G. H. N. Towers 1984. "Biodynamic constituents in *ayahuasca* admixture plants: an uninvestigated folk pharmacopoeia." Unpublished MS.

McKenna, Dennis J., and G. H. N. Towers 1985. "On the comparative ethnopharmacology of malpighiaceous and myristriaceous hallucinogens." *Journal of Psychoactive Drugs* 17, 35-39.

MacKenzie, D. N. 1977. *A Concise dictionary of Pahlavi.* Oxford.

Madan, Dhanjishah Meherjibhai (Editor) 1911. *The Complete text of the Pahlavi Dinkard.* 2 vols. Bombay.

Mahdihasan, S. 1963. "Identifying soma as Ephedra." *Pakistan Journal of Forestry* 13:4, 370-373.

________1974. "Soma in the light of comparative pharmacology, etymology and archaeology." *Janus* 61, 91-102.

________1985. "A Persian painting illustrating Ephedra leading to its identity as soma." *Journal of Central Asia* 8, 171-175.

Majlisī, M. Bāqir ibn M. Taqī 1699. *Ḥulyat al-muttaqīn.* Edition of Tehran 1371 *Qamerī* or of Tehran 1347 *Šamsī.*

Makowiecki, Stefan 1936. *Słownik botaniczny łacinsko-maloruski zebrał ułozył w Latach 1877-1932.* Krakow (*Polska Akademia Umiejetności, Prace Komisji Jzykówej* 24).

Maksimovich, Karl I. 1889. *Enumeratio plantarum hucusque in Mongolia.* Fasc. 1. St. Petersburg.

Malandra, William 1979. "*Atharvaveda* 2.27: evidence for a *soma*-amulet." *Journal of the American Oriental Society* 99, 220-224.

Mallik, A. B., and A. R. Mohajir 1958. "A Survey of the medicinal plants of the Karachi area." *Pakistan Journal of Science and Industrial Research* 1, 66-68.

Manandhar, N. P. 1980. *Medicinal plants of Nepal Himalaya.* Kathmandu.

Marzell, H. 1943-1958. *Wörterbuch der deutschen Pflanzennamen.* 4 vols. Leipzig.

Masclans I Grivés, F. 1954. *Els noms vulgars de les plantes les terres Catalans.* Barcelona.

Massé, Henri 1938. *Croyances et coutumes persanes, suivies de contes et chansons populaires.* 2 vols. Paris (*Les littératures populaires de toutes les nations, n.s.* 6).

Mayer, Thomas John Lee 1909. *English Biluchi dictionary.* Lahore. Reprinted 1975.

Mayrhofer, Manfred 1956-1976. *Kurzgefasstes etymologisches Wörterbuch des Altindischen.* 3 vols. Heidelberg.

_____1977. *Die altiranischen Namen, Faszikel 1. Die avestischen Namen.* Vienna (*Österreichische Akademie der Wissenschaften).*

_____1985. Review of *Cambridge History of Iran, Vol. 2. Die Sprache* 31, 326-327.

Menges, Karl (Editor and translator) 1933. *Volkskündliche Texte aus Ost-Türkestan, aus dem Nachlass von N. T. Katanov.* Berlin (*Sitzungsberichte der Preussischen Akademie der Wissenschaften, Ph.-h. Klasse* 32, 1171-1293).

Meyerhof, M. and G. P. Sobhy (Translators) 1932-1940. *The Abridged version of "The Book of Simple Drugs" of Aḥmad ibn Muḥammad al-Ghāfiqi by Gregoris Abu'l-Farag (Barhebraeus).* Cairo (*Egypt University Faculty of Medicine publication* 4).

Meyerhof, Max 1918. "Der Bazar der Drogen und Wohlgerüche in Kairo." *Archiv für Wirtschaftsforschung im Orient* 1/2, 1-40; 3/4, 185-218.

Migahid, Ahmad Mohammad 1978. *Flora of Arabia.* 2nd edition. 2 vols. Riyadh.

Minorsky, V. 1953. "Addenda to the *Ḥudūd al-ʿālam." Bulletin of the School of Oriental and African Studies* 17, 250-270.

Modi, Jivanji Jamshedji 1921. "An Iranian legend of the use of the plant *sidāb* (rue, order Rutaceae)." *Journal of the Bombay Anthropological Society* 12, 290-300.

_____1937. *Religious ceremonies and customs of the Parsees.* 2nd edition. Bombay.

Moghadam, Mohamad E. 1938. "The Indo-European origins of the Iranian new year festival." Ph.D. dissertation. Princeton.

Molé, Marijan 1951. "Les Implications historiques du prologue du *Livre d'Artā Virāz." Revue de histoire des religions* 1139, 36-44.

_____1963. *Culte, mythe et cosmologie dans l'Iran ancien: le problème zoroastrien et la tradition mazdéenne.* Paris (*Annales du Musée Guimet* 69).

_____1967. *Le Légende de Zoroastre selon les textes pehlevis.* Paris (*Travaux de l'Institut d'études iraniennes de l'Université de Paris* 3).

Monchi-Zadeh, Davoud 1969. *Das Persische im Codex Cumanicus.* Uppsala (*Acta Universitatis Upsaliensis: Studia Indoeuropaea Upsaliensia* 1).

Monier-Williams, Monier 1899. *A Sanskrit-English dictionary.* 2nd edition. Oxford. Reprinted Berkeley 1976.

Mooney, H. F. 1963. *A Glossary of Ethopian plant names.* Dublin.

Moran, E. A., J. F. Couch and A. B. Clowson 1940. "*Peganum harmala*, a poisonous plant in the Southwest." *Veternary Medicine* 35, 234-235.

Morgenstierne, Georg 1927. *An Etymological vocabulary of Pashto.* Oslo.

_____1952. "Feminine nouns in *-a* in western Iranian dialects." In *A Locust's leg: studies in honour of S.H. Taqizadeh.* Edited by W.B. Henning and E. Yarshater. London, 203-208.

_____1954. "A Vedic word in some modern Hindukush languages." In *Sarūpa Bhāratī: the Dr. Lakshman Sarup memorial volume.* Edited by J.N. Agrawal and B.P. Shastri. Hashiarpur. Vol. I, 30-33.

_____1973. *Indo-Iranian frontier languages.* 2nd edition. 4 vols. Oslo (*Institutet for Sammenlignende Kulturforskning Serie B.* 11; 35; 40; 58).

_____1974. *Etymological vocabulary of the Shughni group.* Wiesbaden (*Beiträge zur Iranistik* 6).

Moybayeni, Sadiq 1980. *Rostanihā-yi Irān: flora giyāhā-yi āvandī.* Vol. 1. 2nd ed. Tehran 1359.

Muʿin, Muḥammad (Editor) 1951-1956. *Burhān-i Qāṭiʿ* [by M. Ḥusayn b. Khalaf Tabrīzī Burhān]. 5 vols. Tehran 1330-1335.

Müller, K. O. 1932. "Über die Verbreitung der Harmel-staude in Anatolien und ihre Bindung an die menschlichen Wohnstätten." In *Festschrift zur Feier des 50-jahrigen Bestehens der Deutschen Botanischen Gesellschaft.* Berlin-Dahlem (*Berichte der Deutschen Botanischen Gesellschaft* 50a), 262-275.

Müller, R. E. G. 1954. "Soma in der altindische Heilkunde." In *Asiatica, Festschrift Friedrich Weller zum 65. Geburtstag gewidmet vom seinen Freunden, Kollegen und Schulern.* Leipzig, 428-441.

Munkácsi, Bernat 1907 "'Pilz' und 'Rausch'". *Keleti Szemle* 8, 343-344.

al-Murtaḍā al-Zabīdī (d. 1791) 1868. *Tāj al-ʿarūs min jawāhir al-qāmūs.* 10 vols. Cairo.

Musil, Alois 1927. *Arabia deserta.* New York.

Nabil el-Hadidi, M. 1972. "*Zygophyllaceae.*" In *Flora Iranica.* Edited by K. H. Rechinger. Graz. Liefg. 98.

Nadkarni, K. M. 1954. *Indian materia medica.* 2 vols. Bombay.

Nair, N. C. 1978. *Flora of the Punjab plains.* Hawrah.

Naranjo, Claudio 1967. "Psychotropic properties of the harmala alkaloids." In *Ethnopharmacologic search for psychoactive drugs.* Edited by E. H. Efron. Washington, D. C., 389-391.

_____1973. "Psychological aspects of the *yagé* experience in an experimental setting." In *Hallucinogens and shamanism.* Edited by Michael J. Harner. Oxford, 176-190.

_____1975. "Harmine and the collective unconscious." In Claudio Naranjo, *The Healing journey: new approaches to consciousness.* New York, 119-170.

Naranjo, Plutarco 1983. *Ayahuasca: etnomedicina y mitologia.* Quito.

Narten, Johanna 1986. *Der Yasna Haptaŋhāiti.* Wiesbaden.

Nāṣerī, ʿAbdallah 1971. *Farhang-e mardom-e Bālūč.* Tehran 1358.

Nikitin, V. 1957. "*Ephedraceae.*" In *Flora Tadzhikskoj SSR.* Edited by P. N. Ovčinnikov. Moscow. Vol. 1, 60-83.

Nyberg, H. S. 1964. *A Manual of Pahlavi.* Vol. 1. Wiesbaden.

_____1974. *A Manual of Pahlavi.* Vol. 2. Wiesbaden.

O'Flaherty, W. D. 1968. "The Post-Vedic history of the soma plant." In R. G. Wasson, *Soma: divine mushroom of immortality.* New York. Part II (95-147).

Osadča, M. 1930. "Pro garmalu *Peganum harmala* L. na Ukraini ta vykorystovuvannja ii jak lykars'koi roslyny." *Visnyk Prykladnoi Botaniky* (Cherkow) I, 98-105.

Ossadcha-Janata, Natalice 1952. *Herbs used in Ukrainian folk medicine.* New York (*The New York Botanical Gardens Memeographed Series* 21).

Pakistan Forest Research Institute, Medicinal Plant Branch 1956. *A Note on the plants of medicinal value found in Pakistan.* Abbottabad.

Parsa, Ahmad 1943-1952. *Flora de l'Iran.* 5 vols. Tehran.

Patel, Rajivbhai Manibhai 1963. *Manav mootra (Human urine, an elixer [sic] of life: a treatise on urine therapy for universal health).* Ahmadabad, India.

Patzak, A. 1964. "*Zygophyllaceae.*" In *Flora of lowland Iraq.* Edited by K. H. Rechinger. Weinheim.

Pavry, Cursetji Erachji 1918. "Ancient ceremonies; additions and improvements made in them." In *Dastur Hoshang memorial volume.* Bombay. pp. 165-192.

Payne Smith, Robert 1879-1901. *Thesaurus Syriacum.* 2 vol. Oxford.

Pedersen, Holger 1901. "Przyczynki do gramatyki porównawczej języków słowianskich." *Materiały i Prace Komisyi Jzykówej Akademii Umiejetności w Krakowie* I, 167-176.

Pedrotti, G., and V. Bertoldi 1930. *Nomi dialettali delle plante indigene del Trentino e della Ladinia Dolomitica.* Trento.

Pennes, H. H., and P. H. Hoch 1957. "Psychotomimetics, clinical and theoretical considerations, harmine, Win. 2299, and naline." *American Journal of Psychiatry* 113, 887-890.

Perrin, Bernadotte (Editor and translator) 1914-1926. *Plutarch, life of Artaxerxes. Loeb Classical Library Plutarch Bk. XI.* Cambridge, Mass.

Piddington, H. 1832. *An English index to the plants of India.* Calcutta.

Pinkley, Homer 1969. "Plant admixtures to *Ayahuasca." Lloydia* 32, 205-214.

Pischel, R. 1900. Grammatik der Prakrit-Sprache. Strassburg.

Pokorny, Julius 1959-1969. *Indogermanisches etymologisches Wörterbuch.* 2 vols. Bern.

Polak, J. E. 1874. Review of J. L. Schlimmer, *Terminologie médico-pharmaceutique et anthropologique française-persane.* Tehran 1874. *Zeitschrift der Deutschen Morgenländischen Gesellschaft* 28, 699-703.

Qazilbash, N. A. 1960. "Ephedra of the Rigveda." *The Pharmaceutical Journal* 185, 497-501.

Raehner, Hugo 1963. *Greek myths and Christian mysteries.* London.

al-Rāzī, Abū Bakr M. Ibn Zakariyāʾ (c . 900 C.E.) 1967. *al-Ḥāwī fī al-ṭibb.* Vols. 20-21. Hyderabad (Osmania Oriental Publications Bureau).

Rechinger, K. H. (Editor) 1963-. *Flora Iranica: Flora des iranischen Hochlands und der umrahmenden Gebirge.* Graz.

Redhouse, James 1974. *New Redhouse Turkish-English Dictionary,* 2nd ed. Istanbul

Reichel-Dolmatoff, Gerardo 1971. *Amazonian cosmos: the sexual and religious symbolism of the Tukano Indians.* Chicago.

_____1972. "The Cultural context of *Banisteriopsis caapi.*" In *Flesh of the Gods.* Edited by P.T. Furth. New York, 84-113.

_____1975. *The Serpent and the jaguar: a study of narcotic drugs among the Indians of Colombia.* Philadelphia.

_____1978. *Beyond the Milky Way: hallucinatory imagery of the Tukano Indians.* Los Angeles (*U.C.L.A. Latin American Center Publication*).

Rempis, Ch. 1963. "Qui est l'auteur du *Zartusht-Nāmeh?*" In *Mélanges d'orientalisme offerts à Henri Massé.* Tehran, 337-342.

Renaud, H. P. S., and Georges Colin (Editors and translators) 1934. *Tuḥfat al-aḥbāb, glossaire de la matière médicale marocaine.* Paris (*Publ. de l'Institut des Hautes Études Marocaines* 24).

Riedl, H. 1963. *"Ephedraceae."* In *Flora Iranica.* Edited by K. H. Rechinger. Graz.

Rieu, E. V. (Translator) 1946. *Homer: the Odyssey.* New York.

Rivier, L., and J. Lindgren 1972. "*Ayahuasca,* the South American hallucinogenic drink: ethnobotanical and chemical investigation." *Economic Botany* 29, 101-129.

Rolland, Eugene 1903. *Flore populaire ou histoire naturelle des plantes dans leurs rapports avec la linguistique et le folklore.* Vol. 4. Paris.

Rosenberg, Frederic (Editor and translator) 1904. *Zarātusht Nāma* [by Zartusht Bahrām Son of Paždū.] St. Petersberg. Revised by Muḥammad Dabīr Siyāqī. Tehran 1959.

Rosenthal, Franz 1968. *The Herb: hashish versus medieval Muslim society.* Leiden

Roth, R. 1884. "Wo wächst der Soma?" *Zeitschrift der Deutschen Morgenländischen Gesellschaft* 38, 134-139.

Saad, Farouk (Editor) 1973. *Kitāb ʿAjāʾib al-maxlūqāt* [by Zakariyā' ibn M. al-Qazwīnī (d. 1283)]. Beirut.

Sabeti, Ḥabībollah 1965. *Daraxtān va daraxtčahā-ye Irān.* Tehran 1344.

Sachau, Eduard (Editor) 1878. *Al-Athār al-bāqiya ʿan al-qurūn al-xāliya* [by Abū Rayḥān M. ibn Aḥmad al-Bīrūnī]. Leipzig.

Sachau, Eduard (Translator) 1879. *The Chronology of ancient nations by al-Bīrūnī.* London.

Safina, L. K., R. G. Medvedeva, and L. D. Bryzgalova 1970. "Dinamika alkaloidov v garmale obyknovennoj-*Peganum harmala* L." *Trudy Instituta Botaniki Akademij Nauk Kazakskoj SSR* 28, 226-235.

Ṣafīnažād, Javād 1966. *Monoghrāfī-ye deh-e Ṭālabābād.* Tehran 1345.

Said, Hakim M., and R. E. Elahie (Editors and translators) 1973. *Al-Bīrūnī's book on pharmacy and materia medica.* 2 vols. Karachi.

Sami, S. 1926. *Die Pflanzennamen in der altarabischen Poesie.* Munich.

Sanjana, Darab P. (Editor) 1894. *Nirangistan, a photozincographed facsimile of a MS.* Bombay (*Pahlavi Text Series* 1).

Schapka, U., and O. H. Volk 1979. "Ein Verzeichnis von in Afghanistan gebräuchlichen Pflanzennamen." *Afghanistan Journal* 6:1, 3-14.

Schlerath, B. 1968. *Awesta-Wörterbuch, Vorarbeiten.* 2 vols. Wiesbaden.

____1971. "Zarathuštra im Awesta." In *Festgabe deutscher Iranisten zur 2500 Jahrfeier Irans.* Edited by W. Eilers. Stuttgart, 133-140.

____1976. "*Yasna* 32.8." *Farhang-e Irān zamīn* 21, 133-136.

Schmidt, Hanns-Peter 1969. "Avestan *unā-* and *ūnā-.*" In *K. R. Cama Oriental Institute golden jubilee volume.* Bombay, 124-132.

____1982. "Avestan root(s): homonymy or polysemy?" In *Golden Jubilee Volume.* Edited by T. N. Dharmadhikari. Poona, 265-269.

Schmucker, Werner 1969. *Die Pflanzliche und mineralische Materia Medica in Firdaus al-Ḥikma des Ṭabarī.* Bonn (*Bonner Orientalistische Studien, Neue Serie* 18).

Schultes, R.E. 1957. "The Identity of the malpighiaceous narcotics of South America." *Harvard University Botanical Museum Leaflets* 18, 1-56.

____1982. "The Beta-carboline hallucinogens of South America." *Journal of Psychoactive Drugs* 14, 205-220.

Schutzenberger, M. P. 1867. *Traité des matières colorantes.* 2 vols. Paris.

Schwartz, Martin 1969. Review of H. W. Bailey, *Indo-Scythian studies, being Khotanese texts, Vol. VI: Prolexis to the Book of Zambasta.* Cambridge. *Journal of the American Oriental Society* 89, 444-447.

_____1970. "On the vocabulary of the Khwarezmian *Muqaddimatu l-Adab,* as edited by J. Benzing." *Zeitschrift der Deutschen Morgenländischen Gesellschaft* 120, 288-304.

_____1975. "Cautes and Cautopates, the Mithraic torchbearers." In *Mithraic Studies.* Edited by John R. Hinnells. Manchester. Vol. 2, 406-422.

_____1980a. Review of Manfred Mayrhofer, *Iranisches Personennamenbuch. Band I: Die altiranischen Namen. Faszikel 1: Die avestischen Namen,* 1977. *Orientalia,* 123-126.

_____1980b. "The Etymon of *snake, snail,* and *sneak* in the light of Indo-Iranian." In *American Indian and Indoeuropean studies: papers in honor of Madison S. Beeler.* Edited by Kathryn Klar, Margaret Langdon, and Shirley Silver. The Hague, 461-467.

_____1985a. "Scatology and eschatology in Zoroaster: on the paronomasia of *Yasna* 48.10 and on Indo-European *$*H_2EG$* 'to make taboo' and the reciprocity verbs *$*K^wSEN(W)$* and **MEGH.*" In *Papers in honour of Professor Mary Boyce.* Leiden. Vol. 2 (*Acta Iranica* 25), 473-496.

_____1985b. "Achaemenian Religion." In *Cambridge history of Iran. Vol. 2: The Median and Achaemenian periods.* Edited by I. Gershevitch. Cambridge, 664-698.

_____1986. "Coded sound patterns, acrostics, and anagrams in Zoroaster's oral poetry." *In Studia grammatica Iranica: Festschrift für Helmut Humbach.* Edited by Rüdiger Schmitt and Prods Oktor Skjærvø. Munich (Münchener Studies zur Sprachwissenschaft, Beiheft 13, Neue Folge), 327-392.

Schweinfurth, Georg 1912. *Arabische Pflanzennamen aus Aegypten, Algerien und Jemen.* Berlin.

Shaked, Shaul 1971. "The notions of *mēnōg* and *gētīg* in the Pahlavi texts and their relation to eschatology." *Acta Orientalia* 33, 59-107.

al-Shamma, Ali, and Abdul-Mutalib Abdul-Ghany 1977. "A Comparative study of the alkaloidal contents of *Peganum harmala* L." *Bulletin of the Biology Research Center, Baghdad* 8, 10-16.

Shea, David, and A. Troyer (translators) 1901. *The Dabistan or school of manners.* Edited by A.V. Williams Jackson. Washington and London.

Sheriyar, Khudayar Dastur 1914. "The Funeral ceremonies of the Zoroastrians in Persia." In *Papers on Iranian subjects written by various scholars in honour of the jubilee of Sir Jamsetjee Jejeebhoy Zarthoshti Madressa.* Edited by J. J. Modi. Bombay, 306-318.

Shokurzāde, Ebrāhīm 1967. *ʿAqāyed va rosūm-e ʿāmma-ye mardom-e Khorāsān.* Tehran 1346.

_____1974. "Souvenirs de l'Iran ancien dans le folk-lore du Xorasan." *Acta Iranica* 3, 360-378.

Shrestha, K. 1979. *Nepali names for plants.* Kathmandu.

Sims-Williams, Nicholas 1985. *The Christian Sogdian manuscript C2.* (*Schriften zur Geschichte und Kultur des alten Orients. Berliner Turfantexte XII. Akademie der Wissenschaften des DDR.*) Berlin.

Singh, M., S. Malla, S. Rajbhandari and A. Manandhur 1979. "Medicinal plants of Nepal: retrospect and prospects." *Economic Botany* 33, 185-198.

Skjærvø, Prods Oktor 1983. "'Kirdīr's vision': translation and analysis." *Archaeologische Mitteilungen aus Iran* 16, 269-306.

Słuszkiewicz, Eugeniusz 1977. "La Drogue: notice étymologique." *Indologica Taurinensia* 5, 167-175.

Sontheimer, Joseph von (Translator) 1842. *Grosse Zusammenstellung ueber die Kraft der bekannten einfachen Heil- und Nahrungsmittel von Abu Mhd. Abdallah b. Ahmed aus Malaga bekannt Ebn Baithar.* 2 vols. Stuttgart.

Soroushian, Jamshīd S. 1956. *Farhang-e Behdīnān.* Tehran 1335.

Sotoudeh, M., and Iraj Afshar (Editors) 1973. *Ṣaydana* [by Abū Rayḥān M. ibn Aḥmad al-Bīrūnī]. 2 vols. Tehran 1352.

Sotoudeh, M. 1963. *Farhang-e Semnānī, Sorxeʾī, Lašgerdī, Sangesarī, Šahmirzādī.* Tehran 1342.

Spiegel, Friedrich 1883. "Zur Erklärung des Avesta." *Zeitschrift der Deutschen Morgenländischen Gesellschaft* 27, 649-668.

Srivastava, T. N., and O. P. Gupta 1982. "Medicinal plants used by Amchies in Ladakh." In *Cultivation and utilization of medicinal plants.* Edited by C. K. Atal and B. M. Kapor. Jammu-Tawi.

Staal, J. Frits 1979. *Agni: the Vedic ritual of the fire altar.* 2 vols. Berkeley.

Stannard, Jerry 1967. "The Plant called *moly.*" *Osiris* 14, 254-307.

Stapf, Otto 1889. Die Arten der Gattung *Ephedra.* Vienna (*Denkschriften der Kaiserlichen Akademie der Wissenschaften Math.-Nat. Klasse.* 56).

Steblin-Kamenskij, I. M. 1982. *Ocherki po istorii leksiki Pamirskikh uz'ron.* Moscow.

______1983 *"Venok iz Vakhana:* a wreath from Wakhan." *Acta Iranica* 22, 225-248.

Stein, Aurel 1931. "On the Ephedra, the *hōm* plant and soma." *Bulletin of the School of Oriental Studies* 6, 501-514.

Steingass, F. 1894. *A Comprehensive Persian-English dictionary.* London.

Steinschneider, Moritz 1897. "Heilmittelnamen des Araber." *Wiener Zeitschrift für die Kunde des Morgenlandes* 11, 259-278, 313-330; 12, 1-20, 81-101, 201-229, 319-334; 13, 75-94.

Stewart, J. L. 1869. *Punjab Plants.* Lahore.

Stutley, Margaret 1980. *Ancient Indian magic and folklore.* London.

Sundararaj, D. D., and Giurija Balasubramanyam 1959. *Guide to the economic plants of South India.* Madras.

Täckholm, V. 1969. "Alfred Kaiser's Sinai Herbarium." *Publications of the Cairo University Herbarium* 2, 1-137.

Tavadia, J.C. 1948. "Ordeal in *Yasna Ha* 8." In *Dinshah Irani memorial volume.* Bombay, 2-20.

Thalen, D.C.P. 1979. *Ecology and utilization of desert shrub rangelands in Iraq.* The Hague.

Thieme, Paul 1957. "Vorzarathustrisches bei den Zarathustriern und bei Zarathustra." *Zeitschrift der Deutschen Morgenländischen Gesellschaft* 107, 66-104.

Thomas, Bertram 1930. *The Kumzari dialect of the Shiluh tribe.* London.

Thompson, R. Campbell 1949. *A Dictionary of Assyrian botany.* London.

Thomson, Margaret H. (Editor) 1955. *Textes grecs inédits relatifs aux plantes.* Paris.

Togan, Ahmad Zeki Velidi (Editor) 1941. "Bīrūnī's picture of the world." *Memoirs of the Archaeological Society of India* 53.

Tomaschek, Wilhelm 1894. "Die dakischen Pflanzennamen," pp. 22-36 of *Die alten Thraker, eine ethnologische Untersuchung.* Vienna. (*Sitzungsberichte der Ph.-h. Kl. der Kaiserlichen Akademie der Wissenschaften,* Bd. 103, Abh. 2).

Toporov, Vladimir N. 1981. "Die Ursprünge der indoeuropischen Poetik." *Poetica: Zeitschrift für Sprache- und Literaturwissenschaft* 13, 189-251.

Townsend, C. C. 1965. "*Ruta* L." and "*Haplophyllum* A. Juss." In *Flora of Turkey and the East Aegean.* Edited by P.H. Davis. Edinburgh. Vol. 2, 495-498.

______1966a. "Towards a revision of *Haplophyllum* A. Juss. *(Rutaceae)* I." *Kew Bulletin* 20, 89-102.

______1966b. *"Rutaceae."* In *Flora Iranica.* Edited by K. H. Rechinger. Graz.

Townsend, C. C., and Evan Guest (Editors) 1980. *Flora of Iraq.* Vol. 4. Baghdad.

Trabut, L. 1935. *Flore de nord de l'Afrique, répertoire des noms indigènes des plantes spontanées, cultivées et utilisées dans le nord de l'Afrique.* Algers.

Turner, R. L. 1966. *Comparative dictionary of the Indo-Aryan languages.* London. Reprinted 1977.

Unvala, Jamshedji Maneckji (Editor and translator) 1921. *The Pahlavi text: King Husrav and his boy: published with its transcription, translation and... with an appendix and a complete glossary.* Paris.

______1924. *Neryosangh's Sanskrit version of the Hōm Yašt (Yasn IX-XI): with the original Avesta and its Pahlavi version.* Vienna.

Unvala, Maneckji Rustomji 1908. "A Few Parsee festivals (jashans) according to an old Parsee manuscript." In *Spiegel memorial volume.* Edited by J. J. Modi. London, 201-210.

______(Editor) 1922. *Darab Hormazyar's Rivāyat.* 2 vols. Bombay.

Vasmer, Max 1950-. *Russisches etymologisches Wörterbuch.* Heidelberg.

Venzlaff, Helga 1977. *Der marokkanische Drogenhändler und seine Ware. Ein Beitrag zu Terminologie und volkstümlichen Gebrauch traditioneller arabischen Materia Medica.* Wiesbaden (*Veröffentlichungen der orientalische Kommission* 31).

Viktorov, S. V. 1973. "Man-made indicators and their significance in landscape-indicator investigations." In *Landscape indicators: new techniques in geology and geography.* Edited by A. G. Chikishov. Moscow Society of Naturalists. Translated by J. Paul Fitzsimmon Consultants Bureau. New York, London, 158-165.

Vincett, Betty A. Lipscombe 1979. *Wild flowers of Central Saudi Arabia.* Milan.

Volk, O. H. 1955. "Afghanische Drogen." *Planta Medica* 3, 129-146, 171-178.

____ 1961. "A Survey of Afghan medicinal plants." *Pakistan Journal of Science and Industrial Research* 4, 230-236.

Von Soden, Wolfram 1978. *Akkadisches Handwörterbuch,* Lief. 13. Wiesbaden.

Vonderheyden, M. 1937. "Le Harmel." In *Mélanges de géographie et d'orientalisme offerts à E.-F. Gautier.* Tours, 456-462.

Vries, Herman de 1985. " *L'Hermel, harmel, harmal, Peganum harmala* L., die Steppenraute, ihr Gebrauch in Marokko als Heilpflanze und Psychotherapeutikum." *SALIX* 1, 36-40.

Vullers, Johann August 1855-1867. *Lexicon Persico-Latinum etymologicum.* 3 vols. Bonn. Reprinted Graz. 1962.

Waag, Anatol (Editor and translator) 1941. *Nirangistan: Der Awestatraktat über die rituellen Vorschriften.* Leipzig.

Wasson, R. Gordon 1968. *Soma: divine mushroom of immortality.* New York.

______1970. "Soma of the Aryans: an ancient hallucinogen?" *Bulletin on Narcotics* 22:3, 25-30.

______1971. "Soma of the Rig Veda: what was it?" *Journal of the American Oriental Society* 91, 169-187.

______1978. "Soma brought up to date." *Harvard University Botanical Museum Leaflets* 26:6, 211-223.

______1979. "Soma brought up to date." *Journal of the American Oriental Society* 99, 100-105.

______1982. "The Last meal of the Buddha (with memorandum of Walpola Rahula and epilogue by Wendy Doniger O'Flaherty)." *Journal of the American Oriental Society* 102, 591-604.

Watkins, Calvert 1978. "Let us now praise famous grains." *Proceedings of the American Philosophical Society* 122, 9-17.

Watson, Patty Jo 1979. *Archaeological ethnography in western Iran.* Tucson (*Viking Fund Publications in Anthropology* 57).

Watt, George (Editor) 1889-1896. *A Dictionary of the economic products of India.* 6 vols. Calcutta.

Wellmann, Max (Editor) 1907-1914. *Pedanii Dioscuridis Anazarbei de materia medica libri quinque.* 3 vols. Berlin.

Weryho, Jan 1962. "Seistani Persian folklore." *Indo-Iranian Journal* 5, 276-370.

West, E. W. (Translator) 1904. "Transliteration and translation of the Pahlavi version of *Yasna XXXII,* the fifth chapter of the first Gāthā." In *Avesta, Pahlavi and ancient Persian studies in honour of Shams-ul-Ulama Dastur Peshotanji Behramji Sanjana.* Strassburg, 182-198.

______1882. *Pahlavi texts part II: the Dādistān-ī Dīnīk and the Epistles of Mānūskīhar.* London (*Sacred Books of the East* 18). Reprinted Delhi 1965.

Westermarck, E. 1926. *Ritual and belief in Morocco.* 2 vols. London.

Widengren, Geo 1979. "Révélation et prédication dans les *Gathas.*" In *Iranica.* Edited by Gherardo Gnoli and Adriano V. Rossi. Naples (*Istituto Universitario Orientale Seminario di Studi Asiatici. Series Minor* 10), 339-363.

Windfuhr, Gernot L. 1985. "Haoma/Soma the plant." In *Papers in honour of Professor Mary Boyce.* Leiden. Vol. 2 (*Acta Iranica* 25), 699-726.

Wolff, Fritz 1910. *Awesta, die heiligen Bücher des Parsen, übersetzt auf der Grundlage von Chr. Bartholomae's Altiranischen Wörterbuch.* Strassburg.

Wright, W. Ramsey (Editor and translator) 1934. *The Book of instruction in the elements of the art of astrology (Kitāb at-Tafḥīm li-awā᾽ il ṣinā῾at at-tanjīm)* [by Abū Rayḥān M. ibn Aḥmad al-Bīrūnī]. London.

Wüstenfeld, Ferdinand (Editor) 1849. *Kitāb ῾Ajā᾽ib al-maxlūqāt wa-gharā᾽ib al-mawjūdāt und Athār al-bilād* [by Zakariyā' ibn M. al-Qazwīnī (d. 1283)]. 2 vols. Göttingen.

Zohary, M. 1973. *Geobotanical foundations of the Middle East.* Stuttgart.

INDEX LOCORUM

WORD INDEX

Forms in Tables 1, 2, and 3 are, with few exceptions, not normalized and may be inaccurate, even where unmarked.

✘ Indicates rejected forms.

A. = Attested in Arabic script

GENERAL INDEX

Appendix 5

"The inhibitory effect of norharman on morphine withdrawal syndrome in rats: comparison with ibogaine"

Susanne L.T. Cappendijk*[a], Durk Fekkes[b], Michailo R. Dzoljic[a]

Deparment of [a]Pharmacology [PO Box 1738] and [b]Psychiatry, Faculty of Medicine and Health Sciences, Erasmus University Rotterdam, 3000 DR Rotterdam, The Netherlands

Received 21 June 1994; revised 5 August 1994; accepted 5 August 1994 *Corresponding author

Abstract

Norharman (20 mg/kg, i.p.) and ibogaine (40 mg/kg, i.p.) significantly attenuated naloxone (4 mg/kg, i.p.)-precipitated withdrawal syndrome in morphine-dependent rats. Several withdrawal signs, such as teeth-chattering, chewing, penile licking and diarrhorea were decreased by both norharman and ibogaine. In addition, norharman reduced also the withdrawal grooming and rearing. It is concluded that both norharman and ibogaine are inhibitors of withdrawal syndrome in morphine-dependent rats.

Norharman (β-carboline) is an endogenous occurring substance in brain and other tissues in rats and man [13, 14]. Recently, elevated plasma levels of norharman were detected in chronic alcoholics [17] and heroin addicts [18]. These data favour an idea of involvement of norharman in drug dependence processes. A structurally related substance to norharman is ibogaine. Both, norharman and ibogaine are indole derivatives with psychogenic/hallucinatory properties [2, 9]. It has been shown that ibogaine attenuates morphine withdrawal [8, 12] and interrupts drug dependence [5, 11]. These facts justify a further elucidation of the effects of these two substances in drug dependence phenomena. In order to make a comparison between these two chemically and behaviorally (psychogenic/hallucinatory) similar substances, we studied the effects of both drugs, norharman and ibogaine on naloxone-precipitated withdrawal in morphine-dependent rats.

Male Wistar rats (TNO Zeist), weighing 290-330 g were housed in groups and had a free access to food and water. The room was maintained on a 12-h light/dark cycle (lights on 08.00 h), with constant temperature (21°C) and humidity (55%). Morphine dependence was induced by implantation of a morphine base pellet (75 mg/rat, s.c., n = 30) on the back of the animal under ether anaesthesia [4]. All morphine-dependent animals were used only once. Morphine-dependent rats were divided into three groups, pretreated intraperitoneally with vehicle (distilled water, n = 10), norharman (20 mg/kg, n = 10) or ibogaine (40 mg/ kg, n = 10). The selected doses of norharman and ibogaine are biologically active, shown by previous studies [5, 15]. The withdrawal syndrome in morphine-dependent animals was precipitated by naloxone (4 mg/kg, i.p.), given 30 min after vehicle, norharman or ibogaine. The naloxone treatment occurred 72 h following pellet implantation. The observer was 'blind' to the treatment order and registered the withdrawal symptoms during 30 min following injection of naloxone. The withdrawal signs were scored according to the weighting factors described by Neal and Sparber [16]. In short, the signs observed during a mild withdrawal syndrome were assigned with 1 (diarrhoea, chewing, grooming, irritability on touch, rearing), whereas the sign rhinorrhoea, observed during severe withdrawal was assigned a 3. All other withdrawal signs, teethchattering, wet-dog shakes, penile licking, ptosis and jumping were assigned by a weighting factor 2.

Norharman (Sigma, England) and ibogaine (Sigma, England) were administered in volume of 2.2 ml/injection. Naloxone HCl (Sigma Chemical Co., St Louis, MO) was given in volume of 1 ml/kg. The pH of drug solutions and vehicle were adjusted to 7-8. All drugs were dissolved in distilled water. Data were evaluated by using the nonparametric Kruskall–Wallis one-way analysis of variance, followed by the Mann–Whitney U-test, with a level of $P<0.05$ being considered significant [10].

A decreased locomotion and exploratory behaviour was observed in norharman (20 mg/kg, i.p.)-treated naive (n = 6) and morphine-dependent (n = 10) animals. This effect lasted 5–20 min. In contrast, the ibogaine (40 mg/kg, i.p., n = 10) induced within 4 min tremor and excitatory behaviour (jumping or violent locomotion on touch). The behavioral effects, induced by norharman or ibogaine disappeared within 30 min.

This study is the first demonstration that norharman, a physiological substance significantly attenuates a nalox-one-precipitated withdrawal syndrome in rats (Fig. 1A). Ibogaine, similarly to previous data [8, 12], also reduced naloxone-precipitated withdrawal

Reprinted by permission of Elsevier Science B.V. from *Behavioral Brain Research* 65 (1994) pp.117–119.

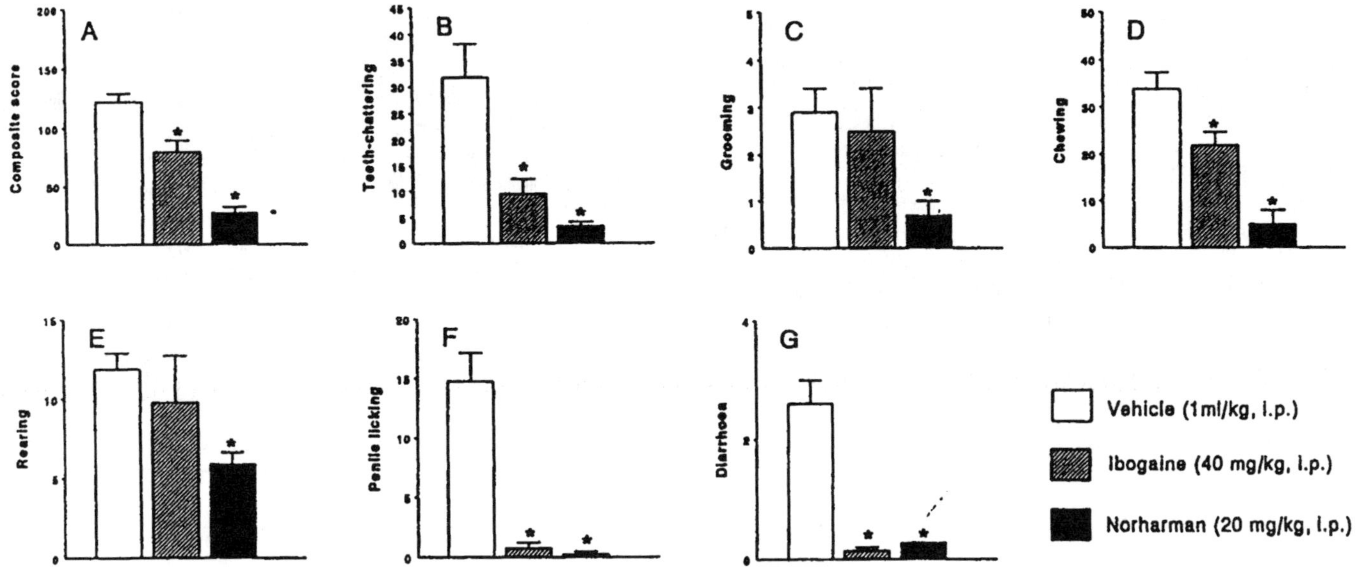

Fig. 1. Effect of norharman and ibogaine on the severity of naloxone (4 mg/kg, i.p.)-precipitated withdrawal syndrome (A) and specific withdrawal signs (B–G) in morphine-dependent rats. Morphine dependence was induced by implantation of morphine pellet on the back of the animal under ether anaesthesia. Animals were treated with vehicle (distilled water, 1 ml/kg, i.p., $n = 10$), ibogaine (40 mg/kg, i.p., $n = 10$) or norharman (20 mg/kg, i.p., $n = 10$), 72 h following pellet implantation and 30 min prior naloxone. Data in Fig. 1A are expressed as composite score, determined by counting the number of all observed withdrawal signs, during the 30-min period of abstinence. The withdrawal signs were scored according to the method described by Neal and Sparber [16]. All data were expressed as mean ± S.E.M. * Significant decrease of withdrawal syndrome or signs (Mann–Whitney U-test, $P < 0.05$) compared to the control group. Note that norharman and ibogaine attenuated the severity of withdrawal syndrome and frequency of withdrawal signs.

syndrome (Fig. 1A). Related to the specific symptoms, both norharman and ibogaine attenuated teeth-chattering, chewing, penile licking and diarrhoea (Fig. 1B, D, F, G). Grooming and rearing response were reduced by norharman only (Fig. 1C, E). These data indicate that norharman and ibogaine induced a similar (but not identical) decrease of opioid withdrawal symptoms.

Although a mechanism of action of norharman and ibogaine is not known, an involvement of the opioid system could be considered, since both drugs interfere with opioid receptors as agonists. Norharman acts as a partial μ–agonist [2], while ibogaine is an agonist of κ-receptors [6]. The binding activity of both drugs to central opioid receptors with possible displacement or preventing the binding of naloxone to opioid receptors may lead to an antiwithdrawal effect. In periphery μ– and κ-agonists can depress the acetylcholine release from the cholinergic neurons of myenteric plexus [3]. This effect may contribute to the decreased intensity of withdrawal diarrhoea, induced by norharman and ibogaine.

The other neurotransmitter system which could be involved in the decreased expression of the opioid withdrawal is the glutaminergic system. Glutamate antagonists may prevent morphine abstinence in mice and guinea pigs [4, 19]. Consistent with this finding, morphine is able to block the glutamate-induced excitation in the monkey [20] and in the mouse [1]. The fact that both norharman and ibogaine have also morphine-like properties [9, 6] favours a hypothesis that blockade of the glutamate-mediated transmission could contribute to thc attenuation of the excitatory character of withdrawal syndrome. This idea has been supported by Dowson [7], showing that harmala alkaloids inhibit the transmission at the glutamate-mediated neurons.

In conclusion, these experiments show that norharman and ibogaine attenuated the opioid withdrawal syndrome and favour an idea of an inhibitory role of both drugs in the expression of morphine abstinence. Although all involvement of the opioid- and/or glutamate-neurotransmitter system could be considered at present as a main underlying mechanism for the attenuation of withdrawal syndrome, the precise mechanisms of action of norharman and ibogaine remain unclear. However, of particular importance would be a further clarification of the role of norharman as a physiological modulator of morphine withdrawal phenomena.

This research was supported by Addiction Research Institute Rotterdam.

[1] Aanonsen, L.M. and Wilcox, G.L., Nociceptive action of excitatory amino acids in the mouse: effects of spinally administered opioids, phencyclidine and *sigma* agonists, *J. Pharmacol. Exp. Ther.*, 243 (1987) 9–19.

[2] Airaksinen, M.M. and Kari, I., β–Carbolines, psychoactive compounds in the mammalian body, *Med. Biol.*, 59 (1981) 190–211.

[3] Burks, T.F., Fox, D.A., Hirning, L.D., Shook, J.E. and Porreca, F., Regulation of gastrointestinal function by multiple opioid reccplors, *Life Sci.*, 43 (1988) 2177–2181.

[4] Cappendijk, S.L.T., De Vries, R. and Dzoljic, M.R., Excitatory amino acid receptor antagonists and naloxone-precipitated withdrawal syndrome in morphine-dependent mice, *Eur. Neuropsychopharmacol.*, 3 (1993) 111–116.

[5] Cappendijk,S.L.T.and Dzoljic,M.R.,Inhibitory effects of ibogaine on cocaine self-administration in rats, *Eur. J. Pharmacol*, 241 (1993) 261–265.

[6] Deecher, D.C., Teitler, M., Soderlund, D.M., Bornmann, W.G., Kuchne, M.E. and Glick, S.D., Mechanisms of action of ibogaine and harmaline congeners based on radioligand binding studies, *Brain Res.*, 571 (1992) 242–247.

[7] Dowson, R.J., Clements, A.N. and May T.E., The action of some harmala alkaloids on transmission at a glutamate-mediated synapse, *Neuropharmacology*, 14 (1975) 235–240.

[8] Dzoljic, E.D., Kaplan, C.D. and Dzoljic, M.R., Effect of ibogaine on naloxone-precipitated withdrawal syndrome in chronic morphine-dependent rats, *Arch. Int. Pharmacodyn.*, 294 (1988) 64–70.

[9] Farnsworth, N.R., Hallucinogenic plants, *Science*, 162 (1968) 1086–1092.

[10] Glantz, S.A., *Primer of Biostatistics: Methods Based on Ranks.* McGraw-Hill, New York, NY, 1989, pp. 291–317.

[11] Glick, S.D., Rossman, K., Steindorf, S., Maisonneuve, I.M. and Carlson, J.N., Effects and aftereffects of ibogaine on morphine self-administration in rats, *Eur. J. Pharmacol.,* 195 (1991) 341–315.

[12] Glick, S.D., Rossman, K., Rao, N.C., Maisonneuve, I.M. and Carlson, J.N., Effects of ibogaine on acute signs of morphime withdrawal in rats: independence from tremor, *Neuropharmacology,* 31 (1992) 497–500.

[13] Greiner, B. and Rommelspacher, H., Two metabolic pathways of tetrahydro-norharmane (tetrahydro-beta-carboline) in rats, *Naunyn Schmiedeberg's Arch. Pharmacol.,* 325 (1983) 349–355.

[14] Honecker, H. and Coper, H., Tetrahydronorharmane (THN) and 6-hydroxy-norharmane: physiological components in platelets and urine of man, *Naunyn Schmiedeberg's Arch. Pharmacol.,* 302 (1978) R63.

[15] Morin, A.M., β—Carboline kindling of the benzodiazepine receptor, *Brain Res.,* 321 (1984) 151–154.

[16] Neal, B.S. and Sparber, S.B., Mianserin attenuates naloxone-precipitated withdrawal signs in rats acutely or chronically dependent upon morphine, *J. Pharmacol. Exp. Ther.,* 236 (1986) 157–165.

[17] Rommelspacher, H., Schmidt, L.G. and May, T., Plasma norharman (β—carboline) levels are elevated in chronic alcoholics. *Alcohol Clin. Exp. Res.,* 15 (1991) 553–559.

[18] Stohler, R., Rommelspacher, H., Ladewig, D. and Dammann, G., Beta-carboline (harman/norharman) sind bei heroinabhängigen erhöht, *Ther. Umschau,* 50 (1993) 178–181.

[19] Tanganelli, S., Antonelli, T., Morari, M., Bianchi, C. and Beani, L., Glutamate antagonists prevent morphine withdrawal in mice and guinea pigs, *Neurosci. Lett.,* 122 (1991) 270–272.

[20] Willcockson, W.S., Kim, J., Shin, H.K., Chung, J.M. and Willis, W.D., Actions of opioids on primate spinothalamic tract neurons, *J. Neurosci.,* 6 (1986) 2509–2520.

Appendix 6

"Ibogaine in the Treatment of Chemical Dependence Disorders: Clinical Perspectives"

Howard Lotsof

THE PRIMARY PURPOSE OF this paper is to provide general information to the clinician who will be using the Lotsof Procedure[SM] (Goutarel, 1993) developed by NDA International, Inc. in which Ibogaine is administered to treat chemical dependence disorders. This is a preliminary report. The patient base upon which my conclusions have been made totals thirty-five treatment episodes. All clinical observations conducted after 1963 have been made on patients treated outside of the United States.

Ibogaine is not a substitute for narcotics or stimulants, is not addicting and is given in a single administration modality (SAM). It is a chemical dependence interrupter. Retreatment may occasionally be needed until the people being treated with Ibogaine are able to extinguish certain conditioned responses related to drugs they abuse. Early data suggests that for many patients, a period of approximately two years of intermittent treatments may be required to attain the goal of long-term abstinence from narcotics and stimulants. The majority of patients treated with Ibogaine remain free from chemical dependence for a period of three to six months after a single dose. Approximately ten percent of patients remain free of chemical dependence for two or more years from a single Ibogaine treatment. An equal percentage return to drug use within two weeks after treatment. Multiple administrations of Ibogaine over a period of time are generally more effective in extending periods of abstinence. It is noteworthy that twentynine of the thirty-five patients successfully treated with Ibogaine had numerous unsuccessful experiences with other treatment modalities.

A Brief History

Ibogaine is a naturally occurring alkaloid found in Tabernanthe iboga and other plant species of Central West Africa. It was first reported to be effective in interrupting opiate narcotic dependence disorders in U.S. patent 4,499,096 (Lotsof,1985), cocaine dependence disorders, U.S. patent 4,587,243 (Lotsof, 1986) and poly-drug dependence disorders, U.S. patent 5,152,994 (Lotsof, 1992). The initial studies demonstrating Ibogaine's effects on cocaine and heroin dependence were conducted in a series of focus group experiments by H. S. Lotsof in 1962 and 1963. Additional data on the clinical aspects of Ibogaine in the treatment of chemical dependence were reported by Kaplan (1993), Sisko (1993), Sanchez-Ramos & Mash (1994), and Sheppard (1994).

Reprinted with permission of publisher from *Bull. MAPS,* 1995, Vol. 5, #3, pp. 16–27.

Dedicated to the work of J. Bastiaans and N. Adriaans; in memory of N. Kribus.

Correspondence: Howard S. Lotsof, NDA International, Inc., PO Box 100506, Staten Island, NY 10310–0506, USA. E-mail: ibogaine@desk.nl.

Prior to Ibogaine's evaluation for the interruption of various chemical dependencies, the use of Ibogaine was reported in psychotherapy by Naranjo (1969, 1973) and at the First International Ibogaine Conference held in Paris (Zeff, 1987). The use of Ibogaine-containing plants has been reported for centuries in West Africa in both religious practice and in traditional medicine (Fernandez, 1982; Gollnhofer & Sillans 1983, 1985). An overview of the history of Ibogaine research and use was published by Goutarel et al. (1993).

Claims of efficacy in treating dependence to opiates, cocaine, and alcohol in human subjects were supported in preclinical studies by researchers in the United States, the Netherlands and Canada. Dzoljic et al. (1988) were the first researchers to publish Ibogaine's ability to attenuate narcotic withdrawal. Stanley D. Glick et al. (1992) at Albany Medical College published original research and a review of the field concerning the attenuation of narcotic withdrawal. Maisonneuve et al. (1991) determined the pharmacological interactions between Ibogaine and morphine, and Glick et al. (1992) reported Ibogaine's ability to reduce or interrupt morphine self-administration in the rat. Woods et al. (1990) found that Ibogaine did not act as an opiate, and Aceto et al. (1991) established that Ibogaine did not precipitate withdrawal signs or cause dependence.

Cappendijk and Dzoljic (1993) published Ibogaine's effect in reducing cocaine self-administration in the rat. Broderick et al. (1992) first published Ibogaine's ability to reverse cocaine-induced dopamine increases and later reported on Ibogaine's reduction of cocaine-induced motor activity and other effects (1994). Broderick et al.'s research supported the findings of Sershen et al. (1992), that Ibogaine reduced cocaine-induced motor stimulation in the mouse. Sershen (1993) also demonstrated that Ibogaine reduced the consumption of cocaine in mice. Glick (1992) and Cappendijk (1993) discovered in the animal model that multiple administrations of Ibogaine over time were more effective than a single dose in interrupting or attenuating the self-administration of morphine and cocaine, supporting Lotsof's findings in human subjects (1985).

Popik et al. (1994) determined Ibogaine to be a competitive inhibitor of MK-801 binding to the NMDA receptor complex. MK-801 has been shown to attenuate tolerance to opiates (Trujillo & Akil 1991) and alcohol (Khanna et al.1993). MK-801 has also shown to blockade "reverse tolerance" of stimulants (Karler et al. 1989). Ibogaine's effects on dopamine and the dopamine system (dopamine is a substance hypothesized to be responsible for reinforcing pleasurable effects of drugs of abuse) were found by Maisonneuve et al. (1991), Broderick et al. (1992) and Sershen et al. (1992). Ibogaine binding to the kappa opiate receptor was reported by Deecher et al. (1992). Thus we begin to see a broad spectrum of mechanisms by which Ibogaine may moderate use of substances as diverse as opiate narcotics, stimulants and alcohol.

CLINICAL PRACTICE

The effects of Ibogaine treatment are viewed in three categories: acute, intermediate and long-term. The acute and intermediate effects have sometimes been referred to as the effects and aftereffects. The two major effects of Ibogaine are the ability to interrupt narcotic and stimulant withdrawal, and the attenuation or elimination of the craving to continue to seek and use opiates, stimulants and alcohol (Lotsof 1985, 1986, 1989). Knowledge concerning the use of Ibogaine in treating alcohol dependence is limited to: 1) a single alcohol-only dependent patient, 2) the attenuation and, in some cases, cessation of alcohol use in persons treated for poly-drug dependence disorders. Ibogaine's ability to treat nicotine dependence (Lotsof,1991) has been observed in poly-drug dependent subjects treated primarily for opiate and/or cocaine use.

There are some general considerations in reviewing the use of Ibogaine. The primary obligations of the treatment team are four-fold: 1) to earn the trust of the patient, 2) to maintain the comfort of the patient, 3) to assist the patient in interrupting their chemical dependence and 4) to supply the psychosocial support network needed by the majority of patients to enable them to develop a sense of personal accomplishment and the ability to function as productive members of society. This is a process the Dutch treatment community refers to as normalization.

In the Lotsof Procedures[SM], for which a manual is now being prepared, the sense of conflict seen in most treatment modalities between the doctor and patient over the immediate cessation of drug use does not exist. The patients have been allowed, if narcotic dependent, to continue their use of narcotics until a certain time prior to treatment with Ibogaine. There is no conflict over opiate use before treatment, as our position has been that Ibogaine will either work to interrupt chemical dependence or it will not. Patients dependent on stimulants are not maintained on stimulants and this has not created a problem for the patients or the medical staff.

Prior to our conducting Ibogaine treatments in hospitals, addicted patients were allowed to use their personal supply of narcotics until the evening before treatment. However, during hospital-administered Ibogaine sessions, the narcotic-dependent patient is maintained on medications prescribed by the principal investigator during the three to five day intake process preceding their treatment with Ibogaine. Even under these circumstances, patient distrust of the medical establishment and extreme fear of going into withdrawal has resulted in the smuggling of narcotics into hospital environments. In order to protect the patient from possible overdose due to narcotics, stimulants or other drugs, a thorough physical examination is performed on all patients upon their admission to hospital environments. The examination and a search of the patient's possessions prior to treatment with Ibogaine serve two important functions. The first, is to limit the possibility of accidental overdose from hidden drugs. The second is to provide a complete understanding of the patient's physical health, since many of the people seeking treatment for chemical dependence have masked various and often numerous medical problems for years or even decades by self-medicating with illicit drugs.

ACUTE EFFECTS REGIMEN

The acute effects of Ibogaine are dramatic. The initial reaction is usually noted within forty-five minutes after the oral administration. Full effects are generally evident within two to two and a half hours.

The earliest subjective indication by patients of Ibogaine's effects is the report of a pervasive oscillating sound. The patient tends to lie down and, if asked to stand or walk, shows signs of ataxia.

The protocol for the Lotsof Procedures[SM] stipulates that the patient remain in bed with as little movement as possible from the time of Ibogaine administration. This is because nausea associated with Ibogaine use has proven to be motion-related and/or, in later stages (those longer than four hours after administration), possibly to be a psychosomatic reaction to previously repressed traumatic experiences. In addition to keeping the patient as still as possible, we use a non-phenothiazine anti-nauseant, since phenothiazines may interfere with the psychoactive properties of Ibogaine. If the patient vomits in less than two and a half hours after the administration of Ibogaine, an examination of the regurgitated material should be made to determine how much Ibogaine may have already been absorbed by the patient. A rectal infusion of Ibogaine to supplement the lost portion of the dose may be provided if it is not possible for this dose to be administered orally. The rectal administration should occur only if the patient has previously consented to this mode of dosing.

VISUALIZATION

One of Ibogaine's principal effects during its first phase of action is to produce a state which emulates dreaming, except that the subject is fully awake and has the ability to respond to the treatment staff's questions. In most cases, people under the influence of a therapeutic dose of Ibogaine do not wish to speak. They prefer instead to pay close attention to the visual presentation of memories or phenomena that they are experiencing. These phenomena have been noted to have both Freudian and Jungian connotations.

The presentation of visual material is rapid. Some patients have described it as a movie run at high speed. Others describe it as a slide show, each slide containing a motion picture of a specific event or circumstance in the viewer's life. In either case, the presentation of visual material is so compressed and fast moving that distracting the patient for even a moment may interfere with the process of abreaction. Therefore, during the primary phase of Ibogaine treatment, the intrusion of the medical staff should be kept to a minimum.

AUTONOMIC RESPONSES

During the first through the fifth hour there is a moderate rise in blood pressure of ten to fifteen percent and, in some cases, an associated decline in the pulse rate. The most significant autonomic changes occur between one and a half and two and a half hours after administration of therapeutic doses of Ibogaine. In many cases pulse rates are elevated due to pre-administration anxiety.

On two occasions, persons with transient hypertension were treated. In one of those instances the patient's blood pressure dropped to normal levels during the primary and secondary stages of treatment. The second hypertensive exhibited little change at a 23 mg/kg therapeutic dose, but showed significant changes on two occasions when provided with only a 1.6 mg/kg test dose. The two 1.6 mg/kg doses were supplied due to our concern over the patient s hypertension. He had been previously treated with an 18 mg/kg dose by Dutch Addict Self-Help (DASH) with no apparent negative results. This alleviated some of our concern for the patient's safety. Variation in individual patient reactions should be anticipated.

Female Patient Safety

One 24-year-old female patient treated with Ibogaine for chemical dependence died from undiagnosed causes in the Netherlands. Although her autopsy did not determine the cause of death, it reported Ibogaine levels of 0.75 mg/liter in blood. This level has not been seen to be toxic in animal research or in our prior human experience. Subsequent to this death and to the previously reported death of a Swiss woman who received Ibogaine during a psychotherapy session in Europe (totally unrelated to NDA's research program), the FDA excluded women from the present clinical trials taking place at the University of Miami. However, the FDA decision is contrary to the gender guidelines of the National Institutes of Health. The guidelines with regard to women call for the inclusion of women at the earliest stages of clinical trials, as this would provide the greatest determination of drug safety for women. Thirty percent of NDA International's patients have been women who have shown no negative effects from taking Ibogaine either during or after treatment. However, considering all of the circumstances, the Procedure should be administered only in a hospital or clinic with the patient under continuous staff observation and electronic monitoring.

An ongoing intemational research program is developing evidence to determine a hypothesis for the cause of death of the woman in the Netherlands. We are additionally seeking Swiss government cooperation concerning the death of the Swiss woman. The results of this research may facilitate either an exclusion criteria or an antidote allowing bogaine safely to treat chemical dependence n women.

Cognitive Evaluation

During the second phase of Ibogaine's action in the Lotsof Proceduressm, the patient experiences the intellectual evaluation of his or her previous life experiences and decisions. This occurs after the visualization phase, which generally ends abruptly in three to five hours. However, individual reactions and variations are the norm and not the exception within the parameters of the Procedure.

When various decisions were made by the patient in the past, those decisions appeared to be the only options available at the time. However, due to Ibogaine's ability to catalyse the reevaluation of one's life, actions and behavior, it is possible for patients to understand that alternatives to their original decisions were available. This knowledge appears to allow the patient to modify their current behavior and cease their drug dependence.

Behavioral Immobility

During the periods of visualization, and extending into the stage of cognitive evaluation, patients will demonstrate a state of behavioral immobility (Depoortere, 1987). Brain wave pattems associated with dreaming and sleep, but distinct from those states, are represented by rhythmic slow activity of 4–6 Hz. These EEG patterns are associated with a state characterized by a lack of movement. Some early observers of the Lotsof ProceduresSM (Kaplan, personal communication, 1990) initially believed that the condition represented paralysis, but when patients were asked to stand and move around, the patients were able to do so, albeit with difficulty.

Attenuation of Narcotic Withdrawl

One of the major acute effects experienced with Ibogaine treatment is the attenuation or elimination of narcotic withdrawal in opiatedependent patients. This is extremely important to the narcotic-dependent patients who live in fear of going into withdrawal.

The treatment team's experience in the field is of the utmost importance in dealing with this aspect of the Procedure. Withdrawal symptoms are a combination of physical and, in many cases, psychosomatic manifestations that are anxiety-driven. Therefore, it is imperative for the medical and paramedical staff to have experience in identifying and distinguishing between these varieties of symptoms. Provided below are examples of psychosomatic withdrawal manifestations demonstrated by two of the patients treated outside the United States.

Example One

On one occasion I was called into the room by a colleague about twenty hours after Ibogaine had been administered to a twentyfive year old male heroin-dependent patient. The patient had been using approximately 1/4 gram of heroin a day, but had increased his daily intake to two grams while in the Netherlands.

I was informed that the patient was complaining of muscle spasms. I asked the patient if this was true, and he responded in the affirmative. I asked if I might see these spasms. The patient agreed, showing me the calf of his leg. He was exhibiting what appeared to be involuntary movements. I checked his pupils and observed that they were not dilated, nor was he exhibiting any other form or manifestation of withdrawal. When I tumed to my colleague for discussion I noticed the patient's spasms had ceased. Upon reexamination of his calf, the spasms returned. I turned away once again, but continued to watch him and the spasms ceased again. I informed the patient that I believed the spasms to be psychosomatic in origin. I placed a pillow under the patient's calf to give it support and covered the patient with a blanket. The spasms did not occur again.

Example Two

On another occasion I received a call from a person involved with Dutch Addict Self-Help (DASH) groups who had been observing a number of treatments. She informed me that a Yugoslavian woman in her mid to late twenties had been complaining of narcotic withdrawal during Ibogaine treatment. However the DASH observer did not believe this to be the case, as there were no observable signs of withdrawal.

When I arrived, the patient was sitting on a couch. I checked her pupils and observed they were not dilated, and asked her if she was in withdrawal. The patient said she was.

"How are you in withdrawal? What are its manifestations?" I asked.

"I'm sick," she said.

I asked her if her eyes were tearing.

"Yes," she said, but her eyes were not tearing.

"Is your nose running?"

"Yes," she said, but her nose was dry.

"Do you have goose bumps?" I asked.

"Yes," she said, but I pointed out to her that she did not have goose bumps, and finally I said, "Do you have diarrhea?"

"Yes," she said, but I had no way to determine the validity of her statement.

The patient requested that I provide her with funds to return home. I told her I did not think it wise for her to leave at this time, but would give her carfare in the morning. The following day the DASH observer told me that the patient had left about four hours after I did informing the observer as she left that she had not been sick, but had only said she was. This example should further demonstrate the importance of hospital administered treatments with a full medical staff of psychiatrists, neurologists, internists, therapists, nurses, peer counselors and patient advocates capable of evaluating and responding to any aspect of the patient's condition at all times.

The complaint of experiencing narcotic withdrawal after leaving the treatment environment has been reported in three cases. We have provided additional treatments six months to a year after the initial treatment to patients who were re-addicted and stated they had experienced some form of withdrawal within a week of their first Ibogaine treatment. Our working group decided to keep patients making such complaints under observation for periods equal to the number of post treatment days during which the patients stated they previously experienced withdrawal symptoms.

Our findings have been that, under the above conditions of monitoring, the reported withdrawal signs are usually symptoms of anxiety or anxiety related conditions that the patients characterized as withdrawal. These symptoms included nausea, diarrhea or increases in blood pressure in one hypertensive patient.

There have been two incidents which did not appear anxiety related, in which diarrhea occurred five to seven days after treatment in patients who had previously used one gram of heroin a day. These episodes were easily controlled with a single administration of an appropriate medication and did not occur again.

AFTEREFFECTS: INTERRUPTION OF CRAVING

The acute interruption of craving to seek and use drugs of abuse is unique to the Lotsof Proceduressm as a treatment modality for chemical dependence disorders. This effect is generally not noticed by the patient until the principal actions of Ibogaine (visualization, cognitive evaluation, behavioral immobility and significant residual stimulation) are no longer evident and the patient has had the opportunity to sleep. The initial recognition of lack of craving is usually noticed forty-eight to seventy-two hours after Ibogaine administration. In a minority of treatments, recovery and the absence of craving may be evident to the person being treated in as little as twenty-four hours. The medical staff, on the other hand, usually notes the absence of craving in the patient in forty-five minutes to one and a half hours after Ibogaine administration.

Our experience gained in recent years through the treatment of twenty persons outside the United States has shown that the majority of patients may need a series of treatments before the conditioned responses (craving) to a long history of chemical dependence can be extinguished. However, for three of these patients, a single treatment interrupted chemical dependence for a minimum of two years. The advantage of Ibogaine is that it allows patients time periods free of craving during which the psychiatrist, social worker, therapist, paraclinician and the patient often bond into a cohesive working group to accomplish a state of long-term non-dependence by the patient to the drug(s) of abuse for which the patient is under treatment.

PSYCHOSOCIAL SUPPORT

All aspects of treatment for chemical dependence disorders common to other treatment modalities are common to the use of Ibogaine. The patient's characteristics in terms of psychopathology and behavior, societal accomplishments, as well as the skills of the treatment team are significant to treatment outcome.

In rare cases, when the patient already has the occupational, educational, and professional skills needed to succeed in society, the task may be somewhat easier. In cases where the patient does not have those societal skills, or lacks medical care for disorders other than chemical dependence, care and training must be provided through psychosocial support structures.

Trauma suffered by the patient during childhood appears to play an important part in the drive for love and the fear of abandonment that are common to many of the patients we have treated (Bastiaans, 1991).

All psychosocial support paradigms should be available for the patient after the completion of an Ibogaine treatment. Their use should be contingent upon the evaluation of the patient's needs and progress.

One of the primary differences that social workers, counselors or therapists offering psychosocial support notice in post-Ibogaine treated patients as compared to untreated subjects, is the rapidity with which the support can and must be provided to aid the patient in accomplishing goals and making decisions. Ibogaine presents a symptom-free window of opportunity, of which the patient and therapist must take advantage. One patient put it this way: "Ibogaine and 12–Step (groups) both help you to get in touch with your soul. Ibogaine is like rocket fuel for that process" (*Village Beat,* 1990). This means moving quickly and dramatically to assist the patient to establish goals while the patient has the ability and desire to do so.

Ibogaine generally produces a receptive psychological state in the patient. This produces a relationship between the patient and the therapist which is mutually rewarding and beneficial, but requires the person providing psychosocial support to work both harder and faster than is the norm for other treatment modalities. Prior to the use of Ibogaine in the treatment of chemical dependence, it may have taken the therapist three to twenty-four months (Judd, personal communication, 1993) using traditional methods to assist the patient in reaching a state of well-being free of drug craving (Kaplan et al., 1993). This advantage that Ibogaine treatment provides enables the psychosocial support staff to assist patients in making decisions which facilitate their normalization and integration into society as self-fulfilled and productive human beings.

Many of the accepted parameters of distance between the therapist and the patient are not effective in Ibogaine treatment. Patients require closer and more intensive guidance, and will generally be more open to it. They will require faster intervention to learn societal skills and to overcome and objectively understand various traumas experienced during their lives. Therefore, Ibogaine is not a treatment modality for clinicians whose preference is to simply administer a pill or tablet and then distance themselves from their patients.

REDUCTION OF THE NEED FOR SLEEP

In all cases, Ibogaine temporally reduces the patient's need for sleep to as few as three or four hours a night. This effect may last a month or more, gradually retuming to what is normal. Two theories have been put forth concerning this effect that are not necessarily contradictory. First. the long-lasting bioavailability of Ibogaine or one of its metabolites, and second, the decrease in the psychological requirements for sleep associated with the necessity to dream, as Ibogaine promotes an intense emulation of dreaming that lasts for many hours during its acute stage of activity.

The reduction in the need for sleep is viewed by the majority of patients as a discomfort, as they have used drugs and sleep as an escape mechanism. These patients may require some mild form of sedation during the first days after treatment with Ibogaine. Normal precautions should be taken in providing sedatives to persons with a history of chemical dependence. In a minority of cases, patients have used this newly available time to advantage in their busy work schedules.

Long-Term Effects

By long-term effects I mean those which may be noticed from one to twenty-four months after treatment, and in some cases even longer. I have provided three examples.

Example One

A heroin-dependent couple was treated. The woman of 26 was a relatively new addict of three months while her 27-year-old husband had a history of over ten years of heroin use. At the time of their treatment we generally followed a protocol of treating one patient at a time, as these were early treatments and the medical and medical support staff were familiarizing themselves with what might be expected during such episodes.

Portions of the treatment episodes were observed by Dr. Carlo Contoreggi, Deputy Medical Director of the Addiction Research Center of the National Institute on Drug Abuse in Baltimore and Dr. Lester Grinspoon of the Harvard School of Medicine.

The husband was treated first, and his wife was completely cooperative and helpful during his treatment. The following day, when the wife was administered her dose of Ibogaine, her husband demanded that he be allowed to leave his room and remain in bed with her. He informed the medical and paramedical staff present that unless he got his way he would create a disturbance to interfere with his wife's treatment. Rather than deal with a belligerent and angry patient, we decided it would be less harmful to let him have his way. He continuously disturbed his wife during her treatment. This resulted in a policy of treating couples simultaneously in separate rooms.

He recovered before his wife, as she had been administered Ibogaine twenty-four hours after his treatment. He complained that he was getting bedsore and was no longer able to stay in bed and asked for permission to go for a bicycle ride. Upon his leaving, his wife broke down and cried in the arms of a female paraclinician, stating she did not know if she could remain with her husband, but she was afraid he would die if she left him. This was a concept he continuously stressed to her during their treatment.

After treatment, he followed a pattern of controlling his wife's contacts with other persons including the treatment team, which was denied access to either of them. We later learned that they both returned to heroin use. However, three months later the wife determined that her husband was incapable of loving himself or her and this was not the life she wished. She stopped using heroin, enrolled in nursing school, filed divorce proceedings against her husband, and is now specializing in psychiatric nursing.

While initially she did not recognize that her decision to stop heroin use was due to her Ibogaine treatment, as the months went by she realized that her determination to change her life was catalyzed by her experience with Ibogaine.

Example Two

A cocaine/cocaine-base dependent patient was treated with the Lotsof Procedure and experienced an acute interruption of his drug use. During his Ibogaine treatment he had a strong impression that if he continued drug use God would punish him. He remained drug-free for about thirty days, after which he increased his drug use over the next months. He was then retreated. The dose he received proved to be inadequate due to his vomiting of the oral dose, and to a bowel movement immediately after the rectal administration of Ibogaine, which he requested to compensate for the loss of his oral dose. His drug use continued, but far below his original pretreatment levels.

About six months after his retreatment, the first Ibogaine therapy group sponsored by the International coalition for Addict Self-Help, directed by psychotherapist Barbara Judd, CSW, was established in New York. The patient attended these sessions until fifteen months after his original treatment, when he recognized that he had to move away from his drug-infested neighborhood. Thereupon he moved to Florida.

In Florida, he has remained drug-free, even though he has access to cocaine. He is employed in the construction industry by a business with strict non-drug use guidelines that is owned and run by former drug users.

Example Three

One of the most important concepts learned by persons treated with Ibogaine is that addiction can be reversed. Persons dependent on drugs such as opiates or cocaine are not able to recognize that chemical dependence is a reversible phenomenon.

This third example is of the only chemically-dependent person from the 1962–1963 study to receive a series of Ibogaine treatments at therapeutic levels. The individual remained free of addiction for approximately three and a half years as a result of his series of treatments.

During that period he moved to California, married, and worked in pharmaceutical sales. He later lost his job and, when offered a ride back to New York, accepted it and returned to a life of minor drug dealing and use that resulted in his arrest and imprisonment.

After his release, he worked for a while as a machinist, then slowly fell back into heroin use and addiction in 1969. Luckily, this was a period when methadone programs were expanding, and he was able to enter one of the better programs run by Beth Israel Hospital. At that time, the programs were well-staffed with doctors, nurses and adequate counselors, and the patient reached a point in his life when he recognized that the life of a heroin addict was not what he wanted. It was not just the heroin, but the scene itself, wherein a human life was without value, where sometimes a human being would be murdered for two cents worth of an innocuous powder in a glassine envelope. The patient was ready to quit heroin, but was a slave to the craving to use opiates for the anxiolytic relief they provided.

Over a period of more than two years, the patient stabilized himself on methadone. He tried heroin once, two weeks after starting methadone, was satisfied with the level of blockage that methadone offered, and never used heroin again.

During the next few years the methadone programs changed. Many of the competent counselors were unable to continue in their positions due to the stress and sense of frustration in their work, a condition common in the treatment community. The Federal government placed more and more restrictions on methadone patients freedom of movement and, though methadone is anticipated to maintain the methadone client for a period of twenty-four hours, in many cases it does not. For this patient, withdrawal signs were setting in at eighteen hours and not twenty-four. The patient began a slow detoxification process from 100 mg of methadone per day that took approximately eighteen months.

The final stage of detoxification was followed by the patient's entry into University-level training, for which he had obtained a scholarship to a prominent university. At the time of the detoxification, the philosophy among methadone patients was that you could not get off methadone. However, having previously had the Ibogaine experience, the patient stated that he knew addiction was reversible. That knowledge allowed him to successfully leave addiction behind.

CURRENT TREATMENTS: A SELF REPORT

The following report is from the type of patient we had been seeking for years: a medical doctor who needed to be treated with Ibogaine. The subject was chemically dependent on 600 mg of Demerol a day, and had attempted to stop his drug use a number of times, without any lasting success. Our particular interest in this subject was the hope that, as a medical doctor, he might provide us with some professional insight into the results of his treatment. He kept notes and prepared a report on the four different doses he received. His report is presented below in its entirety.

This subject proved to be more sensitive to Ibogaine than any other individual in our studies conducted outside the United States, and had a full-blown experience from a 10 mg/kg dose. The patient participated in a research protocol which called for an intermediate dose of 10 mg/kg of Ibogaine. This dose was administered as part of a pharmacokinetic study, and was not expected to have a therapeutic effect, but it did. As part of the protocol, he was also administered a known therapeutic dose of 20mg/kg;

1ST DAY — 100 MG (TEST DOSE #1)

"I've taken my Ibogaine dose and went to bed, and stayed laying down. I felt nothing, until the medical staff arrived to do the 1 hour tests. I was surprised because in my mental measurements, I thought I had taken Ibogaine about 20 minutes earlier. When I stood up, I felt a little drowsiness, and it was difficult to walk in a straight line. I was feeling photophobia and every little noise seemed to be much louder than in reality. The sounds were very disturbing to me.

During the two hour testing, symptoms were worse. It was very difficult to walk in a straight line, and the room seemed to beat, like a heart. I felt very tired, and the only thing I wanted was to rest in bed. Each head movement seemed to make things worse.

When I stood up for the 3 hour test I felt that the symptoms were disappearing. I was very hungry and ate. After eating, I was a little nauseated. Eor the following hours I felt nothing, except for sensation that my mind images were richer in details than before, like a 3-D movie.

I ate with no nausea, slept very well, and awakened in very good condition."

2ND DAY — 25 MG (TEST DOSE #2)

"After this dose of Ibogaine I felt nothing different from my normal state."

3RD DAY — 10 MG/KG (EXPERIMENTAL DOSE)

"For the first two hours I felt a little different, like I had smoked marijuana. I was very calm and relaxed and all the tension of the beginning of the procedure was gone. The room seemed to be a little different and the colors around me sharper than normal. The lights and sounds were disturbing to me, like the first time. Suddenly, with my eyes closed I began to see images that appeared in screens, exactly like TV or cinema screens. These screens were appearing in small sizes and then they would get bigger as I focused my attention on them. Sometimes they appeared small and would then begin to grow, like I was walking in their direction, and sometimes they were going from left to right, in a continuous way.

The images on the screens were moving in slow motion and were very sharp and well defined. I saw trees moving with the wind, a man with bells in his hands, various landscapes with mountains and the sunset. At this time I was a little nauseated, and when the doctors asked me to stand up for some tests, I vomited. Erom all of the hundreds of images I saw this day, I recognized only two: the first, an image of myself as a child, static like a photo. This image began to approach me and get bigger, but something in the room happened and I opened my eyes, losing the image. The second image I recognized was one of some horses dancing in a circus. It was a TV show that I had seen two days before. The time seemed to go very quickly, because after about four hours (in my mind), they told me I had taken Ibogaine nine hours earlier! It was very difficult for me to speak in English or in Spanish. I was only able to speak in my native language. At this time the images started to appear at a slower rate and for another two hours I saw only screens with no images on them. About 10–11 hours after the beginning of the experiment they disappeared.

I ate very well and stayed awake all night long, falling asleep only about 7 AM, almost 24 hours after the medication had been administered. During the night I had some insights about my life and about the things I realized I was doing wrong. I stayed all the following day very tired, sleepy, but very happy and relaxed, in a way I never was before."

5TH DAY — 20MG/KG (THERAPEUTIC DOSE)

"The first 3 hours were similar to the last time; photophobia and a bad sensation with little noises. After that the images began to appear, in a slower rate than the other time. There were less images, but I was recognizing all of them as part of my childhood. I saw myself playing in my father's farm, riding a motorcycle, playing with a cousin, feeding a fish and other things. I saw some recent images, like one of my father, laughing in the living room of my house. This happened about a year ago. I understood that I had a happy childhood, and there was no one to blame for my addiction, only myself. I felt their love coming from my parents and relatives. I was feeling the same time distortion that I felt the other day, and after many hours I suddenly had an insight. It was that my mind and the universe were the same thing, and that all the people in the universe and all things in the universe are only one. I saw many mistakes I was doing in my life, so many attitudes I could not have, and this helped me to decide very strongly that I will never use Demerol again. Now I can see very clearly that I don't need Demerol to live my life. And I feel better if I don't use it. During the first 8 hours after taking the Ibogaine I vomited 4 or 5 times, always when I tried to move. I was able to sleep about 4 AM, and to eat only about 9 AM the following day. I awakened feeling weak, tired and drowsy. As the hours were going, I slept a lot and began to feel better and in the morning of the following day I was normal."

DIFFERENCES IN DAY-BY-DAY LIFE

"I returned to my normal life with absolutely no cravings, with better appetite than before, and highly self-confident. Now I can see differences in some aspects of my personality, things are changed. For example, I used to avoid driving at night, because it reminded me of a car accident I had years ago. Now I can drive anytime, day or night, without anxiety. I'm sure that this is caused by Ibogaine, because now I m not the same very anxious person I was. I'm not as shy as I used to be, too. It's easier now to contradict people when I think they are wrong, and to make them know what I want and what I think. I used to accept all that other people said only to avoid a discussion, even when I was sure that my point of view was the correct one.

These are the main happenings in my Ibogaine experience and the main differences I can perceive in these few days."

Some Months Later

"The most important thing I learned with all that happened is that I can never underestimate the power of the addictive personality I have inside. I can never say I'm cured because if I do this, I will forget to protect myself from drug using thoughts. I must know I have a chronic disease that will be quiet in its place until I decide to give it a chance to grow. This decision, and that's the point, is a conscious decision. If I give in, the disease will be out of control in a few days. But, if I could be strong to take real and honest control of my Demerol using thoughts, I will be free forever.

A few days ago, because of professional needs, I had to keep two Demerol doses with me, in my house, all night long. To protect myself, I gave them to my wife. But, it was amazing to see how I was not anxious to use them but, to give them to the patients that needed them. I clearly felt that Demerol was a strange thing in my environment. I wasn't curious about the place my wife had put them, I wasn't feeling any craving. I was only looking forward to the moment I could give them to the patient and say: I've done it. And I did it, because of all of you from NDA.

I don't want to be boring, but I have no words to say how grateful we, my family and I, are. I will remember you for a lifetime."

Needless to say, this patient provided particular advantages in terms of his treatment outcome. He had a career, was highly motivated, and did not require the significant psychosocial support needed by so many others who do not have his background.

Summary

We have only been able to track a significant minority of patients for follow-up observations, about twenty-five percent. In many cases we have maintained direct contact with the patients for only two months after treatment. In a single case, for five years. The difficulty concerning patient contact has been one of geographic distances, both national and international, as our patients have come from diverse cities and countries. This factor, as well as the normal problems in tracking a chemically dependent population, must be taken into consideration when evaluating the findings of this paper.

General conclusions based on study observations are that a single administration of Ibogaine is an interrupter for chemical dependence disorders. A series of treatments given over a period of time will produce more significant results. It may allow some of the persons treated to free themselves completely, (or for a period of years) from dependence to, or the use of, opiates and stimulants, including cocaine and nicotine. Data on alcohol dependence treatment in human subjects is minimal.

A single treatment of Ibogaine has the ability to significantly attenuate opiate withdrawal in all patients. In ninety percent of cases treated, a single treatment can interrupt an individual's craving to continue drug use for periods of time ranging from as short as two days to as long as two and a half years. Concurrently, Ibogaine has demonstrated the ability to precipitate the release of repressed memories and to foster a process of abreaction. I believe these are important aspects of Ibogaine's ability to interrupt chemical dependence.

In order to obtain the greatest benefit for those treated with Ibogaine, a psychological support structure should be in place. Providers of the Procedure should be knowledgeable in the field of chemical dependence treatment, and patients should be shown kindness and respect. In many cases, such an approach will be the first attentions of this kind the patient may have experienced in decades.

Patients are deserving of kindness and respect, and such care is an important part of the healing process: Ultimately, physicians and support staff should be specifically trained in the Lotsof Procedures[SM], to fully understand the physical and psychological transformation of the patient, the advantages of the Procedure, and the providers responsibilities in administering Ibogaine to treat chemical dependence disorders. Eventually, the understanding of Ibogaine's actions may yield important data about memory, learning, dreams and sleep, as well as chemical dependence, tolerance and abuse.

Acknowledgments

The author acknowledges the editorial assistance of Norma E Alexander; Rick Doblin; William J. Gladstone; David Goldstein; Barbara E Judd, CSW; Daniel Luciano MD; Natalie Chantel Luke; Piotr Popik, MD; Bruce H. Sakow; Bob Sisko; Sylvia Thyssen; Boaz Wachtel and Rommell Washington.

The author thanks: N. Adriaans; N. Alexander; Z. Amit, PhD; J. Bastiaans, MD; P A. Broderick PhD; C. Contoreggi, MD; MR. Dzoljic, MD; E. Della Sera, MD; G. Erenken; W.J. Gladstone; S.D. Glick MD; O. Gollnhofer, PhD; R Goutarel, MD (deceased); C. Grudzinskas, PhD; B.E.Judd, CSW; J.S. Kahan, Esq; C.D. Kaplan, PhD; D. Luciano, MD; D.G Mash, PhD; G.J. Prud'Homme, Esq; L Rolla, PhD; B.H. Sakow; J. Sanchez-Ramos, MD; B. Sisko; H. Sershen, PhD; Erank Vocci, PhD, B. Wachtel; R Washington; Curtis Wright, MD and all of the volunteer patients for their courage, their science and the cooperation they have provided.

Bibliography

1 Aceto M.D., "Biological Evaluation of Compounds for Their Physical Dependence Potential and Abuse Liability", NIDA Research Monograph 119:506,520–523,1991, in *Jacobson, A.E.*

2 Bastiaans J., "The Psychiatric and Psychosomatic Dimensions of Trauma," unpublished paper, 1991.

3 Brodenck P.S., Phelan F.T., & Berger S.P., "Ibogaine Alters Cocaine-Induced Biogenic and Psychostimulant Dysfunction, but Not [3H] GBR–12935 Binding to the Dopamine Transporter Protein, *Problems of Drug Dependence 1991: Proceeding of the 53rd Annual Scientific Meeting, CPDD,* NIDA Research Monograph 119:285,1992.

4 Broderick P.S., Phelan F.T., Eng F. & Wechsler T., Ibogaine Modulates Cocaine Responses which are Altered Due to Environmental Habituation: In Vivo Microvoltammetric and Behavioral Studies, *Pharmacology Biochemlstry and Behavior,* vol. 49, no.3,711–728,1994.

5 Cappendijk S.L.T. & Dzoljic M.R., "Inhibitory Effects of Ibogaine on Cocaine Self-Administration in Rats," *European Journal of Pharmacology,*241:261–265,1993.

6 Deecher, D.C., Teitler M., Soderlund D.M., Bornmann W.G., Kuehne M.E. & Glick S.D., "Mechanisms of Action of Ibogaine and Harmaline Congeners Based on Radioligand Binding Studies," *Brain Research* 571:242–247,1992.

7 Depoortere H, "Neocortical Rhythmic Slow Activity During Wakefulness and Paradoxical Sleep in Rats," *Neuropharmacology* 18:160–168,1987.

8 Dwljic E.D., Kaplan C.D. & Dwljic M.R., Effects of Ibogaine on Naloxone Precipitated Withdrawal Syndrome in Chronic Morphine Dependent Rats," *Archive of International Pharmacodynamics,* 294:64-70,1988.

9 Fernandez J.W., *Bwiti: An Ethnography of Religious Imagination in Africa,* Princeton University Press,1982.

10 Glick SD, Rossman K, Rao NC, Maisonneuve IM and Carlson JN, Effects of Ibogaine on Acute

Signs of Morphine Withdrawal in Rats: Independence From Tremor, Neuropharmacology, 31(5):497-500,1992

11 Glick SD, Rossman K, Steindorf S, Maisonneuve IM and Carlson JN, Effects and Aftereffects of Ibogaine on Morphine SelfAdministration in Rats, European Journal of Pharmacology 195:341-345.1992.

12 Gollnhofer O. & Sillans R., "L'Iboga Psychotrope Africain" ("Iboga, An African Psychotropic Agent"), *Psychotropes,* 1(1):11–27,1983.

13 Gollnhofer O. & Sillans R., "Usages Rituels de l'iboga au Gabbn" ("Ritual Uses of Iboga in Gabon"), *Psychotropes,* 2 (3):95–108,1985.

14a Goutarel R., Gollnhofer O. & Sillans R., "Pharmacodynamics and Therapeutic Applications of Iboga and Ibogaine," *Psychedelic Monographs & Essays,* 6:71–111,1993.

14b Goutarel R., Gollnhofer O & Sillans R. L. "Iboga et l'ibogaine contre la dependence aux stupefiants. Pharmacodynamie et applications psychotherapeutiques," *Psychotropes,* 8 (3), 1993.

15 Kaplan C.D., Ketzer E., deJong J., & de Vries M., "Reaching a State of Wellness: Multistage Explorations in Social Neuroscience," *Social Neuroscience Bulletin* 6 (1), Winter,1993.

16 Karler R., Calder L.D., Chaudhry I.A., Turkanis S.A., "Blockade of 'Reverse Tolerance' to Cocaine and Amphetamine by MK-801," *Life Sciences* 45:599–606,1989.

17 Khanna J.M., Kalant H., Shah G., Chau A., Effect of D-cycloserine on Rapid Tolerance to Ethanol," *Pharmacology Biochemistry Behavior* 45 (4):983–986,1993.

18 Lotsof H.S., U.S. patent 4,499,096; Rapid Method for Interrupting the Narcotic Addiction Syndrome,1985.

19 Lotsof H.S., U.S. patent 4,587,243; Rapid Method for Interrupting the Cocaine and Amphetamine Abuse Syndrome,1986.

20 Lotsof H.S., U.S. patent 4,857,523; Rapid Method for Attenuating The Alcohol Dependency Syndrome,1989.

21 Lotsof H.S., U.S. patent 5,026,697, Rapid Method for Interrupting or Attenuating The Nicotine/Tobacco Dependency Syndrome, l99l

22 Lotsof H.S., U.S. patents 5,l24,994; Rapid Method for Interrupting or Attenuating Poly-drug Dependency Syndromes, 1992.

23 Maisonneuve I.M., Keller R.W. Jr. and Glick S.D., Interactions Between Ibogaine, A Potential Anti-Addictive Agent and Morphine: An In Vivo Microdialysis Study, *European Journal of Pharmacology,* 199:35–42, 1991.

24 Mash D.C., Douyon R., Hearn W.L. Samool N.C. & Sanchez Ramos J., "A Preliminary Report on the Safety and Pharmacokinetics of Ibogaine," *Biological Psychiatry,* 1995 In Press.

25 Naranjo C., "Psychotherapeutic Possibilities of New Fantasy Enhancing Drugs," *Clinical Toxicology,* 2 (2): 209. 1969.

26 Naranjo C., *The Healing Journey,* 174–228, Pantheon Books, Div. Random House, NY, 1973.

27 Popik P., Layer R.T. & Skolnick P., "The Putative anti-addictive Drug Ibogaine is a Competitive inhibitor of [3H] MK-801 Binding to the NMDA Receptor Complex" *Psychopharmacology,* 114: 672–674, 1994.

28 Sanchez-Ramos J. & Mash D.C.; "Ibogaine Research Update: Phase I Human Study," *MAPS,* IV (4): 11, Spring 1994.

29 Sershen H., Hashim A., Harsing L., & Lajtha A., "Ibogaine Antagonizes Cocaine-Induced Locomotor Activity in Mice, *Life Sciences,* 50:1079–1086, 1992.

30 Sershen H., Hashim A., & Lajtha A., "Ibogaine Reduces Preferences for Cocaine Consumption in C57BL/6By Mice," Pharmacology, Biochemistry and Behavior, 47 (1):13–19,1994.

31 Sheppard S.G., "A Preliminary Investigation of Ibogaine: Case Reports and Recommendations for Further Study," *J. Substance Abuse Treatment,* 11(4): 379–385, 1994.

32 Sisko B., "Ibogaine and Substance Abusers: Follow-up on Four Case Histories," *MAPS,* IV (2): 15–23, Summer 1993.

33 Trujillo K.A. & Akil H., "Inhibition of Morphine Tolerance and Dependence by NMDA Receptor Antagonist MK-801," *Science* 2512: 85–87, 1991.

34 *Village Beat,* New York City, May 1990.

35 Woods H.W., Medzihardsky F., Smith C.B., Winger G.D. & Prince C.P., "1989 Annual Report, Evaluation of New Compounds for Opioid Activity," *NIDA Research Monograph* 95:563, 655–656 1990.

36 Zeff L., First International Ibogaine Conference, Paris, January 1987 (video tape).

AUTONOMEDIA BOOK SERIES

THE DAUGHTER
ROBERTA ALLEN

MARX BEYOND MARX: LESSONS ON THE GRÜNDRISSE
ANTONIO NEGRI

MAGPIE REVERIES
JAMES KOEHNLINE

CLIPPED COINS, ABUSED WORDS, CIVIL GOVERNMENT: JOHN LOCKE'S PHILOSOPHY OF MONEY
CONSTANTINE GEORGE CAFFENTZIS

TROTSKYISM AND MAOISM: THEORY & PRACTICE IN FRANCE & THE U.S.
A. BELDEN FIELDS

ON ANARCHY & SCHIZOANALYSIS
ROLANDO PEREZ

SCANDAL: ESSAYS IN ISLAMIC HERESY
PETER LAMBORN WILSON

RETHINKING MARXISM
STEVE RESNICK & RICK WOLFF, EDS.

THE TOUCH
MICHAEL BROWNSTEIN

GULLIVER
MICHAEL RYAN

FILM & POLITICS IN THE THIRD WORLD
JOHN DOWNING, ED.

COLUMBUS & OTHER CANNIBALS: THE WÉTIKO DISEASE & THE WHITE MAN
JACK FORBES

CASSETTE MYTHOS: THE NEW MUSIC UNDERGROUND
ROBIN JAMES, ED.

DEMONO (THE BOXED GAME)
P.M.

POPULAR REALITY
IRREVEREND DAVID CROWBAR, ED.

ENRAGÉS & SITUATIONISTS: THE OCCUPATION MOVEMENT, MAY '68
RENÉ VIÉNET

XEROX PIRATES: "HIGH" TECH & THE NEW COLLAGE UNDERGROUND
AUTONOMEDIA COLLECTIVE, EDS.

ZEROWORK: THE ANTI-WORK ANTHOLOGY
BOB BLACK & TAD KEPLEY, EDS.

THE NEW ENCLOSURES
MIDNIGHT NOTES COLLECTIVE

MIDNIGHT OIL: WORK, ENERGY, WAR, 1973–1992
MIDNIGHT NOTES COLLECTIVE

THE NARRATIVE BODY
ELDON GARNET

THE DAMNED UNIVERSE OF CHARLES FORT
LOUIS KAPLAN, ED.

WILD CHILDREN
DAVID MANDL & PETER LAMBORN WILSON., EDS.

FILE UNDER POPULAR: THEORETICAL & CRITICAL WRITINGS ON MUSIC
CHRIS CUTLER

¡ZAPATISTAS! DOCUMENTS OF THE NEW MEXICAN REVOLUTION
MEMBERS OF THE EZLN

THE OFFICIAL KGB HANDBOOK
USSR COMMITTEE FOR STATE SECURITY

GOD & PLASTIC SURGERY: MARX, NIETZSCHE, FREUD & THE OBVIOUS
JEREMY BARRIS

THE ARCANE OF REPRODUCTION: HOUSEWORK, PROSTITUTION, LABOR & CAPITAL
LEOPOLDINA FORTUNATI

MODEL CHILDREN: INSIDE THE REPUBLIC OF RED SCARVES
PAUL THOREZ

A DAY IN THE LIFE: TALES FROM THE LOWER EAST SIDE
ALAN MOORE & JOSH GOSNIAK, EDS.

GONE TO CROATAN: ORIGINS OF NORTH AMERICAN DROPOUT CULTURE
JAMES KOEHNLINE & RON SAKOLSKY, EDS.

ABOUT FACE: RACE IN POSTMODERN AMERICA
TIMOTHY MALIQALIM SIMONE

HORSEXE: ESSAY ON TRANSSEXUALITY
CATHERINE MILLOT

FORMAT AND ANXIETY:
COLLECTED ESSAYS ON THE MEDIA
PAUL GOODMAN

BY ANY MEANS NECESSARY:
OUTLAW MANIFESTOS & EPHEMERA, 1965–70
PETER STANSILL & DAVID ZANE MAIROWITZ, EDS.

WAR IN THE NEIGHBORHOOD
SETH TOBOCMAN

CAPITAL & COMMUNITY
JACQUES CAMATTE

BLOOD & VOLTS
EDISON, TESLA, & THE ELECTRIC CHAIR
TH. METZGER

DREAMER OF THE DAY
FRANCIS PARKER YOCKEY & THE SECRET NAZI INTERNATIONAL
KEVIN COOGAN

THE IBOGAINE STORY
REPORT ON THE STATEN ISLAND PROJECT

THE ROTTING GODDESS
THE CLASSICAL ORIGINS OF THE WITCH
JACOB RABINOWITZ

CARNIVAL OF CHAOS
SASCHA ALTMAN DEBRUL

AUTONOMEDIA NEW AUTONOMY SERIES
JIM FLEMING & PETER LAMBORN WILSON, EDITORS

TAZ:
THE TEMPORARY AUTONOMOUS ZONE, ONTOLOGICAL ANARCHY, POETIC TERRORISM
HAKIM BEY

THIS IS YOUR FINAL WARNING!
THOM METZGER

FRIENDLY FIRE
BOB BLACK

CALIBAN AND THE WITCHES
SILVIA FEDERICI

FIRST AND LAST EMPERORS:
THE ABSOLUTE STATE & THE BODY OF THE DESPOT
KENNETH DEAN & BRIAN MASSUMI

WARCRAFT
JONATHAN LEAKE

THIS WORLD WE MUST LEAVE & OTHER ESSAYS
JACQUES CAMATTE

SPECTACULAR TIMES
LARRY LAW

FUTURE PRIMITIVE AND OTHER ESSAYS
JOHN ZERZAN

WIGGLING WISHBONE
BART PLANTENGA

THE ELECTRONIC DISTURBANCE
CRITICAL ART ENSEMBLE

X TEXTS
DEREK PELL

WHORE CARNIVAL
SHANNON BELL, ED.

CRIMES OF CULTURES
RICHARD KOSTELANETZ

INVISIBLE GOVERNANCE:
THE ART OF AFRICAN MICROPOLITICS
DAVID HECHT & MALIQALIM SIMONE

THE LIZARD CLUB
STEVE ABBOTT

CRACKING THE MOVEMENT:
SQUATTING BEYOND THE MEDIA
FOUNDATION FOR ADVANCEMENT OF ILLEGAL KNOWLEDGE

SOCIAL OVERLOAD
HENRI-PIERRE JEUDY

MILLENNIUM
HAKIM BEY

ELECTRONIC CIVIL DISOBEDIENCE
CRITICL ART ENSEMBLE

SHOWER OF STARS
THE DREAM & THE BOOK
PETER LAMBORN WILSON

BEYOND BOOKCHIN
DAVID WATSON

SEMIOTEXT(E) NATIVE AGENTS SERIES
CHRIS KRAUS, EDITOR

IF YOU'RE A GIRL
ANN ROWER

THE ORIGIN OF THE SPECIES
BARBARA BARG

HOW I BECAME ONE OF THE INVISIBLE
DAVID RATTRAY

NOT ME
EILEEN MYLES

HANNIBAL LECTER, MY FATHER
KATHY ACKER

SICK BURN CUT
DERAN LUDD

THE MADAME REALISM COMPLEX
LYNNE TILLMAN

WALKING THROUGH CLEAR WATER
IN A POOL PAINTED BLACK
COOKIE MUELLER

THE NEW FUCK YOU
ADVENTURES IN LESBIAN READING
EILEEN MYLES & LIZ KOTZ, EDS.

I LOVE DICK
CHRIS KRAUS

SEMIOTEXT(E) FOREIGN AGENTS SERIES
JIM FLEMING & SYLVÈRE LOTRINGER, EDITORS

INSIDE & OUT OF BYZANTIUM
NINA ZIVANCEVIC

COMMUNISTS LIKE US
FÉLIX GUATTARI & TONI NEGRI

ECSTASY OF COMMUNICATION
JEAN BAUDRILLARD

SIMULATIONS
JEAN BAUDRILLARD

GERMANIA
HEINER MÜLLER

POPULAR DEFENSE & ECOLOGICAL STRUGGLES
PAUL VIRILIO

IN THE SHADOW OF THE SILENT MAJORITIES
JEAN BAUDRILLARD

FORGET FOUCAULT
JEAN BAUDRILLARD

ASSASSINATION RHAPSODY
DEREK PELL

REMARKS ON MARX
MICHEL FOUCAULT

STILL BLACK, STILL STRONG
DHORUBA BIN WAHAD, MUMIA ABU-JAMAL & ASSATA SHAKUR

LOOKING BACK ON THE END OF THE WORLD
JEAN BAUDRILLARD, PAUL VIRILIO, ET AL.

SADNESS AT LEAVING
ERJE AYDEN

NOMADOLOGY: THE WAR MACHINE
GILLES DELEUZE & FÉLIX GUATTARI

PURE WAR
PAUL VIRILIO & SYLVÈRE LOTRINGER

METATRON
SOL YURICK

BOLO'BOLO
P.M.

ON THE LINE
GILLES DELEUZE & FÉLIX GUATTARI